Principles and Management of CANCER

Principles and Management of CANCER

Tejinder Kataria
MD DNB CCST FIMSA
Chairperson
Division of Radiation Oncology
Medanta Cancer Institute
Medanta—The Medicity, Sector-38, Gurgaon
Haryana, India

Hemant Singhal
FRCSED FRCSC MBA
Consultant Breast Surgeon
The Harley Street Breast Clinic
Platinum Medical Centre, Wellington Hospital, UK

Dinesh Chand Doval
MBBS MD
Director Medical Oncology and Research
Rajiv Gandhi Cancer Institute and Research Centre
Rohini, New Delhi, India

Foreword
Karol Sikora

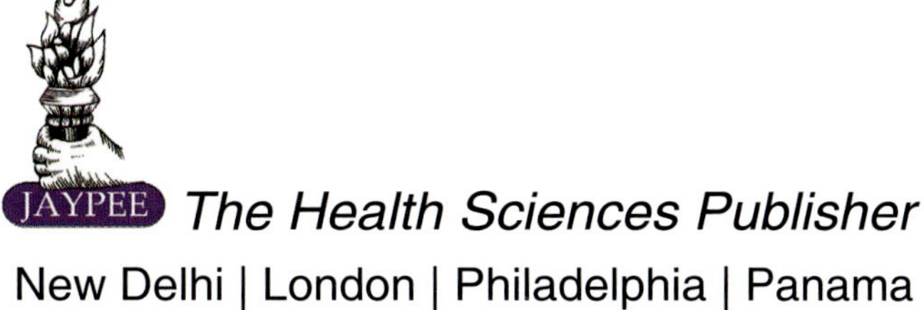

New Delhi | London | Philadelphia | Panama

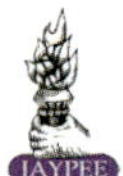

Jaypee Brothers Medical Publishers (P) Ltd.

Headquarters

Jaypee Brothers Medical Publishers (P) Ltd.
4838/24, Ansari Road, Daryaganj
New Delhi 110 002, India
Phone: +91-11-43574357
Fax: +91-11-43574314
E-mail: jaypee@jaypeebrothers.com

Overseas Offices

J.P. Medical Ltd.
83, Victoria Street, London
SW1H 0HW (UK)
Phone: +44-20 3170 8910
Fax: +44(0) 20 3008 6180
E-mail: info@jpmedpub.com

Jaypee-Highlights Medical Publishers Inc.
City of Knowledge, Bld. 237, Clayton
Panama City, Panama
Phone: +1 507-301-0496
Fax: +1 507-301-0499
E-mail: cservice@jphmedical.com

Jaypee Medical Inc.
325 Chestnut Street, Ste 412
Philadelphia, PA 19106, USA
Phone: +215-713-7181
Email: jrusko@jpmedus.com

Jaypee Brothers Medical Publishers (P) Ltd.
17/1-B, Babar Road, Block-B
Shaymali, Mohammadpur
Dhaka-1207, Bangladesh
Mobile: +08801912003485
E-mail: jaypeedhaka@gmail.com

Jaypee Brothers Medical Publishers (P) Ltd.
Bhotahity, Kathmandu, Nepal
Phone: +977-9741283608
E-mail: kathmandu@jaypeebrothers.com

Website: www.jaypeebrothers.com
Website: www.jaypeedigital.com

Inquiries for bulk sales may be solicited at: jaypee@jaypeebrothers.com

Principles and Management of Cancer

First Edition: **2016**

ISBN: 978-93-5152-971-2

Printed at: Ajanta Offset & Packagings Ltd., New Delhi

Dedicated to

Our patients who teach us to perform
to the best of our abilities because life matters and
to our young physicians, who question our beliefs and
make us tread the ever-widening frontiers of science

Contributors

Abhinav Dewan DNB
Senior Resident
Department of Radiation Oncology
Rajiv Gandhi Cancer Institute
and Research Center
Sector-5, Rohini, New Delhi, India

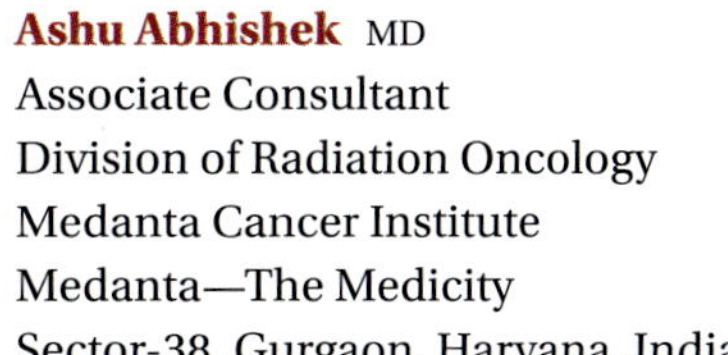

Ajay Kumar Dewan MS MCh (Surgical Oncology)
Medical Director and
Chief of Head and Neck Surgery
Rajiv Gandhi Cancer Institute
and Research Center
Sector-5, Rohini, New Delhi, India

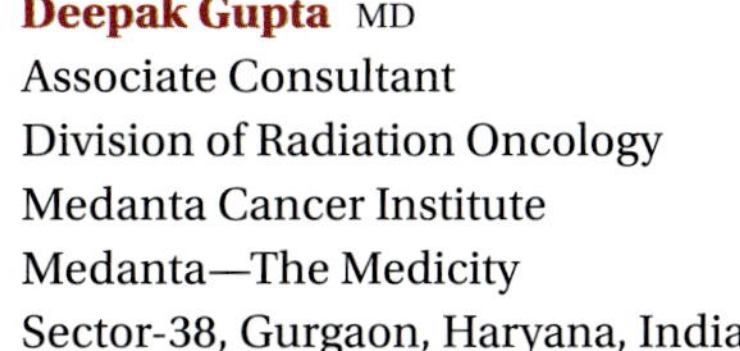

Adarsh Chaudhary MBBS MS FICS FRCS
Chairman and Head
GI and Bariatric Surgery
Medanta—The Medicity
Sector-38, Gurgaon
Haryana, India

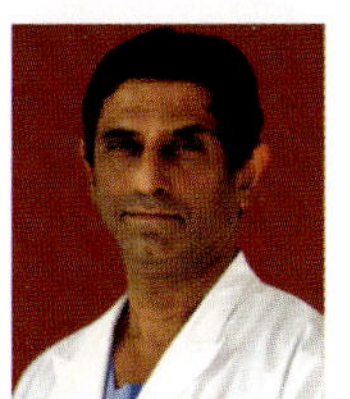

Ajaypal Sandhu MD DMRT
Clinical Professor of Radiation Oncology
Medical Director
Department of Radiation Medicine
and Applied Sciences
University of California San Diego
Moores Cancer Center
3960 Health Sciences Drive, #0865
La Jolla, CA 92093-0865

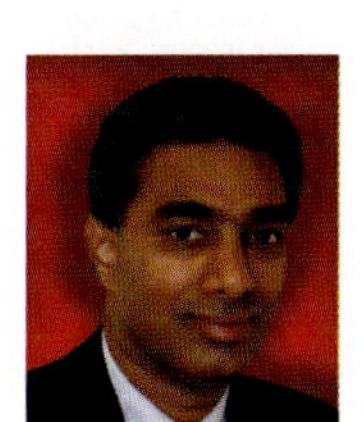

Anurita Srivastava MD DNB
Assistant Professor
Department of Radiotherapy
Maulana Azad Medical College and
Lok Nayak Jai Prakash Narayan Hospital
Bahadur Shah Zafar Marg, New Delhi

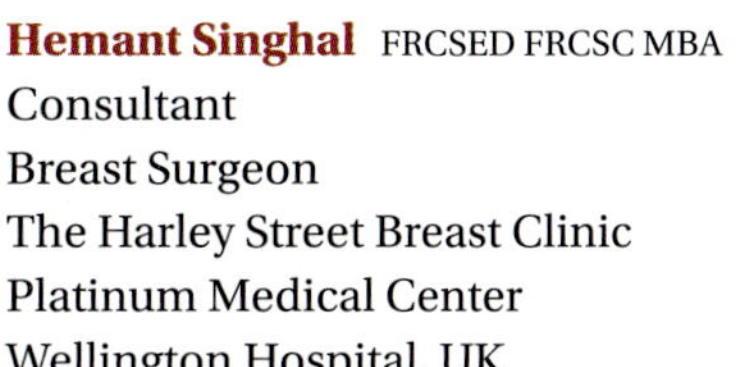

Ashu Abhishek MD
Associate Consultant
Division of Radiation Oncology
Medanta Cancer Institute
Medanta—The Medicity
Sector-38, Gurgaon, Haryana, India

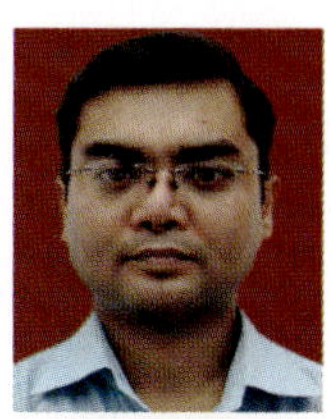

Deepak Gupta MD
Associate Consultant
Division of Radiation Oncology
Medanta Cancer Institute
Medanta—The Medicity
Sector-38, Gurgaon, Haryana, India

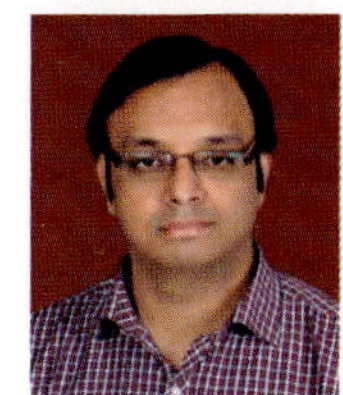

Dilip Kumar Samal
Associate Consultant
Department of ENT and Head and
Neck Surgery,
Medanta—The Medicity, Haryana, India

Dinesh Chand Doval MBBS MD
Director
Medical Oncology and Research
Rajiv Gandhi Cancer Institute and
Research Center
Sector 5, Rohini, New Delhi, India

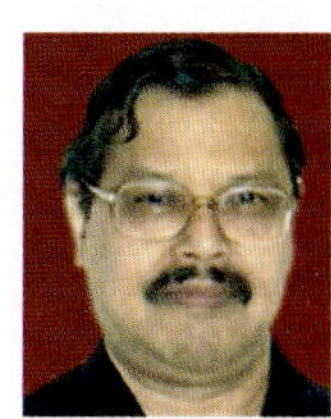

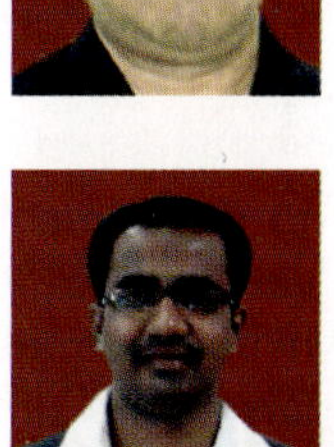

Govardhan HB MD DNB
Assistant Professor
Department of Radiation Oncology
Kidwai Memorial Institute of Oncology
Bengaluru, Karnataka, India

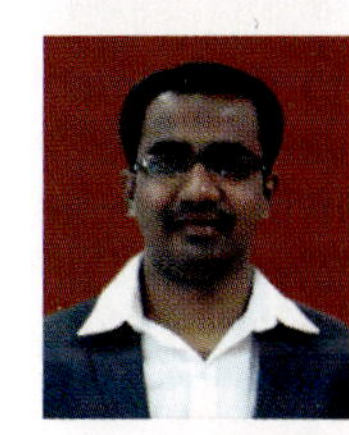

Hemant Singhal FRCSED FRCSC MBA
Consultant
Breast Surgeon
The Harley Street Breast Clinic
Platinum Medical Center
Wellington Hospital, UK

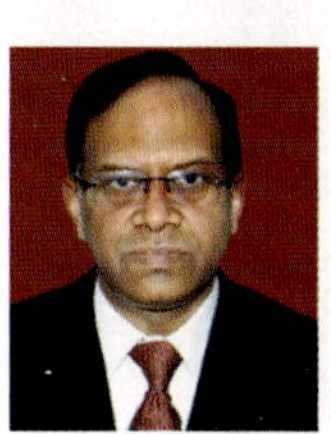

Kajal Pandya Yeptho
PhD (Foods & Nutrition)
Senior Manager
Department of Nutrition and Dietetics
Medanta—The Medicity
Sector 38, Gurgoan, Haryana, India

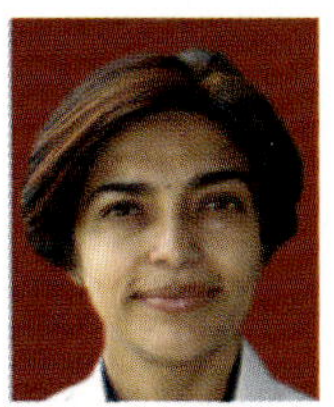

Kanchan Kaur MBBS MS (Gen. Surgery) MRCS (Edin)
Senior Consultant
Medanta Cancer Institute
Medanta—The Medicity
Sector-38, Gurgaon, Haryana, India

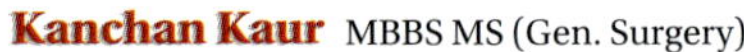

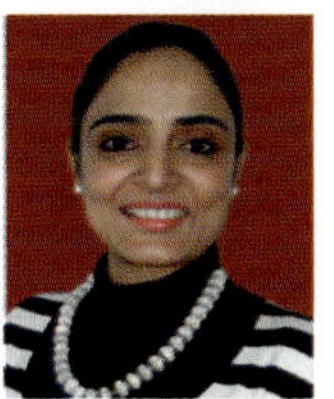

Karrthick KP MSc
Medical Physics
Division of Radiation Oncology
Medanta Cancer Institute
Medanta—The Medicity
Sector-38, Gurgaon, Haryana, India

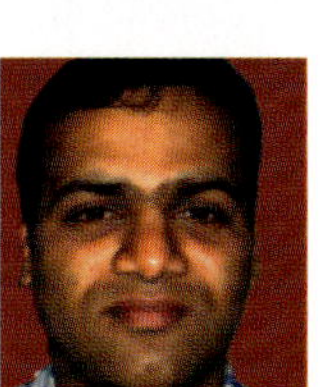

Kuldeep Sharma MD DNB Dip Pall Med (Cardiff, UK)
Consultant
Division of Radiation Oncology
Artemis Hospitals
Gurgaon, Haryana, India

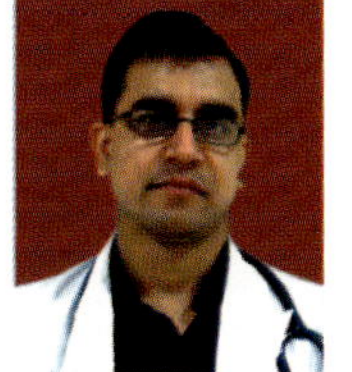

Kumud Kumar Handa MS
Director and Head
Department of ENT and Head Neck Surgery
Medanta—The Medicity
Sector-38, Gurgaon, Haryana, India

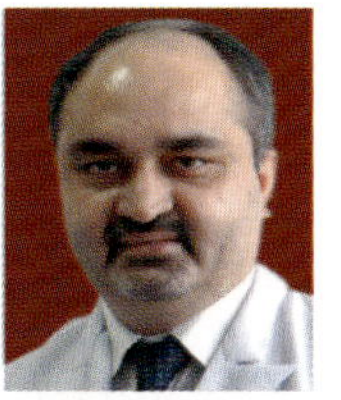

Kushal Narang MD
Attending Consultant
Division of Radiation Oncology
Medanta Cancer Institute
Medanta—The Medicity
Sector-38, Gurgaon, Haryana, India

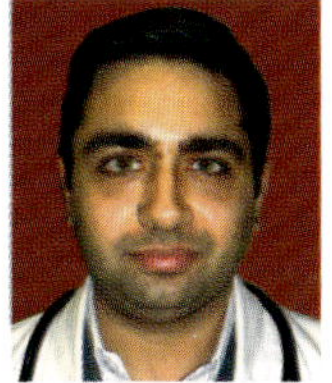

Manoj Tayal MD
Senior Consultant
Radiation Oncology
Medanta Cancer Institute,
Medanta—The Medicity
Sector-38, Gurgaon, Haryana, India

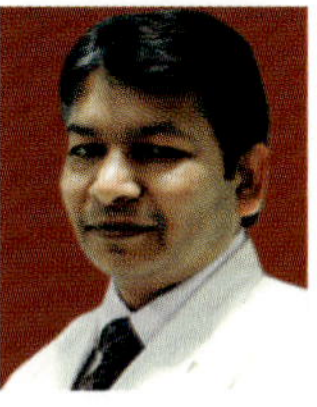

Malolan S Rajagopalan
Department of Radiation Oncology
UPMC Presbyterian Shadyside
5230, Center Ave Rm 215
Pittsburgh, PA 15232, USA

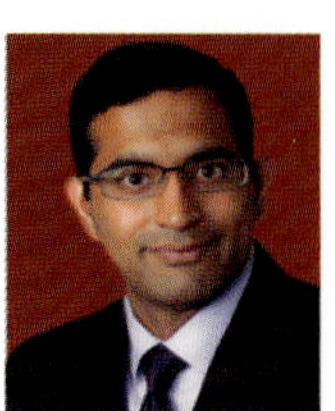

Nimesh Dahima MD
Senior Resident
Division of Radiation Oncology
Medanta—The Medicity
Sector-38, Gurgaon, Haryana, India

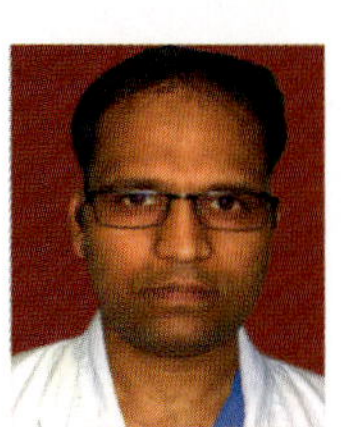

Rahul Patil MD
Dr LH Hiranandani Hospital
Hill Side Avenue, Hiranandani Gardens
Powai
Mumbai, Maharashtra, India

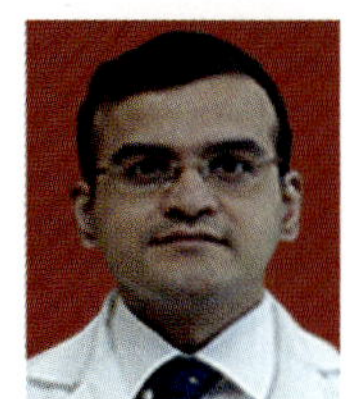

Ramu Mahendran MSc
Jr. Medical Physicist
Division of Radiation Oncology
Medanta Cancer Institute
Medanta—The Medicity
Sector-38, Gurgaon, Haryana, India

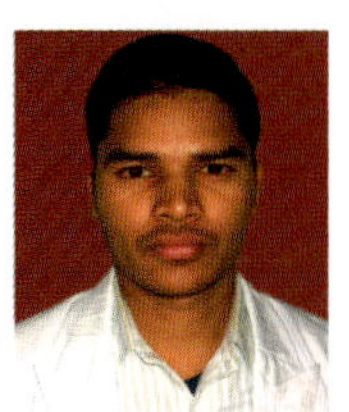

Ruchi Singh MD
Senior Resident
Division of Radiation Oncology
Lok Nayak Jai Prakash Hospital
Maulana Azad Medical College
New Delhi, India

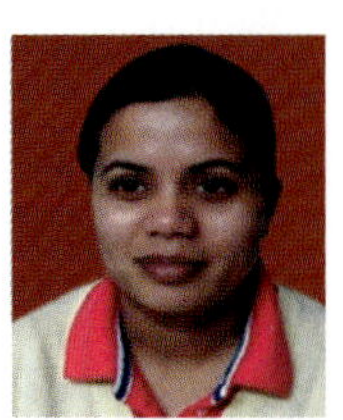

Ruchira Misra DCh DNB (Pediatrics)
Consultant Pediatric Hematology Oncology and Stem Cell Transplant
Fortis Memorial Research Institute
Gurgaon, Haryana, India

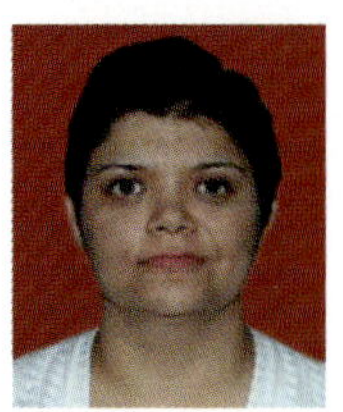

Samba Siva Selli R MSc
Medical Physicist
Narayana Health City
Bommasandra Industrial Area
Anekal Hosur Road
Bengaluru, Karnataka, India

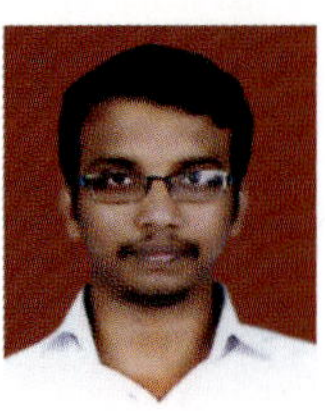

Sandeep Batra MD
Medical Oncology
Medanta—The Medicity
Sector-30, Gurgaon, Haryana, India

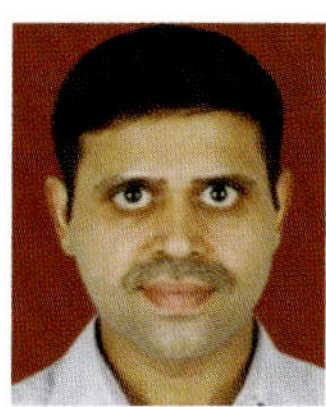

Sandeep Jain MD
Senior Consultant
Division of Radiation Oncology
Jaypee Hospital
Sector 128, Wish town
Nodia, Uttar Pradesh, India

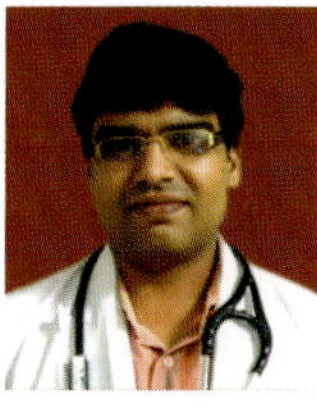

Sanjay Gupta PhD
Managing Director and CEO
Catalyst Clinical Services
New Delhi, India

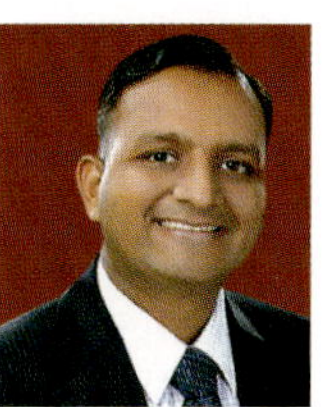

Savio G Barreto
Consultant
Division of GI Surgery
Medanta—The Medicity
Gurgaon, Haryana, India

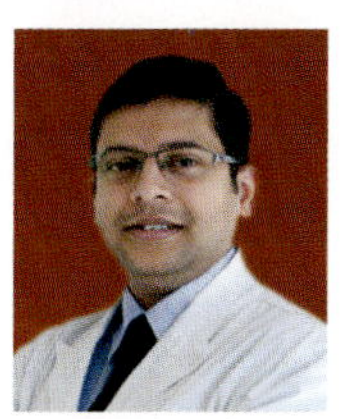

Senni Andavar MSc
Medical Physicist
Narayana Health City
Bommasandra Industrial Area
Anekal Hosur Road
Bengaluru, Karnataka, India

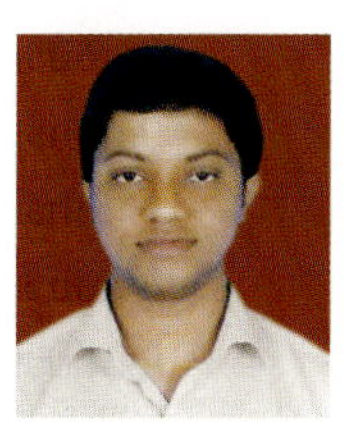

Shikha Goyal MD DNB
Consultant
Division of Radiation Oncology
Medanta Cancer Institute
Medanta—The Medicity
Sector-38, Gurgaon, Haryana, India

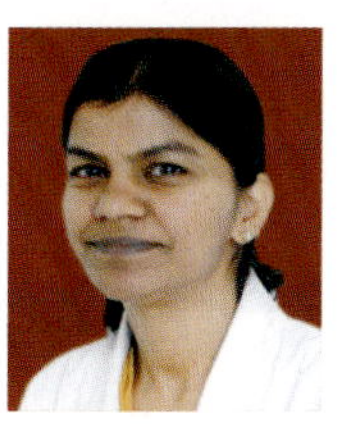

Shyam Singh Bisht MD
Associate Consultant
Division of Radiation Oncology
Medanta Cancer Institute
Medanta—The Medicity
Sector-38, Gurgaon, Haryana, India

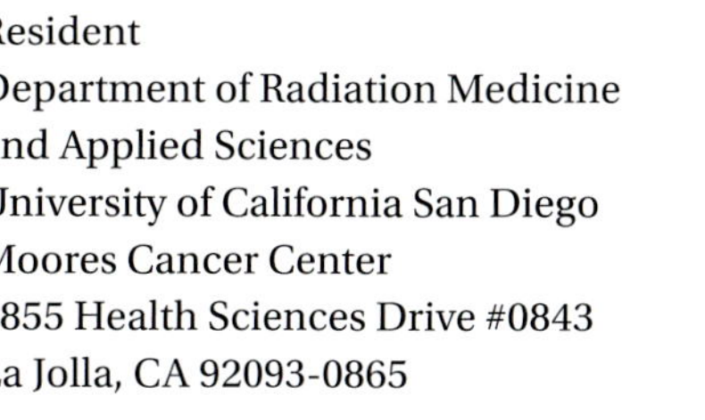

Steven Davis
Resident
Department of Radiation Medicine
and Applied Sciences
University of California San Diego
Moores Cancer Center
3855 Health Sciences Drive #0843
La Jolla, CA 92093-0865

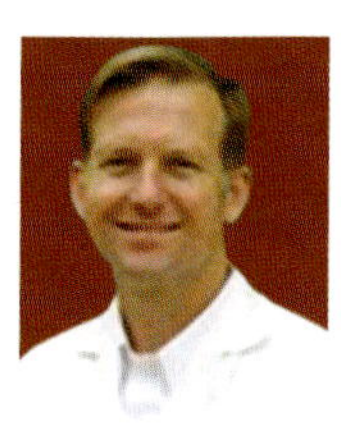

Sushil Beriwal MD
Professor and Medical Director
UPMC Cancer Center
Women's Hospital of UPMC
300 Halket Street
Pittsburgh, PA 1513

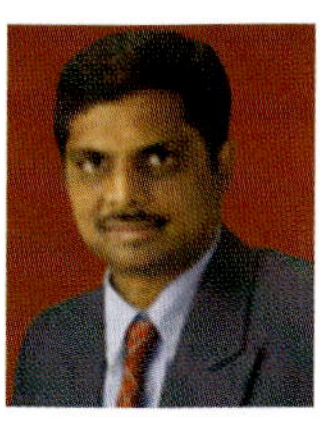

Tejinder Kataria MD DNB CCST FIMSA
Chairperson
Division of Radiation Oncology
Medanta Cancer Institute
Medanta—The Medicity
Sector-38, Gurgaon, Haryana, India

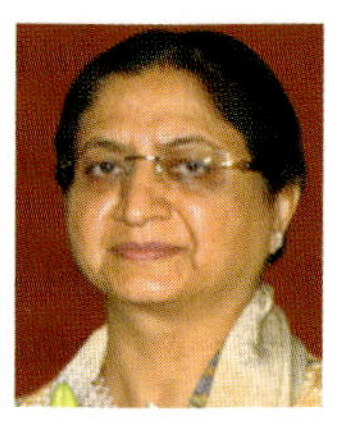

Trinanjan Basu MD
Associate Consultant
Division of Radiation Oncology
Medanta Cancer Institute
Medanta—The Medicity
Sector-38, Gurgaon, Haryana, India

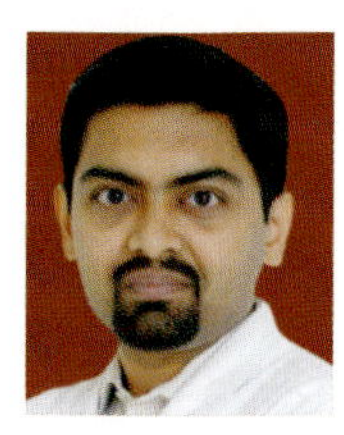

Vikash Kumar MD
Consultant
Division of Radiation Oncology
Jaypee Hospital
Sector-128, Wish Town
Noida, Uttar Pradesh, India

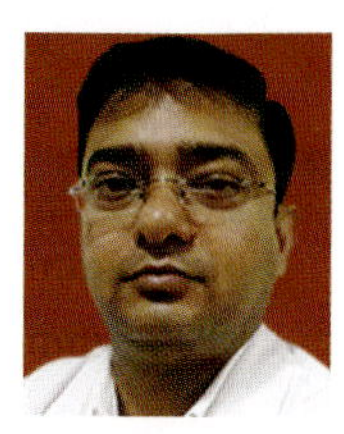

Vikraman Subramani MSc
Medical Physicist
Division of Radiation Oncology
Jaypee Hospital
Sector-128, Wish Town
Noida, Uttar Pradesh, India

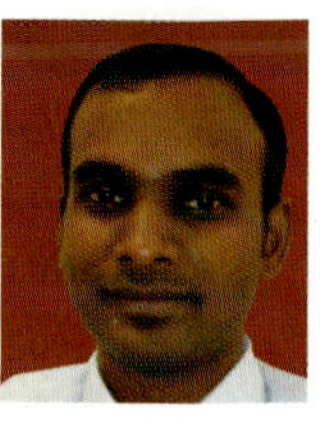

Foreword

The optimal treatment of cancer in every economic environment requires remarkable teamwork. The three main therapeutic modalities—surgery, radiotherapy, and chemotherapy require a seamless integrated approach alongside the equally important psychosocial support of an often distressed human being.

This excellent text is put together by a series of eminent Indian oncologists and it is skillfully edited by Dr Tejinder Kataria from Medanta, The—Medicity, Haryana, India. It summarizes beautifully the current team approach to all major cancers. The epidemiological background to a plethora of malignant diseases is considered, which is followed by the common diagnostic and staging pathways currently used. It is both didactic and pragmatic, and hence provides an excellent basis for trainees in oncology to build-up their knowledge base quickly whilst at the same time learning through their clinical experiences. The text will come to life as the human stories are added to the factual analysis in the book.

It will be particularly useful to those taking training in radiation oncology, but cancer surgeons and medical oncologists will find much of interest too. It teaches a strategy for each tumor type rather than a detailed recipe which can only be concocted when the equipment and resources of a specific treatment center have been identified. The chapters are comprehensive with numerous examples of best practice scattered in-between excellent clinical pathway summaries. Even complex management decisions are explained extremely clearly. The concept of risk of recurrence stratification to determine optimal radiotherapy and chemotherapy is described very clearly for prostate and gynecological cancers in their respective chapters. Maybe one day it will all be carried out by computer algorithm but for now it is clinical judgment that needs to be an acquired skill.

The cost of cancer care has huge effects on the poorer populations around our globe. Some of the new molecular targeted therapies for cancer cost more for one year's supply than many citizens of the world will earn in their whole lifetime. The insertion of cost into the equation to decide on the optimal care for an individual is hugely challenging for clinicians—especially those trained in an era where governments took care of costs. Cancer decisions in the past were based on medical need and not ability to pay. But there is no going back now. This is especially important in low resource environments.

It is clear from these well-thought-out chapters that world class cancer care is being delivered in India. But as in all countries, rich and poor alike, there is a huge variation in the quality of treatment accessed by different patients. Improving the bottom of the pyramid is far more important than the top and this applies throughout the cancer pathway from screening, diagnosis, treatment and palliative care. Seeking to improve the average will have the greatest gain for the most people. This is a task for the educationalist, and Dr Tejinder Kataria and her team have made an exceptionally good start. This book deserves to become a standard text to be found in every resident's bag. Maybe the next edition will be electronic with yearly updates in areas where approaches are rapidly changing. It deserves to become one of Asia's few standard oncology texts.

Professor Karol Sikora MA FRCR FRCP PhD
Chief Medical Officer
Cancer Partners UK and Dean
University of Buckingham Medical School

Preface

Developing countries are facing an ever-increasing incidence of cancer and it is expected that they are going to have a dual burden of infection-related cancers (cervix, liver and stomach) as well as lifestyle-related cancers (lung, colon, breast). Cancer is becoming a major health concern in India, with the number of new cancers projected to double in the next two decades; (Globacon–2012), 1.1 million new cases of cancer are diagnosed every year in a population of 1.2 billion with about 60,000 deaths per year.

An accurate correct diagnosis of cancer is essential for adequate and effective treatment as each disease requires a specific treatment. A patient may need one or more modalities of surgery, radiation, chemotherapy, targeted therapy or immunotherapy. The primary goal of therapy is to cure cancer with minimum toxicity and/or palliate with a good quality of life in advanced disease.

The Human Genome project and subsequent gene mapping, gene sequencing and next generation sequencing have changed the way of cancer diagnosis and treatment, and prognosis of the disease is perceived today. Till the time we can identify and stop the switch that makes cancer cells immortal; we have to approach and treat this malady with an integrated approach. The world has shrunk into a global village with the developments in telecom, computation, analytics, and results of research are available worldwide within a short span of time. Drugs, techniques, equipment, and training thereof, is within the reach of many as compared to a few, till a decade ago. This has revolutionized the way we treat any disease, including cancers, as is evident from the body of work presented in this book.

The book *Principles and Management of Cancer* is an effort to approach cancers site-wise and learn the alphabet of treating the various stages of different cancers using the present-day diagnostic aids and treatment modalities. The first few chapters give an insight on the development of technical nature in the last 100 years, the basics of diet, and emergencies encountered amongst the cancer patients. The site specialized treatments constitute the main body of the book and include stage specific-wise assessment to manage a patient with the best practices of three main therapeutic modalities, namely, viz. surgical, radiation and medical oncology. The final chapters introduce the concepts of Quality assurance, Drug discovery and Clinical trials.

The endeavor of the authors has been to present the standard of care as practised for various cancers and show the case work being done by them in their respective areas. We hope the book is received in the spirit it is written, i.e. to expand the reach of a textbook for cancer to students, teachers and practitioners in developing countries as well as low and middle income countries. We would like to invite the readers to give their feedback to include/exclude any sections, so that the future editions are more inclusive rather than exclusive.

Tejinder Kataria
Hemant Singhal
Dinesh Chand Doval

Acknowledgments

With the deepest gratitude I wish to thank everyone who has touched my life, inspired and guided me through their presence. First and foremost, I am grateful to Dr Naresh Trehan for setting up a world class hospital in Gurgaon, Haryana, India, and giving me an opportunity to be a part of its cancer wing. His vision and insight in medicine at large and deep involvement in planning and execution of the project is unparalleled. The permission to use the pictorial matter and illustrations from Medanta Cancer Institute and Medanta—the Medicity was given by him instantaneously, when I approached him with the proposal to write a book on *Principles and Management of Cancer*.

I have been fortunate in having had excellent teachers during my postgraduation at Postgraduate Institute, Chandigarh, India, BD Gupta and S Ayyagiri were responsible for inculcating a sense of commitment to patient care and coordinating with various surgical subjects to understand the multimodality treatment of cancer. Both of them taught me that I can learn a new way of thinking and perform complex processes required in managing cancer patients not only from doctors but also from our Medical Physicists, Radiotherapy Technologists, Nurses, Pathologists, Surgeons and of course the world of Books ! that is fast disappearing in the electronic era. This book pays a tribute to their dedication to make me learn the Science of Radiation Therapy and develop the Art of Patient Care.

The tutelage of Professor Joslin, Dr DV Ash and Dr Bryan Dixon from UK for Brachytherapy and Radiobiology, formed the alphabet for the syntax of conformal treatments later in life for me. I shall be forever indebted to them for their excellent tutorial skills. Dr Holger Hof at DKFZ, Heidelberg, Germany, taught me the basics of Intensity Modulated Radiotherapy and Professor Frank Lohr at Mannheim, Germany, Image Guided and Volumetric Modulated Radiotherapy. I am obliged to all my teachers to have helped inculcate a sense of wonder and awe, that is brought about by understanding the newer concepts of science.

I am thankful to Dr Hemant Singhal and Dr DC Doval for agreeing to be the Co-Editors to the first issue. Dr Kuldeep Sharma, Dr Vikash Kumar, Dr Shyam Singh Bisht, Dr Deepak Gupta, Dr Trinanjan Basu, Dr Ashu Abhishek, Dr Anurita Srivastava, Dr Govardhan and Dr Manoj Tayal have been my co-authors on different chapters without compromising their clinical duties.

I would like to acknowledge and express my gratitude to Dr AK Dewan, Dr Ajaypal Sandhu, Dr Sushil Beriwal, Dr Kanchan Kaur, Dr Kumud Kumar Handa, Dr Sandeep Jain, Mr Karthick KP, Dr Sandeep Batra and Dr Kushal Narang for their contribution to their areas of expertise. Dr Ishani Mohapatra gave us the histopathology microphotographs and I thank her from the core of my heart.

I am grateful to Dr Rajesh Vashistha, Secretary General AROI, for agreeing to release the book at annual AROICON this year and to Dr Shaleen Kumar, Organising Secretary, to endorse his decision.

This book would not have been possible without—M/s Jaypee Brothers Medical Publishers (P) Ltd, New Delhi, India, their technical support, guidance, manuscript evaluation and patience. I am thankful to Mr Tarun Duneja (Director-Publishing) and Ms Shivangi Pramanik for bearing with us and helping us complete the book.

I would like to thank Mr Reena George and Mr Dinesh Kumar for their secretarial help and collating the text to the photographs.

Last but not least, I am grateful to Rajiv Kataria, my husband and my daughter Shruti Kataria, for their unstinted support during the last 2 years and not begrudging my time away from them, in this academic pursuit.

Tejinder Kataria

Contents

1 CHAPTER

Radiobiology of Radiation Therapy

Govardhan HB, Anurita Srivastava, Tejinder Kataria

INTRODUCTION

Radiobiology is the science that evaluates the effects of radiation in living organisms. "X-rays and Gamma rays are the two important radiation sources that interact with biologic material through Compton effect mainly and result in energetic recoil electrons which traverse through cell and cause ionization along with creation of tracks that remove electrons through a double action. The first one is a "direct effect" where the electrons act on the critical molecules by a straight hit and an "indirect effect" whereby the water molecules are denatured with the production of free radicals to act on critical molecules leading to lethal effects.[1,2]

THE TIME-SCALE OF EFFECTS IN RADIATION BIOLOGY

Irradiation of a tissue generates processes that differ enormously in time-scale and these processes are divided into three phases.[3]

Physical Phase

It consists of interactions between charged particles and the atoms of which the tissue is composed. Physical phase is complete between 10^{-18} s and 10^{-14} s. It includes the interaction of X-ray with orbital electrons, and ejecting some of them from atoms (ionization) and raising others to higher energy levels within an atom or molecule excitation. For 1 Gy of absorbed radiation dose, there will be 10^5 ionizations within 10 μm within cells.

Chemical Phase

It is a period in which the ejected electrons act over water molecules and produce free radicals with a very short half-life. These free radicals are highly reactive and they eventually lead to the restoration of electronic charge equilibrium. This phase is completed within approximately 1 ms of radiation exposure.

Biological Phase

After the physical and chemical phase is the important subsequent process, basically it starts with enzymatic reactions that act on the residual chemical damage. After the radiation effect these cells take time to die and may undergo a number of mitotic divisions before dying. The early manifestations of normal-tissue damage after radiation exposure are the killing of stem cells and the subsequent loss of the progenitor progenies.

After a finite time lag (months to years) from irradiation of normal tissues "late reactions" may appear. Fibrosis and telangiectasia of skin, spinal cord damage (myelitis) and blood vessel damage (endarteritis) are a few of such effects. Appearance of a second primary cancer from 7 to 20 years has also been recorded as a late effect of radiation, although the incidence is <1%. Also the risk versus benefit of cure of first primary cancer needs to be accounted for at the time of giving curative radiation treatment.

DNA DAMAGE

The level and type of DNA damage is established within seconds of irradiation, so that at this point cell signaling pathways are triggered and the biological repair pathways can recognize the problem they have to deal with. The nature and level of initial damage therefore has important implications for the overall biological effects of radiation.

DIRECT ACTION

If any form of radiation (X-rays or Gamma rays), charged or uncharged particles are absorbed in biological material and there is a possibility that it will interact directly with critical target in the cells. The atoms of the target tissue are ionized leading to a biological change called direct action of radiation. It is the dominant process in the high linear energy transfer (LET) radiations like neutrons and alpha particles. It is the dominant process in the high "linear energy transfer" (LET) like neutron and a particle.

INDIRECT ACTION

Alternatively, the radiation may interact with other atom or molecules in the cell, mainly water, to produce the free radicals that are able to diffuse far enough to reach and damage the critical target called "indirect action" on radiation.

Types of Damage

A variety of lesions are produced in DNA by ionizing radiation, including base or sugar damage, DNA single-strand and double-strand breaks (DSB), DNA-protein crosslinks and DNA-DNA crosslinks (Table 1). For most cells it appears that the DNA DSB is the critical lesion, causing cell death by ionizing radiation.[4]

However, DSBs are not a uniform category of lesion. They may vary by virtue of the termini on the free ends of the molecule, also the proximity of other lesions. It has been suggested that a significant number of DSB will have other types of DNA damage nearby. These lesions have been termed clustered damage or locally multiply damaged sites, and they may be particularly significant for radiation cell killing. It is hypothesized that the complexity of these clusters will increase with increasing LET of the radiation. The potential significance of these is that they are formed by single tracks and that they will be more difficult to repair as the complexity of the cluster increases.[4] At the present time, we are unable to distinguish these different kinds of DSB experimentally, however, the reparability of DSB is known to decrease with an increase in LET.[5]

DNA REPAIR

Once damaged, a primary aim for a cell has to be to restore as accurately as possible the structural and functional integrity of the DNA. DNA can be repaired by any one of the following mechanism: Base excision repair, nucleotide excision repair, DNA DSB repair, nonhomologous end joining, homologous recombination repair, single strand annealing, cross link repair and mismatch repair.[4,5]

Table 1 Radiation-induced DNA damage

DNA double-strand breaks	40
DNA single-strand breaks	1,000
DNA-protein crosslinks	150
DNA-DNA crosslinks	30
Base damage	2,000
Sugar damage	1,500

ACUTE AND LATE EFFECTS OF RADIATION

Acute effects of radiation are dose limiting for normal tissues and involve effects on mucosa and hematopoitic system. The effects are predominantly due to apoptosis and loss of reproductive capacity of the cellular systems. Tissues with a rapid cell turnover comprise the early reacting tissues and they recover from the effect of radiation also early as compared to late reacting tissues (spinal cord). The time to recovery is dependent upon the dose delivered and the speed of recovery depends upon the level of stem cell depletion and it may vary from a few days to several months. If the number of surviving stem cells is too low, these acute reaction may turn into sequential late effect. The acute effect depends on the total dose, duration of the treatment and the dose per fraction.

Late effects following radiation occur after months to years and affect the slowly proliferating tissues (lung, kidney, heart, liver and central nervous system). They may also affect the slowly renewing systems like skin causing fibrosis, atrophy or telangiectasia after many years. The most important factor for late effects is the total dose of radiation, dose of radiation per fraction of treatment. The duration of the late effect is not related to the radiosensitivity or tolerance of the relevant normal tissue.

The differentiation between acute and late effects has important clinical implications. The acute reactions are usually observed during conventionally fractionated radiotherapy schedule. The severity depends on the effect on stem cell. It is possible to adjust the dose in the event of unexpectedly severe reactions, allowing a sufficient number of stem cells to survive. Whenever the remaining stem cells are reduced either by reducing overall treatment time or reducing the healing replacing capacity of stem cell, it results in acute reactions which may persist as chronic injury, called consequential late complications.

CELL DEATH

The use of radiation to treat cancer results from its ability to cause the death of tumor cells and its biological consequences are influenced by DNA damage response. The DNA damage response determines both the sensitivity of cells to die following irradiation and type of cell death that occurs and the timing of cell death. The cause of the cell death after irradiation complex process as described below.

Programmed Cell Death (Apoptosis)

Apoptosis is a regulated form of cell death. It can be initiated either as a result of conditions occurring within the cell

(DNA damage) or external signal from a surrounding tissue or immune cell.[6]

Mitotic Catastrophe

Mitotic catastrophe is associated with the accumulation of multinucleated, giant cells with uncondensed chromosomes, chromosome aberrations and micronuclei. This will occur when cells proceed through mitosis in an inappropriate manner and cause entry of cells into mitosis with unrepaired or misrepaired DNA damage. The cells lose their replicative potential called death. This can occur either due to loss of genetic material associated with this process or from a physical inability to replicate and separate the genetic material correctly.[7]

Necrosis

Necrosis is "death by injury". It is most frequently observed in human tumors and can occur following treatment with certain DNA-damaging agents, including radiation.

Senescence

It can be elicited by various cellular stresses, such as those caused by oncogene activation or by radiation-induced DNA damage.[8] In both cases, the cells enter a permanent cell cycle arrest. Senescence does not occur by shortening of the telomeres, but instead are controlled by a number of molecular pathways.

Bystander Death

It is a mechanism in which cell death can occur in cells with irradiation of neighboring cells. The evidences come from studies using high LET α-particles in which a larger fraction of cells die than are estimated. The bystander effects have also been observed for other known biological effects of irradiation, including DNA damage, chromosomal aberrations, mutation, transformation and gene expression.[9]

THE FIVE "RS" OF RADIOBIOLOGY

Clinical observation and experimental radiobiology have identified five factors that are clearly influential in the determination of the outcome of a course of fractionated radiotherapy. These are the five "Rs" of radiobiology and they form the fundamental basis for the application of our molecular knowledge.

Repair

Repair is the increase in surviving fraction of cells when radiation exposure is prolonged or fractionated. It is because of the sublethal damage repair (SLDR). In addition, cells held in a nonproliferating state after irradiation in suboptimal conditions show a reduced sensitivity compared to proliferating cells. This is potentially lethal damage recovery (PLDR). Both of these processes are believed to be a consequence of the repair of radiation damage to DNA. However, SLDR and PLDR are apparently not controlled by the same processes, since they have differing effects on the number of gene mutations that are induced by radiation.[10] The molecular dissection of these processes is still in its infancy but there are data to link the gene *TP53* to PLDR.[11] Of recent interest is the finding that clonogenic cell survival curves may have a steep component at low doses and that some radioprotective processes might be induced by radiation. This could have important implications for cellular recovery in different fractionation regimes and attempts are being made to exploit this in the clinic.

Reassortment

Cells vary in their radiosensitivity as they progress through the cell cycle. For example, cells in mitosis have been found to be approximately twice as sensitive as cells in the latter part of the DNA synthesis phase. Radiation therefore exerts selective damage of cells in the sensitive phase of the cell cycle. If there were no cell cycle progression, then a second radiation dose would be less effective than the first. The effect of cells progressing through the cell cycle in between treatments is that cells that survive the first treatment because of their presence in a resistant phase move into a more sensitive phase before the next fraction is delivered. This movement and redistribution of cells to sensitive phase is called reassortment. Importantly, one of the key cellular responses to DNA damage is the triggering of cell-cycle checkpoints toward the end of G1 and in G2. These have been examined extensively in relation to cellular radiosensitivity but their influence on cell-cycle reassortment during radiotherapy has not been well characterized.

Repopulation

Proliferation of tumor cells during a course of radiotherapy is potentially a major obstacle to the success of treatment. It is apparent that the proliferation of tumor cells can be faster in a treated tumor than in an untreated tumor, and this "accelerated-repopulation" appears to have a significant bearing on the efficacy of radiotherapy.[12] Acceleration may partly be due to physical effects, i.e. the removal of dead cells may lead to an improved nutrient supply to surviving cells. If depopulation within the tumor leads to reduced cell loss, then survivors may proliferate with a doubling time that approaches the "potential doubling time", a process that has been described as the "unmasking" of the high proliferation rate of clonogenic tumor cells.

Reoxygenation

Low oxygen levels render cells relatively resistant to ionizing radiation, largely because of a decreased induction of DNA damage. In some tumors, and to a minor extent in normal tissues such as cartilage, vascular supply is inadequate to maintain good oxygen supply to all regions, so there are cells that are hypoxic and therefore resistant to radiation. Clinically this has been demonstrated to limit the success of therapy.[13] but its influence is reduced when the radiation is fractionated, due to the process of reoxygenation. The death of some tumor cells may lead to improved oxygen supply to others, and thus to an increase in their radiosensitivity. Furthermore, the opening and closing of blood vessels in a tumor is a dynamic process, so that cells adjacent to a closed vessel at the time of one fraction may be oxygenated at the next fraction if the vessel has opened. The effect of a subpopulation of resistant cells at each treatment time may be quite small in some cases, but when amplified over a multiple fraction regime it can result in a significant reduction in the theoretical tumor curability.[14]

Radiosensitivity

It is intuitively reasonable to expect that the inherent radiosensitivity of tumor cells can be a significant factor in the overall level of cell killing induced by radiation. The clinical radioresponsiveness of tumors of different histological origins correlates strongly with radiosensitivity of cells taken from those tumors. To take this one step further, the radiosensitivity of tumor cells from cervix carcinomas has been demonstrated to be predictive of local tumor control.[15] In cervix cancer it therefore appears that cellular sensitivity is a major determinant of the overall response. Not all studies have shown this relationship in other tumor types, and there is still work to be done to determine whether these results are a true reflection of a varied influence of inherent sensitivity or whether technical problems in the assay systems have blurred the situation.

LINEAR ENERGY TRANSFER

Linear energy transfer (LET) is defined as the energy transferred per unit length of the track of radiation passes through. The special unit of LET is kiloelectron volt per micrometer (keV/μm). The International Commission on Radiological Units (ICRU) defined LET as, the charged particles in medium is the quotient of dE/dL, where dE is the average energy locally imparted to the medium by a charged particle of specified energy in traversing a distance of dL.[16]

That is, LET = dE/dL

As radiation is an act over at the microscopic level, LET is an average and the energy per unit length of track varies over such a wide range. There are 2 methods to calculate LET; the most commonly used method is to calculate

- Track average, which is obtained by dividing the track into equal lengths, calculating the energy deposited in each length, and finding the mean
- Energy average is obtained by dividing the track into equal energy increments and averaging the lengths of track over which these energy increments are deposited.[17] The LET for various radiations are given in Table 2.

Table 2 Linear energy transfer values for various radiation types

Type and energy of radiation	*Linear energy transfer*
250 kV X-ray (250 kV)	2
3 MV X-ray (3 MV)	0.2
Cobalt 60 (1.17–133 MV)	0.2
Beta 10 kV (10 kV)	2.3
Beta 1 MV (1 MV)	0.25
Neutron 2.5 MV (2.5 MV)	20
Neutron 19 MV (19 MV)	7
Proton 10 MeV	4.7
Proton 50 MeV	0.5
Alpha 2.5 MeV	166

RELATIVE BIOLOGIC EFFECTIVENESS

In comparing different radiations, it is customary to use X-rays as the standard. The National Bureau of Standards in 1954 defined relative biologic effectiveness (RBE) as follows:

The RBE of test radiation (r) compared with X-rays is defined by the ratio D_{250}/D_r, where D_{250} and D_r are, respectively, the doses of X-rays and the test radiation required for equal biological effect.

This is explained further by the following example. To measure the RBE of some test radiation, one first chooses a biologic system in which the effect of radiations may be scored quantitatively. Suppose, we are measuring the RBE of fast neutrons compared with 250-kV X-rays, using the lethality of plant seedlings as a test system. Groups of plants are exposed to graded doses of X-rays; parallel groups are exposed to a range of neutron doses. At the end of the period of observation, it is possible to calculate the doses of X-rays and that of neutrons that result in the death of half of the plants in a group. This quantity is known as the LD50, the mean lethal dose. Suppose that for X-rays the LD50 turns out to be 6 Gy (600 rad) and that for neutrons the corresponding quantity is 4 Gy (400 rad). The RBE of neutrons compared with X-rays is then simply the ratio 6:4, or 1.5. RBE depends on the following: radiation quality (LET), radiation dose, number of dose fractions, dose rate and biologic system or end point.[18-20]

Relative biological effect (RBE) increases with LET to a maximum to 100 keV/μm, then it start decreases with increasing the LET. At LET of 100 keV/μm, the ionizing events is similar to the diameter of the DNA double helix (2 nm) and can most efficiently produce DSB by a single track. As the dose per fraction decreases, the RBE of high-LET radiations compared with that of low-LET radiations increases. This is a direct consequence of the fact that the dose-response curve for low-LET radiations has a broader shoulder than for high-LET radiations. The RBE values are high for cells or tissues that accumulate and repair a great deal of sublethal damage.[19,20]

OXYGEN ENHANCEMENT RATIO

It is defined as the ratio of radiation doses under hypoxic to aerated conditions to achieve the same biological effect is called the oxygen enhancement ratio (OER). The OER for sparsely ionizing radiations, such as X- and γ-rays is between 2.5 and 3.5. There is some evidence that for rapidly growing cells cultured in vitro, the OER has a smaller value of about 2.5 at lower doses, on the order of the daily dose per fraction generally used in radiotherapy.[21] This is believed to result from the variation of OER with the phase of the cell cycle: cells in G_1 phase have a lower OER than those in S, and because G_1 cells are more radiosensitive, they dominate the low-dose region of the survival curve. For this reason, the OER of an asynchronous population is slightly smaller at low doses than at high doses. The oxygen enhancement ratio has a value of about 3 for low-LET radiations, falls when the LET rises above about 30 keV/μm and reaches unity by an LET of about 200 keV/μm.[22]

DOSE RATE EFFECT IN RADIOTHERAPY

In many experimental model systems it has been demonstrated that irradiations at lower dose rates are less effective for cell killing as compared to high dose rate irradiations. Effectiveness of radiations (in causing cell death) varies remarkably in the dose rate range of 1 mGy min^{-1} to 1 Gy min^{-1}. Ability to recover from sublethal damage has been suggested to be the most important mechanism underlying the dose rate effect.[23]

In radiotherapy a wide range of dose rates are used depending upon the technique of treatment. High dose rates of several Gy min^{-1} is used in external beam therapy, whereas, dose rates as low as 0.5 Gy/hr used in brachytherapy. The dose rate can be as low as 1.3 Gy/day when ^{125}I seeds are used as permanent implants. Response of normal tissues and tumors to variations in dose rate must be clearly understood for designing appropriate strategies for low-dose rate radiotherapy.

Mechanism of Dose Rate Effect and Inverse Dose Rate Effect

Response of the biological system to low-dose rate irradiation is influenced by different complex events, which occur simultaneously. These events include repair from sublethal damage, cell proliferation, redistribution of cells in the cell cycle (G2 block) and reoxygenation. The magnitude of contributions from these different events depends to a great extent on the dose rate used as well as the type of the tissues involved. Final response of the tissue to radiation is a resultant of contributions of these factors. Repair of sublethal damage occurs both in the normal as well as in tumor tissues, but the extent of recovery is generally higher in normal tissues, due to the free availability of nutrients and oxygen. Larger tumors show a lesser repair from sublethal damage compared to smaller tumors.

Repopulation occurs very actively in normal tissues at low-dose rates. Normal cell population can be maintained in intestines up to a dose rate of 14 Gy/day, in bone marrow up to 0.5 Gy/day, and the testis is more sensitive and can maintain normal functioning up to a dose rate of 120 mGy per day. Generally, the repopulation in tumors can be inhibited by a dose rate of 0.3 Gy/hr. On the basis of experimental studies with various cell lines it has been established that the dose required to inhibit repopulation depends upon the cell cycle duration. A dose of 7.5–10 Gy per cell cycle is adequate to inhibit cell division. Since most tumor cells have generation times larger than of 24 hours, repopulation is easily inhibited by a dose rate of 0.3–0.5 Gy/hr. At higher dose rates above 0.5 Gy/hr, the problem of repopulation does not arise. At a critical dose rate 0.37 Gy/hr cells do progress very slowly and tend to accumulate in G_2 phase of the cell cycle. They do not progress further and are effectively killed by radiations. This could possibly be one of the reasons for the less pronounced dose rate effect seen in tumors. Further, in cell cultures (HeLa) it has been demonstrated that a dose rate of 0.37 Gy/hr is more effective than higher dose rates of 0.55, 0.74 or 1.54 Gy/hr. At higher dose rates the cells do not progress in the cell cycle and hence the advantage of cell synchrony and accumulation in the radiosensitive G_2 phase does not occur. This phenomenon is termed as "inverse dose rate effect".[23,24]

In tumors, such as KHT sarcomas, there is no significant dose rate effect in the dose rate range of 1 Gy min^{-1} to 0.41 Gy/hr. It has been suggested that in tumors high-dose rate irradiation may encounter hypoxic cell radioresistance. On the other hand low-dose rates may permit adequate reoxygenation. Hence, the disadvantage of SLD repair occurring in tumors may well be compensated by the reoxygenation and concomitant sensitization of tumor cells.[25]

As compared to the response of tumors, to low-dose rates, normal tissues like the small intestines show an enormous amount of sparing. This forms of biological rationale for brachytherapy at low-dose rates as well as multiple dose fractions daily regimens.[25]

DOSE FRACTIONATION IN RADIOTHERAPY

In radiotherapy, fractionation of the dose was introduced with objective of sparing the normal tissue damage and at the same time eradicating the tumor. Fractionation facilitates repair and repopulation in normal tissues, redistribution of radioresistant cells in the sensitive phases of the cell cycle, and reoxygenation of hypoxic cell fraction which survive the earlier dose fractions.[26-28] Furthermore, quiescent (G0) cells not in the division cycle are recruited into the proliferating compartment. These advantages associated with dose fractionation are generally referred as 4R's of radiotherapy.

Generally, the normal tissue damage is of two types, early reaction and late injury. Late responding normal tissue may have a large number of cells in resting phase. Early responding tissues generally constitute fast proliferating cells. Skin, mucosa, interstitial epithelium, bone marrow, colon, testis, etc. constitute early responding tissues, whereas spinal cord, bladder, lung, and kidneys are late responding tissues. In the recent years there is an improvement in the understanding of proliferation of normal tissues following radiotherapy. Acutely reacting tissues proliferate to compensate the cell loss in these tissues. Tissues like skin and mucosa begin to proliferate 2 or 3 weeks after the start of radiotherapy. In late responding tissues, this type of proliferation occurs only after the end of therapy. As a result, prolongation of therapy could decrease the acute normal tissue reactions without sparing the late damages. However, one of the positive benefits of increasing the intervals between fractions is to allow for adequate reoxygenation. Hence, the use of hypoxic sensitizers and high LET radiations to overcome the hypoxic cell radioresistance may play a critical role in shorter schedules. Since it has been observed that use of large fraction in shorter schedules result in unacceptable levels of late injury, large number of smaller dose fractions (hyperfractionation) can effectively bring about cure, while not increasing the late tissue damage. Hyperfractionation may increase the early tissue damage but not to an unacceptable level.[29,30]

Rationale for Multiple Fractionation Daily

Survival curve of the cells involved in early and late response have different shapes. Survival response of late responding tissues are more curved with a lower response at lower doses, as compared to the sharp fall in surviving fraction with dose observed for early responding tissue. Response curve can be adequately explained on the basis of linear quadratic relationship.

An adequate knowledge of the tissue response enables us to evolve new schemes of fractionation to improve radiotherapy. One of the most important considerations is to understand the tolerance levels of dose for early and late injury for different fractionation schedules. Effect of dose fractionation on the level of damage induced in fast and slow responding tissues. Dose is delivered acutely (single doses) or in fractions of 1,2,3 or 4 Gy each. Fractionation spares both the slow and fast reactions. However, the extent of the sparing is remarkably higher for the late reacting tissues. Further, smaller the fraction size the greater is sparing of damage, particularly so, for the late reacting tissues.[28,31]

Linear Quadratic Model

Concepts of early and late response can be clearly understood by the cell survival response of these tissues. Survival response can be explained on the basis of linear quadratic model. Survival curves have two components, the a component which predominantly operates at low doses and the β component dominates at higher doses. This can be attributed to one hit and two hit mechanisms associated with cell killing. As per this model survival "S" varies with the dose "D".[32]

The α and β are linear and quadratic coefficients. Cells which respond early have a large α value whereas the more curvy late responding cells have a small α value and large β values. Dose at which the linear and the quadratic components contribute equally to the effect is called the α/β value. α/β dose provides a good description of the tissue response. Late responding tissues are characterized by small α/β values 1–3 Gy, whereas the early reacting tissues have large α/β values in the range of 8–10 Gy.

Linear quadratic model can also predict the response for fractionated irradiation. Survival S_n for n fractions of dose "d" equals then, the dose per fraction on X-axis and inverse of the total dose required for a definite level of damage yields a straight line with slope equal to -β/ln Sn and intercept -α/ln Sn. Hence, α/β is the ratio of the intercept to slope. In practice total dose required to produce the same level of damage with different fraction sizes is determined. Such determination is available for skin where it is convenient to score the level of damage. For mouse skin reaction the α/β value is ≈ 10. α/β values available from animal experimental systems for the early and late responding tissues are as shown in Table 3.

There is no reason to believe that the values can be very different for human tissues.

Isoeffect and Dose Fractionation

Using many experimental animal systems and various fraction sizes, variation of the total dose required to produce the same level of injury (isoeffect doses) has been determined

Table 3 α/β values available from animal experimental systems for the early and late responding tissues[33]

A. α/β values for some of the animal tissues*

Early responding tissues	*α/β (Gy)*	*Late responding† tissues*	*α/β (Gy)*
Skin (epithelium)	9–12	Lung	2.3-6.0
Testis	12–13	Kidney	1.9-6.4
Callus	9–10	Spinal cord	1.7-4.9
Colon	10–11	Dermis	1.4-6.2
Jejunum	6–10	Bladder	3.1-7

B. α/β values for medium term reactions

Reactions	*α/β value (Gy)*
Pneumonitis of mouse lung (50% mortality)	2.5–6.0
Breathing rate	3.0–6.0

*α/β values for tumors range from 2.5 to 100

†α/β values for late responding tissues are not very reliable.

Source: Data based on the experiments using rat, mouse, pig and rabbits. Withers 1983 et.al.[33]

for different fraction sizes. The end points scored are response of skin, bone marrow, vertebral growth, fibro sarcoma, small intestine, lung, testis, kidney, colon and spinal cord. The general conclusion from these studies is that for late effects the decrease in dose fraction rapidly increases the isodose. Increase in isodose for many fast responding injuries (and tissues) occur more slowly as compared to that for late injury. From these response curves it is clear that where late damage is the limiting factor in radiotherapy, small dose fractions enable to deliver a higher total dose. Further, large dose per fractions limits the total dose drastically more due to late tissue damage rather than early damage. Hence, large dose fractions can be of use only where small total doses are required for palliation.

α/β Values and Dose Per Fraction

Many efforts have been made to improve the therapeutic gain, viz. by manipulating the biological parameters, selective chemical modifiers, use of high LET radiations, accelerated photon and electron beams. Introduction of fractionation has been one of the most successful methods for improving tumor cure. At present, it is well-known that a standard fractionation schedule may not be adequate for treatment of all the tumors.[28] This is because of the wide variations in the proliferation kinetics of different tumors and also of the surrounding normal tissues. Hence, it should be possible to adopt an appropriate fractionation scheme depending upon the type of neoplasms and improve the therapeutic response.

Choice of the size of fraction should be based on the α/β values of the normal tissues to be spared. Generally, the response curve begins to bend at dose one-tenth of the D/E (flexure dose). Hence, the flexure doses for fast responding tissues range from 0.8 to 1.2 Gy, whereas the same is as low as 0.1–0.5 Gy for late responding tissues such as the spinal cord, kidney, lung and skin contraction. Hence, it must be emphasized that the dose per fraction must be reduced to the lowest possible level and the number of fractions increased up to 4 fractions if possible, to achieve maximum sparing of the late effects. Reducing the dose per fraction to less than 0.8 Gy does not spare either the fast responding tissues or the tumor to the same extent.[34,35]

THE CONCEPT OF THERAPEUTIC INDEX

The "therapeutic index" defined as the tumor control probability (TCP) for a fixed normal tissue complication probability (NTCP) for different doses and type of radiation.[36] First, normal tissues may get more radiation doses that cause more reaction but same dose required to control the tumor; on the other hand, tumor may receive an inadequate dose if, radiation dose is restricted below the normal tissue tolerance. Thus, the main aim in radiotherapy is to achieving the optimal balance between TCP and NTCP, all the recent technologies are directed toward to achieve these aims. TCP and NTCP curves are sigmoid in shape, left curve is TCP and right side is NTCP. The main purpose of radiotherapy treatment is to shift the TCP to the left and the NTCP curve toward right. The therapeutic index also called therapeutic window increases, if the area between the two curves becomes too large then the expected benefit from treatment will increases.

Tumor Control Probability

The effectiveness of radiation-therapy treatment is evaluated by the locoregional TCP and treatment related NTCP.[37] TCP is directly proportional to the dose of radiation and inversely proportional to the number of cells in the tumor tissue or volume of the tumor. The total radiation doses required to control subclinical disease is 40–50 Gy and 60–70 Gy for gross disease. The dose-limiting factor in effectiveness in radiotherapy is the tolerance of the surrounding tissues to radiation.

The factor affecting TCP were divided into:

- *Tumoral factors affecting the TCP:* Intrinsic radio-sensitivity, location and size of tumor, cellular type of tumor and effect of oxygen.
- *Treatment-related factors affecting the TCP:* Dose-time fractionation, radiation quality (RBE, LET), dose rate,

use of radiosensitizers, combination of radiotherapy with surgery and/or chemotherapy, technique (e.g., small field sizes), treatment modality.

Normal Tissue Complication Probability

The NTCP is a function of the total dose (TD), fraction dose (d), fraction number (N) and the volume of normal tissue exposed to the radiation.[37,38]

The Lyman model is used in NTCP calculation and is highly complex mathematical model of biological effects based on the use of algebraic definitions. The tissue types (parallel or serial organs), volume of irradiated normal tissue, its radiosensitivity and functional subunits of tissues make this model more complex.[39]

The factor affecting NTCP were:

Factors related to organ tissue: Tissue radiosensitivity, the volume of organ tissue within the radiotherapy portal and organ type; serial or parallel.

Factors related to treatment: Dose-time fractionation, quality of radiation (RBE, LET), dose rate, use of radioprotectors, combination of RT with surgery and/or chemotherapy, technique (e.g., addition of boost field), treatment modality.

REFERENCES

1. Tobias JS. The role of radiotherapy in the management of cancer—an overview. Ann Acad Med Singapore. 1996;25(3): 371-9.
2. Delaney G, Jacob S, Featherstone C, et al. The role of radiotherapy in cancer treatment: estimating optimal utilization from a review of evidence-based clinical guidelines. Cancer. 2005;104(6):1129-37.
3. Boag JW. The time scale in radiobiology. 12th Failla memorial lecture. In: Nygaard OF, Adler HI, Sinclair WK (Eds). Radiation research. Proceedings of the 5th International Congress of Radiation Research. New York: Academic Press; 1975. pp. 9-29.
4. Jenner TJ, de Lara CM, O'Neill P, et al. Induction and rejoining of DNA double-strand breaks in V79-4 mammalian cells following gamma- and alpha-irradiation. Int J Radiat Biol. 1993;64(3):265-73.
5. Goodhead DT. Initial events in the cellular effects of ionizing radiations: clustered damage in DMA. Int J Radiat Biol. 1994;65(1):7-17.
6. Taylor RC, Cullen SP, Martin SJ. Apoptosis: controlled demolition at the cellular level. Nat Rev Mol Cell Biol. 2008;9(3):231-41.
7. Chu K, Teele N, Dewey MW, et al. Computerized video time lapse study of cell cycle delay and arrest, mitotic catastrophe, apoptosis and clonogenic survival in irradiated 14-3-3sigma and CDKN1A (p21) knockout cell lines. Radiat Res. 2004;162(3):270-86.
8. Campisi J, d'Adda di Fagagna F. Cellular senescence: when bad things happen to good cells. Nat Rev Mol Cell Biol. 2007;8(9):729-40.
9. Mothersill C, Seymour CB. Radiation-induced bystander effects—implications for cancer. Nat Rev Cancer. 2004;4(2):158-64.
10. Thacker J, Stretch A. Recovery from lethal and mutagenic damage during postirradiation holding and low dose rate irradiations of cultured hamster cells. Radiat Res. 1983; 96(2):380-92.
11. Schwartz JL, Rasey J, Wiens L, et al. Functional inactivation of p53 by HPV-E6 transformation is associated with a reduced expression of radiation-induced potentially lethal damage. Int J Radiat Biol. 1999;75(3):285-91.
12. Withers HR, Taylor JMG, Maciejewski B. The hazard of accelerated tumor clonogen repopulation during radiotherapy. Acta Oncol. 1988;27(2):131-46.
13. Overgaard J. Sensitization of hypoxic tumour cells--clinical experience. Int J Radiat Biol. 1989;56(5):801-11.
14. Tannock IF, Hill RP. The basic science of oncology. New York: McGraw-Hill;1998.
15. West CM, Davidson SE, Roberts SA, et al. The independence of intrinsic radiosensitivity as a prognostic factor for patient response to radiotherapy of carcinoma of the cervix. Br J Cancer. 1997;76(9):1184-90.
16. International Commission on Radiation Units and Measurements: The Quality Factor in Radiation Protection. Report 40. Bethesda, MD, ICRU, 1986.
17. Barendsen GW. Responses of cultured cells, tumors, and normal tissues to radiation of different linear energy transfer. Curr Top Radiat Res Q 4:293-356,1968.
18. Field SB. The relative biological effectiveness of fast neutrons for mammalian tissues. Radiology. 1969;93(4):915-20.
19. Field SB, Jones T, Thomlinson RH. The relative effect of fast neutrons and X-rays on tumor and normal tissue in the rat: II. Fractionation: recovery and reoxygenation. Br J Radiol. 1968;41(488):597-607.
20. Broerse JJ, Barendsen GW. Relative biological effectiveness of fast neutrons for effects on normal tissues. Curr Top Radiat Res Q. 1973;8(4):305-50.
21. Palcic B, Skarsgard LD. Reduced oxygen enhancement ratio at low doses of ionizing radiation. Radiat Res. 1984;100(2):328-39.
22. Barendsen GW, Koot CJ, van Kersen GR, Bewley DK, Field SB, Parnell CJ. The effect of oxygen on impairment of the proliferative capacity of human cells in culture by ionizing radiations of different LET. Int J Radiat Biol Relat Stud Phys Chem Med. 1966;10(4):317-27.
23. Hall EJ. Radiation dose-rate: a factor of importance in radiobiology and radiotherapy. Br J Radiol. 1972;45(530):81-97.
24. Hall EJ, Brenner DJ. The dose-rate effect revisited: radiobiological considerations of importance in radiotherapy. Int J Radiat Oncol Biol Phys. 1991;21(6):1403-14.
25. Hall EJ, Bedford JS. Dose Rate: Its effect on the survival of hela cells irradiated with gamma rays. Radiat Res. 1964;22:305-15.
26. Ellis F. Dose time and fractionation: A clinical hypothesis. Clin Radiol. 1969;20(1):1-7.

2

CHAPTER

Radiation Pathology

Shyam Singh Bisht, Tejinder Kataria, Govardhan HB, Deepak Gupta

INTRODUCTION

X-rays interact with biologic material primarily by the Compton effect, producing energetic recoil electrons that traverse the cell and induce ionization events along their tracks by removing orbital electrons, either by direct or indirect effects. Most critical damages are produced in the DNA. The vast majority of lesions are successfully repaired and some lesions fail to repair and it is these that lead eventually to cell death. Cell death, is highly influenced by pathways within the DNA damage response (DDR) system. The DDR determines not only the sensitivity of cells to die following irradiation, but also the type of cell death that occurs, and the timing of cell death. Because the DDR differs among different types of normal and tumor cells (and perhaps even within different populations of tumor cells), the manifestation of cell death can also differ widely among different cell types. It is the killing of stem cells and the subsequent loss of the progenies that causes the early manifestations of normal-tissue damage after radiation exposure. At later times after the irradiation of normal tissues the so-called "late reactions" appear. These include fibrosis and telangiectasia of the skin, spinal cord damage and blood vessel damage.

Pathological changes or alterations that occur in human tissues exposed to radiation can be grouped into three categories: (1) those that occur in the epithelium and parenchymatous tissues, (2) those that occur in the stroma, and (3) those that occur in the blood vessels.[1] Some alterations appear months to years after exposure, i.e. delayed radiation injuries. Radiation does not produce pathognomonic morphologic features. Therefore, none of the alterations that occur are specific to radiation; they may occur as a result of injuries by other various agents also. This is an important consideration, particularly when morphology is used for medicolegal purposes.

PART I
RADIATION PATHOLOGY—GENERAL

EPITHELIAL AND PARENCHYMAL LESIONS

Necrosis and Ulceration

Necrosis and ulceration often coexist and generally precede the atrophic stage. It occurs in many epithelial and parenchymal cells during the "acute phase" of radiation injury. With exception of the skin and mucosa, such early lesions are seldom seen in humans. Examples, include mucosal ulceration and necrosis after intraluminal brachytherapy for carcinoma esophagus and skin ulceration after high dose of radiation. "Delayed necrosis" generally results from ischemia. It causes interruption of the lining epithelia/ulceration in the skin, upper alimentary and respiratory tracts, intestine, urinary tract, and genitalia. One of the most characteristic sites for delayed necrosis without ulceration is the central nervous system, particularly the white matter of the cerebral hemispheres.

Atrophy

Atrophy is one of the most common and consistent delayed effects of therapeutic irradiation. It is characterized by progressive loss of number and volume of epithelial cells.[2] It may occur in all lining epithelia (skin, alimentary, respiratory, and urinary tracts) as well as in all glands, parenchymatous tissues (salivary, pancreatic, mammary, kidney, lung, gonads, etc.). Some tissues/epithelia suffer more often or more severely than others. The distribution, extent and degree of atrophy are characteristically focal and random. It is not uncommon to observe relatively intact minor salivary glands adjacent to totally atrophic ones, all within the same radiation field.[3] Qualitatively such tissues may be separated into three

27. Ellis F. Nominal standard dose and the ret. Br J Radiol. 1971; 44(518):101-8.
28. Withers HR. Biologic basis for altered fractionation schemes. Cancer. 1985;55(9 Suppl):2086-95.
29. Begg AC, Hofland I, Van Glabekke M, et al. Predictive value of potential doubling time for radiotherapy of head and neck tumor patients: Results from the EORTC Cooperative Trial 22851. Semin Radiat Oncol. 1992;2:22-25.
30. Begg AC, McNally NJ, Shrieve D, et al. A method to measure the duration of DNA synthesis and the potential doubling time from a single sample. Cytometry. 1985;6(6):620-6.
31. Fowler JF. Dose response curves for organ function in cell survival. Br J Radiol. 1983;56(667):497-500.
32. Fowler JF. The linear-quadratic formula and progress in fractionated radiotherapy. Br J Radiol. 1989;62(740):679-94.
33. Withers HR, Thames HD, Peters LJ, et al. Normal tissue radioresistance in clinical radiotherapy. In: Fletcher GH, Nervi C, Withers HR (Eds). Biological Bases and Clinical Implications of Tumor Radioresistance. pp 139-152. New York: Masson; 1983.
34. Withers HR. Cell cycle redistribution as a factor in multifraction irradiation. Radiology. 1975;114(1):199-202.
35. Withers HR. Response of tissues to multiple small dose fractions. Radiat Res. 1977;71(1):24-33.
36. Willers H, Held KD. Introduction to clinical radiation biology. Hematol Oncol Clin North Am. 2006;20(1):1-24.
37. Baumann M, Petersen C, Krause M. TCP and NTCP in preclinical and clinical research in Europe. Rays. 2005;30(2):121-6.
38. Baumann M, Petersen C. TCP and NTCP: a basic introduction. Rays. 2005;30(2):99-104.
39. Lyman JT. Normal tissue complication probabilities: variable dose per fraction. Int J Radiat Oncol Biol Phys. 1992; 22(2):247-50.

groups: "severe atrophy" is more commonly observed in radiosensitive organs including epidermis, sebaceous glands (most affected in the skin), alimentary epithelium (especially intestine), urothelium, salivary glands, and germinal cells of the testis; "moderate atrophy" occurs in the epithelia of the upper respiratory and alimentary tracts, lung, mammary glands, prostate, and kidney, and "less severe atrophy" observed in sweat glands, liver, and endocrine glands.

Metaplasia

Metaplasia (the replacement of a normal tissue by another normal tissue) is seen in some organs; a common example is squamous epithelial metaplasia, which often replaces the normal glands of the prostate and urothelium. Hypermaturation and the converse, dedifferentiation of cells as the result of radiation, have been observed in carcinomas and could possibly occur in non-neoplastic epithelia.[4]

Atypia

Atypia of epithelial cells is not only a striking, usually delayed, alteration but also a source of confusion and error. A differential diagnosis can be made between radiation-induced atypia of non-neoplastic epithelium and residual or recurrent tumor with experience. It may affect either nucleus or cytoplasm or both. Most often there is enlargement of both nucleus and cytoplasm of individual cells. The nuclei may appear hyperchromatic but the chromatin is "smudged", i.e. chromatin granules are not distinct.[5] Nucleoli are often prominent. Generally, only some of the cells of a given structure (duct, gland, epithelial surface) show atypia, and architecturally there is no suggestion of neoplasia. Atypia has been observed in epidermis, squamous mucosa (mouth, larynx, vagina, cervix, etc.), bronchi and pulmonary alveoli, stomach, minor salivary glands, endometrial, urothelium, mammary gland, and prostate. In the last three sites this atypia has caused considerable diagnostic difficulty even to experienced pathologists.

Dysplasia

Dysplasia induced by irradiation of epithelia is frequently seen in epidermis and squamous mucosa and is less common in nonsquamous epithelia. It is a late lesion (occurring several years after exposure) characterized by nuclear atypia with hyperchromatism, lack of polarity (directional, organized maturation), involvement of large clones of cells and architectural alterations. Dysplasia implies genetic damage and abnormal ploidy can be documented. It should be distinguished from the benign atypia described above and should be considered premalignant, although not all cases evolve necessarily into neoplasms.[6]

Neoplasia

Neoplasia of epithelia and parenchymatous organs resulting from irradiation is well-documented for a number of tissues and organs. Neoplasia often follows dysplasia in skin and squamous mucosa, years after exposure. Not all radiation-induced neoplasms of these tissues are preceded by dysplasia.[5]

STROMAL LESIONS

Of all the lesions described here, those of the stroma are the ones best recognized by pathologists as radiation-induced or radiation-associated. The most typical combination of the features described below, occur in the submucosa and in the deep soft tissues of the mouth, pharynx, larynx and genitalia. Typical stromal lesions can be seen in the skin, lower urinary tract and alimentary tube.

Fibrosis

Fibrosis is one of the most common and consistent delayed manifestations of radiation injury.[7] It occurs in practically all tissues and organs, but extent and severity vary from site to site. Fibrosis is very much time- and dose-dependent, and, of course, it has been used to evaluate both of these variables. The typical radiation-induced fibrosis is in homogeneous: some areas have very dense, acellular collagen, while next to them other areas have only a few fibrous bands. The fibrous areas are within the irradiated field but do not fill it entirely. Such alterations in adipose tissue, skeletal or cardiac muscle, or parenchymatous organs (lung, kidney) are easy to appreciate.

It is more practical to list the sites where fibrosis does not occur or is rare, than to list the tissues where it is found. In the hemopoietic system, bone marrow replacement by adipose tissue is the result of high doses; fibrosis does not occur unless a neoplasm or an inflammatory lesion had been present prior to the irradiation, in which case the stroma of such a lesion persists in the marrow space. Radiation injury to the bone after a high dose leads to necrosis rather than fibrosis. The delayed hepatic injury shows surprisingly little fibrosis, except in the areas that contained tumor prior to exposure. The same can be said of lymph nodes: when high doses result in lymphocyte depletion, the skeleton of the node remains, with little additional connective tissue, except in the areas that harbored tumor.

Fibrosis is much more than a marker of radiation damage; it leads to deformation of skin resulting in retraction and esophageal, intestinal, or urinary stenosis with obstruction, myocardial failure, restrictive pericardial disease, as well as reduction in pulmonary function.

A very characteristic feature of radiation-induced change is the presence of fibrin in the stroma. Probably it occurs in most irradiated mesenchymal tissues but it is only detectable by light microscopy in some soft tissues. Fibrinous exudate appears as a delicate network of acidophilic fibrils in the midst of collagen and fibroblasts. It is not seen throughout the entire area of fibrosis but rather occurs in widely separate foci. Special stains, such as phosphotungstic acid-hematoxylin or the Fraser/Lendrum techniques, facilitate the recognition of fibrin. This finding is valuable in the differential diagnosis of delayed radiation fibrosis but only in sites that do not have other causes for active inflammatory exudate (particularly ulcers); fibrin is a well-known component of the inflammatory exudate, and, therefore, it is expected to be present wherever there is inflammation. Radiation-associated fibrin is not only deposited in the interstitial tissues, it accumulates also on the serosal surfaces; and typically a carpet-like exudate can be seen on the pericardium in radiation-induced heart disease.

Atypical Fibroblast

Atypical fibroblasts (so-called "radiation fibroblasts") are very characteristic of delayed radiation injury. These are large, bizarre cells, usually basophilic, with angulated and elongated cytoplasm. Triangular or even star shapes are observed, and a common configuration is reminiscent of a "swallow tail". The nuclei are hyperchromatic and "smudged" but mitotic figures are practically never seen. Atypical fibroblasts are found in delayed lesions, predominantly in the submucosa of the upper respiratory tract, the entire alimentary tract, the lower urinary tract and genitalia. They are less common in the nonulcerated skin and in the deep soft tissues. Atypical fibroblasts are not seen in the deep organs, such as lungs, heart, liver or brain.[8] Cells identical to atypical fibroblasts are seen occasionally in nonirradiated chronically inflamed tissues, particularly at the base of chronic pressure ulcers (decubitus ulcers). Necrosis of stromal elements is uncommon in the absence of ulceration, superimposed infection, or tumor. Fat necrosis is also rare. It has been described in the irradiated breast, and in such a location it may present as a mass mimicking a recurrent tumor on clinical examination.[9] Most instances of necrosis in irradiated tissues are associated with radiation-induced ulcers.

A consistent feature of delayed radiation injury in mammalian tissues is the lack or paucity of cellular inflammatory response. With some exceptions (such as ulcers) the stromal reactions described above are devoid of granulocytes and contain only a few lymphocytes or macrophages. This is best seen in deep tissues such as myocardium, pericardium and renal parenchyma. The absence of cellular inflammatory response is helpful in the differential diagnosis of radiation pathology. Furthermore, it supports the concept that radiation injury is not mediated through an immune mechanism.

Vascular Lesions

Vascular lesions are prominent morphologically and play an important role in the pathogenesis of delayed radiation injury. Late vascular injury contributes to secondary organ damage through decreased perfusion leading to tissue ischemia, necrosis, ulceration and fibrosis. Blood vessel damage was recognized by radiation workers as early as 1899. Common morphologic changes of blood vessels include endothelial damage, intimal hyperplasia and vascular wall fibrosis. Blood vessels are described in decreasing order of radiation sensitivity.

Blood Capillaries and Sinusoids

The narrowest and most ubiquitous elements of the vasculature appear to be the most radiosensitive. Capillaries are the most frequent blood vessels to be affected. This is related to the high radiation sensitivity of endothelial cells which constitute the most important part of capillary walls.[10] Only some lesions of these vessels are appreciated by light microscopy: dilatation is common, and, when superficially located, it can be detected clinically as telangiectasia of skin or mucous membranes; asymmetry with irregularity of the wall; focal prominence of endothelial cells; and rarely, thrombosis. Neither light microscopic studies of human tissues nor electron microscopy reveals the most important result of acute damage: a reduction in the microvascular network that ultimately results in ischemia. This has been well-shown by various techniques in some tissues such as myocardium, central nervous system and skin.[11]

Small-Sized Arteries

These (measuring up to 100 µm in external diameter) have a muscular wall, which gives some protection from rupture. These segments may develop necrosis soon after irradiation or in the delayed phase (e.g. "fibrinoid" necrosis of arterioles in the brain). Subendothelial or adventitial fibrosis, "hyalinization" of the media (dense, acellular, acidophilic, collagenous material), the accumulation of lipid-laden macrophages in the intima and thrombosis may occur as a post radiation sequel.

Medium-Sized Arteries

The medium-sized arteries (100–500 µm) develop late lesions and the most common change is intimal fibrosis, characterized by deposition of collagen and fibroblasts (myofibroblasts). Lipid-containing macrophages (foam cells) may accumulate in the intima, in variable numbers, sometimes causing narrowing or complete obstruction. Fibrin may be present among the foam cells, and there may be occlusive thrombosis. By contrast, in spontaneous atherosclerosis the foam cell plaques are usually seen in arteries of large size, but rarely in medium- and small-sized vessels. Therefore, although not specific, foam cell plaques in medium and small arteries are highly suggestive of irradiation-induced changes and can be observed in the vessels of the intestinal wall and in the ovaries.[12] Acute vasculitis may occur as an uncommon, delayed lesion. Although cellular inflammatory exudate is absent or minimal in delayed radiation pathology it can be seen in the active arteritis in the wall of the intestine, in the pelvic adipose tissue and in the irradiated breast. Such radiation-associated vasculitis is self-limited and heals without therapy; hence, it should not be confused with ominous systemic vasculitis. Arterioles adjacent to arteries (coronary or iliac) that have been subjected to endovascular brachytherapy can develop acute vasculitis with fibrinoid necrosis.

Large Arteries

The large arteries (> 500 μm) are less often affected than the smaller vessels, because of their ample lumen and thick wall, which is made of relatively radioresistant cells.[13] The changes that can be seen are: myointimal proliferation, with or without lipid deposits, thrombosis, mural or occlusive, and rupture of large arteries. This is a fatal complication that tends to occur in the carotid or the femoral arteries or in the aorta. It may not result from irradiation alone, and such ruptures can be caused by bacterial infections, exposure to digestive enzymes, or exposure to air. There is experimental evidence indicating that arterial perforations may result solely from high-dose irradiation.[14,15]

Small Veins

The small veins (having only a few layers of muscle) are affected less often than their arterial counterparts. Intimal or medial fibrosis or, thrombosis of the veins can be seen in the wall of the intestines similar to arterial lesions after abdominal irradiation. Irradiation produces predominantly a venous lesion and not an arterial one in the liver.

Large Veins

The (>/500 μm) large veins are least affected by irradiation, although they can be infiltrated and damaged by tumor invasion. The veins that show transmural scars are often in fact vessels that contained neoplasms prior to irradiation.[12]

PART II
RADIATION PATHOLOGY—ORGAN SPECIFIC

HEART

Radiation-induced heart disease includes three clinical entities which differ with regard to latency, radiation exposure and clinical features. Early onset cardiac toxicity is most often seen in the form of acute pericarditis while late complications can range from chronic constrictive pericarditis to radiation cardiomyopathy, myocardial insufficiency, cardiovascular damage/coronary artery disease, valvulopathy to conduction deficit. Cuzick et al. reported excess overall mortality in breast cancer patients postradiotherapy for women surviving more than 10 years.[16] A meta-analysis of 8 randomized controlled trials of breast cancer initiated before 1975, involving 8,000 women found, a 62% increase in cardiac deaths in women who received radiation.

Radiation Pericarditis

Acute Radiation Pericarditis

Pericardium is the most commonly affected heart tissue in cases undergoing radiation to the chest. Acute pericarditis can manifest soon after radiation therapy and symptoms may include fever and chest pain. The incidence of cardiac disease, postradiation is estimated to be around 5%. Radiation-induced pericarditis is characterized by fibrosis and exudates. The exact mechanism is unknown although inflammatory and mesothelial cells are main target in this case. Inhibition of the local fibrinolytic mechanism that would normally lead to reabsorption of any pericardial effusion caused by a radiation-induced increase of capillary permeability is also a contributing factor. Mostly, it starts as exudative pericarditis and is self-resolving, however, some patients may progress to constrictive pericarditis which is quite rare.[17] The risk of pericarditis is higher above a dose of 35 Gy to significant portion of heart. A mean dose of less than 26 Gy to whole pericardium is recommended, if possible.

Chronic Pericarditis

It is a late complication, arising months to years (usually1–2 years) after radiation therapy. The incidence of chronic pericarditis is 1–5% in breast and lung cancer patients but the data are from older series where patients were treated with obsolete techniques. The frequency of chronic pericarditis is estimated to between 2% and 7% for mediastinal doses ranging from 35 to 40 Gy. In a series of Hodgkin's lymphoma patients treated at Stanford University, the mortality rates from pericarditis was 0.7%.[18] Most often it is asymptomatic, it can be diagnosed by pulmonary radiograph, ECG or an ECHO. Majority of patients with chronic pericarditis will resolve spontaneously, with no long-term adverse complication. Some patients develop late constrictive pericarditis with rapidly developing cardiac effusion that may result in cardiac tamponade requiring drainage.

Dose per fraction and total dose constitute the main factors responsible for development of chronic pericarditis. Risk of pericarditis is present at 35 Gy, but increases significantly above 40 Gy when a large volume of the heart (> 30%) is exposed to doses more than 40 Gy (threshold dose).

Myocarditis and Cardiomyopathy

It is mostly seen in patients who already have chronic pericarditis with significant diastolic insufficiency. The incidence of radiation-induced myocarditis is difficult to determine. Autopsy series have found myocardial fibrosis in 50% of patients irradiated at a young age. Older series on Hodgkin's lymphoma have reported a decrease in left ventricular ejection fraction in 30–50%, however, these data are from older techniques and faulty dose calculation.[19] In modern series, for patients treated with newer techniques, normal cardiac function is maintained throughout long-term follow-up.

The mean latency of myocarditis is about 5 years. The myocytes are not directly damaged by doses common in radiotherapy but arterioles or capillaries are injured through damage of the vascular endothelium. This initiates intravascular thrombosis and micro-rupture of arterioles and capillaries, leading to disruption of the vascular network in the myocardium. These changes compromise the microcirculation, ultimately leading to fibrosis and ischemia. Left ventricle is more commonly affected than the right because of its anterior location.[20] Radiation-induced changes manifest as reduced left ventricular function, myocardial perfusion defects, valve dysfunction or conduction defects (due to ischemic fibrosis disturbing the conduction system).

Coronary Artery Disease

Radiation causes endoluminal fibromuscular hyperplasia, aggravating the risk of atherosclerosis, leading to stenosis.[21] Spontaneous atherosclerosis cannot be morphologically distinguished from atherosclerosis due to radiation injury. It manifests as ischemic heart disease including angina pectoris, myocardial infarction and cardiac incompensation. There is a long latency period of more than 10 years for delayed cardiac morbidity. The true incidence of coronary artery disease is underestimated as it is often asymptomatic. A higher incidence of coronary artery stenosis in high-risk radiotherapy (like treating internal mammary) has been reported in many series. Proximal left anterior descending artery is the most common vessel affected in left side breast cancer post-radiotherapy. It has been postulated that hotspot areas of coronary vessels are at risk of stenosis.

Valvulopathies

Perivalvular myocardial and endocardial fibrosis leads to secondary valvular dysfunction. With modern diagnostic techniques, rate of valvulopathies is quiet high (15–30%). The cumulative incidence at 20 and 25 years is reported to be 45% and 60%.[22] Valvular dysfunction usually presents as mitral or aortic insufficiency. Total dose is an important risk factor with a low incidence reported at a dose below 30 Gy but rises sharply to 12% above 31 Gy.

Constraints

Gagliardi G et al.[23] by using NTCP model, have predicted the cardiac morbidity of less than 1% at 15 years follow-up if V25 Gy is kept below 10% (2 Gy fractions). They have also advocated, attempts should be made to keep whole heart to receive less than 15 Gy with adriamycin-based chemotherapy.

LUNGS

Radiation Pneumopathy

Two well-recognized conditions are associated with pulmonary radiation damage, radiation pneumonitis (acute/subacute toxicity) and radiation fibrosis (late toxicity).[24] A less well-known "sporadic radiation pneumonitis" is diffuse lymphocytosis involving whole lung. It also involves the part of lung away from radiation zone.[25]

Radiation Pneumonitis

It has a clinical presentation similar to bacterial pneumonia.

A summary was published by Gross et al. which provides an overview on the sequence of events that lead to pulmonary injury after exposure to radiation.[26] The cells affected by radiation are the capillary endothelial cells, type I/II pneumocytes, macrophages and stromal fibroblasts.

In the "early phase" there is loss of type I pneumocytes that line the alveoli, resulting in a sloughed epithelium, as well as type II pneumocytes, which are the less-differentiated precursors to type I cells and secrete surfactant. On a microscopic level, there is increased capillary permeability and swelling of basement membrane. These changes can be seen with radiation doses of more than 10–20 Gy.[27] No gross histological/light microscopy changes seen in lungs but chemical, ultra-structural and cellular changes (plasma membrane disruption, increased permeability) are seen in endothelial cells and in Type I and II pneumocytes.

In the "intermediate/subacute/exudative phase" protein leaks into alveolar spaces, the alveolar septa are thickened and changes appears in the type II pneumocytes or macrophages.

This reduces the volume of air space, decreasing the gaseous diffusion subsequent to above changes. Reduction in perfusion precedes the signs and symptoms of pneumonitis and usually occurs 3–4 weeks after radiation exposure. Clinical manifestations include mild to severe dyspnea, nonproductive cough and transient fever. Fullness of chest, chest pain and weakness are also seen. Extreme conditions, like severe respiratory insufficiency/cyanosis, are infrequent but not rare.

In the "late phase" of radiation damage, there is a decrease in the number of cells, including endothelial cells of the capillaries and type I, II pneumocytes. Alveolar macrophages are present in the interstitial space and are activated once radiation damage has occurred under stimulus induced by inflammation and growth factor. Activated macrophages along with cytokines, growth factors stimulate the proliferation of fibroblasts which leads to overproduction of collagen fibers ultimately leading to pulmonary fibrosis.

Onset of radiation fibrosis may be manifested by gradually increasing dyspnea, persistent dry cough, or signs and symptoms of cor pulmonale. However, this stage is often asymptomatic, recognized only when an abnormality is seen on radiographs or with the development of secondary infection, bronchiectasis, spontaneous pneumothorax.[28] Often, clinical or radiologic evidence indicates radiation fibrosis, without any clear antecedent radiation pneumonitis. Rubin et al. hypothesized that the cascade of cytokines begins immediately at the time of radiation and persists till the appearance of late injury. Role of TGF-beta, IL-1, IL-6 has been postulated in radiation pneumonitis.

Dosimetric Predictors of Radiation Injury to Lung

Volume of lung receiving 20 Gy (V20) parameter is commonly used to predict rates of radiation pneumonitis, as 20 Gy has been estimated to be a threshold dose at which lung tissue is no longer functional. Graham et al. examined the predictive value of V20 in radiation pneumonitis and stratified patients into four main groups. There was 8%, 13% and 19% risk of grade II pneumonitis when V20 values were 22–31%, 32–40% and more than 40%, respectively.[29]

Radiological Picture

Changes in the lung are usually confined to the irradiated portal and changes in the remainder of the lung may also be seen occasionally. This may be different as the clinics adopt intensity modulated radiation.

Computed Tomography

Computed tomography (CT) is able to better delineate parenchymal changes and often demonstrates the changes restricted to the irradiated field, making the diagnosis much easier. It should be noted, however, that with stereotactic body radiotherapy the shape of the irradiated field will not have straight edges or conform to the traditional conventional radiotherapy portals. In cases of early or subtle radiation-induced pneumonitis, areas of ground-glass opacity may be evident on CT despite a normal chest X-ray. The common findings are ground-glass opacities and airspace consolidation. Other findings may be focal or nodular opacities, tree-in-bud appearances, ipsilateral appearance, atelectasis and pleural effusion. Late changes include loss of volume, linear scarring, and chronic consolidation often with air bronchograms, traction bronchiectasis, mediastinal shift, pleural thickening and ipsilateral pleural effusion. Cavitations are not a usual feature and suggest superimposed infection.

Libshitz and Shuman[30] described four radiologic patterns evident on CT (1) homogeneous, slight increase in attenuation, uniformly involving the irradiated portion of lung; (2) patchy consolidation within the irradiated lung, not necessarily conforming to the shape of the portal; (3) discrete consolidation, conforming to the shape of the portal, but not uniformly outlining it; and (4) solid consolidation, conforming to and totally involving the irradiated region of lung. Patterns 1 and 2 appear to represent generalized and inhomogeneous radiation pneumonitis, respectively. The third pattern may reflect focal organizing pneumonitis or fibrosis. The fourth pattern more clearly represents radiation fibrosis. CT is more sensitive than chest radiography for showing radiation effects.

Fludeoxyglucose-Positron Emission Tomography

Positron emission tomography (PET) performed soon after completion of radiotherapy often demonstrates an increased metabolic activity in both lungs, especially in a peripheral distribution. Only a minority of patient go on to develop clinically or CT evident pneumonitis. Fludeoxyglucose-positron emission tomography (FDG-PET) is useful in differentiating radiation fibrosis from recurrent or radiation-induced malignancy, as the former will not be metabolically active.

TREATMENT AND PROGNOSIS

Steroids can reduce the severity of acute radiation pneumonitis. Depending on the degree of injury changes may be mild and spontaneously resolve or progress to adult respiratory distress syndrome (ARDS) with a high rate of mortality.

QUANTEC Constraints

Marks L et al. have reviewed the three-dimensional dose, volume and outcome data for lung[31] and have suggested to limit V20 to less than 30–35% and mean lung dose less than 14–20 Gy.

LIVER

Radiation-induced liver disease (RILD) typically occurs 4–8 weeks after radiation exposure but can happen as early as 2 weeks and as late as 7 months after completion of radiation therapy. Majority of patients recover completely in 3–5 months, while a minority progress toward a chronic stage, with worsening liver fibrosis and failure, only rarely developing fulminant hepatic failure. The term "radiation hepatitis" is a misnomer, since pathological evaluation fails to reveal inflammation, instead showing nonspecific veno-occlusive disease.[32]

Pathogenic Mechanism

Radiation-induced endothelial damage exposes the subendothelial basement membrane, leading to platelet activation and aggregation, and stimulation of dormant hepatic stellate cells. Fibrin thrombus causes venous occlusion, pan lobular congestion, diffuse hemorrhagic and necrotic foci, and distension of hepatic sinusoids. Prolonged obstruction and activation of hepatic stellate cells results in hepatocyte loss and fibrosis mediated by transforming growth factor-1 release.[32-34]

Histopathology

Veno-occlusion is observed at the tissue level, characterized by severe congestion in the central portion of the parenchymal lobules. It specifically involves the small branches of hepatic veins, unlike Budd-Chiari syndrome, the major hepatic veins and inferior vena cava are not involved. On gross pathology, hyperemia is observed. There is collagen deposition within lumen of afferent sinusoids. TGF-beta is thought to mediate this process by stimulating migration of fibroblasts that proliferate and deposit collagen in the areas of injury. Within 6 months of injury, little congestion is seen and liver ultra-structure is largely restored.[35]

Imaging

The region of radiation damage is hypodense on the portal venous phase and becomes hyperdense on the delayed phase obtained 4 minutes after contrast medium injection compared with the normal surrounding parenchyma. This appearance has been explained by a decreased vascular perfusion and by reduced hepatic venous drainage with subsequent stasis of the contrast medium.[36,37]

Clinical Manifestations

Clinical manifestations include ascites, fatigue, rapid weight gain, increase abdominal girth, anicteric hepatomegaly, and right upper quadrant discomfort. There is a marked increase in alkaline phosphatase (3–10 fold). Moderate transaminase elevation with little or no increase in bilirubin is seen. Majority of patients recover within 3–5 months while minority will progress toward chronic stage.

Constraints

Pan C. et al. have analyzed the liver constraints for conventional fractionations and stereotactic body radiation therapy (SBRT).[38] *Conventional fractionation*: In case of liver metastasis, whole liver dose should be kept below 30 Gy (@ 2 Gy fraction) and below 21 Gy (@ 3 Gy fraction). In case of hepatocellular carcinoma (HCC) whole liver dose should be kept below 28 Gy (@ 2 Gy fraction) and below 21 Gy (@ 3 Gy fraction). *In SBRT*: In HCC, mean liver dose (MLD) should be kept below 13 Gy (for 3 fractions), and less than 18 Gy (in 6 fractions).

KIDNEY

Renal radiation injury can appear within first few months following renal radiation exposure or it can manifest as late or chronic radiation nephropathy, years after radiation exposure and which may not necessarily be a direct outcome of acute renal event.[39]

The Pathogenic Mechanisms

The pathogenic mechanisms responsible for the development of radiation nephropathy remain ill-defined. Experimental studies indicate that primarily glomerular and tubular alterations occur in the primary stages of radiation nephropathy. Glomerular capillary endothelial cell loss with increased permeability can be detected within 1 hour in rats, remaining endothelial cells exhibit increased permeability leading to a subendothelial transudate, mesangiolysis is also observed. Overt proteinuria does not appear until 5 weeks after irradiation and it is followed by azotemia. In contrast, podocytes appear to be relatively unaffected at this stage. The endothelial changes appear to resolve, but the mesangial lesions progress, with hypercellularity and/or hypertrophy, increased mesangial matrix, mesangial sclerosis and ultimately, glomerulosclerosis. These mesangial changes are similar to those observed in other chronic glomerulopathies. Anemia develops along with the azotemia, but at a level disproportionate to azotemia.[40,41] Azotemia becomes progressively worse over several months and can eventually lead to renal failure. Histopathological changes are first observed when the serum urea levels reaches double the normal value.

Histology

The light microscopy appearance of classical radiation nephropathy and nephropathy after radioisotope therapy is same as bone marrow transplant (BMT) nephropathy. Mesangiolysis is always present, there is a limited tubulointerstitial inflammation and there is substantial subendothelial expansion by low-density material that seems mostly to be plasma proteins. Inflammation is not prominent.

Clinical Spectrum

The findings associated with radiation-induced kidney injury can be segregated into subclinical (acute) and clinical (subacute and chronic) type. Acute (within 3 months) radiation-induced kidney injury is generally subclinical. The signs and symptoms develop during the subacute period

(3–18 months). Manifestations of chronic injury are seen after more than 18 months and are characterized by benign or malignant hypertension, elevated creatinine level anemia, and renal failure. If no changes in renal blood perfusion or glomerular filtration rate (GFR) are observed within 2 years after radiation therapy, subsequent chronic injury is unlikely. The long latency for clinical kidney toxicity has been reported and this can reduce a patient's reserve against future renal insults.[42]

Subclinical

Physiological endpoints include elevated blood pressure, increased weight along with biochemical changes including elevated urine β2 microglobulin, elevated serum blood urea nitrogen, serum creatinine, serum renin, reduced glomerular filtration rate, decreased creatinine clearance, proteinuria, hematuria and anemia. Imaging defects include reduced glomerular function manifested on GFR 99mTc-DTPA renography, reduced tubular function seen on 99mTc-DMSA scintigraphy, perfusion deficits on scintigraphy 131 Iodine radiohippurate, asymmetric uptake of intravenous contrast on CT and atrophy of the kidney.

Clinical

Physiological manifestations are malignant hypertension, headache, edema, dyspnea, fatigue, nausea and vomiting.

Imaging

CT scan and MR scan do not have an important role in imaging of radiation nephropathy. Radiation nephropathy-induced parenchymal scarring is evident on ultrasound scans by increased echogenicity and loss of corticomedullary differentiation. Nuclear medicine scans may suggest chronic parenchymal disease by reduced or slowed parenchymal uptake of tracer. The flow part of the nuclear medicine study may show asymmetry of flow, which could point to renovascular disease.

Mitigation and Treatment of Radiation Nephropathy

Antagonism of renin-angiotension system (RAS) has been shown to be highly effective for the mitigation and treatment of experimental radiation nephropathy.[43] Both angiotensin-converting enzyme (ACE) inhibitors and AII receptor blocker (ARB) are effective in reducing the incidence of radiation-induced renal failure when used after irradiation but before there is physiological evidence of injury.[44] Other types of antihypertensive drugs have not been shown to prevent radiation-induced renal injury in animals. Dietary protein restriction and corticosteroids can also reduce the severity of experimental radiation nephropathy.

Constraints

Dawson et al. have reviewed the constraints for the kidney in abdominal radiotherapy.[42] They suggested that mean dose to bilateral kidney should be kept below 1,500c Gy, V12 should be less than 55%, V20 should be less than 32%.

BRAIN

Cerebral Radionecrosis

Radiation-induced CNS injury is associated with a high rate of morbidity and mortality. CNS injury has been well-described in terms of histological and functional criteria as well as radiobiological parameters,[45,46] although the underlying cellular and biochemical processes remain poorly defined. Classically radiation-induced CNS injury has been divided into three categories based on time of expression: Acute, early-delayed and late-delayed. "Acute radiation encephalopathy" is expressed within days to weeks after radiation and is uncommon under current radiotherapy protocols. "Early delayed injury" occurs from 1 to 6 months postradiation and can involve transient demyelination with somnolence (brain radiation) or L'hermitte's syndrome (spinal radiation). Both acute and early delayed effects are normally reversible and resolve spontaneously. In contrast late-delayed effects, which occur more than 6 months after radiation are not completely reversible and may be progressive. They are characterized by demyelination, vascular abnormalities and ultimately cerebral radionecrosis (RN) which is generally restricted to white matter.

Clinical Symptoms

Radionecrosis may be symptomatic or asymptomatic. Symptoms include seizure, headache, vomiting, motor, cognitive and speech deficits.

Latency

The mean interval from the end of radiotherapy until onset of white matter necrosis is about 11 months,[47] though it has been reported to manifest as early as 3 months and as late as 47 years. Latency period for development of necrosis in glioma patients appears to be five times shorter than in other patients (e.g. nasopharyngeal carcinoma) receiving equivalent dose.

Pathophysiology

Various hypotheses have been proposed regarding the primary cell population whose death or inactivation after radiation results in white matter necrosis.

Vascular hypothesis: According to this hypothesis white matter necrosis is considered to be a secondary response to ischemia. There is evidence of radiation-induced vascular abnormalities including vessel wall thickening, dilatation and endothelial cell damage. Time-and dose-related reduction in blood vessel density has been reported prior to development of necrosis in white matter.

Oligodendrocyte hypothesis: RN is typically dominated by demyelination which implies that Oligodendrocytes are the target cell population. Oligodendrocytes provide the myelin sheath for neurons and their loss is a source of demyelination.

Neural stem cell hypothesis: The subventricular zone (SVZ) is the main source of neurons, astrocytes and oligodendrocytes in the late embryonic forebrain of mammals. SVZ persists into adulthood as mitotic stem cell area. It has been suggested that depletion of the SVZ cells could play a role in radiation-induced late delayed effects.

Histology

Radiation necrosis is seen most commonly around blood vessels within white matter. The most frequent histopathological feature is fibrinoid necrosis of blood vessel wall with surrounding perivascular parenchymal coagulative necrosis. It may be peritumoral or distant; unifocal or multifocal. Clusters of abnormally dilated thin-walled telangiectasias are often seen. White matter changes may also be focal or diffuse; in the diffuse pattern, widespread periventricular demyelination is seen. Other histological features include oligodendrocyte dropping out, axonal swelling, reactive gliosis, and disruption of the blood-brain barrier.

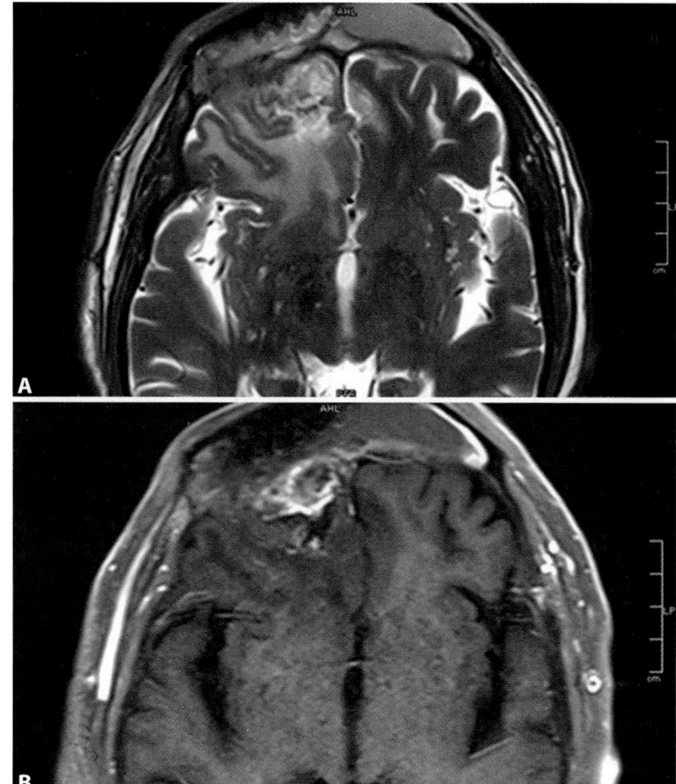

Figs 1A and B MRI images of a patient with frontal sinus carcinoma of treated with conventional radiation with concurrent chemotherapy developed radionecrosis of the frontal lobe ("Swiss cheese" pattern) after one year of treatment

Courtesy: Dr Tejinder Kataria, Division of Radiation Oncology Medanta—The Medicit, Haryana, India

Imaging

Conventional MRI: No MRI radiographic pattern is pathognomonic for RN and supplementary imaging is necessary and sometimes a surgical intervention may give the final verdict.

Radionecrosis can closely resemble recurrent tumor on conventional MRI because of its close proximity to original tumor site, contrast enhancement, progressive enlargement over many months, surrounding edema and mass effect. On T2 weighted images, surrounding edema has high signal intensity, solid portion of the radionecrotic lesion has low signal intensity and central necrotic component shows increased signal intensity.

Lesion quotient (LQ) has been defined by Dequesada et al. as ratio of nodule as seen on T2 imaging to total enhancing area on T1 imaging and suggested that a LQ more than 0.6 correlated with recurrence and less than 0.3 correlates with RN.[48] Kumar et al. cite two MRI features that are consistent with RN, the "Swiss cheese" pattern and "soap bubble" pattern (Figs 1A and B).

Magnetic resonance spectroscopy (MRS): In general, regions of tumor are characterized by N-acetylaspartate (NAA)/ phosphorylcholine (Cho) ratio less than 1 and Lipid(Lip)/ Cho ratio less than 3. In contrast Lip/Cho ratio more than 3 or significant decrease of all metabolite levels within the lesion or surrounding brain are considered characteristic of RN.

Diffusion-weighted imaging (DWI): This technique depends on the diffusion of water molecules within the tissue under study and generates an apparent diffusion coefficient (ADC) map.[49] Areas of high ADC, appears dark on DWI whereas low ADC areas produce increased intensity. Areas with RN have a high ADC than areas of hypercellular tumor.

Perfusion MRI: Dynamic contrast enhanced perfusion MRI (pMRI) of brain provides hemodynamic information that complements the conventional MRI. Contrast enhanced pMRI methods exploit signal changes that accompany the passage of paramagnetic contrast agent through the cerebro-vascular system. Analysis of dynamic data from pMRI yields quantitative estimation of relative cerebral blood flow volume (rCBV) of the lesion versus other region of interest, such as surrounding tissue or contra lateral normal tissue. In a series of 20 cases, the authors found that a normalized rCBV of 2.6 or above indicated tumor recurrence and a ratio of 0.6 or less was suggestive of nonneoplastic contrast enhancing tissue.[50]

Nuclear scans: FDG-PET is often used in differentiating between RN and tumor recurrence.

Amino acid PET: It is a particularly attractive radioactive substance for imaging brain tumors because of high uptake in tumor tissue and low uptake in normal tissue. It is more sensitive than 18F-FDG-PET in visualizing tumor. Most extensively studied amino acid tracer is 11C-methionine (T1/2 20 minutes). 18F-FLT (18F-Fluoroethyl-L-tyrosine) which does not accumulate in macrophages, a common inflammatory cell type in necrosis, may be able to differentiate between RN and tumor recurrence. Absence of 18F-FLT in case of RN has been reported.[51]

Single photon emission computed tomography (SPECT): Tl SPECT. Uptake of thallium by tumor cells relies on a combination of mechanisms including blood brain-barrier disruption, blood flow and Na^+/K^+-ATPase pump activity.[52] It can differentiate between tumor and radiation necrosis and even estimate the grade of a tumor. It reflects viable tumor burden more accurately than CT, MR, or other radionuclide studies. Radiation-induced necrotic tissue does not take up thallium-201 due to lack of the active transport mechanism and absence of Na^+/K^+-ATPase enzyme. Lower spatial resolution compared to PET is one of the main setbacks of SPECT.

Management

Steroids: Anti-inflammatory effect of steroids (dexamethasone) when provided early can modify subsequent vascular and inflammatory changes and reduce, limit or delay the subsequent necrosis. Administration of steroids early in the course of RN is more effective than delayed. Doses must be adequate to control clinical symptoms. Some patients require long-term treatment (6 months) as they become symptomatic when it is withdrawn.

Surgical excision: When steroid therapy is poorly tolerated and when necrosis becomes progressively larger and symptoms are not controlled despite steroids, excision of necrotic mass is indicated. It is more effective for well circumscribed lesions than diffuse lesions.

Dose and volume dependence: A fraction size of more than 225c Gy, shorter overall time, twice daily radiation, re-irradiation and SRS/SRT increases risk of RN.

Constraints

Lawrence et al. have reviewed the data regarding radiotherapy induced brain injury.[53] For fractionated RT with a fraction size of less than 2.5 Gy, an incidence of radiation necrosis of 5% and 10% is predicted to occur at biologically effective dose (BED) of 120 Gy and 150 Gy. There is steep increase in toxicity when twice daily fraction is used beyond 80 Gy BED.

SALIVARY GLANDS

The major salivary glands (parotid, submandibular, and sublingual) produce up to 80% of the salivary secretions with the rest supplied by the minor salivary glands in the oral cavity. The submandibular glands produce saliva during a resting state, while the parotid glands are the main contributors under a stimulated state. Radiation injury to the major salivary glands can be seen in the first 1–2 weeks of a course of radiotherapy. The serous-producing cells appear to be more sensitive than the mucinous-producing cells as the saliva becomes more mucinous, thick, ropey, and sticky. Also there is reduction in baseline and stimulated flow. Interphase death of serous cells occurs resulting in atrophy of the cells without inflammation suggesting apoptosis playing a role during this phase. Progressive reduction in flow rates, pH, and secretory immunoglobulin A is observed as the radiation dose increases. The pathological changes seen in animal models post-radiations are fibrosis, acinar atrophy, parenchymal loss, striated duct dilation, and intercalated duct proliferation and dilation.

The pathohistological changes in the irradiated salivary glands may be classified into three stages.[54] Stage I is characterized by marked swelling and vacuolization of the serous glandular acini. Isolated glandular acini may show moderate atrophy in several regions. Lymphocytic infiltrate may be seen around periductal tissue with moderate fibrosis. In stage II there is atrophy of glandular acini/significant parenchymal reduction. In addition to ectasia of the excretory ducts, moderate ductal proliferation is also observed. Moderate periductal fibrosis and significant lymphocytic infiltration are also observed. Interstitial lipomatosis occurs in some areas. The blood vessels exhibit only minor sclerotic changes. Stage III is characterized by high-grade parenchymal reduction. The periductal tissue exhibits extensive lymphocytic infiltrate. Numerous ductal proliferations are also found. Goblet cell and squamous cell metaplasia may also develop in the ductal epithelium. In addition to an intraluminal accumulation of secretions, isolated periductal mucosal excretion changing over to mucosal granuloma may be observed. The gland lobules exhibit interstitial sclerosis. A further increase in interstitial connective tissue results in a picture of glandular transformation of the cirrhotic salivary gland type. Significant proliferation of the intima with the formation of vascular stenoses may be observed.

The tolerance dose (TD) 50/5 for the parotid gland (uniform dose resulting in a 50% complication probability at 5 years) is 38–46 Gy with gradual improvement in parotid flow after radiotherapy.[55] There is a linear correlation with 5% loss of function per 1 Gy of mean dose to the parotid with no threshold dose. The incidence of xerostomia is significantly reduced when the mean dose of at least one parotid gland is kept less than or equal to 26 Gy and may return back to pretreatment levels when the mean dose is less than 25–30 Gy.[56] For complete salivary production recovery after 24 months, the volume of the contralateral parotid gland receiving more than 40 Gy should be less than 33%.[57] Submandibular gland is more radioresistant in comparison to the parotid gland.[58] Stimulated and unstimulated flow rates recovered at 2 years post-treatment when the mean dose did not exceed 39 Gy.

The parotid glands have been shown to decrease in size (volume) by about 5% per week during a course of radiotherapy. This results in a shift of the lateral superficial lobe medially by about 0.85 mm/week during treatment.

REFERENCES

1. Fajardo LF. The pathology of ionizing radiation as defined by morphologic patterns. Acta Oncol. 2005;44(1):13-22.
2. Fajardo LF. Basic mechanisms and general morphology of radiation injury. Semin Roentgenol. 1993;28(4):297-302.
3. Fajardo LF, Berthrong M. Radiation injury in surgical pathology. Part III. Salivary glands, pancreas and skin. Am J Surg Pathol. 1981;5(3):279-96.
4. Fajardo LF. Morphologic patterns of radiation injury. Front Radiat Ther Oncol. 1989;23:75-84.
5. Fajardo L, Berthong M, Anderson R. Radiation Pathology. Oxford: Oxford University Press; 2001.
6. Ting Liu, Lynn Million. Human Radiation Injury. Philadelphia: Lippincott Williams and Wilkins; 2011.
7. O'Sullivan B, Levin W. Late radiation-related fibrosis: pathogenesis, manifestations, and current management. Semin Radiat Oncol. 2003;13(3):274-89.
8. Maximow AA. Studies on the changes produced by roentgen rays in inflamed connective tissue. J Exp Med. 1923;37(3): 319-40.
9. Clarke D, Curtis JL, Martinez A, et al. Fat necrosis of the breast stimulating recurrent carcinoma after primary radiotherapy in the management of early stage breast carcinoma. Cancer. 1983;52(3):442-5.
10. Fajardo LF, Stewart JR. Pathogenesis of radiation-induced myocardial fibrosis. Lab Invest. 1973;29(2):244-57.
11. Hopewell JW, Campling D, Calvo W, Reinhold HS, Wilkinson JH, Yeung TK. Vascular irradiation damage: Its cellular basis and likely consequences. Br J Cancer Suppl. 1986;7:181-91.
12. Fajardo LF, Bethrong M. Vascular lesions following radiation. Pathol Annu. 1988;23 Pt 1:297-330.
13. Reinhold HS, Fajardo LF, Hopewell JW. The vascular system. In: Altman KI, Lett JT (Eds). Relative Radiosensitivities of Human Organ Systems, Vol II. San Diego: Academic Press; 1990.
14. Fajardo LF, Lee A. Rupture of major vessels after radiation. Cancer. 1975;36(3):904-13.
15. FeeWE, Goffinet DR, Fajardo LF, et al. Safety of 125iodine and 192iridium implants to the canine carotid artery: preliminary report. Laryngoscope. 1985;95(3):317-20.
16. Cuzick J, Stewart H, Rutqvist L, Houghton J, Edwards R, Redmond C, et al. Cause-specific mortality in long-term survivors of breast cancer who participated in trials of radiotherapy [see comment]. J Clin Oncol. 1994;12(3):447-53.
17. Fajardo LF, Stewart JR, Cohn KE. Morphology of radiation-induced heart disease. Arch Pathol. 1968;86(5):512-9.
18. Hancock SL, Hoppe RT. Long-term complications of treatment and causes of mortality after Hodgkin's disease. Semin Radiat Oncol. 1996;6(3):225.
19. Cohn KE, Stewart JR, Fajardo LF, et al. Heart disease following radiation. Medicine (Baltimore). 1967;46(3):281-98.
20. Gagliardi G, Lax I, Rutqvist LE. Partial irradiation of the heart. Semin Radiat Oncol. 2001;11(3):224-33.
21. Corn BW, Trock BJ, Goodman RL. Irradiation-related ischemic heart disease. J Clin Oncol. 1990;8(4):741-50.
22. Glanzmann C, Huguenin P, Lütolf UM, Maire R, Jenni R, Gumppenberg V. Cardiac lesion after mediastinal irradiation for Hodgkin's disease. Radiother Oncol. 1994;30(1):43-54.
23. Gagliardi G1, Constine LS, Moiseenko V, Correa C, Pierce LJ, Allen AM, et al. Radiation dose-volume effects in the heart. Int J Radiat Oncol Biol Phys. 2010;76(3 Suppl):S77-85.
24. Roswit B, White DC. Severe radiation injuries of the lung. AJR Am J Roentgenol. 1977;129(1):127-36.
25. Abratt RP, Morgan GW, Silvestri G, et al. Pulmonary complications of radiation therapy. Clin Chest Med. 2004; 25(1):167-77.
26. Gross NJ. The pathogenesis of radiation-induced lung damage. Lung. 1981;159(3):115-25.
27. Morgan GW, Breit SN. Radiation and the lung: a re-evaluation of the mechanisms mediating pulmonary injury. Int J Radiat Oncol Biol Phys. 1995;31(2):361-9.
28. Coggle JE, Lambert BE, Moores SR. Radiation effects in the lung. Environ Health Perspect. 1986;70:261-91.
29. Graham MV, Purdy JA, Emami B, Harms W, Bosch W, Lockett MA, et al. Clinical dose-volume histogram analysis for pneumonitis after 3D treatment for non-small cell lung cancer (NSCLC). Int J Radiat Oncol Biol Phys. 1999;45(2):323-9.
30. Libshitz Hi, Shuman LS. Radiation-induced pulmonary change: CT findings. J Comput Assist Tomogr. 1984;8(1):15-9.
31. Marks LB, Bentzen SM, Deasy JO, Kong FM, Bradley JD, Vogelius IS, et al. Radiation dose-volume effects in the lung. Int J Radiat Oncol Biol Phys. 2010;76(3 Suppl):S70-6.
32. Sempoux C, Horsmans Y, Geubel A, Fraikin J, Van Beers BE, Gigot JF, et al. Severe radiation-induced liver disease following localized radiation therapy for biliopancreatic carcinoma: activation of hepatic stellate cells as an early event. Hepatology. 1997;26(1):128-34.

33. Jeffrey RB, Moss AA, Quivey JM, et al. CT of radiation-induced hepatic injury. AJR Am J Roentgenol. 1980;135(3):445-8.
34. Da Silveira EB, Jeffers L, Schiff ER. Diagnostic laparoscopy in radiation-induced liver disease. Gastrointest Endosc. 2002;55(3):432-4.
35. Lewin K, Millis RR. Human radiation hepatitis. A mophologic study with emphasis on the late changes. Arch Pathol. 1973; 96(1):21-6.
36. Unger EC, Lee JKT, Weyman PJ. CT and MR imaging of radiation hepatitis. J Comput Assist Tomogr. 1987;11(2):264-8.
37. Okumura T, Itai Y, Tsuji H, Matsueda K, Matsuzaki Y, Tsujii H. Focused radiation hepatitis after bragg-peak proton therapy for hepatocellular carcinoma: CT findings. J Comput Assist Tomogr. 1994;18(5):821-3.
38. Pan CC, Kavanagh BD, Dawson LA, Li XA, Das SK, Miften M, et al. Radiation-associated liver injury. Int J Radiat Oncol Biol Phys. 2010;76(3 Suppl):S94-100.
39. Turesson I. The progression rate of late radiation effects in normal tissue and its impact on dose-response relationships. Radiother Oncol. 1989;15(3):217-26.
40. Robbins ME, Campling D, Rezvani M, et al. Radiation nephropathy in mature pigs following irradiation of both kidneys. Int J Radiat Biol. 1989;56(1):83-98.
41. Prescott DM, Hoopes PJ, Thrall DE. Modification of radiation damage in the canine kidney by hyperthermia: a histologic and functional study. Radiat Res. 1990;124(3):317-25.
42. Dawson LA, Kavanagh BD, Paulino AC, Das SK, Miften M, Li XA, et al. Radiation-associated kidney injury. Int J Radiat Oncol Biol Phys. 2010;76(3 Suppl):S108-15.
43. Moulder JE, Fish BL, Cohen EP, et al. Angiotensin II receptor antagonist in the prevention of radiation nephropathy. Radiat Res. 1996;146(1):106-10.
44. Stone HB, Moulder JE, Voleman CN, Ang KK, Anscher MS, Barcellos-Hoff MH, et al. Models for evaluating agents intended for the prophylaxis, mitigation and treatment of radiation injuries. Report of NCI workshop, December 3-4, 2003. Radiat Res. 2004;162(6):711-28.
45. Gutin PH, LeibelSA, Sheline GE. Radiation injury to the nervous system. New York, NY: Raven Press; 1991.
46. Hopewell JW, Wright EA. The nature of latent cerebral irradiation damage and its modification by hypertension. Br J Radiol. 1970;43(507):161-7.
47. Ruben JD, Dally M, Bailey M, Smith R, McLean CA, Fedele P. Cerebral radiation necrosis: incidence, outcomes and risk factor with emphasis on radiation parameters and chemotherapy. Int J Radiat Oncol Biol Phys. 2006;65(2): 499-508.
48. Dequesada IM, Quisling RG, Yachnis A, et al. Can standard magnetic resonance imaging reliably distinguish recurrent tumor from radiation necrosis after radiosurgery of brain metastasis? A radiographic-pathological study. Neurosurgery. 2008;63(5):898-903; discussion 904.
49. Le Bihan, Breton E, Lallemand D, Grenier P, Cabanis E, Laval-Jeantet M. MR imaging of intravoxel incoherent motions: application to diffusion and perfusion in neurologic disorders. Radiology. 1986;161(2):401-7.
50. Sugahara T, Korogi Y, Tomiguchi S, Shigematsu Y, Ikushima I, Kira T, et al. Post-therapeutic intraaxial brain tumor: the value of perfusion sensitive contrast enhance MR for differentiation tumor recurrence from non-neoplastic contrast-enhancing tissue. AJNR Am J Neuroradiol. 2000;21(5):901-9.
51. Enslow MS1, Zollinger LV, Morton KA, Butterfield RI, Kadrmas DJ, Christian PE, et al. Comparison of 18F-fluorodeoxyglucose and 18F-fluorothymidine PET in differentiating radiation necrosis from recurrent glioma. Clin Nucl Med. 2012;37(9): 854-61.
52. Schwartz RB, Carvalho PA, Alexander E, Loeffler JS, Folkerth R, Holman BL. Radiation necrosis vs high-grade recurrent glioma: differentiation by using dual-isotope SPECT with 201TI and 99mTc-HMPAO. AJNR Am J Neuroradiol. 1991;12(6):1187-92.
53. Lawrence YR1, Li XA, el Naqa I, Hahn CA, Marks LB, Merchant TE, et al. Radiation dose-volumes effects in the brain. Int J Radiat Oncol Biol Phys. 2010;76(3 Suppl):S20-7.
54. Dreyer JO, Sakuma Y, Seifert G. Radiation-induced sialadenitis. Stage classification and immunohistology. Pathologe. 1989;10(3):165-70.
55. Braam PM, Roesink JM, Moerland MA, Raaijmakers CP, Schipper M, Terhaard CH. Long-term parotid gland function after radiotherapy. Int J Radiat Oncol Biol Phys. 2005;62(3):659-64.
56. Blanco AI, Chao KS, El Naqa I, Franklin GE, Zakarian K, Vicic M, et al. Dose-volume modeling of salivary function in patients with head-and-neck cancer receiving radiotherapy. Int J Radiat Oncol Biol Phys. 2005;62(4):1055-69.
57. Meirovitz A, Murdoch-Kinch CA, Schipper M, et al. Grading xerostomia by physicians or by patients after intensity-modulated radiotherapy of head-and-neck cancer. Int J Radiat Oncol Biol Phys. 2006;66(2):445-53.
58. Murdoch-Kinch CA, Kim HM, Vineberg KA, et al. Dose-effect relationships for the submandibular salivary glands and implications for their sparing by intensity modulated radiotherapy. Int J Radiat Oncol Biol Phys. 2008;72(2):373-82.

3

CHAPTER

Brachytherapy

Anurita Srivastava, Tejinder Kataria

INTRODUCTION

Brachytherapy has been variously called as "curietherapy", "internal therapy" or "endocurietherapy". The term "brachytherapy" is derived from the Greek word "brachy" meaning short, based on the distance between the target and the therapeutic radiation source. It is a method of delivering radiation at short distances by placing a sealed radiation source inside or in close contact to the tumor/target area. Unlike external beam therapy where the radiation source is at a distance from the patient and the radiation travels from outside to the deep seated target after traversing the intervening normal tissues, with brachytherapy the radiation source is inside the target and radiation travels from inside to outside. On account of rapid dose fall off, the adjacent normal tissues are preferentially spared. This way large dose can be delivered to the tumor. Inherent to the practice of brachytherapy is precise target localization to achieve treatment accuracy. Brachytherapy can be used in treatment of several cancers and forms an integral form of treatment for some of them.

HISTORY

The year 1895 marked the discovery of a "new kind of radiation" by WC Roentgen. The following year, 1896, was marked by the discovery of natural radioactivity by AH Becquerel. In 1898, Marie Curie successfully announced the discovery of a radioactive element, radium.[1] Within 5 years, brachytherapy was used to successfully treat two histologically proven cases of basal cell carcinoma of the face and an American surgeon, Robert Abbe had used radium applications using a primitive afterloading system to treat cancer in 1905.[2] The term brachytherapy was coined by G Forssell in 1931, he also made considerable contributions in terms of treatment of uterine cancer (Stockholm technique), time-dose fractionation (Strandqvist method) and radiation protection issues.[3] The first 5 decades of the 20th century saw a rapid surge in the use of radium for treatment of cancer. This period saw an equally rapid progress in physics and radiobiology of brachytherapy. During this period dosage systems were formulated and tested for calculation of radiation within a tumor. Next few decades saw rapid developments in use of brachytherapy for gynecological and genitourinary cancer treatments.

PRINCIPLES OF BRACHYTHERAPY

The advantage of brachytherapy lies in delivery of localized dose as compared to external beam therapy. It is feasible only for small localized targets. The radiobiological advantage at cellular level derives from the continuous irradiation of the tumor resulting in a delivery of a much higher biologically effective dose (BED) as compared to the teletherapy. The BED is considered to be 10–20% higher than teletherapy when compared dose for dose.[4]

The correct selection of cases is important. Thus, results of any brachytherapy application depend on the proper placement of the sources within or close to the target area. Since the doses are localized around the source itself, it is mandatory to ensure accurate placement of the source within the area of interest. Several models had been developed governing the distribution of sources within the target volume. It is important to mention the exact model used for placing the sources and for dose calculation, along with the duration of treatment. The source being used needs to be calibrated accurately as per standards of a national or international standard laboratory in order to have consistent dose delivery enabling comparison of outcomes.

CLINICAL APPLICATIONS OF BRACHYTHERAPY

The clinical applications of brachytherapy are given in Table 1.

Table 1 Clinical applications of brachytherapy

Site	*Use of brachytherapy*
Prostate cancer, localized	As primary treatment with implantation of radionuclides with short half-lives emitting low energy photons in range of 30 keV (Iodine 125 or Palladium 103, Gold 198)—permanent implants Can be used for delivering boost doses after a fractionated course of external beam radiotherapy using HDR machines, with Iridium-192 temporary implants
Gynecologic cancers	Intracavitary as part of radical treatment in carcinoma cervix Interstitial implants used for residual/recurrent disease SORBO cylinders or ovoids used for postoperative cases for vault irradiation Radical treatment for early stage vaginal/vulval lesions
Eye plaques	Intraocular melanomas. Usually Iodine-125 seeds (activity 1mCi) are loaded on to plaques of diameters 12–20 mm and placed on surface of the eyeball. Recently, beta-emitting sources like Strontium-90/Yttrium-90/Ruttenium-106 have been used
Head and neck cancers	For early stage oral cavity lesions (lip, tongue, buccal mucosa, floor of mouth). In experienced hands, certain oropharyngeal primaries can also be taken up for boost treatment Certain recurrent head and neck cancers
Breast cancers	As boost treatments in cases of breast conservative surgery along with fractionated external beam radiotherapy As the sole treatment for selective group of patients as accelerated partial breast irradiation
Soft tissue sarcomas	For postoperative treatments—as sole radiation or as boost along with external beam radiotherapy
Anorectal cancers	As boost along with fractionated EBRT or in cases of residual/recurrent disease as role modality of treatment
Lung	Permanent implants placed preoperatively for treatment of early stage tumors Intraluminal brachytherapy can be used as palliation for advanced cases with endobronchial disease
Esophagus	Intraluminal brachytherapy for dysphagia palliation
Hepatobiliary malignancies	For maintaining patency of intraluminal stents placed to relieve biliary obstruction due to disease
Intravascular	Used to delay/prevent restenosis of intravascular stents Radionuclides usually used are Iridium-192, Yttrium-90, and Strontium-90 for afterloading techniques. In case of inflatable balloons, Xenon-133, Rhenium-186 and Rhenium-188 are used In case radioactive stents are placed then the radionuclide used is Phosphorus-32 or Vanadium-48.

Abbreviations: HDR, high-dose-rate; EBRT, external beam radiation therapy.

CLASSIFICATION OF TYPES OF BRACHYTHERAPY

The classification on the types of brachytherapy is given in Table 2.

PROPERTIES OF AN IDEAL SOURCE

- Gamma ray emission energy should be high enough to avoid photoelectric effect-induced energy deposition in bones and prevent scatter while being low enough to have minimal radiation protection requirements
- High specific activity
- Source itself should be available in a nontoxic insoluble form. It should not be in powder/liquid form to avoid spillage in case of breakage of the source capsule
- Charged particle emission should be negligible or be easily screened
- It could be manufactured in various shapes and sizes

Table 2 Types of brachytherapy

Type of implant	• Temporary • Permanent
Placement of sources	• Interstitial • Intracavitary • Intraluminal • Intravascular • Surface molds
Dose rate	• Low-dose rate: 0.4–2 Gy/hr • Medium-dose rate: 2–12 Gy/hr • High-dose rate: greater than 12 Gy/hr • Ultra low-dose rate: 0.01–0.3 Gy/hr • Pulsed dose rate
Source loading	• Hot loading • Afterloading
Emitted rays	• Gamma ray emitter • Beta ray emitters

- Half-life should be long enough to avoid decay correction during treatment duration
- Decay products should not be gaseous
- Should not get damaged during the process of sterilization.

RADIONUCLIDES AND THEIR PROPERTIES

Each radionuclide has certain distinctive properties on the basis of the inherent physical properties. These physical properties are:

- *Radioactive decay:* Type of radiation depends on the radioactive decay scheme of the particular radionuclide, i.e. whether it is a photon or beta particle or neutron emitting source and this in turn determines the possible form and general design of the source.
- *Half-life:* Time taken for the source to decay to half strength (half-life) determines whether it can be used as a temporary implant or a permanent implant. Duration of half-life has economic implications also, as it determines the number of times source renewal is needed in any department. Half-life and maximal specific activity are inversely related.
- Specific activity determines the maximal dose rate and also the extent of miniaturization of the source physically.
- Energy basically refers to the energy of the emitted radiation, which in turn determines linear energy transfer (LET) value, the biological effectiveness, the depth of penetration in the tissues and thus the amount of shielding required. Thus, energy too has economic implications for any department.
- Density and atomic number determines the radiographic visibility of the source and also the extent of attenuation and absorption within the source, thus affecting the isotropy of the dose distribution.

Brachytherapy sources in clinical use are given in Table 3.

Radium

This was the first radioactive source to be used for brachytherapy. It is naturally occurring and emits 49 photons with energies varying from 0.184 to 2.45 MeV. The average energy of an encapsulated radium source (filtered with 0.5 mm Platinum) is 0.83 MeV. The high energy beta and alpha particles emitted are stopped by the encapsulation material.

Cesium-137

It is a gamma ray emitting radioisotope with energy 0.662 MeV. It has a long half-life and requires less shielding than radium. It is available in the form of insoluble powders or microspheres. The beta rays and characteristic X-rays are absorbed by the stainless steel container.

Iridium-192

It is used as a temporary implant radioisotope with a half-life of 73.8 days and has a complex gamma ray spectrum with an average energy of 0.38 MeV. It is available in the form of thin flexible wire and series of tiny seeds (3 mm long, 0.5 mm diameter) contained in nylon ribbon. It is used for high-dose-rate (HDR) brachytherapy.

Iodine-125

It is used for permanent implants and emits gamma rays of energy 35.5 keV.

Palladium-103

It is used for permanent prostate implants and decays by electron capture with emission of characteristic X-rays in energy range of 20–23 keV and Auger electrons.

Table 3 Brachytherapy sources in clinical use

Radionuclide	*Half-life*	*Photon energy [MeV]*	*Half-value layer (mm Pb)*	*Tenth-value layer (cm of concrete)*
Ra-226	1600 years	0.047–2.45 (0.83 avg)	12.0	Approx 25.0
Rn-222	3.83 days	0.047–2.45 (0.83 avg)	12.0	Approx 25.0
Cs-137	30.0 years	0.662	5.5	Approx 15.0
Co-60	5.26 years	1.17, 1.33 (1.25 avg)	11.0	Approx 20.0
Ir-192	73.7 days	0.136-1.06 (0.38 avg)	2.5	14.7
I-125	59.4 days	0.028 avg	0.025	Approx 2.0
Pd-103	17.0 days	0.021 avg	0.008	< 1.0
Au-198	2.697 days	0.412	2.5	Approx 14.0

Abbreviations: Avg, average; Approx, approximate.

TYPES OF SOURCES

Brachytherapy sources are sealed sources in contrast to the nonsealed ones like Iodine-131, Phosphorus-32, Strontium-89, Yttrium-90, etc. that can be ingested or administered intravenously. The double encapsulation of sources provides rigidity to the source; prevents leakage of radioactive materials and absorbs alpha rays and beta rays. A brachytherapy source can produce gamma rays (through gamma decay), characteristic X-rays (electron capture and internal conversion), characteristic X-rays and bremsstrahlung from the source capsule.

These sealed sources can be further classified on the basis of the type of emission, viz.:

- Predominantly photon sources emit gamma rays and characteristic X-rays: Cobalt-60, Cesium-137, Iridium-192, Iodine-125, Palladium-103
- Beta sources emit electrons: Strontium-90, Yttrium-90
- Neutron source emit neutrons following spontaneous nuclear fission: Californium-252.

Selecting the appropriate photon emitting radionuclide depends on the photon energy and its penetration depth, the half-life of the radiation source, specific activity and source strength. Apart from the clinical considerations, the radiation safety requirement also depend on the photon energy, half-value layer of shielding materials and the inverse square fall off of dose with distance.

Photon emitting brachytherapy sources are available in various physical forms, viz.:

- Cesium-137: Needles, tubes, pellets
- Cobalt-60: Pellets
- Iridium-192: Wires, seeds
- Palladium-103, Gold-198
- Iodine-125: Seeds

ROOM SHIELDING

Shielding requirements for the general public, the limit is 0.1 rem (1 mSv) in 1 year and for occupational exposure, the limit is 5 rem (50 mSv) in 1 year. Less than 2 mrem (20 mSv) in any 1 hour in any unrestricted area.

DOSIMETRY UNITS AND SOURCE SPECIFICATION

Early brachytherapy was practiced with Radium-226 and its daughter product Radon-222. Till early 1950s, the source strength was specified in terms of mass of radium in mg (mgRa). Time factor was not specified as it was regarded to be unnecessary given the long half-life of radium, thus mass specification rectification was not needed during a period of approximately less than 20 years, i.e. during normal working life of the source. Dosimetry at that time was in terms of milligram-hours (mgh) for Radium or millicuries-destroyed (mcd) for radon.

With advent of artificial nuclides, source strength was defined in terms of activity content expressed in mCi. However, this was limited by the fact that there was autoabsorption and filtration of emitted gamma rays by the source and its sheath.

To overcome these shortcomings, the concept of apparent activity was introduced. Apparent activity was defined as the activity of a hypothetical ideal point source that had no self-absorption or attenuation and had the same radionuclide that delivered the same exposure rate in air at the specified distance equal to that of the actual source under consideration. The distance was to be large enough to enable the source to be considered as a point source (taken to be 1 m). Apparent activity took into account effects of attenuation, filtration, self-absorption and production of bremsstrahlung X-rays in the source and its capsule.

The vast experience available with radium and the availability of dosage and dosimetry charts was helpful when using radium substitute nuclides. Thus, the term milligram-radium equivalent (mgRa equivalent) was formulated. Radium equivalent mass was defined as the mass in milligram of radium filtered by 0.5 mm Platinum resulting in the same exposure rate as that from the source at a distance of 1 m in air.

These terms were adequate to specify the source itself, but for reporting dose rates in tissue there was a need for a unit that could link the radiation output to the activity. The term specific gamma ray constant and exposure rate constant were thus coined. However, these quantities were characteristic of the radionuclide itself, but not for the source and did not take into account self-absorption or filtration due to encapsulation.

SOURCE SPECIFICATION

Gamma ray sources can be specified in terms of reference air kerma rate in air, air kerma strength, exposure rate in air, air kerma rate in air. Gamma ray sources are specified in terms of reference air kerma rate in air at 1 meter, corrected for air attenuation and scattering. The reference point is perpendicular to the length of the source at its central point. The SI unit for reference air kerma rate is Gy/s.

Beta ray sources can be specified in terms of reference absorbed dose rate in water at a reference distance from the source. The reference distance can vary with type of source however; it is generally between 0.5 mm and 2 mm from the source.

Exposure rate constant is defined as the exposure rate at a distance "d" from a point radioactive source of activity "A". Exposure is the total charge of ions of same sign produced in air when all electrons liberated by photons in air of mass are completely stopped in air. Unit is R and 1R = 2.58×10^{-4} C/kg of air (Table 4).

Table 4 Exposure rate constant for various sources

Source	*Exposure rate constant ($R\ cm^2/mCi\ h$)*
Ra-226, Pt-filtered	8.25 R cm^2/mgRa h
Co-60	13.07
Au-198	2.35
Ir-192	4.69
Cs-137	3.26
I-125	1.46

DOSE RATES

Initially radium was the only isotope available for brachytherapy. The dose rate was low and the treatment time was measured in terms of days. Much later, with development of technology, the International Commission of Radiological Units (ICRU) proposed well-defined criteria for dose rates, viz. low-dose-rate (LDR) as 0.4–2 Gy/hour, medium-dose-rate (MDR) as 2–12 Gy/hour, and HDR as more than 0.2 Gy/minute.

IMPLANT DOSIMETRY SYSTEMS

Treatment planning entails determining the type and distribution of radioisotopes to achieve an optimum dose distribution so as to provide the planned dose distribution in the irradiated volume. Many dosimetric systems have been formulated in the past for interstitial implant treatment planning. These systems were formulated in the era when computers were not available for routine treatment planning and tables were provided with details of total dose delivered as a function of area or volume to be treated. This information was then used to plan the procedure by manually calculating the required number of sources and their arrangement so as to achieve the desired treatment. Two of these, Paterson-Parker and Quimby system were the most commonly used ones. These systems were developed for radium sources (unfiltered) in air. Tables were also available for 0.5 mm and 1.0 mm Platinum filtered sources. Oblique filtration, photon scattering and attenuation in tissue were not taken into account. They were applicable for radioactive sources emitting photons of energy more than 200 keV.

With availability of computers, isodose distributions could be calculated for each patient individually, thus, allowing greater degree of freedom for planning brachytherapy. These systems are used today as guiding principles for implanting sources.

Manchester System

This system was envisaged to deliver a uniform dose (within ± 10%) to a plane or volume. There were rules for source distribution so as to achieve a uniform dose, and dosage tables were provided for dose calculation. The tables were designed to provide milligrams-hours per 1,000 roentgens (mg-h/1000R) for implants. Patterson-Parker roentgens in tables could be converted to cGy in tissue after correction (using exposure rate constant and roentgen-cGy factor 0.957). Apart from gynecological treatments, three different types of implants were described: molds, interstitial planar and volume implants.[5,6]

Molds

Radioisotopes were positioned outside the patient, usually at a distance "d" from the patient's skin called the treatment distance. Dose prescription is to the plane at a distance "d" from the sources and dose within this plane was supposed to be ± 10% accurate. Sources could be arranged either in circles (preferable) or squares. Loading of source activity was dependent on the ratio of the circle diameter to the treatment distance, while in case of squares it was dependent on the ratio of the side of square to the treatment distance.

Planar Implant

Dose uniformity was achieved in parallel planes at a distance of 5 mm from the plane of implantation and within the area bounded by the peripheral needles. Depending on the size of the implanted area, the ratio of radium in periphery versus the area varied. The space between needles was not to exceed 1 cm and if the ends of the implant were not crossed by a needle then the effective area of dose uniformity was reduced by 10% for each uncrossed end. For multiplane implants the planes were supposed to be parallel to each other.

Volume Implants

When 3D distribution was akin to a cylinder, sphere or cuboid, then the distribution rules were different from those of a planar implant. The distribution for cylinder was—4 parts in belt, 2 parts in core, 1 part on each end; for sphere—6 parts in shell and 2 parts in core while for cuboid it was 1 part for each side and 2 parts in core. For uncrossed ends of volume implants, deduction of 7.5% volume was done for table reading.

Quimby System

Basically, Quimby system was an adaptation of the Manchester system. It was formulated to overcome the problem faced by radiation oncologists in fulfilling the requirement of lower linear source strength in the center of implants as mandated in Manchester system. The distribution rules were relaxed so that uniform linear source strength sources could be used and the activity be uniformly distributed. Although the dose homogeneity was not as good as Manchester system, the inhomogeneity was considered clinically acceptable.

Therefore, uniform strength needles were used throughout the implant and the desired activity was achieved by increasing the source separation in the center of the implant. Rules were same as those of Manchester for uncrossed ends.[7-9]

Paris System

This system was designed for modern radioisotopes, especially Iridium-192, that were flexible, had narrow diameter and may be formulated in any desired length. Sources were distributed as per specified rules, over a predefined treatment volume and dose was calculated at specified points (basal dose rate points) within the target volume. Calculating 85% of the average basal dose rate denoted the isodose that would encompass the target volume. The sources were implanted equidistantly and in parallel to each other. Ideally, centers of all linear sources were supposed to be in a single plane that bisects the sources perpendicularly, called the central plane. The source separation for short wires (≤ 50 mm) to be in the range of 8–15 mm and 8–22 mm for longer lengths (≥ 70 mm). The reference air kerma per unit length of source was constant for all sources within the implant.[1,10,11]

Gynecologic Cancers: Manchester System

Cancer Cervix

It was initially formulated for radium tubes and was later adapted for afterloading systems also. Within the system rules specify the spatial distribution of sources, the relative activity and the points for dose calculation. The applicators were specially designed for the purpose of intracavitary applications and consisted of a central tandem that could be inserted into the uterine cavity with an outside flange that abuts against the cervix and a pair of ovoids that were placed in both fornices. Different sizes of tandem and ovoids were available and the key feature was the uniform dose rate that could be achieved at point A with any combination. Point A defined as a point situated 2 cm cranial to the lateral fornices in the plane of the uterine tube and 2 cm lateral to the center of the uterine canal. Doses were prescribed to point A.[12]

Uterine Body Cancers

Similar applicator, with a uterine tube (1 cm diameter) and ovoids were used in conjunction. The loading patterns were different from intracavitary cervix ones and higher dose was delivered by the uterine sources.

Computerized Treatment Planning

Historically, treatment planning in brachytherapy involved use of systems that specified source distribution and provided lookup tables for dose calculation. This was quite empirical and deviations from the system rules resulted in major uncertainties. With availability of computers, the resultant isodoses could be visualized in three dimensions. Additionally, the dose distributions could be evaluated by means of dose volume histograms and not visual display alone. Use made of uniform strength sources that were spaced uniformly at a distance of 1–1.5 cm. The active length of sources kept at 30–40% longer than the target length as the ends were uncrossed. The target volume was defined prior to the procedure and the appropriate length of needles and spacing decided beforehand. Dose prescription based on the isodose surface that completely encompassed the target volume.

The major steps involved in computerized treatment planning were:

- Source localization: Source localization to be done by any of the three available methods; orthogonal imaging method, stereo-shift method or recently by use of CT scan
- Dose calculation around sources
- Evaluation of target volumes, critical organs and dose distributions in 3D format
- Dose optimization
- Plan evaluation using dose volume histograms.

Interstitial Brachytherapy

Alexander Graham Bell first suggested implanting radiation sources into tumor tissues for treatment. The technique involves directly implanting sealed radioactive sources into the tumor in specified fashion, the geometric distribution dictated by the existing dosimetric systems. Interstitial brachytherapy could be either temporary or permanent implants. Usually, Paris system rules are used for interstitial implants.

This can be further classified as "hot loading" when sources are directly implanted into the tissues or "afterloading" when hollow tubes/needles are implanted into the target tissue initially and then these are connected to remote afterloading machines that load the hollow tubes and needles. Remote afterloaders could be LDR, HDR or pulsed dose rate (PDR). Remote afterloaders entail use of a safe housing assembly for storing the radioisotopes, a system that controls the source and the driving mechanism remotely, a source transfer tube and treatment applicators that are hollow and source can be placed inside them. The entire assembly is controlled by a remote operating console and the treatment plans are generated on a dedicated treatment planning computer. Radiation exposure to personnel is negligible when using the afterloading technique.

The usual radionuclides used in remote afterloaders are Cobalt-60, Cesium-137 and Iridium 192; of these, Iridium-192 is used most widely because of its medium gamma ray energy (400 keV) and its high specific activity.

DOSE SPECIFICATION AND REPORTING

As per ICRU report 38 and 58, recommendation is made for use of uniform and standardized methodology for dose reporting so as to enable data comparisons between different centers. The following needs to be reported for all implants:

- Implant description
- Volume of interest
- Prescribed dose
- Delivered dose
- Reference air kerma rate in air (cGy/h at 1 m).

For gynecological brachytherapy treatments, ICRU 38 mandates reporting of the following:

- Description of technique
- Description of reference volume and its dimensions
- Dose at reference points
- Time and dose
- Reference air kerma rate in air (cGy/h at 1 m).

For interstitial implants, as per ICRU 58, the following parameters need to be reported:

- Clinical target volume
- Type of source, technique and treatment time
- Prescribed dose and achieved dose distribution
- Mean central dose and minimum dose required for tumor control
- Description of the low dose (regions receiving less than 90% of the peripheral dose) and high-dose regions (regions receiving more than 150% of the mean central dose) and indices of dose uniformity
- Dose volume histogram data
- Reference air kerma rate in air (cGy/h at 1 m).

ADVANCES IN BRACHYTHERAPY

Image-Assisted Brachytherapy

Imaging is used to acquire 3D volumetric information of the target. The imaging modalities in use are CT scans, MRI scans, USG, PET CT scans. This information enables generation of a provisional treatment plan prior to procedure. This same information is used to place the sources appropriately. Subsequent imaging enables generating a 3D dose distribution and accuracy can be ensured during treatment delivery. This can be subdivided as follows:

Image-based Brachytherapy

Information from imaging modalities is incorporated into assessment of target volume and for planning volumetric dose delivery.

Image-Guided Brachytherapy

Imaging techniques are used for guiding placement of the radiation sources and for planning volumetric dose delivery.

Electronic Brachytherapy (AXXENT)

It comprises of a 30–50 KV miniature X-ray tube that is attached to a high voltage cable and the assembly is retractable and flexible akin to HDR source assembly.

Pulsed Dose Rate Brachytherapy

Continuous LDR brachytherapy had been in use for cancer cervix for many decades and the results have been outstanding. At the time of conversion to HDR brachytherapy, for the ease of delivery to patient and personnel as well as better radiation safety profile, several trials were conducted against the "gold standard" LDR treatment. Only when the outcomes were reported to be equivalent, HDR brachytherapy became routine practice in most hospitals. Given the excellent results of LDR and the ease of delivery of HDR, it was envisaged to combine the advantageous points of both dose rates and hence PDR was derived. The PDR system uses a single stepping Iridium-192 source, which has a lower activity (37–74 GBq at installation) as compared to about 370 GBq activity of a HDR source at installation. The technique involves delivering a "pulsed" dose for about 10–40 minutes every hour, so that a fraction of the total prescribed dose is delivered in pulses every hour over a 48-hour time period. This imitates the biologic effectiveness of classical LDR treatments while improving the delivery technique by using computerized optimization.

Gliasite Radiation

It is a liquid source brachytherapy system used for treating intracranial metastatic or recurrent tumors. It is a balloon-shaped device filled with "lotrex", i.e. liquid iodine (I-135), that is implanted into the tumor cavity and can deliver radiation doses to the wall of the cavity. The catheter at the other end of the balloon is implanted outside the cranium into a distal inflatable balloon. Lortex can be delivered in several small doses or as a single dose into the balloon.

Accelerated Partial Breast Irradiation

With acceptance of breast conserving surgery (BCS) as a standard of care in cancer breast, whole breast radiotherapy (WBRT) followed by local boost became established as an integral part of treatment protocol. Results of BCS + WBRT + boost were equivalent to those of mastectomy. Accelerated partial breast irradiation (APBI), as radical treatment in place of WBRT + boost, has been found to have comparable outcomes with limited toxicity in select group of patients.

CONCLUSION

Brachytherapy is the most conformal treatment that can be delivered. It requires expertise at all steps and with proper application and planning, it has contributed toward improving local control rates at many sites. Modern brachytherapy utilizes the currently available imaging modalities and such a practice has resulted in dramatic improvements in treatment of cancer cervix and prostate. Careful handling of the radionuclides and proper disposal of these sources is the need of the hour. Stringent rules and regulations have been formulated to ensure that radiation accidents do not occur. The major impediment for widespread use of brachytherapy is the rising cost of the radionuclides. With availability of superior linear accelerators that can deliver highly conformal treatments that are nearly comparable to brachytherapy, the high maintenance cost of brachytherapy needs to be addressed, in order to ensure that the practice of brachytherapy continues to be in use.

Specific brachytherapy techniques have been described in the specific chapters.

REFERENCES

1. Pierquin B, Wilson JF, Chassagne D. Modern Brachytherapy,. New York, USA: Masson Publishing USA, Inc.; 1987.
2. Del Regato J A, Brachytherapy. Front. Radiat. Ther. Onc. 1978;12:5-12.
3. Forssell G. "La lutte sociale contre le cancer". J de Radiol et d'Electrol, 1931;15: 621-34.
4. Dale RG, Coles IP, Deehan C, et al. Calculation of integrated biological response in brachytherapy. Int J Radiat Oncol Biol Phys. 1997;38(3):633-42.
5. Patterson R, Parker HM. A dosage system for gamma ray therapy. Br. J Radio 1934;7:592.
6. Meredith WJ. Radium Dosage. The Manchester System, 2nd edition. Edinburgh: Livingstone, Ltd; 1967.
7. Quimby EH. Dosage tables for linear radium sources. Radiology. 1944;43:572-7.
8. Quimby EH, Castro V. Calculation of dosage in interstitial radium therapy. Am J Roentgenol Radium Ther Nucl Med. 1953;70(5):739-49.
9. Quimby EH. Grouping of radium tubes in packs or plaques to produce the desired distribution of radiation. Am J Roentgenol, 1932;27(1):18-39.
10. Pierquin B, Dutreix A. [For a new methodology in curietherapy: the system of Paris (endo- and plesioradiotherapy with non-radioactive preparation). A preliminary note]. Ann Radiol (Paris). 1966;9(9):757-60.
11. Pierquin B, Dutrex A, Paine C, Chassagne D, Marinello G, Ash D. The Paris system in interstitial radiation therapy. Acta Radiol Oncol Radiat Phys Biol. 1978;17(1):33-48.
12. Tod M, Meredith WJ. Treatment of cancer of the cervix uteri, a revised Manchester method. Br J Radiol. 1953;26(305):252-7.

4 CHAPTER

Advances in Radiotherapy Techniques

Anurita Srivastava, Tejinder Kataria, Ashu Abhishek, Govardhan HB, Ruchi Singh

INTRODUCTION

As per the International Agency for Research on Cancer (IARC) estimates, 7.6 million deaths worldwide were due to cancer with 12.7 million new cases per year being reported worldwide. Majority (nearly 63%) of the cancer deaths were reported from the developing countries.[1,2] Cancer treatment increasingly uses a multimodality approach with a judicious combination of surgery, chemotherapy and radiotherapy (RT). RT was first used for cancer more than a hundred years ago (in 1903). It can be used as curative approach or for palliation either alone or in combination with other modalities. Depending on the dose fractionation schedule, total dose and technique the expected outcomes as well as the side effects vary. Of all three modalities, RT is the most cost effective single treatment modality, accounting for only 5% of the total cost of cancer care.[3] Though RT alone is curative in about 40% of cancer cases,[5] approximately 50% of all cancer patients will need RT at some point during their planned course of treatment.[6]

Radiotherapy has seen dramatic changes over the last few decades[4] and this rapid progress can be attributed to incorporation of advanced imaging modalities and modern computer technology for treatment planning. Additionally availability of well-engineered linear accelerators has made the practice of RT more precise. Simultaneously, advances in the understanding of cancer biology itself have improved management decisions.[7,8]

HISTORY

Since the discovery of X-rays by WC Roentgen in 1895, field of RT or radiation oncology has witnessed rapid developments. X-rays were used for clinical use as early as 1896. The earlier methods used low energy X-rays that were limited by the superficial tissue reactions. Gradual improvements in the energy of the X-rays allowed treatment of deep seated tumors also. Simultaneously, scientists started working on the radiobiological effects of radiation, leading to the understanding of the concept of fractionation, normal tissue toxicity, induction of skin, mucus membrane reactions, etc. By 1938, 1 MV X-rays were generated and in 1951, the first Cobalt machine was put into use. In the 1950s, the concept of conformal RT (CRT) was first put forward by Takahashi et al. and the first multileaf collimator (MLC) was constructed in 1959.[9] The next 2 decades saw the advent of more powerful machines[10] as well as rapid changes in the field of imaging and the replacement of radium with alternative radioactive sources for clinical use.[4,10] Year 1972 saw the launch of the first computed tomographic scanner by Godfrey Hounsfield that totally changed the concept of RT that was being practiced at that time.

The ultimate aim of RT has always been maximal tumor cell kill with minimal normal tissue injury. Improved methods for disease assessment using biological imaging—positron emission tomography (PET) scans and improved radiological imaging (CT and MRI) have greatly helped in precise delineation of tumor, which can then be accurately targeted by advanced linacs with pinpoint accuracy thereby decreasing the dose delivered to adjoining normal tissue. Eventually all the precision translates toward improving the therapeutic ratio for the treatment enabling possibility of decreasing the normal tissue toxicity while delivering tumoricidal doses and also enabling dose escalation in selected scenarios. This article/chapter attempts to briefly describe the various technological advances that have changed the field of RT.

Radiation can be delivered in a number of ways, either externally or internally. External beam radiotherapy (EBRT) is the usual method of delivering radiation wherein the radiation source is placed at a distance from the patient while brachytherapy is the term used for describing RT when the radiation source is placed close or inside the patient's body in close proximity to the tumor itself.

TWO-DIMENSIONAL (2D) RADIOTHERAPY (CONVENTIONAL RADIOTHERAPY)

This is based on the use of orthogonal radiographs that are used to locate the target and plan the locoregional irradiation using combination of fields placed at different angles. Conformality is attempted with use of field blocks, wedges, compensators, etc. Delivery of radiation is by means of a number of relatively uniform intensity coplanar beams. The field shapes are customized with help of lead blocks and cutouts of heavy metal alloys of low melting point. The availability of MLCs, has obviated the need for blocks/cutouts for field shaping and use of wedges or compensators for compensating missing tissue.

These treatments are still in use in some centers for different sites. The problem with such an approach is that the entire irradiated area including the nontumor regions receives similar dose resulting in significant toxicities as seen in 2D RT portal of Figure 1D.

THREE-DIMENSIONAL (3D) RADIOTHERAPY

Transition from 2D RT to three-dimensional conformal radiotherapy (3D CRT), which is based on the CT-based volumetric data has improved the RT outcomes immensely

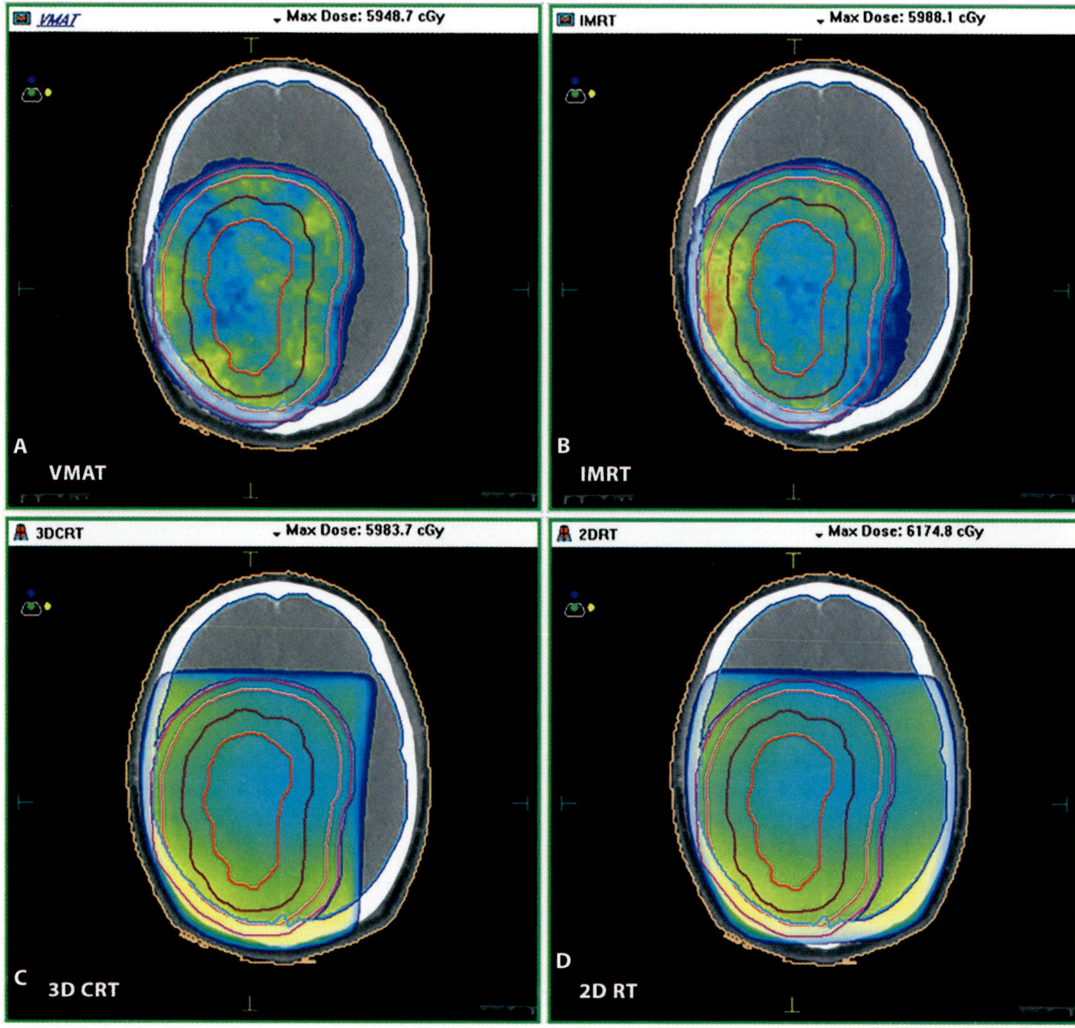

Figs 1A to D Axial views of treatment planning with: (A) VMAT: tightly molded doses around the planning target volume; (B) IMRT: dose conformity around the PTV with minor dose splash in areas outside PTV; (C) 3D CRT: shaped beams used for delivering dose with increasing dose slash in the normal tissues; (D) 2D RT: Parallel pair beam arrangement results in treating the entire volume to a uniform dose

Abbreviations: PTV, planning target volume; VMAT, volumetric modulated arc therapy; IMRT, intensity modulated radiotherapy; CRT, conformal radiotherapy; RT, radiotherapy.

Courtesy: Dr Tejinder Kataria, Division of Radiation Oncology, Medanta—The Medicity, Haryana, India

by allowing sparing of the normal tissues due to the decreased irradiated volume. CRT aims to exploit the potential biological improvements consequent on better localization of the high-dose volumes.[11,12] As described by Tubiana et al. 3D CRT is based on the presumption that achieving higher rate of local control may improve survival, increased local control may be achieved with dose escalation and that such high doses can be delivered only if late toxicity can be decreased.[13] The aim is to deliver radiation to the delineated gross tumor volume (GTV) with a margin for subclinical extension called the clinical target volume (CTV). A further margin is added to the CTV accounting for organ motion and setup uncertainties, referred to as the planning target volume (PTV).[11]

Treatment delivery verification involves verification of patient position prior to treatment performed using electronic portal imaging devices (EPID), that are then matched to the digital radiograph reconstruction (DRR) generated from the axial CT data used for treatment planning.

Conformation around target is to avoid the adjacent normal tissues/organs at risk (OAR) from radiation exposure. Alternatively "conformal avoidance" of OARs can be practiced when the critical normal tissue is very close to the target and priority is given to saving the normal structure. Conformation can be practiced by two methods, viz. field shaping alone (as shown in 3D CRT panel of Figure 1C where the dose distribution can be shaped around the target) or by modulation of the intensity of fluence across a geometrically shaped field. The former is addressed as 3D CRT while the latter is intensity-modulated radiotherapy (IMRT).

INTENSITY-MODULATED RADIOTHERAPY

A step further to 3D CRT is the institution of IMRT aimed to overcome the limitations of 3D CRT. With IMRT it was feasible to treat irregularly shaped targets covered by irregular shaped dose distributions tightly conformed to the shape of the target, multiple targets could be treated simultaneously (with varying dose fractionation schedules if so required). Multiple beams from multiple directions could be designed to produce a homogeneous dose distribution within the target with superior conformality.[14] IMRT technique is the basic method used in modern RT. The basic concept is that in order to achieve a desired dose distribution, the fluence within any of the beams need not be uniform across the PTV.[15] The nonuniformity of each beam is driven by anatomic features specific to the patient. This way the normal structures receive only low doses and even concave dose distributions can be created to better spare the adjacent critical structures (Fig. 1B).

Several subtypes of IMRT can be defined based on:

- Technique of planning (forward planned, aperture based, inverse planned, Monte Carlo based)
- Delivery systems (MLC based, micro-MLC based or tomotherapy device based), or
- Treatment techniques (step and shoot, sliding window, cinematic sequential, intensity modulated arc therapy or tomotherapy).

Intensity modulated radiotherapy uses an inverse planning software and intensity modulation of multiple radiation beams to achieve its goal. Intensity modulation is done by the use of MLCs. Segmental MLC or step and shoot IMRT can be delivered with conventional MLCs by dividing the field into multiple segments, though only limited intensities are feasible.[16] Dynamic MLC (DMLC) leaf pairs, on the other hand move across the field at a varying rate and deliver 'sliding window IMRT.[17,18] With segmental MLCs, the MLC is placed in varying configurations, such that each configuration defines a separate beam aperture from the same beam direction. DMLCs can move at varying rates and the time dependent position of each leaf determines the intensity pattern delivered (Fig 1B).

INTENSITY MODULATED ARC THERAPY

Conventional MLC leaves moves continuously as the gantry rotates around the patient, is the basic technique employed for intensity modulated arc therapy (IMAT) or tomotherapy. For IMAT, several rotational arcs around the patient may be needed for delivering the plan. Arc therapies can achieve highly conformal distributions with reduction of treatment delivery times. Each rotational arc will have different patterns of irradiation, with each rotational arc delivering increasing step-wise intensities in order to deliver the planned intensity levels.[19]

Definite improvement in the outcomes have been documented in several sites, such as head and neck cancers,[20-23] prostate cancers[24] as well as cervical cancers.[25] In fact the clinical results are in keeping with the expectations. However, several new issues, like patient immobilization, internal organ movement, tumor tracking and treatment reproducibility, have to be addressed keeping in view the precise nature of the resultant dose distributions.

The advantages of IMRT are weighed against the increased complexities of treatment planning and execution as compared to the simple approach of 3D CRT. Over the past decade both the technique and the delivery of IMRT have become more efficient and that has reflected in decrease in time required for planning, quality assurance processes and treatment times. This has increased the throughput of patients in busy departments.

VOLUMETRIC MODULATED ARC THERAPY

Volumetric modulated arc therapy (VMAT) technique is different from routine IMRT by delivering dose to the whole volume of the tumor, rather than slice by slice treatment. Dose delivery is arc based this way the algorithm can use biological

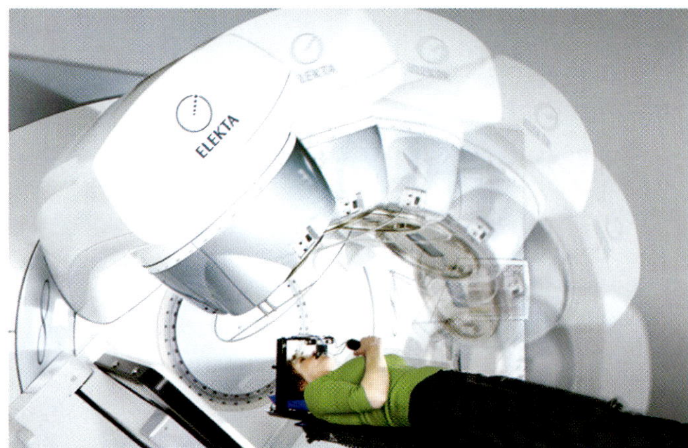

Fig. 2 Volumetric arc therapy: rotation of gantry around the patient

Courtesy: Elekta®

optimization for planning by altering either the speed of rotation of the gantry, the aperture shape, the velocity of MLCs or the dose rate in order to generate biological superior plans with better sparing of normal tissues (Figs 1A and 2).[26,27]

IMAGE-GUIDED RADIOTHERAPY

With precise delineation of the targets, the gains can be consolidated only if the irradiated volumes are limited to the target regions alone. Till date cross-sectional imaging data is used for treatment planning. The planning scans are acquired with the patients adequately immobilized with the help of accessories. Subsequent treatments are delivered by setting up the patient in the same position as on the day of acquiring planning scans. This reproducibility is aided by the help of markings on the skin or on the immobilization aids used (like masks or vacuum bags). This repositioning can be checked with the help of 2D X-rays or digital imaging, providing reproducibility within certain limits. Depending on the repositioning accuracy of the immobilization device the positional variations over the treatment course can range up to several millimeters. These variations are accounted for in the treatment planning process by incorporating additional safety margins beyond the delineated target so as to ensure target positioning within the prescribed dose. These additional margins add to the normal tissue irradiated volume contributing to normal tissue toxicity. Considerable reductions in the irradiated normal tissue volume can be achieved by decreasing the PTV margins (for setup uncertainties). However, with such narrow margins, there is always risk of "precisely missing" the target itself.[28,29] IMRT dose distributions have sharp dose gradients at boundaries of the PTV and the OARs, making these treatments considerably sensitive to setup errors and geometric uncertainties when compared to 2D or 3D CRT treatments. Both inter- and intra-fraction geometric uncertainties gain importance in IMRT treatments given the sharp dose gradients as well as the prolonged treatment times.

Consequently stringent measures are required to tackle these uncertainties in any IMRT treatment. IGRT, as a principle has been in use for last few decades in the form of simulators, megavoltage (MV) port films, EPIDs, ultrasound imaging systems, implanted radioopaque markers, or optical tracking systems. The term IGRT is used to denote modern IMRT delivery systems with integrated imaging capability that can provide 3D volumetric imaging of the soft tissues. The integrated systems can provide daily monitoring of the patient position as well as changes in the anatomy.

Image-guided radiotherapy can thus help to reduce setup uncertainties, better manage internal organ motion as well as detect anatomic variations during treatment (due to weight loss, tumor shrinkage, etc.) and allow the treating physician to modify the treatment plan accordingly. This increased accuracy of verification can be translated for establishing dose escalation protocols aimed at improving local controls. However, it should be borne in mind that the supplemental imaging exposes the patient to an additional dose of radiation ranging between 0.1 and 3% of the treatment dose depending on the imaging modality used.

Common methods employed in IGRT include planar X-rays, ultrasonography- (USG) based imaging, video-based imaging, cone beam CT [MV CT (Siemens) OR KV CT (mobile C arm/Varian OBI, Elekta) or fan beam CT for tomotherapy OR In room CT] or MRI-based.[30]

ADAPTIVE RADIOTHERAPY

The principle of adaptive RT uses feedback data from patient-specific anatomical and biological variations observed during the course of RT treatment. These variations could be categorized as occurring during a single fraction or changes occurring between successive fractions of treatment. The former are called intrafractional and the latter interfractional variations. The issues of intrafractional and interfractional movement of the target have been known for long. The earlier methods to address them were by adding an additional margin around the target to ensure that it is not missed by the directed beam. With the presently available methods of better defining the target, ensuring accurate delivery of the planned dose is of foremost importance. Developing automated mechanisms to identify and manage such changes is called adaptive RT and was started first in 1997. The basic concept of adaptive RT deals with incorporation of systematic measurements of treatment variations within a closed loop and provides feedback for early re-optimization of the treatment plan during the treatment process and ultimately delivering a treatment that has been customized as per the daily target volume. The starting point is image acquisition by a CT scan to have soft tissue localization. This image is registered with the DRR using deformable registration. This way, the regions of interest are aligned according to a common coordinate system. After recalculation, the daily delivered doses are known and can be used to reach the accumulated dose that is then used to evaluate the plan. If significant discrepancies are noted in the dose delivery, then plan needs to be re-optimized in order to compensate for the discrepancies. Daily documentation of the changes in the position of the target yields information about the systematic and the random variations. Systematic variations are more detrimental and need to be addressed early in the course of treatment to ensure delivery of the planned dose. Random errors on the other hand are more forgiving as the dose variations get blurred on a day to day basis. However, major random variations are not acceptable as in the absence of image guidance the margins need to be increased.

Completely implementing adaptive RT needs to incorporate treatment dose assessment, treatment variation identification, decision-making regarding treatment modification and ultimately adaptive treatment modification. The treatment modification can be performed both online or offline and the steps taken to implement the same can involve any or combination of the following: patient position correction, beam aperture adjustment, margin modification for target or critical organs or plan reoptimization by intensity modulation.

STEREOTACTIC RADIOTHERAPY

Stereotactic radiotherapy (SRT) personifies the rapid transition seen in the field of RT. As per the linear quadratic model (LQ) the teaching was that high dose fractions result in increased late toxicity. However, current practice delivers high doses fractions that a decade ago would have been not feasible with the techniques available then. Park et al. concluded that the LQ model over estimates cell kill at SBRT range doses and that the LQ model is inadequate for explaining the SBRT tumor dose effects. SBRT is a technique that builds on the strengths of IMRT and IGRT where high doses of radiation are precisely delivered in few treatment sessions (usually 1-6).[31] This is used for small, well-defined targets that are then ablated. Despite the high doses, the normal tissue toxicity is low as volume of normal tissue irradiated is kept to the minimum by treating only the gross target without incorporating the prophylactic irradiation of the subclinical disease (CTV).[31] The treatment process involves precise immobilization with incorporation of accessories for motion management followed by meticulous treatment planning that involves multiple image fusion and dose calculations. The treatment delivery involves localization and verification prior to treatment (Figs 3A to D). SBRT can be delivered either with 3D CRT, IMRT or arcs, the main difference being the high dose per fraction that is delivered. Given the high doses that are delivered, considerations of normal tissue constraints that need to be followed is of prime importance. Several authors have published the dose constraints that are being followed, including quantitative analyses of normal tissue effects in the clinic (QUANTEC) data that was recently published.[32] However, most of these come from retrospective series and case studies. Data from prospective studies is now emerging which needs to be incorporated into treatment planning for better optimization and improved outcomes.

Stereotactic radiotherapy has been used for both intracranial and extracranial sites. For intracranial treatment initially the treatment was performed with invasive frames screwed to the patients skull (Figs 3A and 6), however with increasing position verification accuracy with use of IGRT the era is now of frameless SRT. Extracranial sites commonly treated are primary and secondary tumors of lung, liver, kidney, adrenal gland or pancreas as well as for pelvic and head and neck tumors that have recurred after primary irradiation.

Tomotherapy

Tomotherapy literally means "slice therapy" (Greek prefix "tomo" means "slice"). The basic idea is to install a linear accelerator or a radiation emitting source on a CT-like ring gantry configuration and deliver therapeutic radiation using a rotating fan beam that is modulated by means of a binary collimator while the couch slides through the gantry. The first implementation of this concept was performed by NOMOS Corporation® and was provided as an add-on accessory to existing linear accelerators. This accessory consisted of a set of MLCs that provided a fan-shaped beam. The leaves could either be open or closed (the beam is either on or off for that segment, i.e. binary beam delivery). After two simultaneous slices had been treated by the rotating linear accelerator, the patient on the couch was translated by two slice thicknesses and then the next two slices were treated and so on and so forth till the entire treatment volume had been treated. This is called "serial tomotherapy".

Traditional linear accelerators could use "serial tomotherapy" alone on account of limited rotation possible (approx 370°) and due to inability to translate the couch smoothly and automatically during radiation delivery. With this treatment delivery, it was not possible to image the patient in the treatment position in totality, and hence, high dose treatments were not feasible. "Helical tomotherapy" aimed to surmount these very issues. The machine encompasses the slip ring technology of diagnostic CT scanners and is thus, capable of continuous rotation around the patient while the

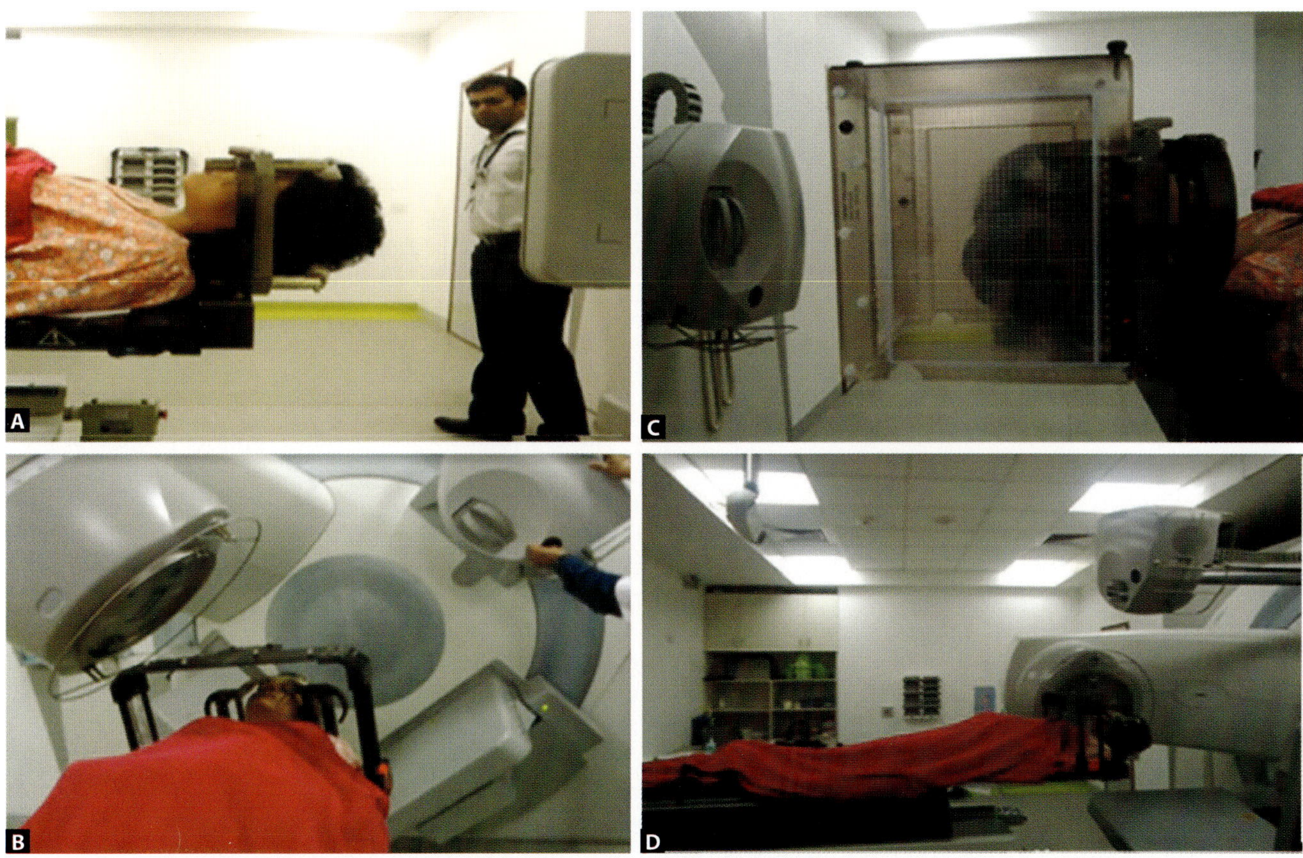

Figs 3A to D Frame-based radiosurgery: (A) Patient with rigid frame screwed to skull; (B) Localiser frame; (C and D) Acquisition of volumetric data on the treatment table prior to treatment for position verification with XVI (Elekta)® and hexapod in situ for correction of the mismatch between the acquired and planned position

Courtesy: Dr Tejinder Kataria, Division of Radiation Oncology, Medanta—The Medicity, Haryana, India

couch moves into the gantry, thus providing smooth helical dose delivery. The 6 MeV S band (3GHz) linear accelerator is about 40 cm long and generates a 6 MV photon beam.

Collimation is done by multileaf binary collimators consisting of 64 leaves. The collimators are specifically designed to minimize leaf transmission and interleaf leakage; ensuring superior dose conformality for narrow beam multislice delivery procedures. The on-board MV CT detection system is used for patient setup verification and repositioning, verification of leaf positions during treatment and reconstruction of the actual dose delivered, making it possible to make corrections in subsequent fractions.[33,34]

Cyberknife

The cyberknife includes a compact linear accelerator that is mounted on a robotic arm and a robotic couch enabled with 5° of movement, viz. craniocaudal, left-right, superior-inferior, and pitch and roll. For image guidance it has a pair of X-ray source mounted on the roof and an additional infrared camera. The X-rays are used for real time imaging while the infrared camera aids the synchrony system to provide information regarding respiratory tracking. The size of the linear accelerator is compact as the operational frequency range (X band) is 3 times (Fig. 4) higher than that of conventional accelerators. It produces a 6 MV beam with dose rate of up to 400 monitor units. The dose distributions are very conformal such that the adjacent normal tissues receive minimum possible doses. Figures 5A to C illustrates the superiority of the dose distribution as compared to linac-based SRT that is depicted in (Fig. 6).

PARTICLE THERAPY/HADRON THERAPY

Hadrons are subatomic particles, made up of quarks; they are divisible and, by atomic standards, are heavy. In contrast to hadrons, photons (X-rays) are without mass. The term "hadron" comes from the Greek word for "strong," based

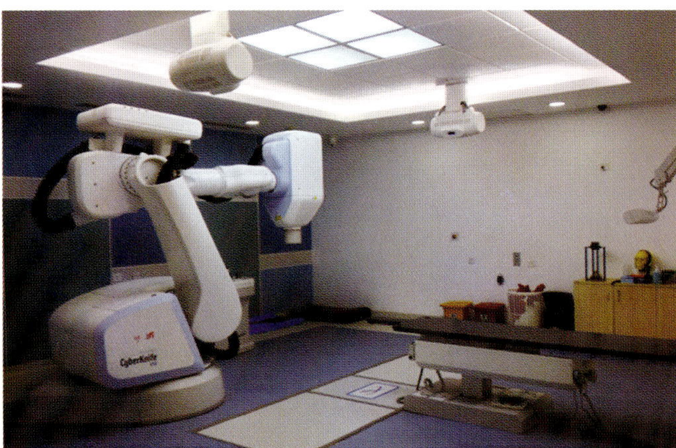

Fig. 4 Cyberknife (CK)

Courtesy: Dr Tejinder Kataria, Division of Radiation Oncology, Medanta—The medicity, Haryana, India

on the fact that these particles interact via strong nuclear force.[35] Protons, neutrons, pions, atomic nuclei heavier than hydrogen including light ions (e.g. carbon, helium, oxygen) and heavy ions (e.g. neon, argon), all belong to the class of particles called hadrons. Thus, the terminology particle therapy and hadron therapy is often used interchangeably.[36]

Clinical, physical and biological properties of protons differ from those of heavier particles, hence, particle/hadron therapy is divided into 2 categories: "proton therapy" characterized by low linear energy transfer (LET) and "heavy ion therapy" with high LET. Thus, for clarity it is preferable to differentiate proton therapy from heavy ion therapy.[37]

Clinical use of proton was investigated after the publication of Robert Wilson's paper in 1946.[38] Protons offer better dose distribution due to their unique physical dose deposition characteristics.

The highly conformal dose distribution and the inherent properties make this modality Specially appropriate for situations where the target is lying in close proximity with the critical organs and in pediatric tumors where maximal normal tissue sparing is needed. Clinical studies have been conducted at base of skull tumors.[37,39,40] Paraspinal tumors, intraocular melanoma,[41] localized prostate cancer,[42-44] breast cancer, nonsmall cell lung cancer (NSCLC) and gastrointestinal malignancies. However, as yet clinical advantage of particle therapy over conventional photon therapy remains to be proven except in selected sites, like

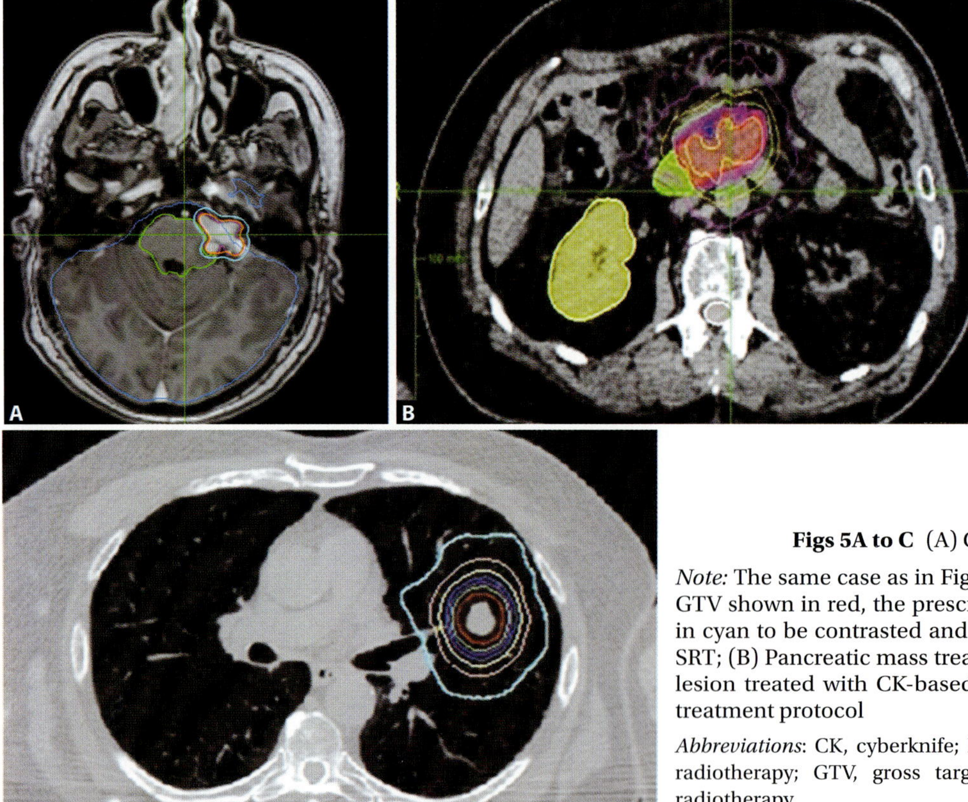

Figs 5A to C (A) CK-based (FSRT)

Note: The same case as in Figure 6 was replanned for CK, GTV shown in red, the prescribed dose isodose is shown in cyan to be contrasted and compared with linac-based SRT; (B) Pancreatic mass treated with CK FSRT; (C) Lung lesion treated with CK-based FSRT with lung optimized treatment protocol

Abbreviations: CK, cyberknife; FSRT, fractionated stereotactic radiotherapy; GTV, gross target volume; SRT, stereotactic radiotherapy

Courtesy: Dr Tejinder Kataria, Division of Radiation Oncology, Medanta—The Medicity, Haryana, India

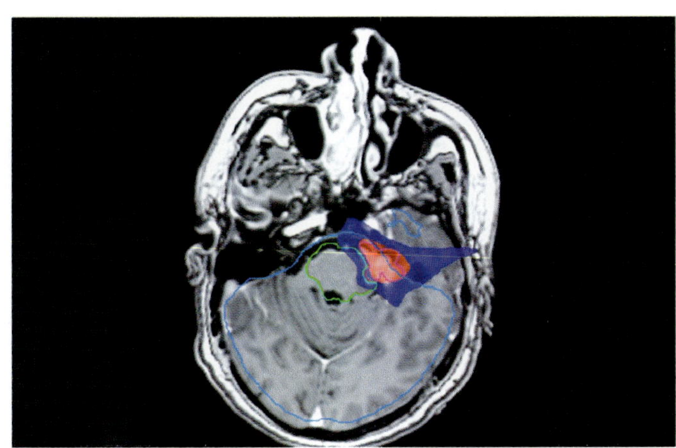

Fig. 6 Linac-based stereotactic radiotherapy (SRT). The gross target volume (GTV) is outlined in red, the prescribed dose is depicted in blue

Courtesy: Dr Tejinder Kataria, Division of Radiation Oncology, Medanta—The Medicity, Haryana, India

uveal melanoma. Given the dosimetric properties there is a general consensus that the expected therapeutic gain is maximal for base of skull chordomas and chondrosarcomas, eye melanomas, medulloblastoma, meningioma and pediatric tumors; average gain for bone sarcomas, soft tissue sarcomas, recurrent previously irradiated head and neck tumors and paranasal sinus tumors; while minimal gain in the case of glioblastoma, primary head and neck tumors, unresectable hepatocellular tumors, low-grade gliomas, NSCLC, pancreatic tumors, prostate adenocarcinomas, pelvic recurrences, uterine tumors and salivary gland tumors. Role of protons is well-established for base of skull chordomas and chondrosarcomas. Certain intracranial tumors have also been considered as potential sites that may benefit which include meningioma, pituitary adenoma, vestibular schwannoma, craniopharyngioma. As per the recently published evaluation report by American Society for Therapeutic Radiology and Oncology (ASTRO),[45] recent developments in the field of proton therapy, signal of a better potential for the use of protons in future. However, they do concede that as per the current evidence there is insufficient evidence to recommend protons for lung cancer, head and neck cancer, gastrointestinal malignancies (except HCC) and in pediatric non-CNS tumors outside of a clinical trial. Despite the availability of evidence of a superior dose distribution in pediatric CNS tumors, it was stated that as yet evidence is insufficient to recommend it as a standard of care. A similar report was published in Europe,[46] which had almost similar conclusions in terms that currently evidence is limited and both reports emphasized the need to generate more scientific evidence before protons can be accepted as a treatment modality outside of the trial settings.

BRACHYTHERAPY

Brachytherapy as a term takes its origin from the Greek word "brachys" meaning "short distance". In this form of RT source of radiation is placed in close vicinity/inside the tumor target. The characteristic of brachytherapy is the relatively sharp dose fall off, conferring the advantage wherein high local doses can be delivered to the tumor while sparing the surrounding normal tissues. The use of brachytherapy is well-established for gynecological malignancies, rectal cancers, anal canal cancers, prostatic carcinomas and soft tissue sarcomas.

The International Commission on Radiation Units report 38 defines low dose radiotherapy (LDR) as 0.4–2 Gy per hour, medium dose rate (MDR) as 2–12 Gy per hour whereas high dose rate (HDR) brachytherapy is delivered at more than 12 Gy per hour.[47]

Gynecological Malignancies

Brachytherapy for gynecological malignancies is an integral part of radical RT regimens as well as for treating postoperative cases. It could be delivered as LDR or HDR or pulse dose rate (PDR). With recent technological advances, majority of centers use HDR brachytherapy given the lower risk of radiation exposure to personnel and the superior safety and comfort of the patient with equivalent results. In most centers brachytherapy is delivered based on radiographic prescriptions to point A. This entails using 2 D orthogonal radiographs taken after insertion of the applicator with dummy sources in situ to help reconstruct the applicator. After applicator placement, the integrated brachytherapy unit (IBU) provides the facility of taking orthogonal radiographs without shifting the patient to another room. Additionally, once the treatment has been planned it can be delivered on the same table, minimizing chances of applicator shifts inside the patient on the same, thus ensuring accuracy of delivering the planned treatment (Figs 7 and 8).

Dramatic changes have been documented in field of intracavitary brachytherapy for cervix cancers over the last few years. From 2D radiograph-based prescriptions to applicator-based prescriptions to point A, brachytherapy has followed and incorporated the radiological developments. Now tumor is better defined by using ultrasounds or CT scans or MRI scans and attempt is made to prescribe dose to the target rather than to point A. Recently Groupe Européen de Curiethérapie/European Society for Therapeutic Radiation and Oncology (GEC ESTRO) guidelines have been formulated and the reported outcomes are superior than those reported with conventional brachytherapy.[48,49]

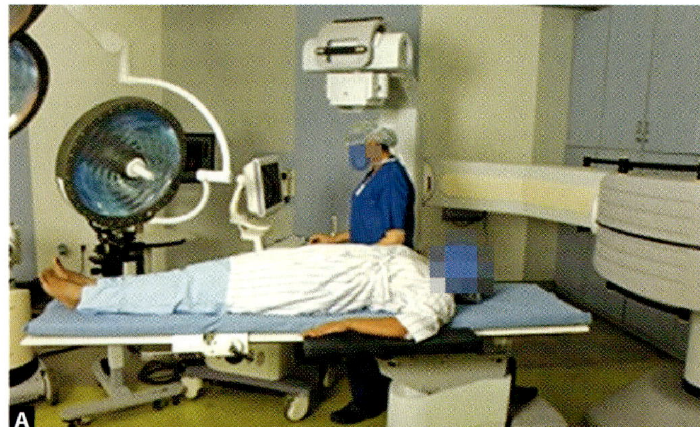

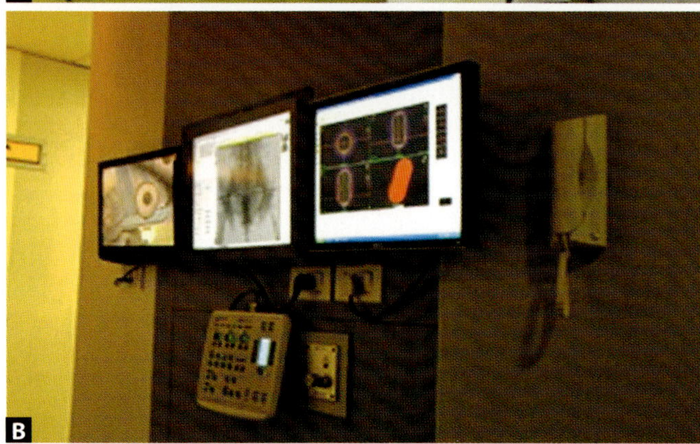

Figs 7A and B (A) The integrated brachytherapy unit (IBU); (B) The control monitors showing the 2D radiograph and the final dose plan

Courtesy: Dr Tejinder Kataria, Division of Radiation Oncology, Medanta—The Medicity, Harya na, India

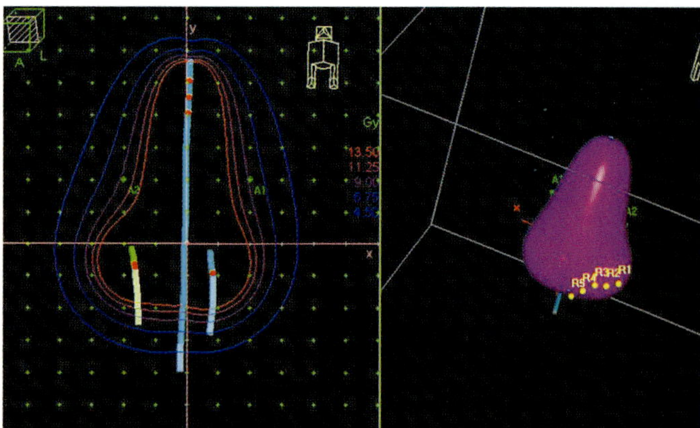

Fig. 8 High dose rate intracavitary radiotherapy (ICRT). The applicator consisting of one intrauterine tandem (blue) and two lateral ovoids (blue and green) reconstructed on treatment planning system and the resulting isodose lines indicated by "A" (A1) dose cloud (A2) with dose being prescribed to ICRU point A.

Courtesy: Dr Tejinder Kataria, Division of Radiation Oncology, Medanta—The Medicity, Harya na, India

Prostate Cancer

In cases of localized cancer prostate, LDR brachytherapy using radioactive permanent seeds implanted inside the prostate is an effective means of delivering RT. This is a onetime procedure and is appropriate for small localized tumors. The radioactive seeds continue to emit radiation over the subsequent few months depending on the half-life of the specific isotope used (Figs 9A to C).

High dose rate brachytherapy too can be used for delivering radiation for prostatic malignancies. It can used as a boost along with EBRT or can be used as the sole treatment in localized cases. This entails placement of transperineal interstitial needles under anesthesia through which radiation can be delivered using afterloading technique. Treatment is delivered over a period of 2–3 days with high dose per fraction being delivered at each session and the patient needs hospitalization during the course of treatment. The needles are retained inside the patient for the entire duration under analgesic cover. At treatment completion, the needles are removed and the patient is discharged.

CONCLUSION

The advancements in RT techniques have undoubtedly contributed to increased control rates for some sites while decreasing toxicity rates uniformly across the board. These advances come with increasing complexities and require longer man-hours with extensive quality assurance tests to deliver treatments as accurately as planned. There is increased possibility of errors at every step if adequate care is not taken, which emphasizes the need for greater responsibility on part of the entire radiation oncology team involved in patient treatment.

Additionally it has been found that all these factors result in escalation of health care costs. The rising cost of cancer care all over the world is a matter of concern and the innovative technologies need to be weighed against the outcomes. There is tremendous need for cost effective analysis and comparative effectiveness research in order to evaluate cost of the gains from newer techniques in order to make prudent and judicious cancer care management decisions.

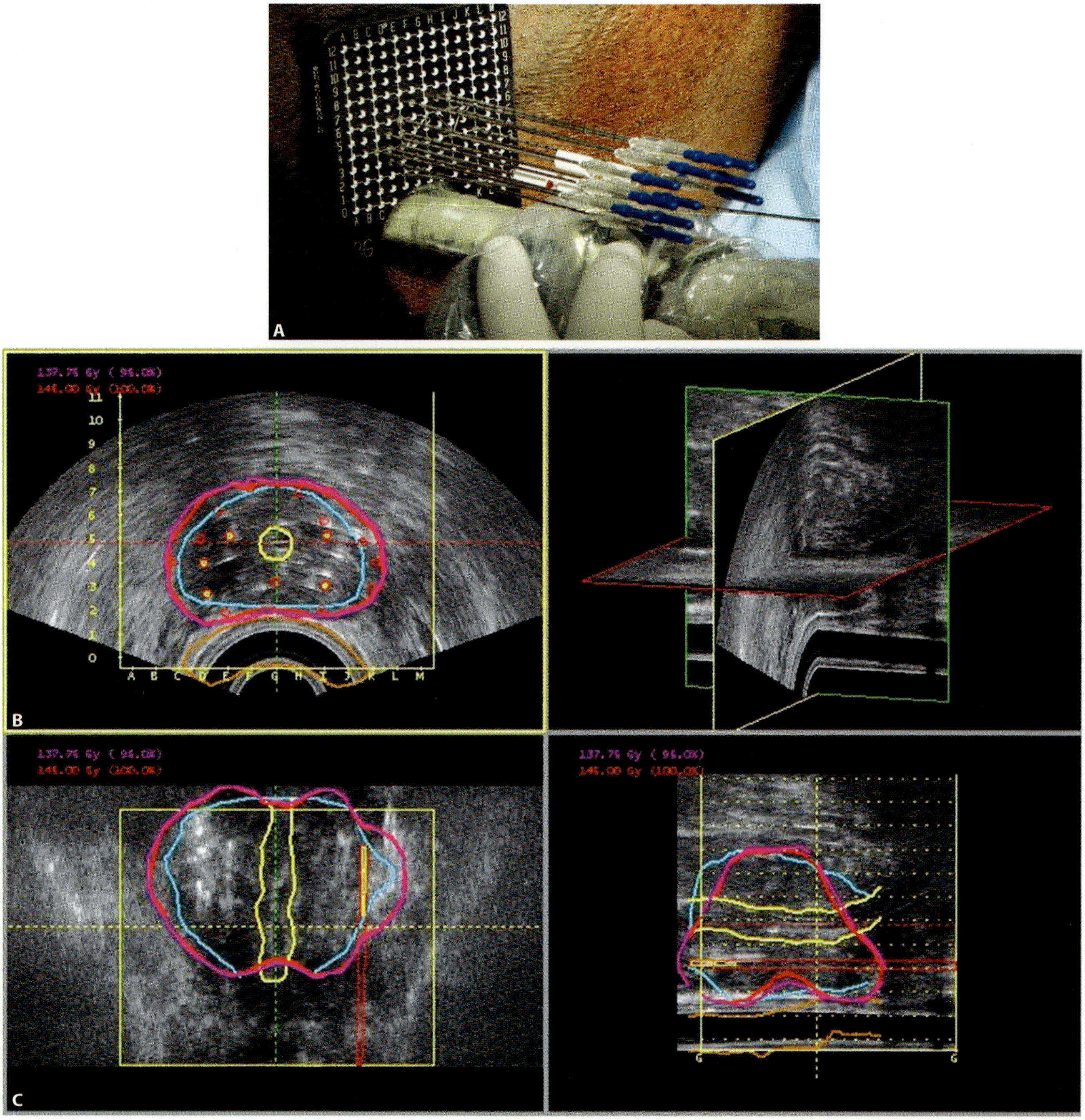

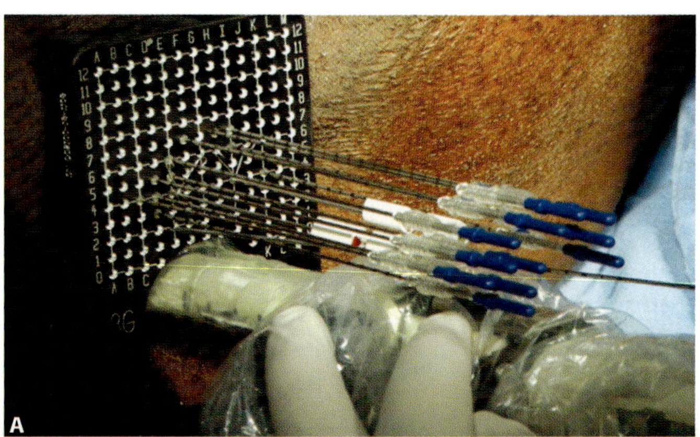

Figs 9A to C (A) Prostate seed implant; (B) Transperineal placement of seeds with help of interstitial needles; (C) The seeds are delineated with red circles and the prescription dose isodose is depicted in red while the delineated prostatic gland is outlined in pink

Courtesy: Dr Tejinder Kataria, Division of Radiation Oncology, Medanta—The Medicity, Haryana, India

REFERENCES

1. Jemal A, Bray F, Center MM, Ferlay J, Ward E, Forman D. Global cancer statistics. CA Cancer J Clin. 2011;61(2):69-90.
2. Ferlay J, Shin HR, Bray F, Forman D, Mathers C, Parkin DM. Estimates of worldwide burden of cancer in 2008: GLOBOCAN 2008. Int J Cancer. 2010;127(12):2893-917.
3. Ringborg U, Bergqvist D, Brorsson B, Cavallin-Ståhl E, Ceberg J, Einhorn N, et al. The Swedish Council on Technology Assessment in Health Care (SBU) systematic overview of radiotherapy for cancer including a prospective survey of radiotherapy practice in Sweden 2001--summary and conclusions. Acta Oncol. 2003;42(5-6):357-65.

4. Thwaites DI, Tuohy JB. Back to the future: the history and development of the clinical linear accelerator. Phys Med Biol. 2006;51(13):R343-62. Epub 2006 Jun 20.
5. Begg AC, Stewart FA, Vens C. Strategies to improve radiotherapy with targeted drugs. Nat Rev Cancer. 2011;11(4):239-53.
6 Delaney G, Jacob S, Featherstone C, Barton M. The role of radiotherapy in cancer treatment: estimating optimal utilization from a review of evidence-based clinical guidelines. Cancer. 2005;104(6):1129-37.
7. Barnett GC, West CM, Dunning AM, Elliott RM, Coles CE, Pharoah PD, et al. Normal tissue reactions to radiotherapy: towards tailoring treatment dose by genotype. Nat Rev Cancer. 2009;9(2):134-42.
8. Bernier J, Hall EJ, Giaccia A. Radiation oncology: a century of achievements. Nat Rev Cancer. 2004;4(9):737-47.
9. Takahashi S. Conformation radiotherapy. Rotation techniques as applied to radiography and radiotherapy of cancer. Acta Radiol Diagn (Stockh). 1965;(Suppl) 242:1+.
10. Ginzton EL, Nunan CS. History of microwave electron linear accelerators for radiotherapy. Int J Radiat Oncol Biol Phys. 1985;11(2):205-16.
11. Webb S. The Physics of Three Dimensional Radiation Therapy: Conformal Radiotherapy, Radiosurgery and Treatment Planning. Bristol: IOP Publishing; 1993.
12. International Commission on Radiation Units. Prescribing, recording and reporting photon beam therapy. Supplement to ICRU report 50. Bethesda: International Commission on Radiation Units and Measurement. MD: ICRU; 1999.
13. Tubiana M, Eschwège F. Conformal radiotherapy and intensity-modulated radiotherapy--clinical data. Acta Oncol. 2000;39(5):555-67.
14. Intensity Modulated Radiation Therapy Collaborative Working Group. Intensity-modulated radiotherapy: current status and issues of interest. Int J Radiat Oncol Biol Phys. 2001;51(4):880-914.
15. Goitein Michael. Radiation Oncology: A physicist's eye-view. New York: Springer-Verlag; 2008. p.171.
16. Bortfeld TR, Kahler DL, Waldron TJ, et al. X-ray field compensation with multileaf collimators. Int J Radiat Oncol Biol Phys. 1994;28(3):723-30.
17. Convery DJ, Webb S. Generation of discrete beam-intensity modulation by dynamic multileaf collimation under minimum leaf separation constraints. Phys Med Biol. 1998;43(9):2521-38.
18. Ling CC, Burman C, Chui CS, Kutcher GJ, Leibel SA, LoSasso T, et al. Conformal radiation treatment of prostate cancer using inversely-planned intensity-modulated photon beams produced with dynamic multileaf collimation. Int J Radiat Oncol Biol Phys. 1996;35(4):721-30.
19. Prescribing, Recording, and Reporting Photon-Beam Intensity-Modulated Radiation Therapy (IMRT): Contents. J ICRU. 2010;10(1).
20. Nutting CM, Morden JP, Harrington KJ, Urbano TG, Bhide SA, Clark C, et al. Parotid-sparing intensity modulated versus conventional radiotherapy in head and neck cancer (PARSPORT): a phase 3 multicentre randomised controlled trial. Lancet Oncol. 2011;12(2):127-36.
21. Eisbruch A, Kim HM, Terrell JE, Marsh LH, Dawson LA, Ship JA. Xerostomia and its predictors following parotid-sparing irradiation of head-and-neck cancer. Int J Radiat Oncol Biol Phys. 2001;50(3):695-704.
22. Eisbruch A, Schwartz M, Rasch C, Vineberg K, Damen E, Van As CJ, et al. Dysphagia and aspiration after chemoradiotherapy for head-and-neck cancer: which anatomic structures are affected and can they be spared by IMRT? Int J Radiat Oncol Biol Phys. 2004;60(5):1425-39.
23. Chao KS, Majhail N, Huang CJ, Simpson JR, Perez CA, Haughey B, et al. Intensity-modulated radiation therapy reduces late salivary toxicity without compromising tumor control in patients with oropharyngeal carcinoma: a comparison with conventional techniques. Radiother Oncol. 2001;61(3):275-80.
24. Wang-Chesebro A, Xia P, Coleman J, et al. Intensity-modulated radiotherapy improves lymph node coverage and dose to critical structures compared with three-dimensional conformal radiation therapy in clinically localized prostate cancer. Int J Radiat Oncol Biol Phys. 2006;66(3):654-62.
25. Mundt AJ, Lujan AE, Rotmensch J, Waggoner SE, Yamada SD, Fleming G, et al. Intensity-modulated whole pelvic radiotherapy in women with gynecologic malignancies. Int J Radiat Oncol Biol Phys. 2002;52(5):1330-7.
26. Otto K. Volumetric modulated arc therapy: IMRT in a single gantry arc. Med Phys. 2008;35:310-7.
27. Palma DA, Verbakel WF, Otto K, et al. New developments in arc radiation therapy: a review. Cancer Treat Rev. 2010;36(5):393-9.
28. Gill S, Thomas J, Fox C, Kron T, Rolfo A, Leahy M, et al. Acute toxicity in prostate cancer patients treated with and without image-guided radiotherapy. Radiat Oncol. 2011;6:145.
29. Duma MN, Kampfer S, Wilkens JJ, Schuster T, Molls M, Geinitz H. Comparative analysis of an image-guided versus a non-image-guided setup approach in terms of delivered dose to the parotid glands in head-and-neck cancer IMRT. Int J Radiat Oncol Biol Phys. 2010;77(4):1266-73.
30. Sterzing F, Engenhart-Cabillic R, Flentje M, et al. Image-Guided Radiotherapy: A New Dimension in Radiation Oncology. Deutsches Ärzteblatt International. 2011;108(16): 274-80. doi:10.3238/arztebl.2011.0274.
31. Lo SS, Fakiris AJ, Chang EL, Mayr NA, Wang JZ, Papiez L, et al. Stereotactic body radiation therapy: a novel treatment modality. Nat Rev Clin Oncol. 2010;7(1):44-54.
32. Bentzen SM, Constine LS, Deasy JO, Eisbruch A, Jackson A, Marks LB, et al. Quantitative Analyses of Normal Tissue Effects in the Clinic (QUANTEC): an introduction to the scientific issues. Int J Radiat Oncol Biol Phys. 2010;76(Suppl 3):S3-9.
33. Piotrowski T, Skórska M, Jodda A, Ryczkowski A, Kamierska J, Adamska K, et al. Tomotherapy - a different way of dose delivery in radiotherapy. Contemp Oncol (Pozn). 2012;16(1):16-25.
34. Mackie TR, Holmes T, Swerdloff S, Reckwerdt P, Deasy JO, Yang J, et al. Tomotherapy: a new concept for the delivery of dynamic conformal radiotherapy. Med Phys. 1993;20(6):1709-19.
35. Welsh JS. Basics of particle therapy: introduction to hadrons. Am J Clin Oncol. 2008;31(5):493-5.
36. Hug EB, Loredo LN, Slater JD, DeVries A, Grove RI, Schaefer RA, et al. Proton radiation therapy for chordomas

and chondrosarcomas of the skull base. J Neurosurg. 1999;91(3):432-9.
37. Munzenrider JE, Liebsch NJ. Proton therapy for tumors of the skull base. Strahlenther Onkol. 1999;175 (Suppl) 2:57-63.
38. WILSON RR. Radiological use of fast protons. Radiology. 1946; 47(5):487-91.
39. Hug EB, Loredo LN, Slater JD, DeVries A, Grove RI, Schaefer RA, et al. Proton radiation therapy for chordomas and chondrosarcomas of the skull base. J Neurosurg. 1999;91(3):432-9.
40. Noël G, Feuvret L, Calugaru V, Dhermain F, Mammar H, Haie-Méder C, et al. Chordomas of the base of the skull and upper cervical spine. One hundred patients irradiated by a 3D conformal technique combining photon and proton beams. Acta Oncol. 2005;44(7):700-8.
41. Damato B. Treatment of primary intraocular melanoma. Expert Rev Anticancer Ther. 2006;6(4):493-506.
42. Zietman AL, DeSilvio ML, Slater JD, Rossi CJ, Miller DW, Adams JA, et al. Comparison of conventional-dose vs high-dose conformal radiation therapy in clinically localized adenocarcinoma of the prostate: a randomized controlled trial. JAMA. 2005;294(10):1233-9.
43. Slater JD, Rossi CJ, Yonemoto LT, Bush DA, Jabola BR, Levy RP, et al. Proton therapy for prostate cancer: the initial Loma Linda University experience. Int J Radiat Oncol Biol Phys. 2004;59(2):348-52.
44. Shipley WU, Verhey LJ, Munzenrider JE, Suit HD, Urie MM, McManus PL, et al. Advanced prostate cancer: the results of a randomized comparative trial of high dose irradiation boosting with conformal protons compared with conventional dose irradiation using photons alone. Int J Radiat Oncol Biol Phys. 1995;32(1):3-12.
45. Allen AM, Pawlicki T, Dong L, Fourkal E, Buyyounouski M, Cengel K, et al. An evidence based review of proton beam therapy: the report of ASTRO's emerging technology committee. Radiother Oncol. 2012;103(1):8-11.
46. Lodge M, Pijls-Johannesma M, Stirk L, Munro AJ, De Ruysscher D, Jefferson T. A systematic literature review of the clinical and cost-effectiveness of hadron therapy in cancer. Radiother Oncol. 2007;83(2):110-22.
47. ICRU Report 38. Dose and volume specification for reporting intracavitary therapy in gynaecology. International Commission on Radiation Units and Measurements, Bethesda, Maryland; 1985.
48. Haie-Meder C, Pötter R, Van Limbergen E, Briot E, De Brabandere M, Dimopoulos J, et al. Recommendations from Gynaecological (GYN) GEC-ESTRO Working Group (I): concepts and terms in 3D image based 3D treatment planning in cervix cancer brachytherapy with emphasis on MRI assessment of GTV and CTV. Radiother Oncol. 2005;74(3):235-45.
49. Pötter R, Haie-Meder C, Van Limbergen E, Barillot I, De Brabandere M, Dimopoulos J, et al. Recommendations from gynaecological (GYN) GEC ESTRO working group (II): concepts and terms in 3D image-based treatment planning in cervix cancerbrachytherapy-3D dose volume parameters and aspects of 3D image-based anatomy, radiation physics, radiobiology. Radiother Oncol. 2006;78(1):67-77.

CHAPTER

Image-guided Radiation Therapy

Shikha Goyal, Tejinder Kataria

INTRODUCTION

With increasing emphasis on reducing the volume of radiation therapy fields while maintaining or improving precision of treatment and reducing radiation-related normal tissue toxicity, treatment position verification and correction before delivering radiotherapy has gained major importance. A variety of techniques have been developed that can accomplish this goal with aplomb, albeit each with its own set of limitations. The best method that eliminates uncertainties in treatment without a huge cost remains to be defined, but it is clear that carrying out "high precision radiotherapy" without periodic image guidance is as accurate as shooting in a dark room. This review discusses the concept of image guidance in radiotherapy, various techniques available along with expected benefits and pitfalls of these systems.

ROLE OF IMAGING IN RADIATION ONCOLOGY

Right from its inception, radiotherapy has relied on the inputs from imaging for treatment planning as well as execution. For tumors that are not amenable to direct inspection or visual confirmation, use of anatomic surface landmarks as well as radiologic correlates from 2D imaging, either in the form of port films or fluoroscopic imaging has been commonplace. Broadly, there are two aspects of imaging inputs in radiotherapy: (1) inputs from sophisticated technologies such as contrast CT scans, MRI, PET scans and angiography, incorporating structural and biologic information to help define the target better, and thus aid precise and accurate treatment planning, and (2) in-room imaging methods, which may be planar, volumetric, video or ultrasound-based and can obtain periodic information on target position and movement (intrafraction or interfraction), subsequently comparing with reference imaging to provide feedback on correcting patient setup and optimizing target localization. The technology can also potentially provide feedback to adapt successive treatment sessions to tumor response. In more specific terms, it is the latter use with regard to in-room imaging that is regarded as "image-guided radiation therapy" (IGRT) in modern day radiotherapy. 3D data acquired using volumetric CT, MR and angiographic studies are used for planning highly conformal radiotherapy with shaped beams in isocentric or nonisocentric geometry.

Routine use of newer techniques such as intensity-modulated radiation therapy (IMRT), volumetric-modulated arc therapy (VMAT), stereotactic radiosurgery (SRS) or stereotactic radiotherapy (SRT) using a host of delivery methods has enabled the reduction of safety margin around the target volumes thus, allowing for reduced normal tissue doses without compromising delivery of tumoricidal doses. However, a great deal of uncertainty exists in accurately defining the position of radiotherapy targets during the process of fractionated radiotherapy, both during a given fraction and between consecutive fractions, thus highlighting the need to develop and implement strategies to measure, monitor and correct these uncertainties. This need has led to evolution of various in-room imaging technologies which help evaluate and correct the setup errors, anatomic changes related to weight loss, or deformation or internal organ motion related to respiration, peristalsis or rectal/bladder filling.

Another use of imaging exists in the use of orthogonal X-ray imaging, CT and MRI for optimizing brachytherapy planning and delivery, increasing safety as well as efficacy of the procedure. The imaging techniques used for interventional radiology (orthogonal images, fluoroscopy) may be used to guide the placement of the brachytherapy catheters/applicators. After applicator insertion, volumetric images such as CT scan or MRI are acquired and the catheters identified and reconstructed on transverse sections. Isodose distribution is reviewed and optimized on visualizing dose distribution to the target as well as critical structures.

IMAGE-GUIDED RADIATION THERAPY: THE CONCEPT

Unlike other forms of local therapy such as surgical resection where the target in question can be visualized and handled under direct guidance, traditional radiation therapy techniques are inherently fraught with the disadvantage of making quite a few assumptions. The 3D image dataset acquired at simulation is a single time snapshot of the tumor, its relation to normal structures and the patient shape and position, and this model is used for plan development and dose calculation. A lot of information is fed into the planning system including assumptions of microscopic spread around the visible tumor, expected range of internal organ motion and setup errors. We then proceed to treat the actual patient with the belief that nothing would have changed since the time of simulation and the patient anatomy on any given day would be in keeping with the original snapshot. However, the assumption that the calculated doses would actually match those delivered through each fraction or through the entire radiation therapy course is grossly in error. Wider margins are taken around the targets to assure that our assumptions do not compromise the dose delivered to the intended target, thus including a large volume of normal tissues in the irradiated volume as well. IGRT provides a method for capturing this information in the form of serial "snapshots" taken through the treatment course, and is a means of verifying accurate and precise radiation delivery. In simple terms, the IGRT process ensures that the delivered treatment matches the intended treatment in accurately targeting the tumor while minimizing "collateral damage". Changes to the composite delivered dose and their impact on disease control as well as toxicity may be minimized by use of appropriate localization devices and planning target volume (PTV) margins. Occasionally, replanning may be required if gross deviations beyond predetermined tolerances are observed.[1-3]

Image-guided radiation therapy allows assessment of geometric accuracy of the "patient model" during treatment delivery. It provides a method whereby deviations of anatomy from initial plan are determined, and this information is used to update dosimetric assumptions. Correction strategies may include daily repositioning to register patient position in accordance with the base plan or recalculation of treatment delivery in real time to reflect the patient's presentation during a given fraction. This philosophy of reevaluating treatment and accounting for the differences between actual patient anatomy on a given day and the snapshot of planned treatment is known as adaptive radiotherapy.[4] The eventual goal is to reevaluate and in certain situations redefine daily positioning for treatment to keep it on the same track as the intended treatment. Future applications may include dose titration for maximizing effect or mitigating side effects.

ERRORS AND MARGINS

An error in radiotherapy delivery is defined as any deviation from intended or planned treatment. A great degree of uncertainty is inherent to radiotherapy practices and may be in the form of mechanical uncertainties related to treatment unit parameters such as couch and gantry motion, patient uncertainties related to ability to lie comfortably in a certain position and cooperate during the treatment time, geometric uncertainties related to position and motion of target, and dosimetric uncertainties. IGRT deals with the *geometric* uncertainties, which may be either intrafractional or interfractional.[5,6]

Both interfractional and intrafractional uncertainties may be a result of a combination of systematic and random errors.

A systematic error is essentially a treatment preparation error and is introduced into the chain during the process of positioning, simulation or target delineation. This error, if uncorrected, would affect all treatment fractions uniformly. A random error, on the other hand, is a treatment execution error, is unpredictable and varies with each fraction. Systematic errors shift the entire dose distribution away from the clinical target volume (CTV), while random errors blur this distribution around the CTV. Of the two, systematic error is more ominous since it would have a much larger impact on treatment accuracy and hence the therapeutic ratio.

Margins are added to the CTV to take these errors into account. These margins are geometric expansions around the CTV and may be nonuniform in all dimensions depending on the expected errors. These margins ensure that dosimetric planning goals are met despite the variations during and between fractions. ICRU-62 defines the expansion of PTV around the CTV as a composite of two factors: internal target motion (internal margin) and setup variations (setup margin).[7] Depending on observed systematic and random errors in a given setup for a particular treatment site, a variety of recipes for calculating PTV margins exist in literature.[8,9] To enhance the therapeutic ratio, a host of correction strategies may be applied to reduce these margins and may include online or offline correction of interfraction errors or real-time correction of intrafraction motion. Tracking and correcting organ motion helps reduce internal margin while improved accuracy of positioning reduces setup margins, thus reducing the required PTV margin.

OFFLINE VERSUS ONLINE CORRECTIONS

Offline and online IGRT correction strategies refer to the fact whether the patient is on the treatment couch while the verification is being done and whether the correction would be applied to the same or subsequent sessions.

In the offline strategy, images are acquired before treatment and matched to the reference image at a later time point. This strategy aims to determine the individual systematic setup error and thus reduce it. When combined with setup data of other patients treated under the same protocol, it helps define the population standard error for that treatment in that institution. Widely used offline correction protocols include Shrinking action level and No action level protocols.[10,11] PTV margins in an institution depend on these determinations of individual and population systematic errors.

An online strategy, on the other hand, employs acquisition of images, and their verification and correction prior to the day's treatment. It aims to reduce both random and systematic errors. The treatment site and the expected magnitude of error may determine the frequency of online imaging. Sites where large daily shifts are anticipated (abdomen, pelvis and thorax) or where even slight shifts will alter the dose distribution within adjacent critical structures (paraspinal tumors, intracranial tumors in close proximity to optic structures) are best managed with daily imaging. Our experience with online corrections showed the maximum errors in thorax followed closely by abdomen and pelvis. The minimum errors were observed in head and neck region.[12] Additionally, treatments such as VMAT and stereotactic body radiation therapy (SBRT) carry the potential to translate minor shifts into major alterations in dose distribution, and hence require daily online verification. For daily online correction, systematic and random errors may be calculated from the matched data. Post-treatment imaging is required to quantify both intrafraction motion and residual errors. If evaluated for a patient population, these data may help check the PTV margin for that treatment protocol. In fact, the use of daily online imaging with corrections in conjunction with use of automatic couch with 6° of freedom has obviated the need for invasive frames for stereotactic radiosurgery treatments.[13]

IGRT TECHNOLOGY SOLUTIONS

Depending on the imaging methods used, the IGRT systems may broadly be divided into radiation-based and nonradiation-based systems.[14,15]

Nonradiation-based Systems[16-22]

These may employ ultrasound, camera-based systems, electromagnetic tracking and MRI systems integrated into the treatment room.

Ultrasound-based systems such as BAT, SonArray, and Clarity acquire 3D images that may help align targets to correct for interfractional errors. Geometric accuracy is 3–5 mm and the greatest advantage is lack of any ionizing radiation. Sites of common application include prostate, lung and breast radiotherapy.

Camera-based (infrared) or optical tracking systems identify the patient reference setup point positions in comparison to their location in the planning CT coordinate system, which aids in computing the treatment couch translation to align the treatment isocenter with plan isocenter. Optical tracking may also be used for intrafraction position monitoring for either gating (treatment delivery only at a certain position of target) or repositioning for correction. Tools, such as AlignRT, image the patient directly and track the skin surface to give real-time feedback for necessary corrections. These systems have found application in treatment of prostate and breast cancer and for respiratory gating using external surrogates. Geometric accuracy is 1–2 mm, but application is limited only to situations where external surface may act as a sufficient surrogate for internal position or motion.

Electromagnetic tracking systems (Calypso) make use of electromagnetic transponders (beacons) embedded within the tumor, and motion of these beacons may be tracked in real time using a detector array system. Beacons need to be placed through a minimally invasive procedure, their presence may introduce artifacts in MR images, and there are limitations to the patient size. This system has a geometric accuracy of less than 2 mm, but its use at present is limited to prostate radiotherapy.

MRI-guided IGRT (e.g. ViewRay) helps real-time assessment of internal soft tissue anatomy and motion using continual soft tissue imaging and allows for intrafractional corrections. Geometric accuracy is 1–2 mm, but the limitations applicable to MRI including distortions with nonuniform magnetic fields, motion artifacts and exclusion of patients with pacemakers or metallic implants who would be otherwise unsuitable for MRI. A wide application potential exists in treatment of prostate, liver, and brain as well as for brachytherapy.

Radiation-based Systems

These include static as well as real-time tracking, using either kilovoltage (KV), megavoltage (MV) or hybrid methods.

Electronic portal imaging devices (EPIDs): EPID was developed as a replacement of film dosimetry for treatment field verification and is based on indirect detection active matrix flat panel imagers (AMFPIs). They are offered as standard equipment by nearly all linear accelerator (LINAC) vendors as both field verification and quality assurance (QA) tools. Image acquisition is 2D, with a geometric accuracy of 2 mm. Bony landmarks on planar images are used as surrogates for defining positional variations respective to the digital reconstructed radiographs (DRRs) developed from the planning CT dataset. Different systems may use either KV or MV X-rays for imaging, the image contrast being superior with KV images while there is lesser distortion from metallic implants (dental, hip prostheses) in MV images. System is unable to detect or quantify rotations. Average dose per image

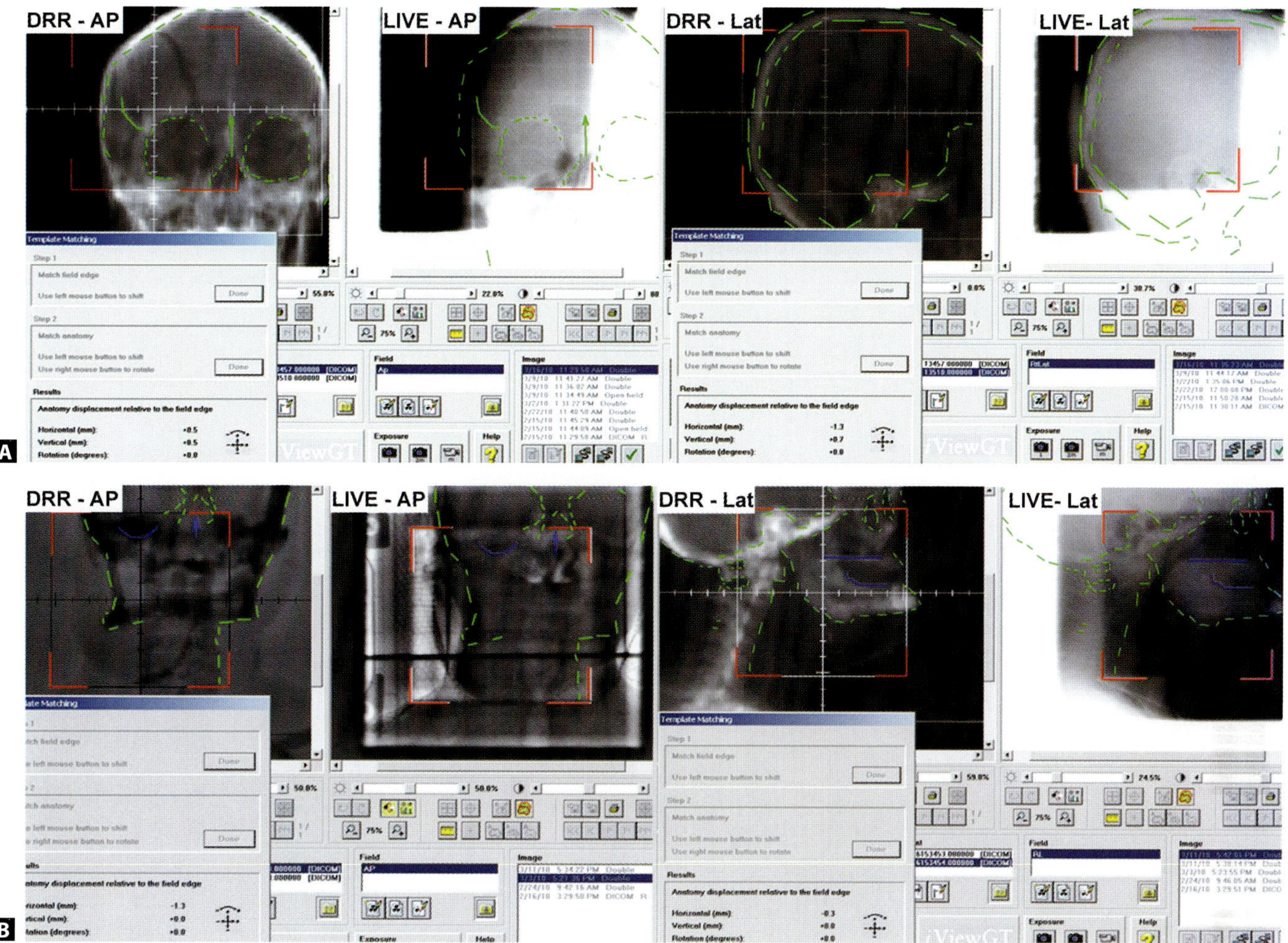

Figs 1A and B Use of MV EPID for online correction using orthogonal 2D images (anteroposterior and lateral). Both the field and the bony anatomy are matched sequentially to give an estimate of error. The comparison of live image with reference DRR helps assess and correct translational shifts, but does not estimate rotational errors. (A) Right parietal glioma and (B) Head and neck cancer

Abbreviations: DRR, digital reconstructed radiographi; AP, anteroposterior; Lat, Lateral
Courtesy: Dr Tejinder Kataria, Division of Radiation Oncology, Medanta—The Medicity, Haryana, India

is 1–3 mGy for KV systems while it is as high as 30–70 mGy for MV systems[23-25] (Figs 1A and B).

Cone beam CT (CBCT)—KV or MV: These systems consist of retractable X-ray tube and amorphous silicon detectors mounted either orthogonal to (Elekta Synergy, Varian OBI) or along the treatment beam axis (Siemens Artiste). These have capability of 2D, fluoroscopic and CBCT imaging. Another system (Vero, BrainLAB) consists of a gimbaled X-ray treatment head mounted on an O-ring with 2 kV X-ray tubes, two flat panel detectors, and an EPID. The O-ring can be rotated 360° around the isocenter and can be skewed 60° around its vertical axis. Geometric accuracy is 1 mm or lesser with possibility of 2D and 3D matching with DRRs or X-ray volumetric images generated from planning CT data sets. Scanning is done through a continuous partial or complete gantry rotation around the couch, acquiring the "average" position of organs with respiratory motion. Both interfraction setup changes and anatomical changes related to weight changes or organ filling (bladder, rectum) may be monitored. Repeat scans at the end of treatment may give an estimate of intrafractional changes. For tumors discernible separately from surrounding normal tissue, treatment response may also be monitored and these scans may be used for dose recalculation or treatment plan adaptation after necessary image processing. KV CT gives better contrast resolution compared to MV CT but may be limited by artifacts from prostheses and scatter from bulky patient anatomy. Average dose per image is 30–50 mGy[26-29] (Figs 2A to C).

Fan beam KV CT (CT-on-rails): This system has an in-room CT scanner and gantry that moves across the treatment couch/ patient, which can be rotated either toward the scanner or the gantry for imaging and treatment, respectively. 3D images are taken with the patient immobilized on the couch, the

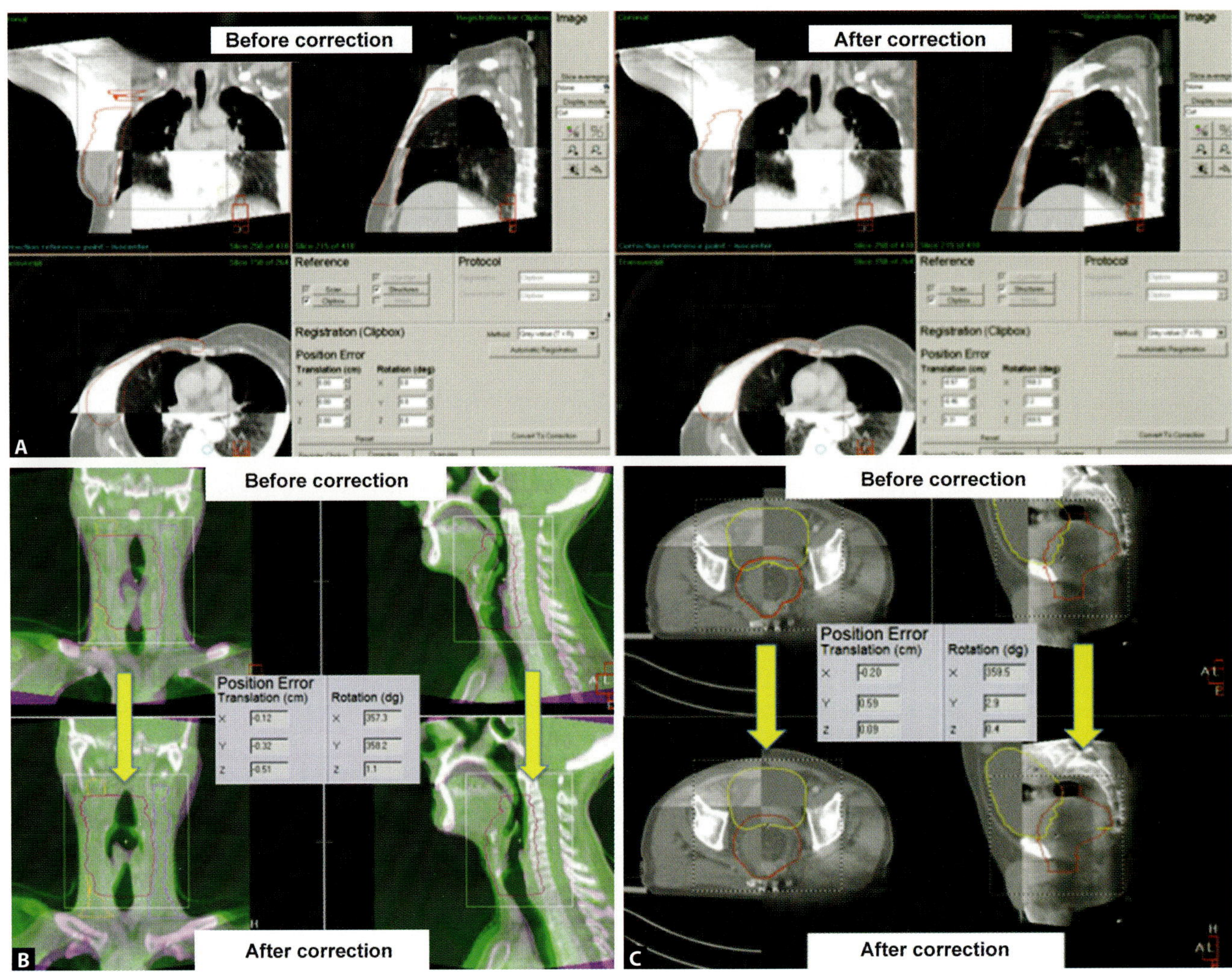

Figs 2A to C The KV CBCT volumetric imaging. Both translational and rotational errors may be estimated. Translational errors are easily corrected whereas few systems have provisions for correcting rotational errors with couch rotations. (A) CBCT compared with reference scan before and after correction of setup error in a case of Carcinoma right breast, postmastectomy; (B) CBCT correction in a case of carcinoma larynx; (C) CBCT in a case of Carcinoma prostate not only corrects for setup errors but also provides an estimate of reproducibility of prostate position with respect to bladder filling. In this particular case, the live image shows negligible bladder filling and treatment was delayed to allow for optimum bladder position for obtaining a reproducible position of prostate as well as moving the bowel out of treatment field

Courtesy: Dr Tejinder Kataria, Division of Radiation Oncology, Medanta—The Medicity, Haryana, India

difference from a diagnostic CT being a larger bore size (>80 cm diameter) to accommodate bulky immobilization devices, and a multislice detector. Accuracy and applications are similar to CBCT with average dose of 10–50 mGy per image.[30]

Fan beam MV CT (TomoTherapy Hi ART II): This includes an on-board imaging system to obtain MV CT images of the patient in treatment position. The same LINAC is used to generate both the treatment (6 MV) and imaging beam (3.5 MV). A xenon detector located on the gantry opposite the LINAC collects exit data for generation of MV CT images. Patient dose from imaging varies with pitch setting, and is typically 10–30 mGy per scan.[31]

Hybrid Systems for Real-time 4D Tracking

2D KV stereoscopic imaging (CyberKnife): The accuray CyberKnife robotic radiosurgery system consists of a compact LINAC mounted on an industrial robotic manipulator arm, which directs the radiation beams to the desired target based on inputs from two orthogonal X-ray imaging systems mounted on the room ceiling with flat panel floor detectors on either side of couch, integrated to provide image guidance for the treatment process. Images are acquired throughout the treatment duration at periodic intervals ranging from 5 seconds to 90 seconds, and the couch and robotic head movements are guided through an automatic process.

Several tracking methods may be used depending upon the treatment site. Skull, skull base or brain tumors may be treated using 6D skull tracking, paravertebral tumors whose movements parallels that of spine may be treated with X-Sight spine tracking, and lung tumors that are surrounded by normal lung parenchyma may be tracked with X-Sight lung tracking. Lung tracking may employ automatic generation of internal target volume depending upon visibility of tumor through both, one or none of the X-ray imaging systems in the treatment position. For all other tumors (e.g. prostate, liver, neck nodes, abdominal masses, etc.), internal surrogates or fiducial markers may need to be placed within or in direct contact with the tumor and the tumor motion is tracked and corrected for through monitoring the fiducial position including translations, rotations and deformation. Respiratory motion is also monitored and accounted for when correcting for target position and motion through a synchrony model generated in real time. The system also has a couch that has 6° of freedom to correct for positional variations. Treatment may be limited by patient position and size, and posterior treatment beams cannot be used. A semi-invasive procedure may be required if fiducial markers are needed for tracking. This system can be employed both for cranial (frameless) and extracranial radiosurgery or SRT[32,33] (Figs 3A to C).

Real-time tumor-tracking system: This system is designed for real-time tracking of tumors by imaging implanted fiducial and using this information for gating. It consists of four X-ray camera systems mounted on the floor, a ceiling-mounted image intensifier and a high-voltage X-ray generator. The LINAC is gated to irradiate the tumor only when the marker is within a given tolerance from its planned coordinates relative to the isocenter.[34,35]

VERO: This system has two X-ray tubes and corresponding flat panel detectors, and uses a combination of initial couch motion and a pair of radiographs for patient alignment. The couch is capable of 3D alignment for initial coarse setup and then the on-board imaging subsystem helps fine-tuning. A pair of radiographs is acquired and registered with prior DRRs using bony landmarks to evaluate the translational and rotational shifts. The system can also compensate for organ motion.[36]

Combination Alignment Systems: Optical Imaging and 2D KV Orthogonal Imaging

ExacTrac X-ray 6D stereotactic IGRT system: It uses a combination of optical positioning and KV radiographic imaging for online positioning corrections. There are two main subsystems: an infrared-based system for initial patient setup and precise control of couch movement using a robotic couch, and a radiographic KV X-ray imaging system for position verification and re-adjustment based on internal anatomy or implanted markers. Infrared system may also be used for respiratory monitoring and signaling to LINAC for beam

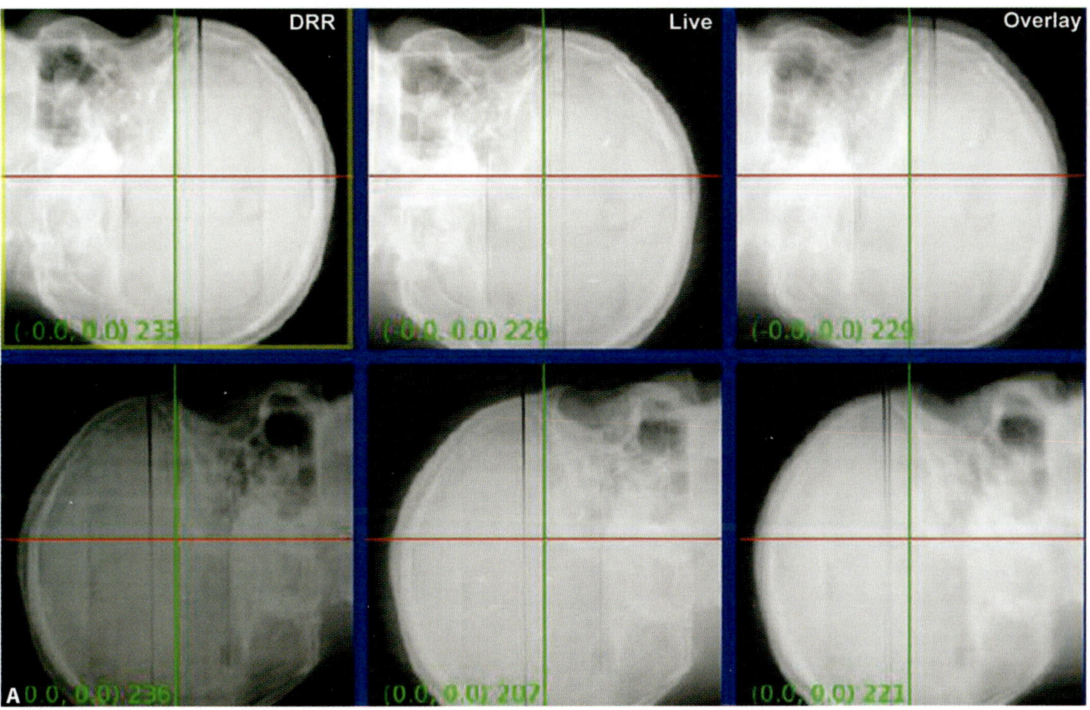

Fig. 3A

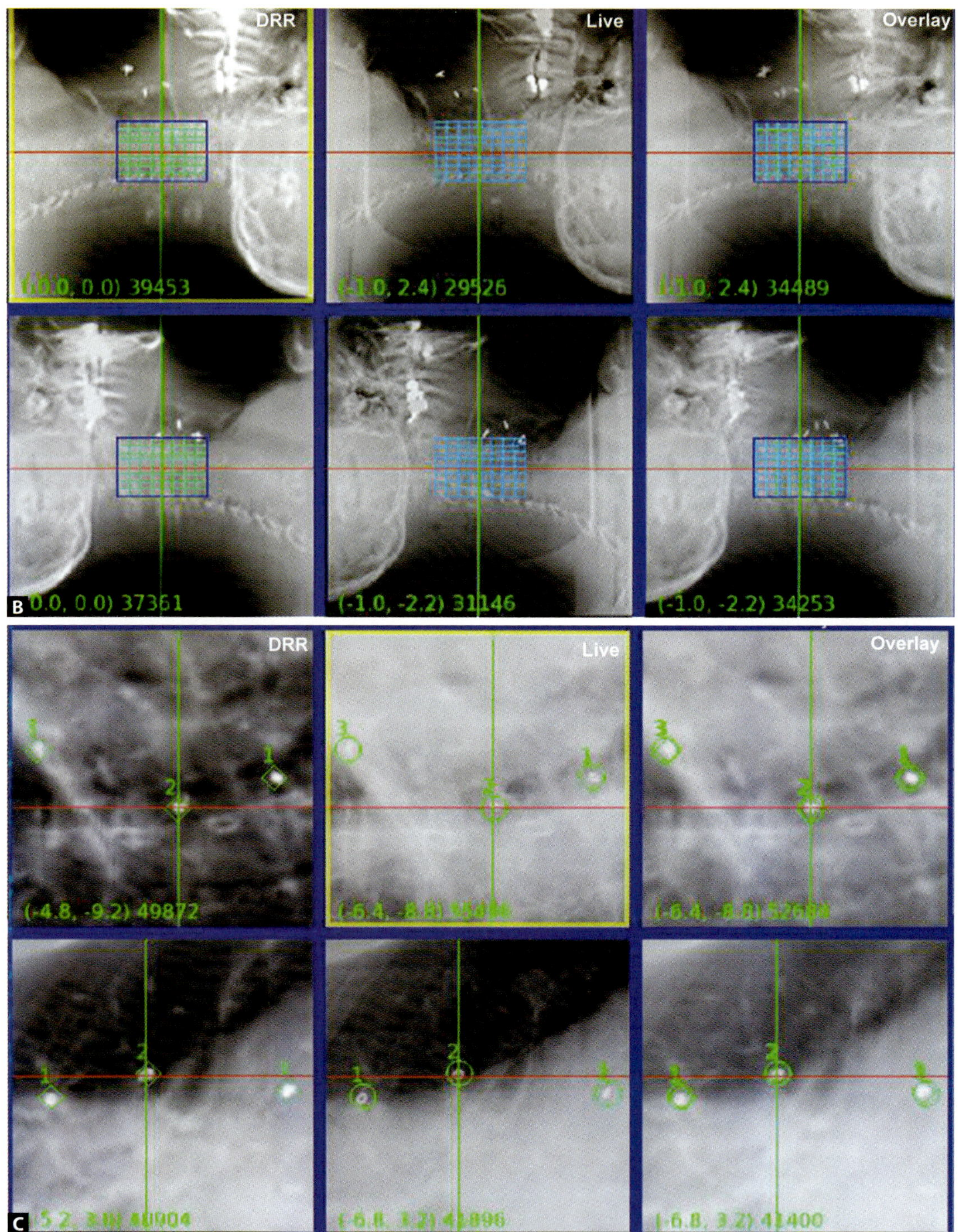

Figs 3B and C

Figs 3A to C CyberKnife console showing the tumor tracking options in a case of head and neck malignancy. (A) 6D skull for skull base lesions; (B) Spine tracking for paravertebral tumors; (C) Fiducial tracking for all other lesions whose motion is independent of skull or spine position, such as base of tongue or neck nodes

Courtesy: Dr Tejinder Kataria, Division of Radiation Oncology, Medanta—The Medicity, Haryana, India

tracking and gating. Novalis Tx combines this system with an additional on-board imaging system (MV, KV X-rays, and KV CBCT) on a multiphoton/electron beam LINAC.[37,38]

GUIDELINES FOR MEDICAL PERSONNEL AND IMPLEMENTATION

American College of Radiology and the American Society for Radiation Oncology jointly developed guidelines for IGRT that define the qualifications and responsibilities of personnel including radiation oncologists, medical physicists, dosimetrists and radiation therapists, QA standards, clinical implementation and suggested documentation. Similar guidelines have also been proposed by European agencies.[39-41] A summary of the key points is given below:

Qualifications

Appropriate certification with specific training in IGRT before performing any stereotactic procedures.

Responsibilities

Radiation Oncologist

- Conduct of disease-specific treatment, staging, evaluation of comorbid conditions and prior treatments, exploration of all available treatments including discussion of pros and cons of IGRT, treatment and subsequent follow-up.
- Determination of the most appropriate patient positioning method, recommendation of the appropriate approach to manage organ motion, supervision of simulation paying particular attention to positioning, immobilization and appropriate motion management, determination and delineation of target volumes and relevant normal critical structures using available imaging techniques, communication of expected goals and constraints and collaboration with the physicist in the iterative process of plan development to achieve the desired goals, supervision of treatment delivery and determination of acceptable day-to-day setup variations, and participation in the QA process and subsequent approval.

Medical Physicist

- Acceptance testing and commissioning, assuring mechanical, software, and geometric precision and accuracy, as well as image quality verification and documentation in a given IGRT system.
- Implementation and management of a QA program.
- Development and implementation of standard operating procedures (SOPs) for IGRT use, in collaboration with the radiation oncologist.

Dosimetrist

- Normal structure delineation under the guidance of radiation oncologist.
- Management of volumetric patient image data (CT and other fused data sets) on radiation treatment planning system.
- Generation of a treatment plan under oncologist's and physicist's guidance.
- Generation of all technical documentation for IGRT plan implementation.
- Assisting with treatment verification.

Radiation Therapist

- Understanding and appropriate use of immobilization/repositioning systems.
- Performance of simulation and generation of imaging data for planning, implementation of treatment plan, acquisition of periodic verification images under supervision and periodic evaluation of stability and reproducibility of the immobilization/repositioning system and reporting inconsistencies immediately.

IGRT Implementation

Fiducial markers: These serve as surrogates to soft tissue targets when they are difficult to visualize and their alignment cannot be related to bony anatomy. These may be tracked in real time to obtain 3D coordinates of the target for subsequent corrections.

Moving targets and delineation: Intrafraction target motion or interfraction displacement, deformation, or alteration of targets and other tissues should be accounted for during determination of PTVs. Appropriate motion management methods should be chosen depending on available expertise, and degree and type of motion. This process starts at the time of simulation and continues through to the end of therapy.

Patient positioning: Ensure accuracy of patient position and its reproducibility for fractionated treatments relative to the chosen IGRT device as well as treatment unit.

Image acquisition: Calibration of the IGRT system to ensure high imaging quality with attention to slice thickness uniformity, image contrast, spatial resolution, isocenter alignment between imaging and treatment planning and delivery systems, accuracy of software used for identification and correction of couch misalignments. Relevant QA procedures should ensure reliability and reproducibility of the entire process.

Treatment verification: Image review by radiation oncologist at the first fraction and then periodically is necessary to ensure treatment accuracy and reproducibility. Each department should determine its own threshold of couch positioning changes that would necessitate setup review or change before treatment delivery.

Quality assurance and documentation: A documentation of all the necessary QA procedures throughout the course of simulation, treatment and periodic verification should be maintained. These would help determine departmental thresholds for action as well as serve as guides for modification of the processes involved following review of findings.

IMAGE-GUIDED RADIATION THERAPY: CLINICAL BENEFITS

Use of the IGRT process has improved our awareness and understanding of daily interfractional and intrafractional setup variations and motion. Real-time tracking has helped quantify interpatient and intrapatient variations in lung and liver tumor motion related to breathing and complexities of such motion have become clearer. We now understand that even when breath-holds are repeated, the relative position of soft tissue and skeletal structures may vary, rendering use of bony landmarks useless for such endeavors. Changes in prostate position (translation, rotation as well as shape) have been quantified, and we can better correct for these errors as well as tailor PTV margins to these findings, thus allowing more accurate targeting. Understanding of the various IGRT techniques, their applicability, limitations, additional radiation hazards help the radiation oncologist take an educated decision on the method best suited to a particular clinical situation for maximizing benefit from radiation therapy. Changes in parotid position relative to the tumor in head and neck cases, change in body contour due to weight loss, seroma or body fluid collections, change in prostate position relative to bladder or rectal filling and effect of bowel gas, reduction of tumor size during treatment and changes in spinal position during spinal or head and neck radiotherapy are situations which were never even considered of significance in the pre-IGRT era and their respective roles and solutions are being developed as we are understanding their roles during treatment. With better geometric precision, volume of irradiated healthy normal tissue can be significantly reduced with reduction in toxicity risks. Adaptation to reduction in tumor volume may lead to additional gains in normal tissue toxicity reduction.

Results from ongoing and future trials will hopefully demonstrate the net gain in therapeutic ratio from application of IGRT technologies and the onus lies on the radiation oncology community to take up the challenge of demonstrating the benefit of these potentially expensive approaches.

Image guided radiation therapy is most likely to benefit clinical situations where the tumor is in close proximity to sensitive healthy tissues, when doses required for disease control exceed the tolerance levels of adjacent normal tissues, or when large organ motion and setup errors may result in severe consequences of positional errors. All patients treated with conformal radiotherapy, IMRT, and SBRT should, in theory, benefit from IGRT. Thoracic and upper abdominal targets with significant respiratory motion, obese patients, head and neck cancers, paraspinal and retroperitoneal sarcomas, and prostate cancer are situations that are expected to derive maximum benefit with some clinical experience forthcoming. Clinical situations where even low dose irradiation produces excellent local control, palliative radiotherapy delivered using large fields and superficial tumors that are amenable to direct visual inspection are likely to derive least benefit from IGRT.

CONCERNS WITH IGRT

Limited availability of experienced trained staff is a major hurdle in wide application of the technique despite its demonstrable benefits, even with the simplest approaches. Other factors that need consideration include quality control, algorithms that define the decisions whether to change a plan or continue with original plan, and need for commercial development of software as well as hardware to match clinical needs and demands. Another major concern regarding frequent on-treatment imaging is the radiation dose to normal tissues. Although the doses from IGRT appear insignificant, only long-term follow-up will define any potential risk of second malignancies from low dose exposure. Thus, there is an ongoing debate on the necessary frequency of verification imaging especially when using ionizing radiation. Recent developments in MR-LINACs have tried to address these concerns while allowing daily imaging for treatment verification. Another concern is that of treatment safety since the technologies available in the clinic require integration of hardware and software from different vendors. Clinical use of any system should be preceded by proper acceptance testing, commissioning, and routine QA used to assure accurate regular functionality. Education of all users (oncologists, physicists, technologists) on safe use and clinical utility is mandatory, along with knowledge of additional dose and possible risks associated with use. No single technology is ideal in every scenario and no single institution can manage to integrate all or most technologies in one place, hence it remains to be seen which of these methods gain wider popularity and acceptance.

CLINICAL APPLICATIONS: CURRENT AND FUTURE

Use of IGRT systems is essential to treatment of any site where setup deviations and organ motion are anticipated. Additional gains are monitoring of treatment response, weight changes and organ filling on day-to-day basis. With improved precision of planning systems, use of stereotactic radiosurgery or radiotherapy and high-dose hypofractionated regimens, the chances of small deviations leading to significant errors in treatment delivery are much higher, and the use of IGRT is far more critical in these situations. Integration of LINACs with MR-based soft tissue imaging and PET-based biological imaging may help even further improve targeting accuracy in the future.[42,43] However, use of such technology and its integration into routine use would mandate that proper QA and training be put in place before undertaking such procedures.

REFERENCES

1. Dawson LA, Jaffray DA. Advances in image-guided radiation therapy. J Clin Oncol. 2007;25:938-46.
2. Beavis AW. Image-guided radiation therapy: what is our Utopia? Br J Radiol. 2010;83:191-3.
3. Jaffray DA. Image-guided radiation therapy: from concept to practice. Semin Radiat Oncol. 2007;17:243-4.
4. Wu QJ, Li T, Wu Q, et al. Adaptive radiation therapy: technical components and clinical applications. Cancer J. 2011;17:182-9.
5. van Herk M. Errors and margins in radiotherapy. Semin Radiat Oncol. 2004;14:52-64.
6. Rasch C, Steenbakkers R, van Herk M. Target definition in prostate, head, and neck. Semin Radiat Oncol. 2005;15:136-45.
7. Stroom JC, Heijmen BJ. Geometrical uncertainties, radiotherapy planning margins, and the ICRU-62 report. Radiother Oncol. 2002;64:75-83.
8. van Herk M, Remeijer P, Rasch C, et al. The probability of correct target dosage: dose-population histograms for deriving treatment margins in radiotherapy. Int J Radiat Oncol Biol Phys. 2000;47:1121-35.
9. Stroom JC, de Boer HC, Huizenga H, et al. Inclusion of geometrical uncertainties in radiotherapy treatment planning by means of coverage probability. Int J Radiat Oncol Biol Phys. 1999;43:905-19.
10. Bel A, van Herk M, Bartelink H, et al. A verification procedure to improve patient set-up accuracy using portal images. Radiother Oncol. 1993;29(2):253-60.
11. de Boer HC, van Os MJ, Jansen PP, et al. Application of the No Action Level (NAL) protocol to correct for prostate motion based on electronic portal imaging of implanted markers. Int J Radiat Oncol Biol Phys. 2005;61(4):969-83.
12. Kataria T, Abhishek A, Chadha P, et al. Set-up uncertainties: online correction with X-ray volume imaging. J Cancer Res Ther. 2011;7(1):40-6.
13. Kataria T, Gupta D, Karrthick KP, Bisht SS, Goyal S, Abhishek A, et al. Frame-based radiosurgery: is it relevant in the era of IGRT? Neurol India. 2013;61(3):277-81.
14. Balter JM, Cao Y. Advanced technologies in image-guided radiation therapy. Semin Radiat Oncol. 2007;17:293-7.
15. De Los Santos J, Popple R, Agazaryan N, et al. Image guided radiation therapy (IGRT) technologies for radiation therapy localization and delivery. Int J Radiat Oncol Biol Phys. 2013;87:33-45.
16. Fuss M, Salter BJ, Cavanaugh SX, Fuss C, Sadeghi A, Fuller CD, et al. Daily ultrasound-based image-guided targeting for radiotherapy of upper abdominal malignancies. Int J Radiat Oncol Biol Phys. 2004;59:1245-56.
17. Bert C, Metheany KG, Doppke KP, Taghian AG, Powell SN, Chen GT. Clinical experience with a 3D surface patient setup system for alignment of partial-breast irradiation patients. Int J Radiat Oncol Biol Phys. 2006;64:1265-74.
18. Brahme A, Nyman P, Skatt B. 4D laser camera for accurate patient positioning, collision avoidance, image fusion and adaptive approaches during diagnostic and therapeutic procedures. Med Phys. 2008;35:1670-81.
19. Litzenberg DW, Willoughby TR, Balter JM, Sandler HM, Wei J, Kupelian PA, et al. Positional stability of electromagnetic transponders used for prostate localization and continuous, real-time tracking. Int J Radiat Oncol Biol Phys. 2007;68:1199-206.
20. Willoughby TR, Kupelian PA, Pouliot J, Shinohara K, Aubin M, Roach M 3rd, et al. Target localization and real-time tracking using the Calypso 4D localization system in patients with localized prostate cancer. Int J Radiat Oncol Biol Phys. 2006;65:528-34.
21. Dempsey J, Dionne B, Fitzsimmons J, Haghigat A, Li J, Low D, et al. A real-time MRI guided external beam radiotherapy delivery system. Med Phys. 2006;33:2254.
22. Fallone BG, Murray B, Rathee S, Stanescu T, Steciw S, Vidakovic S, et al. First MR images obtained during megavoltage photon irradiation from a prototype integrated linac-MR system. Med Phys. 2009;36:2084-8.
23. Herman MG. Clinical use of electronic portal imaging. Semin Radiat Oncol. 2005;15:157-67.
24. Hurkmans CW, Remeijer P, Lebesque JV, et al. Set-up verification using portal imaging; review of current clinical practice. Radiother Oncol. 2001;58:105-20.
25. Walter C, Boda-Heggemann J, Wertz H, Loeb I, Rahn A, Lohr F, et al. Phantom and in-vivo measurements of dose exposure by image-guided radiotherapy (IGRT): MV portal images vs. kV portal images vs. cone-beam CT. Radiother Oncol. 2007;85:418-23.
26. Jaffray DA. Kilovoltage volumetric imaging in the treatment room. Front Radiat Ther Oncol. 2007;40:116-31.
27. McBain CA, Henry AM, Sykes J, Amer A, Marchant T, Moore CM, et al. X-ray volumetric imaging in image-guided radiotherapy: The new standard in on-treatment imaging. Int J Radiat Oncol Biol Phys. 2006;64:625-34.
28. Morin O, Gillis A, Chen J, Aubin M, Bucci MK, Roach M 3rd, et al. Megavoltage cone-beam CT: system description and clinical applications. Med Dosim. 2006;31:51-61.
29. Pouliot J, Bani-Hashemi A, Chen J, Svatos M, Ghelmansarai F, Mitschke M, et al. Low-dose megavoltage cone-beam CT for radiation therapy. Int J Radiat Oncol Biol Phys. 2005;61:552-60.
30. de Crevoisier R, Kuban D, Lefkopoulos D. Image-guided radiotherapy by in-room CT-linear accelerator combination. Cancer Radiother. 2006;10:245-51.
31. Ruchala KJ, Olivera GH, Schloesser EA, et al. Megavoltage CT on a tomotherapy system. Phys Med Biol. 1999;44:2597-621.
32. Adler JR Jr, Chang SD, Murphy MJ, Doty J, Geis P, Hancock SL. The Cyberknife: a frameless robotic system for radiosurgery. Stereotact Funct Neurosurg. 1997;69:124-28.

33. Antypas C, Pantelis E. Performance evaluation of a Cyberknife G4 image-guided robotic stereotactic radiosurgery system. Phys Med Biol. 2008;53:4697-718.
34. Shirato H, Shimizu S, Kitamura K, Nishioka T, Kagei K, Hashimoto S, et al. Four-dimensional treatment planning and fluoroscopic real-time tumor tracking radiotherapy for moving tumor. Int J Radiat Oncol Biol Phys. 2000;48:435-42.
35. Shirato H, Shimizu S, Kunieda T, Kitamura K, van Herk M, Kagei K, et al. Physical aspects of a real-time tumor-tracking system for gated radiotherapy. Int J Radiat Oncol Biol Phys. 2000;48:1187-95.
36. Kamino Y, Takayama K, Kokubo M, Narita Y, Hirai E, Kawawda N, et al. Development of a four-dimensional image-guided radiotherapy system with a gimbaled X-ray head. Int J Radiat Oncol Biol Phys. 2006;66:271-8.
37. Chang Z, Wang Z, Wu QJ, Yan H, Bowsher J, Zhang J, et al. Dosimetric characteristics of Novalis Tx system with high definition multileaf collimator. Med Phys. 2008;35:4460-3.
38. Jin JY, Yin FF, Tenn SE, et al. Use of the BrainLAB ExacTrac X-ray 6D system in image-guided radiotherapy. Med Dosim. 2008;33:124-34.
39. Potters L, Gaspar LE, Kavanagh B, Galvin JM, Hartford AC, Hevezi JM, et al. American Society for Therapeutic Radiology and Oncology; American College of Radiology. American Society for Therapeutic Radiology and Oncology (ASTRO) and American College of Radiology (ACR) practice guidelines for image-guided radiation therapy (IGRT). Int J Radiat Oncol Biol Phys. 2010;76:319-25.
40. Korreman S, Rasch C, McNair H, Verellen D, Oelfke U, Maingon P, et al. The European Society of Therapeutic Radiology and Oncology-European Institute of Radiotherapy (ESTRO-EIR) report on 3D CT-based in-room image guidance systems: a practical and technical review and guide. Radiother Oncol. 2010;94:129-44.
41. White E, Kane G. Radiation medicine practice in the image-guided radiation therapy era: new roles and new opportunities. Semin Radiat Oncol. 2007;17:298-305.
42. Rusten E, Rødal J, Bruland Ø, Malinen E. Biologic targets identified from dynamic 18FDG-PET and implications for image-guided therapy. Acta Oncol. 2013;52:1378-83.
43. Geets X. 4D PET-CT guided radiation therapy. JBR-BTR. 2013;96:155-9.

6

CHAPTER

Lasers in Head and Neck Surgery

Kumud Kumar Handa, Dilip Kumar Samal

INTRODUCTION

The first working light amplification by stimulated emission of radiation (laser) was a ruby laser made by Theodore Harold. "Ted" Maiman at Hughes Research Laboratories on May 16, 1960. By stimulating ruby crystals he developed laser which was a red laser light in the visible spectrum.[1] Further, advancement came after invention of carbon dioxide (CO_2) laser by Patel with the principle that at 10,600 nm wave length CO_2 absorbs water well.

In 1967, Jako pioneered the use of laser in microlaryngeal surgery by demonstration on a cadaver larynx.[2] Strong and Jako presented a 12 patient series of CO_2 laser microsurgery coupling CO_2 laser with microscope in treating laryngeal pathologies in 1972 (Fig. 1).[3]

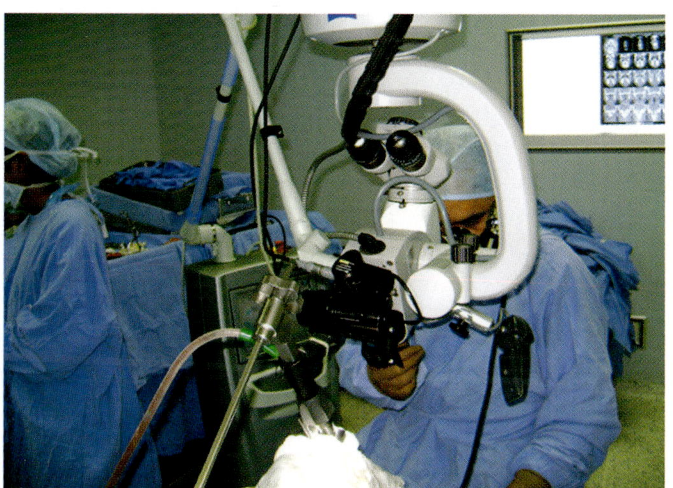

Fig. 1 CO_2 laser, coupling of the microscope with micromanipulator for transoral microlaryngeal surgery

Courtesy: Dr KK Handa, Director and Head, Department of ENT and Head Neck Surgery, Medanta—The Medicity, Haryana, India

Table 1 Type of lasers in ENT and, head and neck

Type of lasers	*Rod/fiber*	*Wavelength*
CO_2	Rod	10,632 nm
Nd-YAG	Fiber	1,064 nm
KTP	Fiber	532 nm
Diode	Fiber	785–980 nm

Lasers constitute an important treatment option in the management of benign lesions, vascular lesions and malignancy in head and neck. Various laser options available for otolaryngology practice are shown in Table 1.

The lasers may be delivered through rod delivery system, articulated arms, fiber optic fibers and the latest one is equipped with robotic scanner and acublade. Currently, CO_2 laser with a rod delivery system is the most commonly and most widely used laser in otolaryngological practice. The type of surgical laser use depends upon its availability, the characteristic of laser beam, the specific tissue absorptive characteristics, target lesion/pathology and not the least, expertise of the concerned surgeon.

TYPES OF SURGICAL LASERS

Carbon Dioxide Laser

It is one of the most widely used lasers in otolaryngology practice since its first introduction by Strong and Jako in 1972.[2,3] CO_2 laser emits light at wave length of 10.6 microns that lies in the invisible infrared region of electromagnetic spectrum. A helium-neon/diode coaxial beam is used as aiming beam along with this laser for the visualization of the laser. For treatment of laryngeal and pharyngeal lesions, the standard CO_2 laser delivery system is mounted on a microscope with fine manipulator and the laser light is fired in a straight line. Recently the fiber version the new acupulse

CO_2 laser with flexible fiber optic delivery system (CO_2 fiber laser flexible wave guide, Lumenis, CA) has become available and is a safe and reliable tool for transoral laser surgery. It can be delivered through flexible bronchoscope.[4]

The principle of laser surgery is that the emitted light is converted into thermal energy within the tissue and causes vaporization of water content. It delivers maximal energy at the center of the focus and fades toward the periphery causing a predictable deep tissue injury. Initially, CO_2 laser was delivered at continuous mode with more collateral thermal damage. To minimize the adverse effects, a pulse delivery mode was developed and in advanced super pulse mode, a high energy is delivered with each peak with a pause to dissipate the thermal energy.

Carbon Dioxide Laser, Neodynium

ND-YAG laser, potassium titanyl phosphate (KTP) laser and diode lasers are most commonly used lasers in head and neck. Broadly they are classified into photoangiolytic [e.g. KTP and pulsed dye laser (PDL), which selectively targets hemoglobin] and ablating or cutting lasers (CO_2, thulium laser). Lasers can be delivered through rod delivery system, with micromanipulators or through flexible fiber optic system and a few newer ones have both the rod delivery and fiber optic delivery system incorporated in one machine. The latest generation CO_2 lasers are incorporated with robotic scanner and AcuBlade. The cutting beam can be manipulated to a desired shape of a spot, straight knife, a curvilinear shape or a ring.

KTP and Argon Lasers

KTP and argon lasers have similar properties. They emit light in the visible spectrum of electromagnetic radiation. They can be delivered through flexible fiber as well as with micromanipulators and are preferably absorbed by hemoglobin and pigmented lesions.

Argon laser is used in photocoagulation of pigmented lesions like port-wine stains and superficial telangiectasias. The localized thermal reaction causes extensive damage to epithelium, subepithelium, postoperative edema and scarring; thus, its use should be avoided in the tracheobronchial tree and esophagus.[5] During stapedotomy it is focused by a small focal spot to increase the power delivery with a blood drop kept over the foot plate to reduce scattering of ray and to potentiate light absorption.

KTP laser is more strongly absorbed by hemoglobin than argon. It may be used for tonsillectomy, excision of pigmented lesions, benign laryngeal lesions like respiratory papillomatosis, ectasias, dysplasia, keratosis and early glottic cancer.[6] As an office-based procedure, it can be used for treatment of laryngeal papillomatosis and dysplasia.[7] In the treatment of Reinke's edema, it has an advantage of histologic preservation of vocal fold along with preservation of mucosal waves.[8] The recently developed pulsed mode use of KTP laser has an advantage of thermal relaxation over the continuous mode and thus reduces the collateral tissue damage.

Neodynium YAG Laser

This laser emits light at wave length of 1.064 micron near the infrared range of electromagnetic radiation. It penetrates into the tissues deeply with an increased absorption by the pigmented lesions. It can be delivered through flexible quartz fibers and hence can be used with both rigid as well as fiber optic bronchoscopes. It is primarily used for ablation of tracheobronchial lesions, subglottic hemangiomas, palliation of obstructive esophageal lesions and photocoagulation of lymphatic and vascular malformations endoscopically, although multiple sitting may be needed in some cases.[9,10] The disadvantage is an unpredictable depth of tissue penetration.

In endoscopic laser treatment of glottic laryngeal carcinoma, it can cause complications like postoperative bleeding, infection, dyspnea, aspiration pneumonia, fistula formation and cord fixation compared to CO_2 laser.[11]

LASER SAFETY

Laser safety protocol is an important and integral part of the laser surgery. There should be a training session for all the involved operation theater staff including the surgeon, the anesthetist and operating room nurses.

Laser use may cause combustion during use and the risk is higher with a collimated laser light like CO_2 laser, more so in continuous mode use; as there is less time for heat dissipation between the bursts. The surgeon should have an adequate knowledge regarding the physics of laser, its use, laser-tissue interaction and should have adequate expertise for the laser use and management of its complications. Accidental exposure may cause various complications ranging from minor eye and skin injury to devastating endotracheal tube burning and laser fire.[3]

- Eye care is a must. All operation theater staff should wear laser protective goggles—depending upon the wave length of laser used (Fig. 2). Patient's eye and face should be covered with goggles and/or saline-moistened eye pads.
- The operation theater should be closed during the procedure with a warning sign at the entrance (Fig. 3).

Endotracheal tube should be cuffed, with non-polyvinyl chloride (PVC) or with noncombustible material (called laser tubes) which separates the anesthetic gases from reaching the surgical field. The endotracheal tube cuff should be protected and avoided from laser fire. Laser protective endotracheal tubes as per the respective wave length of laser should be used. The cuff should be filled up with saline or methylene blue, so that cuff rupture can be diagnosed immediately (Fig. 4).

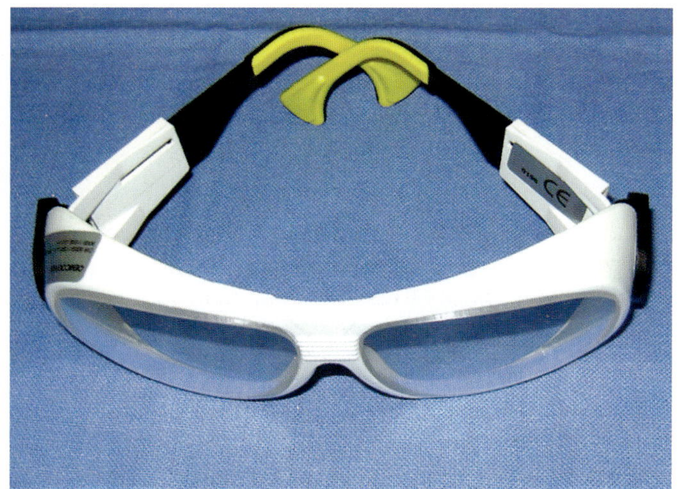

Fig. 2 Eye protection during laser surgery

Courtesy: Dr KK Handa, Director and Head, Department of ENT and Head Neck Surgery, Medanta—The Medicity, Haryana, India

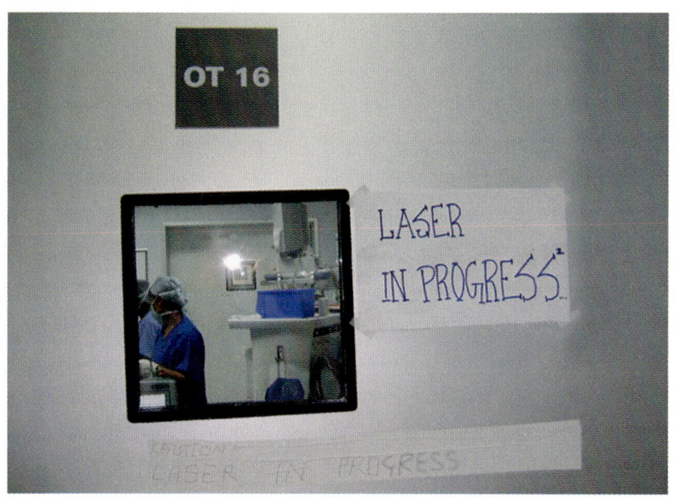

Fig. 3 OT signage during laser surgery

Courtesy: Dr KK Handa, Director and Head, Department of ENT and Head Neck Surgery, Medanta—The Medicity, Haryana, India

- The anesthesia may be a total intravenous anesthesia with air/oxygen mixture with fraction of inspired oxygen (FiO_2) less than 30. Inflammable gases like nitrous oxide should be avoided to decrease the FiO_2.
- Saline soaked neurocottons should be placed in the subglottic area and the surgeon should change it in intervals to avoid laser contact with the subglottic tissue. The surgical field should be free of any dry neurocottons and charred tissue.
- Charred tissue must be cleaned periodically from the field of laser fire and the smoke should be evacuated continuously with scope fitted suction. Endotracheal tube should be protected from any direct or indirect laser beam fire.

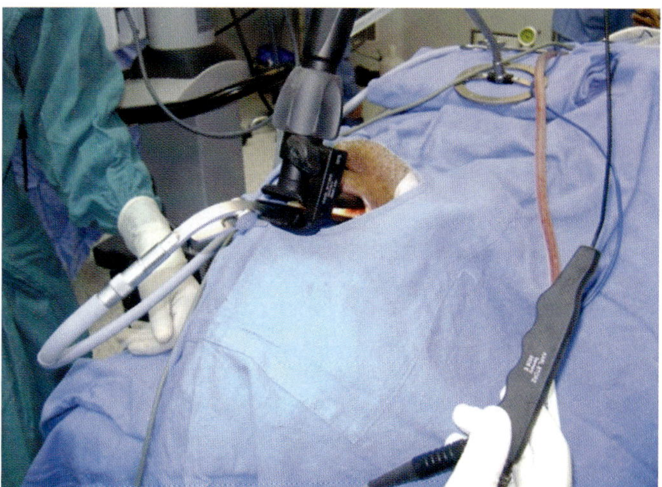

Fig. 4 Use of Steiner expandable laryngoscope for exposure of larynx

Courtesy: Dr KK Handa, Director and Head, Department of ENT and Head Neck Surgery, Medanta—The Medicity, Haryana, India

- Laser fire is a devastating complication of laser use with mortality risk. If happens, extubation should be done immediately with removal of all burning material and patient should be reintubated and ventilated with high oxygen flow. Then patient should be shifted to intensive care unit for proper management with ventilator support, if required and intravenous antibiotics. Patient has to be watched very carefully in the postoperative period, especially for complications like chest infection or septicemia.

LARYNGEAL MALIGNANCIES

Early Laryngeal Cancer

Transoral laser surgery for early laryngeal cancer is an accepted modality today and as an alternative to radiation therapy. The benefits are a short treatment duration, lower costs, oncological control similar to radiotherapy (RT) and possibility of successive treatments. Types of laser cordectomies classified as per European laryngological society classification[12] are as follows:

- Type 1 Subepithelial
- Type 2 Sub-ligamental
- Type 3 Transmuscular
- Type 4 Total cordectomy
- Type 5 Extended cordectomy
  - Involvement of contralateral cord
  - Involvement of arytenoid
  - Involvement of ventricle and false cord
  - Involvement of subglottis

The oncological controls are considered to be equal with both modalities. The voice results with Type 1 to Type 3 laser cordectomies are equal as compared with RT. However for Type 4 and Type 5 cordectomies the initial voice outcomes are inferior to RT, however with voice therapy or augmentation with fat or other materials comparable voice results are obtained with time. In the series of G Peretti et al.[13] no statistical difference in voice was noted after Type 1 and Type 2 cordectomies as compared to normal subjects.

In lesions which mandate Type 3–5 cordectomies initial dysphonia arises because of loss of muscle mass and formation of anterior synechiae. In patients with Type 3 cordectomy immediate or staged injection laryngoplasty using autologous fat is done in our center to optimize voice results. In case of Type 4 or Type 5 cordectomy staged medialization thyroplasty or anterior commissure laryngoplasty may be done after 1 year of primary resection. These patients are also given intensive voice therapy to cause compensation by the other true vocal cord and also the false cords.

At our center we use uses the frozen section intraoperatively to check the margins for all cases (Figs 5A and B).

Elisabeth V Sjögren et al.[14] carried out a study to compare voice quality after RT or endoscopic laser surgery in patients with similar T1a midcord glottic carcinomas according to a validated multidimensional protocol. Approximately half of the patients had mild to moderate voice dysfunction in the perceptual analysis [53% (8 of 15)] in the RT group and [61% (11 of 18)] in the laser surgery group and on the voice handicap index [44% (7 of 16)] in the RT group and [56% (10 of 18)] in the laser surgery group. The voice profile in the laser surgery group was mainly breathy; in the RT group, it was equally breathy and rough, with a trend for more jitter in the acoustic analysis. There was no statistical difference in the severity of voice dysfunction between the groups for any of the variables.

In another study the authors[15] concluded that both oncologic outcomes and self-rated voice-related quality of life are similar in patients treated with RT and transoral laser microsurgery (TLM) for early glottic carcinoma.

Peretti et al.[13] did a cost analysis comparison of voice results and the curative results between external beam radiation and laser surgery for early cancer larynx. The study concluded that cure rates are equal, voice results are comparable and the total cost of external RT significantly higher as compared to the laser surgery for early cancer larynx. Perreti et al.[13,16] also confirmed good surgical outcomes for T1, Tis and selected T2 and T3 glottic tumors with laser. They also achieved high rates (65%) of rescue endoscopic retreatment in cases of early detected local failure, achieving an ultimate local control with laser alone of 93.4%, 95%, 85.6% and 71.6% for Tis T1, T2, and T-3 respectively. Another study[16,17] from the same center concluded that selected recurrences after primary RT for T1 and T2 glottic carcinoma are eligible for endoscopic salvage surgery with oncologic results comparable to those with open neck procedures but with a lower complication rate and a favorable functional outcome.

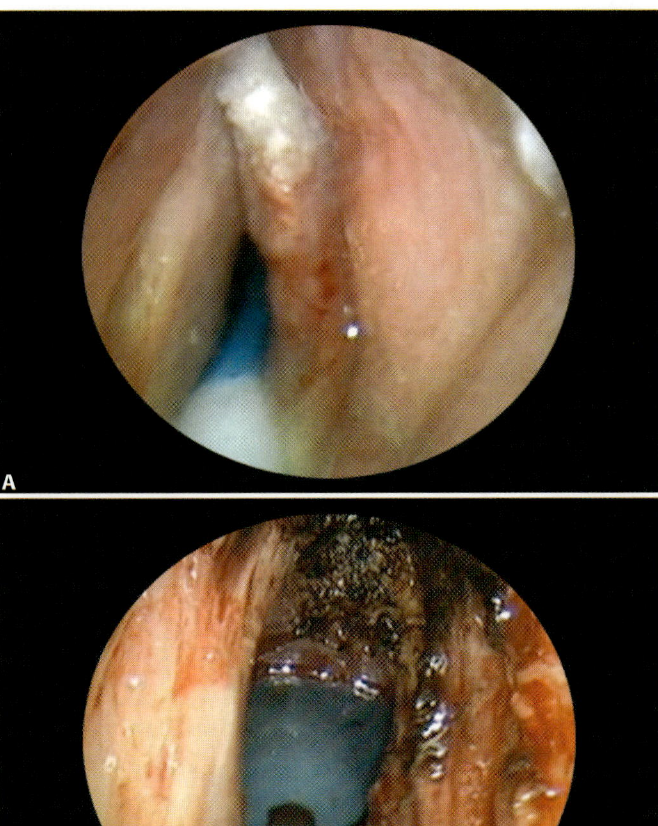

Figs 5A and B Laser excision of early cancer larynx confined to one cord

Courtesy: Dr KK Handa, Director and Head, Department of ENT and, Head Neck Surgery, Medanta—The Medicity, Haryana, India

Early Supraglottic Cancer

A detailed preoperative work up using CT, MRI and office endoscopies including rigid and flexible fiber optic is essential to accurately stage the tumor and also plan the extent of primary resection and how to address the neck. The role of CT/MRI is more important in cord tumors to know the exact deep extension of the tumor including the base of tongue, involvement of cartilages and involvement of pre-epiglottic and paraglottic space. The intraoperative findings need to be carefully recorded. The neck nodes need to be addressed on merit. At times a piecemeal resection may be done and is acceptable and, does not have significant effect on tumor control.[18] The surgical procedures carried out for early supraglottic cancer include:

- Ventriculectomy
- Suprahyoid and infrahyoid epiglottectomy

- Vertical hemi-epiglottectomy with false cord and aryepiglottic resection
- Complete supraglottic laryngectomy.

Endoscopic supraglottic resections are technically more demanding than vocal cord resections and need use of expandable bigger lumen scopes, e.g., Steiner scope. An attempt should be made to give a unimodal treatment by laser resection and keep RT in reserve for recurrent disease. Ambrosch et al. reported control of 100% for T1 and 89% for T2 supraglottic cancer with endoscopic laser resections[19] which compares equally with open procedures.

Oral Cavity and Oropharyngeal Cancer

The main advantage of laser application is to perform a transoral resection with precise margins, minimal tissue manipulation, less scarring and very little postoperative edema or pain. The major determining factor for the excision of a particular lesion by laser is whether all the margins can be visualized and excised with a safety margin of about 1 cm. Erythroplakia and leukoplakia both pre-malignant lesions and along with keratosis, carcinoma in situ and superficial malignant lesions without neck nodes are most amenable to laser resection.

The subsites of oral cavity and oropharynx that are easily accessible areas in certain select situations (depending on the site and the extent of tumor) can be very aptly handled with laser. Laser provides a good cutting tool which is precise and the healing is with very little functional deficit without scarring.[20]

Tongue

Early lesions of the anterior tongue T1 and T2 are very amenable to primary laser resection provided, one leaves about 1.5 cm of disease free margin. Preoperative radiological assessment by contrast MRI is of help in assessing the depth of involvement. Smaller lesions can be left for secondary intention healing without any reconstruction.

Buccal Mucosa

Superficial early lesions of buccal mucosa are very easily excised by laser. The parotid duct needs to be protected and may have to be marsupialized. A large defect may need an inner lining of skin or flap.

Floor of Mouth

Superficial lesions of the floor of the mouth are aptly dealt by the laser surgery. However the submandibular duct and sublingual glands need to be identified and protected in this area.

Base of Tongue

A mandibulotomy may be required to access the base of tongue area. Special scopes, e.g., Steiner may have to be used when transoral exposure is being done.

Palate

Early, superficial lesions on the soft palate can be excised by laser. In certain inaccessible areas fiber laser can be helpful. However the depth of the lesion needs to be assessed with a preoperative MRI.

Tracheal Lesions

Tracheal tumors, especially benign ones viz., neurogenic tumors, papillomas, amyloidosis and lipomas can be dealt with a fiber optic laser without the need for open procedures or tracheostomy. However, the treatment of choice for malignant tracheal tumors is tracheal resection and end to end anastomosis.

BENIGN LARYNGEAL LESIONS

Benign Vocal Cord Lesions

Epithelial lesions like vocal cord polyp and vocal nodule need a precise surgery of the free edge of vocal cord to maintain the integrity of vocal cord functions after failed conservative measures, with either cold instruments or CO_2 laser. In 2000, Benninger et al. demonstrated no significant difference of surgical time, recovery time and surgical outcomes based on acoustic and aerodynamic measurements between microdissection method and microspot CO_2 laser excision of benign vocal cord lesions like nodules, polyps and mucous retention cysts. This study however showed significant improvements in perceptual audio recordings in CO_2 laser treated groups compared to cold instruments in treating benign vocal fold lesions in a blinded randomized control study.[21] After surgical treatment patients are advised for voice rest and vocal hygiene maintenance should be explained followed by speech therapy a week later.

Reinke's Edema

Reinke's edema is defined as subepithelial accumulation of exudative fluid and pseudomyxomatous tissue in whole length of vocal cord at its superficial lamina propria or Reinke's space with dysphonia. It can be treated effectively by combined use of CO_2 laser and cold instruments with removal of redundant mucosa of the vocal fold to reduce the risk of recurrence.[22] Reinke's edema can also be treated with 532 nm pulsed KTP laser.[23]

Recurrent Respiratory Papillomatosis

This is the most common benign tumor encountered in the endolarynx, caused by human papilloma virus type 6 and 11 mainly. There are two types of presentations: One is juvenile aggressive form, seen in pediatric age group with multiple polyps at presentation and the second one less common adult form, less aggressive one. The available treatment options are mainly surgical (e.g., cold instruments/ microdebrider-assisted laser) with adjuvant medical management to decrease the recurrence rate. CO_2 lasers are being increasingly used nowadays for papillomatosis. Our center uses microdebrider to perform an initial debulking of the papillomas followed by CO_2 laser for fine work close to the vocal cords.[24] Also office-based 585-nm pulsed dye laser has been described in literature as a safe and effective surgical treatment option. Proper precautions with continuous suction of plumes should be done during laser surgery to avoid any contamination, although contamination is possible during cold instrument surgery.

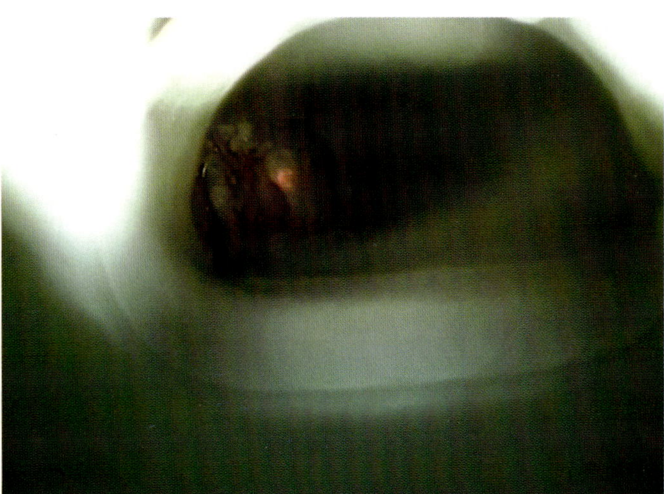

Fig. 6 Keratosis of vocal cords, CO_2 laser being used in an ablative mode

Courtesy: Dr KK Handa, Director and Head, Department of ENT and Head Neck Surgery, Medanta—The Medicity, Haryana, India

Laryngotracheal Stenosis

Laser can be used in treatment of limited laryngotracheal stenosis, glottis and supraglottic webs with the application of CO_2 laser, Nd-YAG laser and KTP lasers. CO_2 laser application has advantages of surgeon's familiarity of use and precise cutting property with disadvantage of difficulty in delivery, that has been overcome by fiber optic delivery system in recent times. Monnier P et al. have described CO_2 laser to be the first choice of treatment in a select group of patients with laryngeal stenosis and found it to be less invasive, less risky and with shorter hospital stay, although less favorable outcome compared to open surgery for laryngotracheal stenosis were reported.[25] Although Nd-YAG laser with a flexible fiber delivery system has facilitated its use through bronchoscopes, the surrounding thermal damage is more as compared to CO_2 laser. We do not recommend laser in treatment of long segment stenosis, stenosis involving cricoid cartilage and extensive posterior glottic stenosis.

Bilateral Abductor Cord Palsy

It is a life-threatening condition requiring urgent intervention to maintain the airway and may sometimes need tracheostomy. Endoscopic CO_2 laser surgery is the treatment of choice at present. Dennis and Kashima had first described posterior transverse laser cordotomy as a treatment modality to maintain the posterior glottic airway with satisfactory outcome.[26] It is a safe, minimally invasive, effective technique with short operation time and rarely requires bilateral cordotomy or revision surgery.[27] Endoscopic laser medial arytenoidectomy, combined laser total arytenoidectomy with posterior cordectomy are other effective procedures for this entity. Endoscopic posterior cordotomy with microdissection radiofrequency electrodes can be used as an alternative to laser also.[28]

Hemangioma and Vascular Lesions

Lasers can be used for the management of other benign laryngeal lesions like laryngomalacia, vocal cord cysts, sulcus vocalis, laryngeal cleft, vocal cord keratosis (Fig. 6) and other premalignant lesions.

OFFICE-BASED USE OF LASERS

Unsedated office-based laryngeal surgeries (UOLS) of larynx and trachea are gaining popularity nowadays. The commonly used lasers in this practice are pulsed dye laser, CO_2 laser, thulium: yttrium-aluminum-garnet laser and KTP lasers delivered by flexible nasopharyngoscopes with a working channel. Adequate laryngeal anesthesia is of utmost importance after selecting the patient and specific laser. Kaufman et al. in 2007 had demonstrated UOLS to be a safe and an effective treatment modality with an experience of 443 cases, with 406 cases performed with pulsed dye laser, 10 cases with CO_2 laser and 27 cases with thulium: YAG laser for recurrent respiratory papillomatosis, granulomas, leukoplakia, and polypoidal degenerations without any significant complications.[29]

RECENT ADVANCES

The prior difficulty of CO_2 laser rod-based delivery has been overcome by flexible fiber optic delivery system,

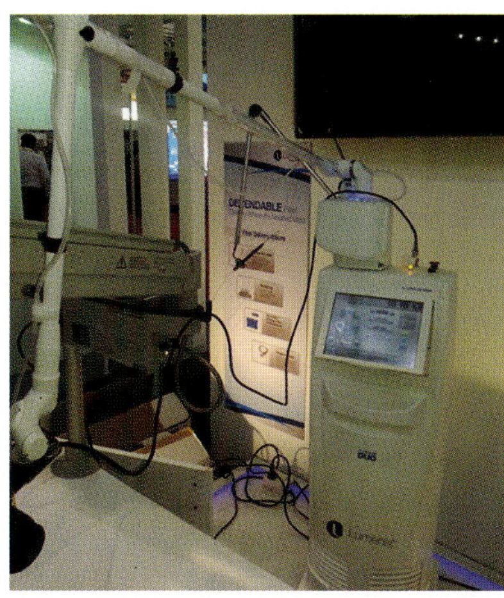

Fig. 7 Combo CO_2 laser machine with both rod delivery and the laser fiber

Courtesy: Dr KK Handa, Director and Head, Department of ENT and Head Neck Surgery, Medanta—The Medicity, Haryana, India

which has enabled the use of this laser through the rigid or flexible bronchoscope also. The advanced micropoint micromanipulator (acuspot) and super pulse laser fire delivery system add to advantage of better precision, regulated power and low surrounding thermal damage. The use of unsedated office-based laser in advanced centers as outpatient procedure is a safe and effective treatment option. The latest has been the introduction of combo CO_2 laser machine which has combined rod delivery system and the fiber in one machine (Fig. 7).

CONCLUSION

Transoral laser surgery offers a very good option for early glottic, supraglottic laryngeal cancers, tracheal lesions, oral and oropharyngeal lesions and certain benign lesions. Proper patient selection is a must and one must take help of radiological investigations including CT and MRI and above all endoscopic assessment wherever required. Proper mouth opening is an essential criterion for transoral laser endoscopic laser treatment of laryngeal pathology. Safety issues and proper training of the personnel are of paramount importance. Advanced understanding of laser tissue interaction and mode of delivery has made it an emerging technique for head and neck cancer surgeries.

REFERENCES

1. Maiman TH. Stimulated optical radiation in ruby. Nature. 1960;187:493
2. Jako GJ. Laser surgery of the vocal cords. An experimental study with carbon dioxide lasers on dogs. Laryngoscope. 1972;82(12):2204-16.
3. Strong MS, Jako GJ. Laser surgery in the larynx. Early clinical experience with continuous CO 2 laser. Ann Otol Rhinol Laryngol. 1972;81(6):791-8.
4. Remacle M, Ricci-Maccarini A, Matar N, Lawson G, Pieri F, Bachy V, et al. Reliability and efficacy of a new CO2 laser hollow fiber: a prospective study of 39 patients. Eur Arch Otorhinolaryngol. 2012;269(3):917-21.
5. Gillis TM, Strong MS, Shapshay SM, Incze J, Simpson G. Argon laser and soft tissue interaction. Otolaryngol Head Neck Surg. 1984;92(1):7-12.
6. Xie X, Young J, Kost K, McGregor M. KTP 532 nm laser for laryngeal lesions. A systematic review. J Voice. 2013;27(2):245-9.
7. Zeitels SM, Burns JA. Office-based laryngeal laser surgery with the 532-nm pulsed-potassium-titanyl-phosphate laser. Curr Opin Otolaryngol Head Neck Surg. 2007;15(6):394-400.
8. Pitman MJ, Lebowitz-Cooper A, Iacob C, Tan M. Effect of the 532nm pulsed KTP laser in the treatment of Reinke's edema. Laryngoscope. 2012;122(12):2786-92.
9. Fu CH, Lee LA, Fang TJ, Wong KS, Li HY. Endoscopic Nd:YAG laser therapy of infantile subglottic hemangioma. Pediatr Pulmonol. 2007;42(1):89-92.
10. Glade R, Vinson K, Richter G, Suen JY, Buckmiller LM. Endoscopic management of airway venous malformations with Nd:YAG laser. Ann Otol Rhinol Laryngol. 2010;119(5):289-93.
11. Gao YJ, Xiao SF, Wang QG, Qin Y, Zhao EM, Shen H, et al. [A comparative study of complications in transoral CO2 and Nd:YAG laser surgery for glottic carcinoma]. Zhonghua Er Bi Yan Hou Tou Jing Wai Ke Za Zhi. 2011;46(8):658-63.
12. Remacle M, Eckel HE, Antonelli AR,Brasnu D, Chevallier D, Friedrich G, et al. Endoscopic cordectomy, a proposal for a classification by the Working Committee, European Laryngological Society. Eur Arch Otorhinolaryngol. 2000;257(4):227-31.
13. Peretti G, Piazza C , Balzanelli C , Cantarella G , Nicolai P. Vocal outcome after endoscopic cordectomies for Tis and T1 glottic carcinoma. Ann Otol Rhinol Laryngol. 2003;112(2):174-9.
14. Sjögren EV, van Rossum MA, Langeveld TP, Voerman MS, van de Kamp VA, Friebel MO, et al. Voice outcome in T1a midcord glottic carcinoma: laser surgery vs radiotherapy. Arch Otolaryngol Head Neck Surg. 2008;134(9):965-72.
15. Osborn HA, Hu A, Venkatesan V, Nichols A, Franklin JH, Yoo JH, et al. Comparison of endoscopic laser resection versus radiation therapy for the treatment of early glottic carcinoma. J Otolaryngol Head Neck Surg. 2011;40(3):200-4.
16. Peretti G, Piazza C, Ansarin M, De Benedetto L, Cocco D, Cattaneo A, Nicolai P, Chiesa F. Transoral CO_2 laser microsurgery for Tis-T3 supraglottic squamous cell carcinomas. Eur Arch Otorhinolaryngol. 2010 Nov;267(11):1735-42. Epub 2010.
17. Puxeddu R1, Piazza C, Mensi MC, Ledda GP, Argiolas F, Peretti G. Carbon dioxide laser salvage surgery after radiotherapy failure in T1 and T2 glottic carcinoma. Otolaryngol Head Neck Surg. 2004;130(1):84-8.
18. Steiner W, Ambrosch P. Endoscopic laser surgery of the upper aerodigestive tract. With special emphasis on cancer surgery. Stuttgart: Thieme 2001.
19. Ambroch P, Kron M, Steiner W. Carbon dioxide laser microsurgery for early supraglottic carcinoma. Ann Otol Rhinol Laryngol. 1998;107(8):680-8.
20. Schuller DE. Use of laser in the oral cavity. Otolaryngol Clin North Am. 1990;23(1):31-42.

21. Benninger MS. Microdissection or microspot CO_2 laser for limited vocal fold benign lesions: a prospective randomized trial. Laryngoscope. 2000;110(2 Pt 2 Suppl 92):1-17.
22. Pitman MJ, Lebowitz-Cooper A, Iacob C, Tan M. Effect of the 532nm pulsed KTPlaser in the treatment of Reinke's edema. Laryngoscope. 2012;122(12):2786-92.
23. Avelino MA, Zaiden TC, Gomes RO. Surgical treatment and adjuvant therapies of recurrent respiratory papillomatosis. Braz J Otorhinolaryngol. 2013;79(5):636-42.
24. Monnier P, George M, Monod ML, Lang F. The role of the CO_2 laser in the management of laryngotracheal stenosis: a survey of 100 cases. Eur Arch Otorhinolaryngol. 2005;262(8):602-8.
25. Dursun G, Gökcan MK. Aerodynamic, acoustic and functional results of posterior transverse laser cordotomy for bilateral abductor vocal fold paralysis. J Laryngol Otol. 2006;120(4):282-8.
26. Özdemir S, Tuncer Ü, Tarkan Ö, Kara K, Sürmelioglu Ö. Carbon dioxide laser endoscopic posterior cordotomy technique for bilateral abductor vocal cord paralysis: a 15-year experience. JAMA Otolaryngol Head Neck Surg. 2013;139(4):401-4.
27. Oysu C, Toros SZ, Tepe-Karaca Ç, Sahin S, Sahin-Yilmaz A. Endoscopic posterior cordotomy with microdissection radiofrequency electrodes for bilateral vocal cord paralysis. Otolaryngol Head Neck Surg. 2014;150(1):103-6.
28. Oysu C, Toros SZ, Tepe-Karaca Ç, Sahin S, Sahin-Yilmaz A. Endoscopic posterior cordotomy with microdissection radiofrequency electrodes for bilateral vocal cord paralysis. Otolaryngol Head Neck Surg. 2014;150(1):103-6.
29. Koufman JA, Rees CJ, Frazier WD, Kilpatrick LA, Wright SC, Halum SL, et al. Office-based laryngeal laser surgery: a review of 443 cases using three wavelengths. Otolaryngol Head Neck Surg. 2007;137(1):146-51.

CHAPTER

Emergencies in Cancer

Sandeep Jain, Kuldeep Sharma

INTRODUCTION

Patients suffering from cancer may have many associated medical comorbidities such as diabetes, chronic obstructive pulmonary disease, heart disease, etc. Additionally, cancer itself as well as its treatment-related toxicities can lead to acute conditions requiring rapid intervention to avoid permanent damage or death; therefore, management of oncological emergencies is quiet challenging and requires a team effort from multiple specialties. Initial management requires a quick assessment according to main presenting symptoms, vital signs and general physical examination.

Oncological emergencies can be classified as:

- Structural or obstructive emergencies caused by a space-occupying tumor
- Emergencies due to metabolic or hormonal imbalance
- Emergencies secondary to complications arising from treatment.

Structural or obstructive emergencies: These may include following conditions:

- Spinal cord compression
- Superior vena cava (SVC) syndrome
- Acute airway obstruction
- Increased intracranial pressure
- Cardiac tamponade
- Urinary obstruction
- Massive hemoptysis.

STRUCTURAL OR OBSTRUCTIVE EMERGENCIES

Spinal Cord Compression

Spinal cord compression is one of the most important oncological emergencies and requires quick intervention because any undue delay in the treatment can lead to grave consequences like paraplegia. Approximately, 10% of the cancer patients may present with the features of spinal cord compression, often due to extradural metastasis to spine.[1] Patients usually present with backache, spinal tenderness and weakness. There may be sudden increase in intensity of pain that may not be relieved with common analgesics. Any cancer patient having persistent backache should be evaluated for cord compression. Early diagnosis is of utmost value and if the diagnosis of cord compression is made before any muscle weakness sets in and the patient is mobile, chances are that over 80% patients will remain mobile after the treatment. On the other hand, only 10% of the patients will be able to walk again if paralysis is present at the time of presentation. Urinary retention and constipation are manifestations of late stage of damage and possibly irreversible paraplegia. Patients with cord compression need a thorough neurological examination including assessment of sensory, motor, bowel and bladder functions. MRI of the spine is the best radiological investigation for assessment of cord compression. Treatment goals include pain relief as well as restoration of neurologic deficit.[2]

Initial treatment includes administration of corticosteroids with high dose methyl-prednisolone or dexamethasone.[3] Surgical decompression is considered if acute onset neurologic deficit is the presenting feature; if there is need for obtaining histopathological proof or in case of fractured vertebrae or tumor hemorrhage requiring urgent decompression and stabilization of spine.[4] In most cases, spinal cord compression due to metastases is managed with steroids and radiation therapy. Patients with cord compression and less than 24 hours of immobility require urgent attention. They should be started on corticosteroids immediately and radiation therapy should be started within 24 hours of the diagnosis if surgery is not considered. Common dose schedules include 20 Gy in 5 fractions or 30 Gy in 10 fractions.

For patients with established paraplegia for more than 24 hours, radiotherapy is usually given for pain relief (8 Gy in a single fraction) and chances of neurological recovery are rare. After surgery for spinal cord compression, postoperative radiation therapy is indicated and the dose recommended is 30 Gy in 10 fractions or 20 Gy in 5 fractions.[5] For patients with recurrent spinal cord compression, retreatment within the tolerance dose of spinal cord (biologically effective dose < 100 Gy) can be considered with maximal sparing of spinal cord by using conformal techniques like stereotactic body radiotherapy.[6]

Superior Vena Cava Syndrome

Superior vena cava (SVC) syndrome is caused by obstruction to the flow of blood from SVC to right atrium, resulting in reduced flow of blood from head and neck and upper extremities. Obstruction of SVC may be caused by extrinsic nodal or tumor compression, tumor infiltration, embolism, thrombus or fibrosis. Carcinoma of lung, lymphoma and metastatic carcinoma are responsible for more than 90% of all cases of SVC syndrome. Non-malignant causes of SVC syndrome are rare and include retrosternal goiter, tuberculosis, sarcoidosis, or SVC thrombosis due to long-term use of central venous catheter in cancer patients.[7] Usually, SVC syndrome develops over a period of time resulting in some mechanism to compensate. Often the collateral channels of azygos system open up for compensation. Most patients present with facial and periorbital puffiness, cough, dyspnea, and dilated veins over neck and chest. Patients may also have central nervous system symptoms like headache, dizziness or syncope. SVC syndrome is usually a clinical diagnosis. Thoracic CT scan with contrast is the most useful radiological investigation as it can show us the site of obstruction or extrinsic compression by tumor or nodes or any thrombus in SVC. Once the diagnosis of SVC syndrome is established, the patient should be started on corticosteroids, diuretics, head elevation and oxygen inhalation for symptomatic relief.[8] If the patient is stable, a biopsy should be considered as it is of utmost importance for management of primary disease. Once histopathological proof of malignancy is available, the patient can be started on specific treatment for underlying cancer. Chemotherapy is preferred modality for small-cell carcinoma or lymphoma, otherwise radiation therapy is the usual initial treatment. Radical or palliative radiation may be planned depending on extent of the disease. Nearly, 70–85% of patients report symptomatic improvement after 3–4 days of starting radiation therapy and most patients remain symptom-free for prolonged periods. If SVC obstruction is related to central venous catheter, catheter removal in combination with anticoagulant therapy should be started to prevent embolization.

Acute Airway Obstruction

Acute airway obstruction is sudden obstruction of airway above main stem bronchus and may be caused by malignant or non-malignant conditions. It can be caused by either intraluminal tumor growth or from extrinsic compression of the airway by tumor or nodes. Tumors that block the upper airway by direct extension are usually primary tumors of the head and neck or lung. Non-malignant causes of airway obstruction include food or foreign body aspiration, airway edema, hemorrhage, tracheal stenosis and infections. Dyspnea is the most common presentation in such condition. If diameter of airway is more than 8 mm, patients develop dyspnea on exertion. On the other hand, if diameter of airway is less than 5 mm then stridor may develop. Patient with airway obstruction should be started on steroids and oxygen as soon as possible. For upper airway obstruction, direct visualization by direct laryngoscopy or bronchoscopy can be performed. For lower airway obstruction, thoracic CT scan or X-ray may be useful. For obstruction proximal to larynx, urgent tracheotomy is lifesaving. For distal airway obstruction, bronchoscopy with clearing of airway by laser, photodynamic therapy or by stenting can provide immediate relief.[9] Brachytherapy or external beam radiotherapy along with steroids can be quite useful in opening up obstructed airways.

Increased Intracranial Pressure

The most common cause of raised intracranial pressure is metastatic disease to brain, resulting in surrounding edema or tumoral bleed. Nearly one-fourth of all cancer patients die of brain metastases. The common primary sites include lung and breast malignancies, and melanomas. Patients with raised intracranial pressure may present with headache, nausea, vomiting, seizures and behavioral changes, and sometimes with focal neurological deficits. A large mass with surrounding edema may lead to various herniation syndromes. All unstable patients with suspected raised intracranial pressure should undergo quick clinical assessment followed by an urgent CT scan of brain to make a diagnosis. MRI of brain, though more accurate may take prolonged time and may not be possible in emergency situations. However, it should be considered once the patient is stable. Treatment with corticosteroids and diuretics (mannitol) should be started immediately to prevent life-threatening herniation.[10] Hypertonic mannitol is effective within minutes of intravenous administration and steroids are helpful in reducing vasogenic edema. Once the patient is stable, treatment for brain metastasis is instituted and usually includes whole brain radiotherapy up to 30 Gy with or without simultaneous or sequential boost. Neurosurgery or stereotactic radiosurgery may be indicated in case of oligometastases with controlled extracranial disease.

Cardiac Tamponade

Cardiac or pericardial tamponade is caused by accumulation of pericardial fluid resulting in hemodynamic instability. Pericardial effusion can result from either excessive secretion or by obstruction of lymphatic drainage by tumor cells, or by non-malignant causes such as drugs, pericarditis, hypothyroidism, uremia, infection or autoimmune diseases. Rarely, radiation-induced acute inflammatory pericardial effusion may occur within months of receiving radiation and usually resolves spontaneously. On the other hand, chronic pericarditis accompanied by thick pericardium usually appears after many years of completion of radiation and requires surgical removal. Patients with pericardial tamponade present with breathlessness, chest pain, orthopnea and demonstrate signs of tachycardia, hypotension, jugular vein distension and edema indicating reduced cardiac output. 2D echocardiography is the most useful investigation in assessing pericardial effusion and its hemodynamic impact or the presence of tamponade. Pericardial tamponade requires pericardiocentesis with instillation of sclerosing agents like bleomycin or tetracycline. Creation of pericardial window or complete pericardial stripping may be required in some situations.[11]

Urinary Obstruction

Urinary obstruction can occur in patients having gynecological tumors such as carcinoma cervix, urological malignancies like carcinoma of prostate or metastatic disease to pelvis. Patients may present with oliguria or anuria and sometimes with alternating polyuria and progressive rise in serum creatinine levels. CT scan or ultrasound abdomen may help establish the diagnosis. CT scan is more useful as it can detect the exact location of obstruction. Urinary obstruction associated with pain, infection or renal failure requires urgent intervention. Ureteral stents may be placed under local anesthesia and may relieve the obstruction. If stenting is not possible, percutaneous nephrostomy can be done. Once obstruction is relieved, patient may develop polyuria resulting in dehydration and electrolyte imbalance, especially hypokalemia, requiring adequate rehydration and correction of fluid and electrolyte imbalance.

Massive Hemoptysis

Massive hemoptysis is expectoration with loss of blood ranging from one single episode of 100 mL or more than 600 mL of blood loss during 24–48 hours. Hemoptysis associated with breathlessness needs urgent attention. Bleeding into airways can lead to life-threatening airway obstruction, aspiration, anemia or hypovolemic shock.[12] Massive hemoptysis may be fatal in one-third of patients and the risk of death is directly associated with the amount of blood loss. Blood grouping, crossmatching, blood transfusion, management of shock, oxygen and other supportive care measures are usually needed. Urgent bronchoscopy may be performed in unstable patients to facilitate the introduction of balloon-tip catheters into the bleeding bronchus for tamponade of the hemorrhagic artery. It can also protect contralateral lung or nonbleeding bronchi from blood aspiration. In stable patients, thoracic CT scan should be ordered before any bronchoscopic exploration, and it can give useful information regarding site of tumor, lung or airway collapse, consolidation or airway obstruction. Bronchial artery embolization, if possible, is an excellent nonsurgical procedure to achieve hemostasis.[12] Patients should be assessed for hemostatic radiation therapy. For central lesions, a single fraction of intraluminal radiation while doing bronchoscopy can help control bleeding, while for peripheral parenchymal lesions, external beam radiotherapy can stop bleeding in most of the patients. The most common schedule being used in such condition is 20 Gy in 5 fractions. Finally, patients should be assessed for definitive treatment according to disease stage and extent.

METABOLIC EMERGENCIES

Hypercalcemia

Hypercalcemia is one of the most common emergencies related to paraneoplastic syndromes, leading to significant morbidity and mortality in cancer patients. It is most commonly associated with advanced solid cancers like lung, breast, head and neck and renal cancer. Hematological malignancies like malignant lymphoma and myeloma can also produce hypercalcemia.

The main cause of cancer-related hypercalcemia is bone metastases causing increased release of calcium from bone. Bone resorption is largely stimulated by the activation and proliferation of osteoclasts. Bone resorption may also be related to the production of several cytokines (tumor necrosis factor, lymphotoxin, endothelin, and interleukin 1 and 6) that may stimulate osteoclast activity by unknown mechanisms.[13] Hypercalcemia may also be caused by excessive production and release of parathyroid hormone-related protein by tumor cells, and this may be the most common cause of hypercalcemia in cancer patients in the absence of bone metastases, particularly in patients having squamous-cell carcinoma. Malignant lymphoma cells can produce vitamin D derivative (calcitriol), which can increase the gastrointestinal absorption of calcium, leading more frequently to hypercalciuria thereafter leading to frank hypercalcemia.

Initial symptoms of hypercalcemia include fatigue, malaise, anorexia, nausea, vomiting, confusion, bone pain, polydipsia, polyuria, constipation and weakness.[14] If serum calcium rises above 3.5 mmol/L, neurological symptoms are more prevalent and patients may have confusion, sleepiness, lethargy and coma, which may also lead to death.

Dehydration is commonly associated with hypercalcemia, and it may be due to concentration defects in renal tubules due to calcium deposits. Persistent vomiting and reduced fluid intake can worsen dehydration. Severe hypercalcemia is also a prognostic indicator and is quite often associated with a short survival from a few weeks to a few months only.

For management of hypercalcemia, we should always correlate serum calcium levels to serum albumin levels using the formula:

Corrected calcium (mmol/L) = Measured calcium (mmol/L) + [0.02 × (40 – measured albumin g/L)].[15]

Initial therapy of hypercalcemia includes intravenous fluids and a bisphosphonate. Dehydration should be corrected by infusing normal saline at 100–300 mL/h. After 6–12 h of intensive hydration, serum calcium levels may fall by 20–40%. However, in patients with severe hypercalcemia (>13 mg/dL) or patients presenting with neurological symptoms or renal failure secondary to high calcium levels, treatment with a bisphosphonate needs to be started together with vigorous hydration. Bisphosphonates, which are potent inhibitors of bone resorption, are very effective in rapidly lowering serum calcium levels with minimal toxic effects. Zoledronate (4 mg) by intravenous infusion lasting 15–20 minutes is quite effective in the treatment of severe, acute hypercalcemia.[16] Treatment with corticosteroids, gallium nitrate or calcitonin is needed when the serum calcium levels are more than 15 mg/dL. However, in patients with lymphoma, glucocorticoids may be more useful.

Syndrome of Inappropriate Secretion of the Antidiuretic Hormone

The syndrome of inappropriate secretion of the antidiuretic hormone (SIADH) is not uncommon in cancer patients. This should be considered whenever a cancer patient presents with persistent hyponatremia. This condition arises due to the production of arginine vasopressin by the tumor cells. In SIADH, hyponatremia is associated with plasma hyposmolarity and inappropriately high urinary osmolarity, which occurs due to higher sodium loss in the urine. Other findings include a high level of excretion of urinary sodium without plasma volume depletion. While making this diagnosis, other causes of hyponatremia, like renal failure, hypothyroidism or adrenal insufficiency, should be excluded. Certain drugs such as antidepressants, angiotensin-converting enzyme inhibitors and antineoplastic agents (cyclophosphamide, vincristine, melphalan, cisplatin, vinorelbine) may also cause SIADH.

The tumor most frequently associated with this syndrome is small-cell carcinoma of lung. Hyponatremia often confers a poor prognosis in patients with small-cell lung cancer. Although most patients with SIADH are asymptomatic, clinical manifestations are directly related to the severity of hyponatremia. Early symptoms may include anorexia, depression, irritability, lethargy, muscle cramps, weakness and behavioral changes. When plasma sodium levels fall below 110 mEq/L, patients may have neurological signs like depressed deep tendon reflexes, pseudobulbar palsy, seizures and coma. If SIADH is caused by a tumor, optimal therapy is related to the treatment of the underlying malignancy. In the case of small-cell lung cancer, chemotherapy should be started as soon as possible to control the situation. Hyponatremia can be corrected with water restriction and increased salt intake. Serum sodium level should always be raised in a controlled manner, the rate of correction should be kept 12 mEq/L in 24 hours and 18 mEq/L in 48 hours as rapid correction make the brain susceptible to osmotic demyelination.

Treatment of symptomatic hyponatremia in patients with SIADH or other euvolemic states or hypervolemia includes correction of sodium by administering hypertonic (3%) saline if serum sodium levels are below 114 mEq/L. Treatment with hypertonic saline should be discontinued once symptoms resolve, and a safe serum sodium concentration is achieved. Asymptomatic patients with euvolemic or hypervolemic hyponatremia are usually managed initially by attaining negative water balance by restricting fluid intake.[17] Fluid (but not sodium) should be restricted to approximately 500 mL below the average daily urine output. At the same time, any drug known to cause SIADH should be discontinued and replaced with another agent that does not cause hyponatremia. Tolvaptan acts by increasing the urinary water excretion by blocking the effects of endogenous arginine vasopressin on V2 receptors in the renal collecting duct. Thus, increasing free water clearance in urine, reducing urine osmolality and finally elevating sodium concentration in the serum. Tolvaptan therapy should be started and continued while patients are admitted, which allows monitoring of response in a controlled manner.[18] The starting dose is 15 mg once daily, which is first increased to 30 mg once daily and subsequently to 60 mg once daily. The dose increments are done at 24-hours intervals if desirable sodium is not achieved. Demeclocycline is another agent that needs to be considered in refractory cases.

TREATMENT-RELATED EMERGENCIES

Tumor Lysis Syndrome

Tumor lysis syndrome is caused by the destruction of a large number of actively proliferating tumor cells as a consequence of cancer chemotherapy or radiotherapy. Tumor lysis syndrome may manifest as a combination of several electrolyte disorders such as hyperuricemia, hyperkalemia, hyperphosphatemia, hypocalcemia and lactic acidosis, which can lead to acute renal failure. Therefore, assessment of any fluid and electrolyte disturbances and prompt correction is essential to avoid serious complications of this syndrome. Tumor lysis syndrome is often observed in patients with chemosensitive or radiosensitive tumors and may appear shortly after initiating treatment in acute leukemia, Burkitt's lymphoma and diffuse aggressive lymphomas. This syndrome is also seen in patients with chronic lymphocytic leukemia, low-grade lymphomas or solid tumors like ovarian, breast or small-cell lung cancers. Factors that contribute to the development of tumor lysis syndrome include the type of malignancy, responsiveness to treatment, rapid cell turnover and overall tumor burden. High pretreatment serum lactate dehydrogenase concentrations more than 1,500 U/L tend to correlate with tumor burden. Symptoms of tumor lysis syndrome are non-specific and include nausea, vomiting, fatigue, weakness, myalgia and dark urine. Electrolyte alterations can lead to muscle weakness, neuromuscular irritability, arrhythmias, seizures and even sudden death. Massive release of cell contents and degradation products of destroyed neoplastic cells into the bloodstream cause the metabolic abnormalities associated with tumor lysis syndrome. Destruction of malignant cells can lead to increased serum uric acid levels. Uric acid precipitates in the presence of acidic medium in the kidneys inducing renal failure. Hyperphosphatemia is also caused by the release of intracellular phosphate by tumor cell lysis and produces lowering of serum calcium. Hypocalcemia can lead to severe neuromuscular irritability and tetany. Potassium, as the main intracellular cation, is also liberated into the bloodstream when tumor cells are destroyed. Hyperkalemia, especially in the presence of renal failure, can lead to life-threatening ventricular arrhythmias.[19]

Routine uric acid and electrolyte measurements are indicated in patients with high tumor burden, particularly, if they have acute leukemia or aggressive lymphomas, in which a rapid response to chemotherapy may be predicted. Prevention should include hydration with normal saline up to 3 L/m^2/day, to induce a urinary output of at least 100 mL/h with or without diuretics. Oral sodium bicarbonate should be given to avoid acidic urine. Allopurinol, a xanthine oxidase inhibitor is often used to prevent hyperuricemia in a dose of 200–300 mg/day (in two to three divided doses). Rasburicase, a recently developed recombinant form of urate oxidase, is also an effective drug for preventing hyperuricemia. It acts by catalyzing the enzymatic oxidation of uric acid to allantoin, a metabolite that is five to ten times more soluble in urine than uric acid.

Whenever a patient presents with severe tumor lysis syndrome, an intensive care approach, including monitoring of hemodynamic, electrolyte and electrocardiographic parameters, should be started promptly. Adequate hydration, allopurinol or rasburicase and sodium bicarbonate, together with electrolyte correction and dialysis (in case of renal failure) are the key issues of management. Dialysis is recommended in cases presenting with conditions like severe hyperphosphatemia (> 10.2 mg/dL), symptomatic hypocalcemia, azotemia, hyperuricemia, refractory acidosis, uncontrollable hyperkalemia, oliguria, anuria and volume overload.[20]

Anaphylactic Reactions

Anaphylactic reactions, commonly known as allergic reactions related to drug administration or blood transfusion may sometimes create medical emergencies in oncology. Angioedema and urticaria are the most common manifestations of anaphylaxis and are associated with more than 90% of allergic reactions to drugs. Other frequent manifestations include abdominal pain, chest tightness, upper airway obstruction, bronchospasm and low blood pressure. Laryngeal edema followed by hypotension is the most frequent cause of death related to anaphylactic reactions.[21]

The important steps of treating anaphylactic reactions includes:

- Early recognition of the condition
- Airway maintenance during the episode
- Hemodynamic support during and after the allergic episode.

Immediate management of anaphylaxis involves removing the drug or agent considered to be responsible for the allergic reaction. This is followed by immediate assessment of the airway and administration of epinephrine subcutaneously depending on the severity of the condition. The patient should be monitored closely and intravenous fluids should be given in case of hypotension. Glucocorticoids and antihistamines should also be added to reduce the severity of the allergic reaction. In case of resistant hypotension, intensive care unit management should be promptly started. Multiple cytotoxic drugs can produce anaphylactic reactions. The most common being the L-asparaginase, taxanes and platinum derivatives. Risk factors for adverse reactions are high dosage, previous exposure to the similar agents, intravenous administration at a faster rate and a personal history of allergy. Taxane (paclitaxel and docetaxel) induced major hypersensitivity reactions are seen in almost 30% of treated patients and some minor reactions in around 40% patients. The major reactions are of anaphylactoid type. Reactions occur more often when fast infusion rates and short infusion schedules are used. Most reactions happen in the first cycle itself and rarely thereafter. Reactions start within 2–10 min of intravenous infusion and most of them resolve after 15–20 min of stopping the infusion. Most common presenting features are dyspnea, urticaria, angioedema, hypotension or bronchospasm. The most useful ways of preventing reactions are prolongation of infusion or the use of prophylactic medication with corticosteroids and antihistamines. There is a substantial risk of the development of hypersensitivity reactions with prolonged use of carboplatin. Most of these reactions are mild and limited to skin rashes. Occasionally, more serious signs and symptoms, such as hypotension, intense anxiety, dyspnea or cardiovascular collapse, may develop.

REFERENCES

1. Spinazzé S, Caraceni A, Schrijvers D. Epidural spinal cord compression. Crit Rev Oncol Hematol. 2005;56:397-406.
2. Bilsky M, Smith M. Surgical approach to epidural spinal cord compression. Hematol Oncol Clin North Am. 2006;20:1307-17.
3. Higdon ML, Higdon JA. Treatment of oncologic emergencies. Am Fam Physician. 2006;74:1873-80.
4. Patchell RA, Tibbs PA, Regine WF, Payne R, Saris S, Kryscio RJ, et al. Direct decompressive surgical resection in the treatment of spinal cord compression caused by metastatic cancer: a randomised trial. Lancet. 2005;366:643-8.
5. Rades D, Stalpers LJ, Veninga T, Schulte R, Hoskin PJ, Obralic N, et al. Evaluation of five radiation schedules and prognostic factors for metastatic spinal cord compression. J Clin Oncol. 2005;23:3366-75.
6. Rades D, Stalpers LJ, Veninga T, et al. Spinal reirradiation after short-course RT for metastatic spinal cord compression. Int J Radiat Oncol Biol Phys. 2005;63:872-5.
7. Baker GL, Barnes HJ. Superior vena cava syndrome: etiology, diagnosis, and treatment. Am J Crit Care. 1992;1:54-64.
8. Rowell NP, Gleeson FV. Steroids, radiotherapy, chemotherapy and stents for superior vena caval obstruction in carcinoma of the bronchus: a systematic review. Clin Oncol (R Coll Radiol). 2002;14:338-51.
9. Colt HG, Harrell JH. Therapeutic rigid bronchoscopy allows level of care changes in patients with acute respiratory failure from central airways obstruction. Chest. 1997;112:202-6.
10. Weissman DE. Glucocorticoid treatment for brain metastases and epidural spinal cord compression: a review. J Clin Oncol. 1988;6:543-51.
11. Colleoni M, Martinelli G, Beretta F, Marone C, Gallino A, Fontana M, et al. Intracavitary chemotherapy with thiotepa in malignant pericardial effusions: an active and well-tolerated regimen. J Clin Oncol. 1998;16:2371-6.
12. Jean-Baptiste E. Clinical assessment and management of massive hemoptysis. Crit Care Med. 2000;28:1642-7.
13. Theriault RL. Hypercalcemia of malignancy: pathophysiology and implications for treatment. Oncology (Williston Park). 1993;7:47-50; discussion 52-5.
14. Bajorunas DR. Clinical manifestations of cancer-related hypercalcemia. Semin Oncol. 1990;17:16-25.
15. Murphy K, Nakashima L, Khoo K. BCCA protocol summary guidelines for the diagnosis and management of malignancy related hypercalcemia. June 1999. Revised Jan 2006.
16. Berenson JR, Hillner BE, Kyle RA, Anderson K, Lipton A, Yee GC, et al. American Society of Clinical Oncology clinical practice guidelines: the role of bisphosphonates in multiple myeloma. J Clin Oncol. 2002;20:3719-36.
17. Verbalis JG, Goldsmith SR, Greenberg A, et al. Hyponatremia treatment guidelines 2007: expert panel recommendations. Am J Med. 2007;120:S1-21.
18. Salahudeen AK, Ali N, George M, et al. Tolvaptan in hospitalized cancer patients with hyponatremia: a double-blind, randomized, placebo-controlled clinical trial on efficacy and safety. Cancer. 2014;120:744-51.
19. Davidson MB, Thakkar S, Hix JK, Bhandarkar ND, Wong A, Schreiber MJ. Pathophysiology, clinical consequences, and treatment of tumor lysis syndrome. Am J Med. 2004;116:546-54.
20. Tiu RV, Mountantonakis SE, Dunbar AJ, Schreiber MJ Jr. Tumor lysis syndrome. Semin Thromb Hemost. 2007;33:397-407.
21. Gomes ER, Demoly P. Epidemiology of hypersensitivity drug reactions. Curr Opin Allergy Clin Immunol. 2005;5:309-16.

8 CHAPTER

Nutrition and Cancer

Kuldeep Sharma, Kajal Pandya Yeptho

INTRODUCTION

Nutrition is the intake of food considered in relation to the body's dietary needs. Good nutrition, defined as an adequate, well-balanced diet combined with regular physical activity, is cornerstone of good health. Poor nutrition can lead to reduced immunity, increased susceptibility to disease, impaired physical and mental development and reduced productivity. While diet is just the sum of food a person consumes on daily basis, nutrition involves more than simply eating a "good" diet—it is about nourishment at every level. Nutrition plays an important role in management of patients with cancer, right from the time illness is first diagnosed and through various phases of treatment and recovery. Compromised nutrition can be considered a complication of disease or treatment process and can have far-reaching consequences. The prevalence of cancer-related malnutrition ranges from 30% to 74% for inpatients and outpatients, and is related to an increased risk of adverse clinical outcome.[1,2]

Although, the exact mechanism is unknown, nutrition may modify the carcinogenic process at any stage including the carcinogen (a physical, chemical or viral agent that induces cancer) metabolism and processing, cellular and host defense system, and response to treatment. Some cancers, particularly esophageal, pancreatic and liver cancer, affect an individual's nutritional status even before he is diagnosed. Is it that a lack of some nutritional factor aids progression to frank cancer or the cancerous process causes nutritional deficiencies—it is still not answered. In addition, treatment of cancer including surgery, chemotherapy and radiotherapy (RT) can have a significant impact on the individual's nutritional status.

Primarily a wasting disease, cancer produces loss of body fat and skeletal proteins. Since the cancer cells also need nutrition, they take it from the body and lead to muscle wasting and weight loss, resulting in cachexia and lowered immunity thus resulting in repeated infections. Weight loss, anorexia, alterations in metabolism and lean body mass wasting that often occur in cancer patients can have a profound impact on the ability of an individual to tolerate treatment and maintain quality of life. These challenges can be met with prompt and appropriate nutritional management.

Despite limitations in research design, epidemiologic studies have provided a strong and consistent data to support an inverse relationship between cancer risk and consumption of fruits and vegetables.[3] This means that as the intake of fruits and vegetables increases, the risk of cancer decreases. Research also supports inverse relationship between cancer risk and whole-grain consumption. Grains contain fibers rich in certain micronutrients and certain types of fat (e.g. omega-3 fatty acids and omega-3 fatty acid/omega-6 fatty acid), which protect against cancer.

Research supports direct relationship between cancer risk and intake of total fat/saturated fat and alcohol, obesity (as measured by a high body mass index) and certain food preparation methods such as smoked foods, salting, pickling and cooking meat at a high temperature.[4] Planned nutritional therapy can minimize nutrition-related deficiencies, help improve the tolerance for treatment and enhance indices of quality of life. Even in patients with advanced cancer, where nutritional therapy may not make a significant difference in eventual outcome, it plays a distinct role in palliative care.

GOALS OF NUTRITION THERAPY IN CANCER

Nutrition plays a significant part in the overall clinical management, be it a newly diagnosed illness, ongoing active treatment, recovery phase, or the terminal phase.[5]

The primary goal of nutrition therapy for cancer patients is to prevent malnutrition and provide a framework to offset the catabolic stress due to cancer or its treatment, as once malnutrition sets in, reversing it may be very difficult.

Nutrition treatment relies heavily on screening of those patients who are at risk of developing malnutrition which may result from either cancer or its treatment including surgery, chemotherapy and RT. The effects of anticancer therapy impair the intake, digestion and absorption of food and tend to produce a nutritional deficit. Hence, the goals for therapy should be to reverse or retard the nutrition depletion, preserve lean body mass, control side effects of the anticancer therapy and improve the indices of quality of life.

Nutrition Screening and Assessment

Early nutrition intervention is an essential part of comprehensive cancer care. Nutrition screening and assessment for risk of nutritional problems should be interdisciplinary and instituted at the time of diagnosis and should be re-evaluated and monitored throughout the treatment and recovery.[6]

Nutritional status is evaluated by taking a careful review of patient's weight chart, dietary history including appetite and intake, nutrition impact symptoms (e.g. nausea, vomiting and diarrhea), weight loss, comorbid conditions and laboratory studies. Nutrition focused physical examination of the individual's body including assessment of subcutaneous fat, muscle mass and fluid status provides vital information to fully evaluate the individual nutrition status and degree of risk.[7]

If the nutritional therapy is not initiated early, meeting the nutrition goals becomes increasingly difficult. Maintenance of adequate nutritional intake and preservation of body weight are important from several perspectives even in situations where it does not alter the natural history of the illness.

Body Weight

Best practices dictate that individuals who are able to maintain their body weight and nutrient stores are able to tolerate the treatment better and recover more quickly from the therapy-related aftereffects. Thus, patients should be advised to consume sufficient energy and proteins to maintain their nutrition store and appropriate weight for height. Therefore, even if the individual is overweight, the maintenance of the lean body mass should be encouraged throughout the treatment and recovery.[8]

Energy Intake

Provision of adequate calories is essential to maintain current weight and/or prevent treatment or disease-associated weight loss. Methods used to estimate energy requirements for individuals diagnosed with cancer include standardized equations such as Harris Benedict or Mifflin-St Jeor and Ireton Jones,[9] and indirect calorimetry using a metabolic chart (Table 1). Close monitoring and follow-up are essential to ensure adequate energy is being provided.

Protein Intake

An individual's need for protein increases during the time of illness and stress. Additional proteins are required by the body to repair and rebuild the tissues affected by cancer therapy and to maintain a healthy immune system.[10] For the body to use the protein effectively, adequate energy through carbohydrates and fats should be provided, else the body starts using its lean body mass as a source of energy. Protein needs are especially elevated in patients with severe diarrhea and/or malabsorption. Protein needs may be calculated based on body weight (kg) (Table 2), using the available guidelines.[9]

Micronutrients

Vitamins and minerals act as cofactors for essential processes both in health and illness. Many individuals may have pre-existing nutritional deficiencies when they are diagnosed with cancer because of poor diet and lifestyle choices and the metabolic effects of the cancer itself.[11] Thus, for individuals experiencing difficulty with eating or treatment-related side effects, use of multivitamin and mineral supplements that

Table 1 Energy requirements in different conditions[9]

Condition	*Energy requirements (kcal/kg)*
Obese	21–25
Nonambulatory or sedentary	25–30
Slightly hypermetabolic or those who need to gain weight	30–35
Hypermetabolic or severely stressed	> 35

Table 2 Protein requirements in various conditions

Condition	*Protein requirements (g/kg)*
Normal individual or patients on maintenance	0.8–1.0
Nonstressed cancer patients	1.0–1.5
Transplant patients	1.5
Increased protein needs (protein losing enteropathy, hypermetabolism, extreme wasting)	1.5–2.5
Hepatic or renal compromise including BUN approaching 100 mg/dL or elevated ammonia	0.5–0.8

Abbreviation: BUN, blood urea nitrogen.

provide no more than 100% recommended daily allowances is generally effective and safe.[12]

Fluid

Water forms an integral part of the body composition and may vary between 65% and 70% of the total body mass. The goal of fluid management is to ensure the maintenance of adequate hydration, tissue perfusion and electrolyte balance. Individuals undergoing chemotherapy and/or RT can become dehydrated easily. There is a need to identify possible causes for alteration in fluid balance such as fever, ascites, edema, profuse vomiting or diarrhea, multiple concurrent intravenous therapy, impaired renal function, or medications (diuretics), etc. Fluid needs can be calculated using the same formula used for most other patients without renal disease (30–35 mL/kg).

Antioxidants

Controversy over whether the use of antioxidant supplements such as vitamin A, C, E and beta-carotene, zinc, and selenium actually inhibits or enhances the antitumor effects of radiation therapy and chemotherapy continues. Currently, antioxidants are not a part of routinely prescribed nutritional therapy in cancer patients,[13,14] over and above the natural foods during treatment; however, they are prescribed after completion of treatment to help the recovery processes.

CANCER TREATMENT AND ITS NUTRITIONAL IMPLICATIONS

Nutrition therapy is used to help cancer patients in getting the required nutrients to maintain their body weight and strength, keep body tissues healthy, and to fight potential infections effectively.

Cancer can Change the Way the Body Uses Food

Some tumors express chemicals that change the way the body uses certain nutrients. The mechanism of body to use protein, carbohydrates and fat may be affected, especially by tumors of the stomach or intestines. A patient may seem to be eating enough, but the body may not be able to absorb all the nutrients from the food, either due to shortening of the absorptive surface due to surgery or mucosal reactions due to chemotherapy/radiotherapy.

Cancer and its Treatment may Affect Nutrition

The effects of cancer and cancer treatments make it difficult to eat well. Cancer treatments that affect nutrition include:

- Surgery
- Chemotherapy
- Radiotherapy
- Immunotherapy
- Stem cell transplant.

The side effects of cancer and cancer treatments that can affect nutrition include:

- Anorexia (loss of appetite)
- Mouth sores
- Dry mouth
- Difficulty in swallowing (dysphagia)
- Painful swallowing (odynophagia)
- Nausea/vomiting
- Diarrhea
- Constipation
- Pain
- Depression/anxiety
- Structural deformity.

Cancer treatments may affect taste, smell, appetite and the ability to eat enough food or absorb the nutrients from food. This can cause malnutrition. Malnutrition can cause the patient to be weak, tired and unable to fight infections or get through cancer treatment.

Chemotherapy and Nutrition

Chemotherapy affects cells all through the body, especially the fast-growing cells. This also includes the healthy cells that divide quickly, e.g. cells in the mouth, digestive tract, hair follicles, etc.

While on chemotherapy, the following side effects are common which have implication on nutrition:

- Loss of appetite
- Inflammation and sores in the mouth
- Changes in the way food tastes
- Feeling full after only a small amount of food
- Nausea/vomiting
- Diarrhea
- Constipation.

Patients who have side effects from chemotherapy may not be able to eat normally and get all the required nutrients to restore health during treatments. Nutrition therapy can help relieve side effects and thus help in preventing delay in treatment, weight loss, and maintain general health.

Radiotherapy and Nutrition

Radiotherapy selectively destroys the dividing cells which include the cancer cells and healthy cells surrounding them. The advanced techniques of radiation planning and delivery have made it possible to spare the surrounding structures and/or reduce the dose to these tissues and prevent acute radiation toxicity. The amount of damage depends on the following:

- The part of the body being treated
- Total dose of radiation and the size of each treatment fraction

- The precision with which RT is delivered
- Respecting the tolerance of the surrounding tissues as they may be able to tolerate a dose less than that required to control the cancer.

Radiotherapy to any part of the digestive system often produces side effects that may compromise nutritional intake. Usually, the side effects begin in the first few weeks after RT starts and go away a few weeks after it is finished. Some chronic side effects like malabsorption may persist for months to years.

The following are the expected side effects of RT:

- Radiotherapy to the head and neck
  - Loss of appetite
  - Changes in taste
  - Pain during swallowing
  - Dry mouth or thick saliva
  - Sore mouth and gums.
- Radiotherapy to the chest
  - Inflammation of the esophagus leading to trouble in swallowing
  - Worsening of symptoms in case of pre-existing gastric esophageal reflux disease (GERD)
  - Nausea/vomiting
  - Loss of appetite.
- Radiotherapy to abdomen or pelvis
  - Diarrhea
  - Tenesmus
  - Abdominal pain
  - Nausea/vomiting
  - Inflamed intestines and rectum
  - Malabsorption (decrease in the amount of nutrients absorbed by the intestinal mucosa).

This may also cause tiredness and fatigue which can lead to decrease in appetite.

Nutrition therapy during RT can help the patient get enough protein and calories to get through treatment, prevent weight loss, help wound and skin healing, and maintain general health.

Ways to Supplement Nutrition

The goal of oral intake is to achieve more than 75% of the daily energy requirements. If this objective cannot be met, other types of nutritional support have to be evaluated.[15] Nutrition support for such patients can be given in following ways:

- *Oral nutritional supplements*: They are suggested to supplement nutrition in patients who are still able to eat food. It includes supplements containing proteins, lipids, carbohydrates and essential micronutrients. They are available as ready-to-use preparations in the form of powder, granules, etc.
- *Enteral nutrition:* It is also called tube feeding. It involves giving the patient nutrients in liquid form (formula) through a tube that is placed into the stomach or small intestine. This tube can be placed as a nasogastric or nasojejunal tube or as percutaneous endoscopic gastrostomy (PEG).
- Parenteral nutrition: It is a way to directly deliver the nutrients into the bloodstream. It is an extremely useful method for supporting nutrition in patients when food cannot be taken by mouth or by enteral feeding due to any reason. Parenteral feeding thus bypasses the digestive tract in the time of crisis. Nutrients are delivered into the blood through a catheter/line inserted into a vein. Almost all nutrients can be delivered using this approach including proteins, fats, vitamins, and minerals. Various commercial preparations are available in various combinations and can be chosen as per the specific requirement of a patient.

NUTRITION MANAGEMENT OF SYMPTOMS

When side effects of cancer or cancer treatment affect normal nutrition, changes can be made to provide the patient with required nutrients. A few of the common conditions seen during cancer illness or its treatment and the strategies to control or overcome them are described in the following paragraphs.

Anorexia: It is described as the loss of appetite or desire to eat. It is one of the most common complaints observed in cancer clinics. The following measures may help cancer patients who have a loss of appetite:

- Eating in a calm, clean and comfortable dining space along with regular exercise may improve appetite.
- Eating small and frequent meals every 2 hourly or so instead of fixed large meals may improve the condition.
- Extra calories and protein may be added to food for compensating the calorie loss. It can be done by using butter, purified butter (ghee), fats in the form of edible oils, skim milk powder, honey, or brown sugar.
- Soft and pureed foods when solid food intake is compromised, e.g. porridge, suji or rice kheer, halwa, custard, ice-cream, thick soups, blenderized pulses. The food should be homogenized such that the grains do not irritate the acutely inflamed tissue surfaces.
- Drink liquid supplements (special drinks that have nutrients), soups, milk, juices, shakes, butter milk and smoothies, if eating solid food is a problem.
- Eat breakfasts that have one-third of the calories and protein needed for the day.
- Eat snacks that have plenty of calories and protein.
- Eat food that smells good. Strong odors can be avoided.
- Try new foods and new recipes, flavorings, spices, and foods with a different texture or thickness. Food likes and dislikes may change day-to-day.
- Plan menus ahead of time and get help in preparing meals.

- The following are high-calorie, high-protein food choices:
  - Cheese slices
  - Muffins
  - Puddings
  - Nutritional supplements
  - Milkshakes
  - Yogurt
  - Ice-cream
  - Powdered milk added to foods such as pudding, milkshakes, or any recipe using milk
  - Halwa.

Altered/loss of taste: Changes in food taste may be caused by radiation treatment, chemotherapy, dental problems, mouth sores, infections and medicines. This can cause a loss of appetite, weight loss, and a decreased quality of life. The following tips may help cancer patients facing such problem:

- Eat small meals and healthy snacks several times a day
- Eat meals when hungry rather than at set mealtimes
- Eat citrus fruits (oranges, tangerines, lemons, grapes), unless mouth sores are present
- Add spices and sauces to foods
- Eat meals with something sweet such as jelly, applesauce or stew apple
- Rinse mouth with water before eating.

Xerostomia/dry mouth: Dry mouth is often caused by RT to the head and neck region and by certain medicines. Dry mouth may affect speech, taste and the ability to swallow or to use dentures or braces. There is also an increased risk of cavities and gum diseases because less saliva is made to wash the teeth and gums.

The main treatment for dry mouth is drinking plenty of liquids. Other ways to help relieve dry mouth include:

- Keeping water handy at all times to moisten the mouth
- Eating moist food with extra sauces, gravies, butter, or margarine
- Eating food and drinks that are sweet or tart (to increase saliva)
- Eating ice chips or frozen desserts (such as frozen grapes and ice pops)
- Drinking fruit nectar instead of juice
- Sucking on hard candy or chew gum
- Cleaning teeth (including dentures) and rinsing mouth regularly (after eating and at bedtime). Avoiding mouth rinses that contain alcohol.

Mouth sores and infections: Mouth sores can be caused by chemotherapy and RT. Mouth sores can be painful and may get infected and cause difficulty in eating. The following measures can help patients who have mouth sore and infections:

- Eat soft foods that are easy to chew and swallow such as:
  - Soft fruits like bananas, applesauce and watermelon
  - Peach, pear and apricot nectars
  - Cottage cheese
  - Mashed potatoes (paste form)
  - Macaroni and cheese
  - Custards and puddings
  - Gelatin
  - Milkshakes
  - Scrambled eggs
  - Dalia, oatmeal or other cooked cereals
  - Suji or wheat flour halwa in thin consistency
  - Ice-creams
  - Suji kheer or seviyan kheer
  - Lassi or yogurts.
- Use a blender to make vegetables (such as potatoes, peas and carrots) and meats smooth
- Add gravy, broth or sauces to food
- Drink high-calorie, high-protein drinks in addition to meals
- Cook food until soft and tender
- Eat food at room temperature. Hot and warm foods can irritate a tender mouth
- Cut food into small pieces
- Use a straw to drink liquids
- Numb the mouth with ice chips or flavored ice pops before eating
- Clean teeth (including dentures) and rinse mouth at least four times a day (and after eating and at bedtime)
- Avoid the following:
  - Citrus fruit and juices if they hurt or they can be sweetened with sugar/sugar free preparations
  - Spicy food
  - Rough, coarse, or dry food including raw vegetables, granola, toast and crackers.

Nausea: Nausea caused by cancer treatment can affect the amount and type of food eaten by patient. The following measures may help cancer patients control nausea:

- Eat before cancer treatment sessions
- Rinse out mouth before and after eating
- Eat foods that are bland, soft and easy to digest
- Eat small meals several times a day rather than heavy meals
- Eat dry food such as crackers, breadsticks, or toast throughout the day
- Slowly sip fluids throughout the day
- Suck on hard candies such as peppermints or lemon drops if mouth has a bad taste
- Sit up or lie with the upper body raised for 30–45 minutes after eating
- Avoid food that aggravates nausea like spicy food, greasy food, and food having strong odor.

Diarrhea: It may be caused by cancer treatment, surgery on the stomach or intestines, or by emotional stress. Long-term diarrhea may lead to dehydration or electrolyte derangement.

The following measures may help cancer patients having diarrhea:

- Taking broth, soups, bananas and canned fruits to replace electrolytes lost by diarrhea. Sport drinks may also help
- Drinking plenty of fluids during the day. Liquids at room temperature may cause fewer problems than hot or cold liquids
- Drinking at least 1 cup of liquid (ORS/Electral/Coconut water/Salted lassi/Shikanji) after each loose bowel movement.
- Avoiding the following:
  - Greasy foods, hot or cold liquids, or caffeine
  - High-fiber foods—especially dried beans and cruciferous vegetables (such as broccoli, cauliflower and cabbage)
  - Plain milk until the cause of diarrhea is known. Curd, milk in tea and cottage cheese can be taken during diarrhea.
  - Food and beverages that cause gas (such as peas, lentils, cruciferous vegetables, chewing gum and soda)
  - Sugar free candies or gum made with sorbitol (sugar alcohol).

Dehydration: The body needs plenty of water to replace the fluids lost everyday. Nausea, vomiting and pain may keep the patient away from drinking and eating adequately. Long-term diarrhea causes a loss of fluid from the body. One of the first signs of dehydration is feeling of tiredness. The following measures may help cancer patients in preventing dehydration:

- Drinking 8–12 cups of liquids a day. This can be water, juice, milk, or any food containing liquid such as ice pops, flavored ice and gelatin
- Limiting intake of drinks having caffeine such as soda, coffee and tea (both hot and cold)
- Taking a water bottle whenever leaving home. It is important to drink even if not thirsty
- Drinking liquid between meals
- Using medicines that help to prevent or treat nausea and vomiting.

Constipation: It is very common for cancer patients to have constipation (fewer than three bowel movements a week). Constipation may be caused by the following:

- Too little water or fiber in the diet
- Reduced movements
- Certain medicines used to treat nausea, vomiting or pain.

General dietary measures to prevent constipation:

- Eat fiber-containing foods. Taking 25–35 g of fiber a day is best. Food labels show the amount of fiber in a serving. Good source of fiber include:
  - Legumes (beans and lentils)
  - Vegetables
  - Cold cereals (whole grain or bran)
  - Hot cereals
  - Fruits
  - Whole-grain breads.
- Addition of more fibrous diet on daily basis helps in this condition. Fibrous diet should be accompanied by plenty of fluids. The fluid helps in propelling the fiber through the intestines.
- Fluid should include drinking 10–15 cups of fluid each day. This may include water, prune juice, warm juices, lemonade and tea. Aerated drinks and fluids containing caffeine should be avoided.
- Regular walks and exercise as per the individual capacity are also important.

Low white blood cell counts: This is a common condition caused by chemotherapy, RT or cancer itself. Patients with low white blood cell count remain at increased risk of infection including food and water-related infections. The following measures help such patients in preventing infections under this situation:

- The food items to be avoided include:
  - Raw eggs, meat or fish
  - Stale, moldy or damaged fruits and vegetables
  - Food procured from open counters or stored in open containers
  - Food from salad bars and buffets when eating out.
- Washing hands properly by patient and attendants helps in preventing the spread of infection.
- Cold foods should be thawed in a refrigerator or microwave and should be cooked immediately after thawing. Never thaw foods at room temperature.
- Keeping hot food hot and cold food cold prevents emergence/growth of germs.
- Meat, poultry and fish need to be stored and cooked well.
- Refrigerating all leftover food within 2 hours of cooking and consuming those within 24 hours prevent them to become a source of infection. Buying food packed as single servings to avoid leftovers may be another measure.
- To avoid consuming food that has crossed the date of expiry mentioned over.
- To avoid consuming packed food from cans that are swollen, dented or damaged.

Stem cell transplant patients: These patients have special nutritional requirements. Chemotherapy, RT and medicines used during stem cell transplant may cause side effects which compromises patient from eating and digesting food as usual. Common side effects include the following:

- Changes in the way food tastes
- Dry mouth or thick saliva
- Mouth and throat sores
- Nausea/vomiting

- Diarrhea.
- Constipation
- Weight loss and loss of appetite
- Weight gain.

Transplant patients are on immunosuppressive drugs which render them susceptible to infection. In addition, treatment with radiation and chemotherapy decreases the number of white blood cells and further increases the risk of infection. Thus, it is very important for transplant patients to avoid infections.

Patients who have undergone a transplant need sufficient protein and calories to recover from the treatment, prevent excessive weight loss, fight infection and maintain general health. Nutrition therapy in post-transplant cases undergoing cancer treatment needs following dietary measures:

- Their diet should include properly cooked and processed food only, as inadequately cooked food may be a source of infection
- The guidelines on safe food handling should be followed at home and hospital
- A specific diet plan based on the type of transplant and the type of cancer should be followed
- Parenteral nutrition during the initial period after the transplant should be considered to help patient in recovery.

Nutrition plays an important role throughout the continuum of cancer care—right from reducing the cancer risk to withstanding the stress associated with cancer diagnosis to overcome the effects of cancer therapies. Prompt and appropriate nutritional management may help to improve patients' tolerance of treatment, minimize nutrition impact symptoms and maximize quality of life.

REFERENCES

1. Fearon KC, Barber MD, Moses AG. The cancer cachexia syndrome. Surg Oncol Clin N Am. 2001;10(1):109-26.
2. Isenring E, Cross G, Kellett E, et al. L. Nutritional status and information needs of medical oncology patients receiving treatment at an Australian public hospital. Nutr Cancer. 2010;62(2):220-8.
3. Chen DA. Neoplastic disease. In: Nelms M, Sucher K, Long S (Eds). Nutrition Therapy and Pathophysiology. Belmont: Thomson Brooks; 2007. pp. 751-79.
4. Greenwald P, Clifford CK, Milner JA. Diet and cancer prevention. Eur J Cancer. 2001;37(8):948-65.
5. Eldridge B, Rock CL, McCallum PD. Nutrition and the patient with cancer. In: Coulston NM, Rock CL, Monsen ER (Eds). Nutrition in the prevention and treatment of disease. San Diego, CA: Academic Press; 2001.p. 397-412.
6. McCallum PD. Nutrition screening and assessment in oncology. in: L. Elliott, LL Molseed, PD McCallum, B. Grant (Eds) The Clinical Guide to Oncology Nutrition. 2nd ed. American Dietetic Association, Chicago, IL. 2006;89-90.
7. Fuhrman MP. Nutrition-focused physical exam. In: Charney P, Malone A (Eds). ADA Pocket Guide to Nutrition Assessment. Chicago, Ill: American Dietetic Association; 2004:41-62.
8. Grant B. Medical nutrition therapy in cancer. In: Mahan LK, Escott-Stump S (Eds). Krause's Food and Nutrition Therapy, 12th edition. Philadelphia (AA): Saunders Elsevier; 2000 pp. 959-90.
9. Martin C. Calorie, protein, fluid and micronutrient requirements. In: McCallum PD, Polisena CG (Eds). The Clinical Guide to Oncology. Nutrition. Chicago: American Dietetic Association. 2000;45-52.
10. Hurst JD, Gallagher AL. Energy, macronutrient, micronutrient and fluid requirements. In: Elliott L, Molseed. LL, McCallum PD (Eds). The Clinical Guide to Oncology Nutrition. 2nd ed. American Dietetic Association, Chicago, IL. 2006;54-71.
11. Kucuk O, Ottery FD. Dietary supplements during cancer treatment. Oncology Issues. 2002;17(S):27.
12. Brown JK, Byers T, Doyle C, Coumeya KS, Demark-Wahnefried W, Kushi LH, et al. Nutrition and physical activity during and after cancer treatment: an American Cancer Society guide for informed choices. CA Cancer J Clin. 2003;53(5):268-91.
13. Conklin KA. Dietary antioxidants during cancer chemotherapy: impact on chemotherapeutic effectiveness and development of side effects. Nutr Cancer. 2000;37(1):1-18.
14. Prasad KN, Cole WC, Kumar B, et al. Scientific rationale for using high-dose multiple micronutrients as an adjunct to standard and experimental cancer therapies. J Am Coll Nutr. 2001;20(5 Suppl):450S-463S; discussion 473S-75S.
15. Bozzetti F, Arends J, Lundholm K, Micklewright A, Zurcher G, Muscaritoli M, et al. ESPEN Guidelines on Parenteral Nutrition: non-surgical oncology. Clin Nutr. 2009;28(4):445-54.

CHAPTER

Central Nervous System Tumors

Vikash Kumar, Deepak Gupta, Tejinder Kataria, Kushal Narang

INTRODUCTION

Intracranial brain tumors are relatively rare tumors and constitute only 3.3% of all cancers in India as per the GLOBOCAN 2012 report. The recorded incidence amongst the males is 11,000/year as compared to approximately 6,000/year for females. Intracranial space occupying lesions cause symptoms by pressure effect on the normal brain structures leading to functional anomalies that may not be corrected even after the tumor has been removed in some cases. The tough cranium prevents any displacement of brain tissue and the resultant edema secondary to tumor, surgery, medications and/or radiation may at times mimic symptoms similar to an intracranial tumor precipitating seizures, headache and vomiting in many instances. The first treatment of choice for any intracranial pathology is resection followed by microscopic histopathology of the resected brain lesion. Depending upon the histology, brain tumors have been classified by the World Health Organization (WHO) classification.[1] Some of the tumors have been further studied using immune-histochemical markers that may have a guidance value for therapeutic decisions.

WHO CLASSIFICATION

Tumors of Neuroepithelial Tissues

Astrocytic Tumors

- WHO grade I
  - Pilocytic astrocytoma
  - Subependymal giant cell astrocytoma
- WHO grade II
  - Pilomyxoid astrocytoma
  - Pleomorphic xanthoastrocytoma
  - Diffuse astrocytoma
    - Fibrillary astrocytoma
    - Protoplasmic astrocytoma
    - Gemistocytic astrocytoma
- WHO grade III
  - Anaplastic astrocytoma
- WHO grade IV
  - Glioblastoma
  - Giant cell glioblastoma
  - Gliosarcoma
- Gliomatosis cerebri

Oligoastrocytic Tumors

- Oligoastrocytoma
- Anaplastic oligoastrocytoma

Oligodendroglial Tumors

- Oligodendroglioma
- Anaplastic oligodendroglioma

Ependymal Tumors

- Subependymoma
- Myxopapillary ependymoma
- Ependymoma
- Anaplastic ependymoma

Choroid Plexus Tumors

- Choroid plexus papilloma
- Atypical choroid plexus papilloma
- Choroid plexus carcinoma

Other Neuroepithelial Tumors

- Astroblastoma
- Chordoid glioma of the third ventricle
- Angiocentric glioma

Neuronal and Mixed Neuronal-Glial Tumors

- Dysplastic gangliocytoma of cerebellum (Lhermitte-Duclos)
- Desmoplastic infantile astrocytoma/ganglioglioma
- Dysembryoplastic neuroepithelial tumor
- Gangliocytoma
- Ganglioglioma
- Anaplastic ganglioglioma
- Central neurocytoma
- Extraventricular neurocytoma
- Cerebellar liponeurocytoma
- Papillary glioneuronal tumor
- Rosette-forming glioneuronal tumor of the fourth ventricle
- Paraganglioma

Tumors of the Pineal Region

- Pineocytoma
- Pineal parenchymal tumor of intermediate differentiation
- Pineoblastoma
- Papillary tumor of the pineal region

Embryonal Tumors

- Medulloblastoma
- CNS primitive neuroectodermal tumor (PNET)
- CNS neuroblastoma
- CNS ganglioneuroblastoma
- Medulloepithelioma
- Ependymoblastoma
- Atypical teratoid/rhabdoid tumor

Tumors of Paraspinal and Cranial Nerves

- Malignant peripheral nerve sheath tumor (MPNST)
- Perineurioma
- Neurofibroma
- Schwannoma

Tumors of the Meninges

- Meningioma
- Atypical meningioma
- Anaplastic meningioma

Lymphomas and Hematopoietic Neoplasms

- Malignant lymphomas
- Plasmacytoma
- Granulocytic sarcoma

Germ Cell Tumors

Germinoma
Embryonal carcinoma
Yolk sac tumor
Choriocarcinoma
Teratoma
- Mature
- Immature
- Teratoma with malignant transformation

Mixed germ cell tumor

Tumors of the Sellar Region

- Craniopharyngioma
- Granular cell tumor
- Pituicytoma
- Spindle cell oncocytoma of the adenohypophysis

LOW-GRADE GLIOMAS

Epidemiology

Low-grade gliomas (LGGs) are slow-growing tumors accounting for approximately 20% of patients with gliomas and approximately 10% of all primary intracranial tumors in adults. 1/100,000 is diagnosed with LGGs every year. An increased incidence of LGG is seen with neurofibromatosis type I and tuberous sclerosis (Von Hippel-Lindau disease).[2,3]

Pathology

Low-grade gliomas are divided into non-infiltrative and diffusely infiltrative. Pilocytic astrocytomas are usually non-infiltrative and are defined as grade I glioma and more common in children. The diffusely infiltrative tumors are defined as grade II tumors as per WHO grading. They usually occur in the 3rd or 4th decade of life.

The cell of origin of LGG is the specialized supportive cell in central nervous system (CNS): astrocytic, oligodendrocytic cells or rarely other cells that may have features of these or other histological lineage. LGGs in adults tend to occur in both cerebral hemispheres, although they can occur in any part of brain.

Presentation

Most common symptoms at presentation are seizures, headache and focal neurological defect. However, LGGs can present in any number of ways.

Radiological Features

Computed tomography (CT) typically demonstrates an ill-defined, diffuse, nonenhancing low-density region, often in the frontal or temporal lobes. Calcifications are commonly seen with oligodendrogliomas. On magnetic resonance imaging (MRI), there will be hypodensity relative to normal brain parenchyma on T1-weighted image and bright area on T2 or fluid-attenuated inversion recovery (FLAIR) sequence. Infiltrative LGGs are usually nonenhancing on contrast imaging and are associated with a more aggressive behavior.

Treatment

Low-grade gliomas are usually slow growing and nonaggressive. An early treatment with surgery and radiation therapy may be able to eradicate tumor clonogens. However, some scientists have argued for a nonaggressive treatment approach because of morbidity associated with surgery and radiation therapy. Treatment, in particular the timing of intervention, for patients with diffusely infiltrative low-grade tumors remains controversial. In general, early intervention is indicated for patients with increasing symptoms, radiographic progression, and high-risk features suggestive of transformation to a higher-grade tumor.

Surgery

Although surgery is considered an integral part of treatment, the goal of surgery and its timing are debated. Complete resection of pilocytic astrocytoma is associated with excellent survival, with the majority (> 90%) of patients cured of the tumor. No adjuvant therapy is necessary. Incomplete resection is associated with long-term survival rates of 70–80% at 10 years. However, even under the best circumstances, total resection in diffuse infiltrative glioma with an adequate margin is rarely achieved due to the diffusely infiltrative nature of these tumors and involvement of eloquent regions. No class I evidence exists that shows that maximal safe resection in LGGs is associated with an improved survival. Although controversial, most studies have found total or subtotal (> 90%) resection to be associated with improved outcome. In a study by Claus EB et al. an improved survival associated with the use of intraoperative guidance for complete resection[4] has been reported. Another study by Berger et al. concluded that near complete resection was associated with a low recurrence rate.[5]

Adjuvant Radiotherapy

Two important issues exist—the need and timing of radiotherapy (RT) and dose of radiation in LGGs. Radiation Therapy Oncology Group (RTOG) 98-02 trial supports the deferral of RT in LGGs. The study includes an observation arm for completely resected patients less than 40 years of age. The overall survival (OS) and progression-free survival (PFS) has been reported to be 97% and 73% respectively at 3 years. A useful scoring system predicting survival for LGGs has been derived from European Organisation for Research and Treatment of Cancer (EORTC) data. The factors identified for recurrence were age >/40 years, astrocytoma histology, maximum tumor dimension more than 6 cm, tumor crossing midline and presence of neurological deficit at the time of surgery.[6] The recent phase III trials by EORTC 22,845, 22,844 and North Central Cancer Treatment Group (NCCTG) provide the best evidence with respect to the indications for RT as well as the dose. In EORTC 22,844, 379 patients were randomized to receive 45 Gy in 5 weeks or 59.4 Gy in 6.6 weeks postoperatively.[7] With a median follow-up of 74 months, OS (58% vs 59%) and PFS (47% vs 50%) were similar in both arms. In a joint NCCTG, RTOG and Eastern Cooperative Oncology Group (ECOG) study, 203 patients were randomized to low-dose RT to 50.4 Gy in 28 fractions (n = 101) or high-dose RT to 64.8 Gy in 36 fractions. There was no significant difference in PFS or OS. Survival at 2 years and 5 years was 94% and 72%, respectively, with low-dose RT and 85% and 64% with high-dose RT. Grade 3–5 neurotoxicity occurred in 5% of patients in the high-dose cohort and 2.5% of patients in the low-dose cohort.[8]

Radiotherapy Techniques

Adverse effect of RT on CNS is related to dose, treatment duration and fraction size. Therefore, a conformal treatment would decrease normal tissue irradiation and thus decrease morbidity. There is no class I data to guide RT treatment portal design.

Simulation

A three clamp Orfit as an immobilization device is appropriate. A volumetric contrast enhanced CT of head and neck with 3 mm slice to be taken with immobilization device. Postoperative contrast and T2-weighted or FLAIR MRI is to be co-registered with volumetric CT scan.

Target Volume Delineation

As per RTOG 98-02 to include T2 signal abnormality from a postoperative MRI with a 1.5–2 cm margin to make a clinical target volume (CTV) (CTV should respect anatomical barrier such as bone or dural surface, etc.). For planning tumor volume (PTV) add 0.3–0.5 mm margin to CTV.

Treatment Planning Technique

A conformal treatment is preferred as it decreases irradiation of normal tissue and thereby results in decreased morbidity. However, no clinical studies have compared three-dimensional conformal radiotherapy (3DCRT) and intensity-modulated radiotherapy (IMRT) for LGGs.

Dose

Recommended dose is 5,040 cGy–5,400 cGy at 180–200 cGy per fraction 5 days a week.

Chemotherapy

Role of chemotherapy in LGG remains investigational. There is lack of data which support concomitant use of chemotherapy and RT.

HIGH-GRADE GLIOMAS

High-grade gliomas (HGGs) constitute almost 50% of all primary brain tumors in adults. It comprises glioblastoma (GBM) which accounts for 75% and anaplastic gliomas which accounts for the remaining 25% of HGGs. The main treatment modalities are surgery, radiation therapy, and chemotherapy in the curative treatment of HGGs. Various genetic alterations have been identified in the pathogenesis of HGGs (Fig. 1). Apart from that all HGG express oligodendrocyte lineage transcription factor 2 (OLIG2) and vascular endothelial growth factor (VEGF).[9] Hereditary disorders like neurofibromatosis, Li-Fraumeni syndrome, von Hippel-Lindau disease, and Turcot's syndrome[2,3] are also associated with CNS tumors.

Pathology

Treatment and prognosis varies with the grade and subtype of glioma identified in histopathology of the resected specimen. Newer imaging modalities facilitate stereotactic biopsy and have allowed access to eloquent locations. Glioblastoma multiforme shows nuclear atypia, mitotic activity, neovascularization and necrosis (Fig. 2B). Anaplastic gliomas show nuclear atypia and mitotic activity (Fig. 2A).

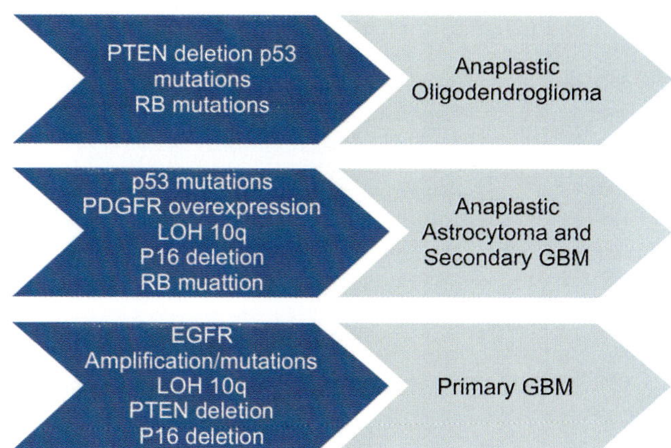

Fig. 1 Genetic alterations in high grade glioma[9]

Diagnosis, Staging

Clinical Presentation

General signs and symptoms include alteration in mental status, headache, vomiting, motor deficits, sensory deficits, speech deficit, gait disturbance and cranial nerve palsies. Patients present with signs and symptoms relevant to the location of the tumor and the resulting mass effect (Table 1).

Physical Examination

Complete history and physical examination with a thorough neurological examination including a baseline mini-mental status examination (MMSE) will help define the initial neurological deficits and help in rehabilitation and physiotherapy. Particular attention should be given to

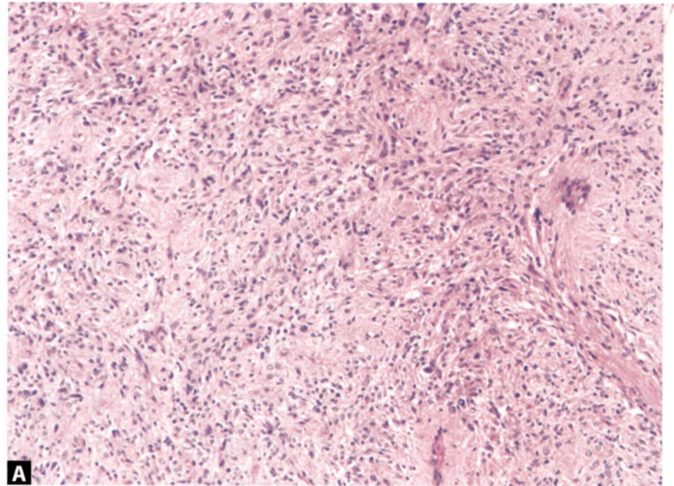

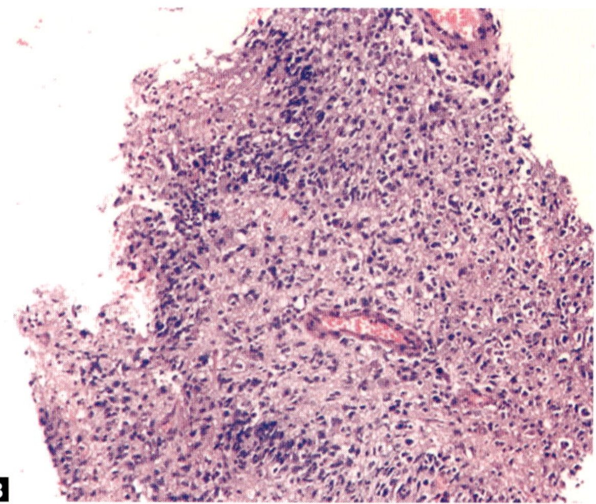

Figs 2A and B Histologic features of high-grade glioma showing atypia, mitotic activity, neovascularization and necrosis. (A) Anaplastic astrocytoma; (B) Glioblastoma

Courtesy: Dr Ishani Mohapatra, Neuropathology, Medanta—The Medicity, Haryana, India

Table 1 Signs/symptoms related to tumor location

CNS location	*Signs/symptoms*
Frontal lobe	Hemiparesis, seizures, alteration in mental status, urinary incontinence
Occipital lobe	Visual changes, seizures, morning headache and vomiting
Parietal lobe	Seizures, spatial disorientation, difficulty with reading and calculations, language disturbances
Temporal lobe	Seizures, emotional disturbance, hearing and memory disturbances
Thalamus	Altered motor and sensory function, behavioral changes
Hypothalamus	Impaired thirst, sleep, eating patterns, urination, temperature intolerance and emotional changes
Optic tract	Impaired vision, abnormal pupil reactions
Basal ganglia	Hemiparesis

ophthalmological and endocrine findings, depending on the tumor location and age of the patient.

Imaging

The gold standard imaging modality for evaluation of malignant brain tumors is contrast MRI due to unparalleled resolution. T1-weighted images help in defining anatomy and T2-weighted images and FLAIR aid in evaluating edema or infiltration of brain parenchyma. Computed tomography is useful for identifying calcifications as seen in oligodendrogliomas and in patients who cannot undergo MRI.

Magnetic resonance (MR) spectroscopy, perfusion MRI, and positron emission tomography (PET) are useful guide for discriminating radiation necrosis from tumor recurrences or progression. Diffusion tensor imaging (DTI) gives better understanding of white matter tracts along which HGGs can infiltrate and may be useful for guiding surgical approaches and RT planning. Oligodendrogliomas are noninfiltrating and shows calcification on CT. Anaplastic astrocytomas (AAs) are usually infiltrative, may show a mass effect and may or may not enhance. GBMs show peripherally enhancing tumor with a central necrotic region and surrounding FLAIR/T2 signal change indicative of edema or tumor infiltration. The recursive partitioning analysis (RPA) and RTOG classifies patients with HGGs into six classes:[10]

Class I–II: Anaplastic astrocytomas with age < 50 years and normal mental status or age > 50 years and Karnofsky Performance Scale (KPS) > 70, and symptom duration > 3 months. Median survival: 40–60 months.

Class III–IV: Anaplastic astrocytomas with age < 50 years and abnormal mental status or age ≥ 50 years, KPS ≥ 70, and symptom duration < 3 months. Median survival: 11–18 months. GBM with age < 50 years or age ≥ 50 years, KPS ≥ 70, surgical resection, and good neurologic function status.

Class V–VI: GBM with age ≥ 50 years, KPS < 70 or GBM with age ≥ 50 years, KPS ≥ 70 surgical resection but a poor neurologic function status or GBM with age ≥ 50 years, KPS ≥ 70 biopsy only. Median survival: 5–9 months.

Prognosis

The prognosis for high-grade brain tumors is generally poor and varies by histologic subtype and molecular markers (Tables 2 and 3). In general, an oligodendroglial component confers an improved survival. Codeletion of chromosomes 1p and 19q has been identified as a good prognostic factor in oligodendrogliomas. Clinical and prognostic factors include duration of symptoms, age, KPS, extent of surgery and neurologic status. Stupp et al. published their 5-year results from the landmark EORTC evaluating the effect of concurrent temozolomide and radiation therapy in the treatment of GBM. In this study, the O6-methylguanine-DNA methyltransferase (MGMT) methylation status was the most important prognostic factor for survival. MGMT codes for an enzyme, and if it is methylated, it becomes inactive, impairing the tumor cell's ability to repair the damage caused by the temozolomide.[11] A newer molecular marker isocitrate dehydrogenase 1 (IDH1) may affect the prognosis and predict response to therapy in patients with GBM.[9]

Treatment

Principles and Practice

The treatment of HGGs involves the multimodality approach of surgery, RT, and chemotherapy. Temozolomide is the current drug of choice, and more recently, targeted agents are also being explored in the treatment of HGGs like bevacizumab, cilengitide, etc.

Table 2 Survival by tumor type[10,11]

Tumor type	*Median-survival (months)*	*5-year overall survival (%)*
Glioblastoma multiforme	12–16	5–10%
Anaplastic gliomas	24	25–30%
Anaplastic oligodendroglioma	60	50–60%

Table 3 Impact of molecular markers on survival[9]

Tumor	*Marker*	*Status*	*Survival median (months)*	*2-year (%)*	*5-year (%)*
Glioblastoma	MGMT	Methylated	15.3–23.4		5.2–13.8%
		Unmethylated	11.8–12.6		0–8.3%
	IDH1	Mutated	30		
		Wild type	12		
Anaplastic oligoastrocytoma	1p/19q	Codeleted	> 84	65.4–71.7%	
		Nondeleted	33.6	31.3–46.7%	

Abbreviations: MGMT, O6-methylguanine DNA methyltransferase; IDH1, isocitrate dehydrogenase 1

Surgery

Surgery ranges from diagnostic biopsy to debulking and gross total resection (GTR).

Tumor biopsy

Biopsies are minimally invasive, well tolerated and suitable for lesions of any site or size except for the brainstem gliomas. Biopsy is usually considered when the risks of resection outweigh the benefit. It is best utilized in cases where initial diagnosis may influence subsequent management. To reduce the risk of non-diagnostic biopsies, image-guidance or stereotactic biopsy is routinely used.[12]

Tumor resection

Tumor decompression reduces the mass effect and tumor load and thereby effects of raised intracranial pressure and provides a histological sample. Extent of resection is one of the important prognostic factors.[13] Studies have shown that more than 98% of gross tumor resection has shown a better quality of life and PFS.[14] The median survival, according to one study, improved from 8 months for subtotal resection (STR) to 13 months after GTR.[15]

5-aminolevulinic acid (5-ALA) fluorescence-assisted surgery is helpful in identifying glioma tissue under blue light. 5-ALA is taken up by the glioma cells and is converted in the normal heme biosynthesis pathway. Due to the deficiency of the enzyme ferrochelatase, there is accumulation of the fluorophore protoporphyrin IX that fluoresces under blue light. The use of 5-ALA enables more complete resection of contrast enhancing tumor, leading to improved PFS in patients with malignant glioma. Studies have shown a better resection rate and a higher 6 months PFS than the white light group (41% vs 21.1%).[16]

Intraoperative placement of bis-chloroethylnitrosourea (BCNU) wafers delivers a high concentration of chemotherapeutic agent to the tumor cavity bypassing the blood-brain barrier (BBB). These agents are still controversial due to the lack of translation of their use into survival benefit and a higher complication rate.[17,18]

Radiotherapy

Radiobiological Considerations

The process of radiation response in the brain is dependent on a variety of factors including dose, volume, fraction size, and the specific target cell population, as well as secondary mechanisms of expression such as vascular leak causing edema, vascular endothelial loss resulting in hypoxia, and reactive gliosis. Historically, late effects from RT have been reported as the dose at either the 5% or 50% risk level at 5 years (TD 5/5 or TD 50/5). The values for whole-brain fractionated RT at 2 Gy per fraction are 60 Gy and 70 Gy, respectively. Even focal lesions may result in widespread radiographic and/or functional manifestations. The effect on endothelial cells often becomes manifest as an early T2 signal abnormality on MRI, possibly due to disruption of the BBB and resultant edema.[19] Metabolic changes observed with PET may reflect demyelination of oligodendroglial cells. Further, vascular changes and regeneration in response to radiation shows as an enhancing lesion on imaging.

Treatment Delivery

Randomized trials have demonstrated a clear survival benefit to the use of RT after surgery.[20] External-beam RT commonly is started 2–4 weeks after surgery to allow for wound healing. The use of IMRT may yield even more conformal dose distributions and better avoidance of organs at risk. For HGGs [GBMs, AA, anaplastic oligodendrogliomas (AOs), anaplastic oligoastrocytoma (AOA)], external-beam RT to a total dose of 60 Gy at 2 Gy per fraction (or 59.4 Gy at 1.8 Gy per fraction) is delivered. A cone down is performed in case of proximity to critical structures like brainstem and optic nerve after 46 Gy (or 45 Gy).[20]

Older patients (> 65 years), especially those with poor performance status, have been shown to have limited post-treatment improvement or rapid neurological deterioration following conventional RT, hence, a shorter course of treatment may provide good palliation.[21] Phillips et al. randomized 68 such patients to standard RT to 60 Gy in 30 fractions or a shorter course to 35 Gy in 10 fractions. There was no significant survival difference between the two arms.[22]

CT Simulation and Target Volume Definition

Computed tomography-based treatment planning with MR fusion is used for defining gross tumor volume (GTV) and PTV. Other imaging modalities like PET, perfusion imaging, spectroscopy or DTI are not in routine use. Recent evidence neural stem cells in the region of subventricular zone and in the subgranular zone of the dentate gyrus may affect RT planning in the future. For target volume delineation, postoperative images are used because they provide anatomic shifts that have occurred during and after surgery. Clinical target volume may be modified in the regions of natural barriers that would likely preclude microscopic tumor extension, such as the cerebellum, the contralateral hemisphere, the tentorium cerebri, and the ventricles. Wallner KE et al.[23] have shown that 78% of unifocal tumors recur within 2 cm of the initial tumor volume, defined as the enhancing edge of the tumor on CT scan, and 56% of tumors recur within 1 cm of the initial tumor margin.

Target Volume Definition

GTV1: Contrast-enhancing lesion, the surgical resection cavity and surrounding edema (T2/FLAIR abnormality).

PTV1: GTV1 plus 2.0 cm margin (PTV1 was treated to 46 Gy in 23 fractions, and after that there was a cone down to PTV2 that was treated for an additional 14 Gy in 7 fractions).

GTV2: Contrast-enhancing lesion and surgical cavity.

PTV2: GTV2 plus 2.5 cm margin (Figs 3A and B).

Chemotherapy

During the duration of RT, temozolomide 75 mg/m^2 is administered concurrently for the full duration of RT, typically 42 days. Temozolomide is given approximately 1 hour before radiation therapy, and at the same time on the days that no RT is scheduled. Postradiation a gap of 4 weeks is followed by MR assessment and complete blood counts and adjuvant temozolomide 150 mg/m^2, in a 5/28 days schedule, is recommended for cycle 1, followed by 5 cycles if well tolerated for a total of six cycles.[11] The dose is increased to 200 mg/m^2 at cycle 2 if well tolerated.[20] Weekly monitoring of blood counts is advised during chemoradiation therapy in all patients. *Pneumocystis carinii* pneumonia has been reported, and prophylaxis should be considered.

Follow-up

The recommended follow-up schedule is as follows:
First follow-up: 4 weeks after completion of RT
Year 1–3: Every 3 months
Year 4–5: Every 6 months
> 5 year: Annually.

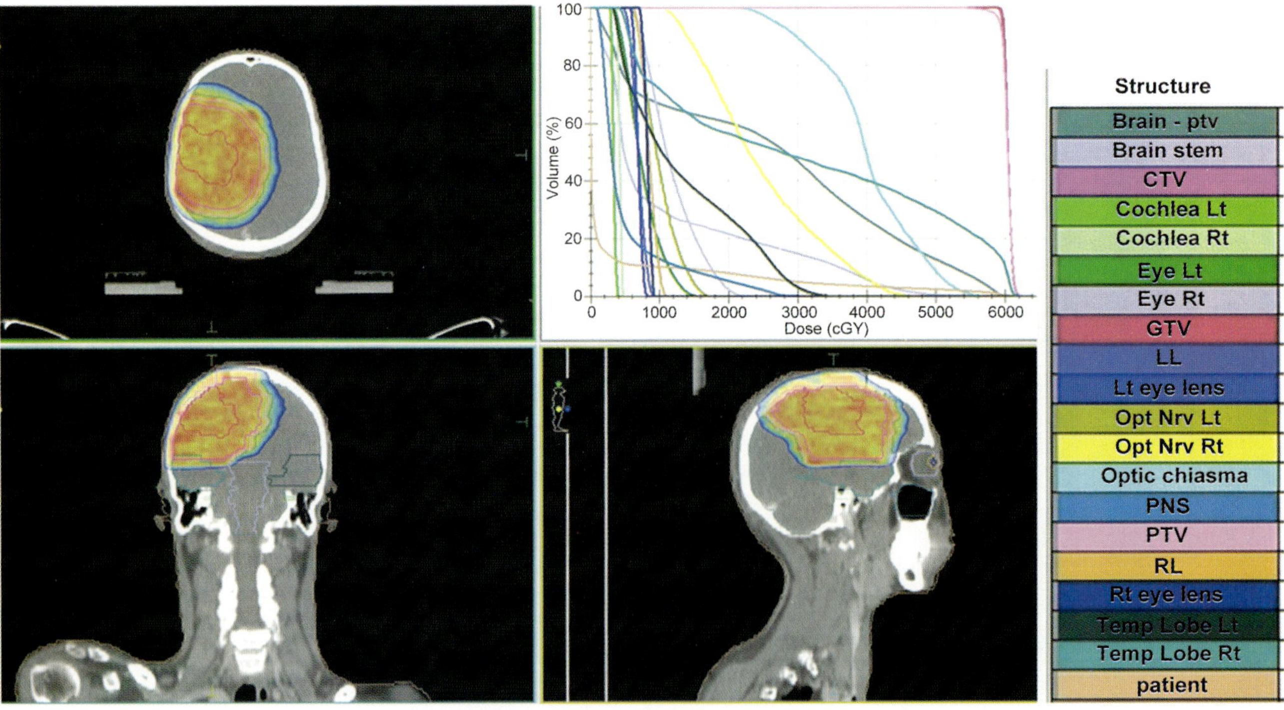

Fig. 3A Target volume and dose distribution in a case of right frontal lobe glioblastoma with proximity to the right optic nerve and optic chiasma, hence, the cone down technique was used

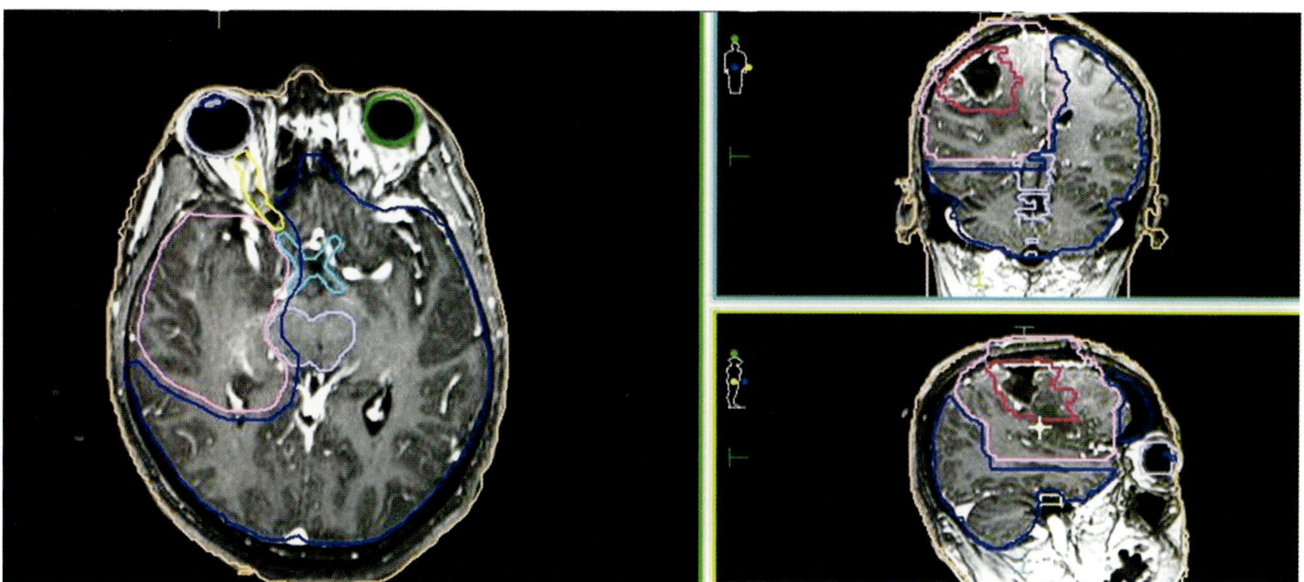

Fig. 3B MRI for the same case showing proximity of the planning tumor volume (PTV) (magenta) to the critical structures like optic chiasma (cyan), right optic nerve (yellow) and brainstem (light blue)

Courtesy: Dr Tejinder Kataria, Division of Radiation Oncology, Medanta—The Medicity, Haryana, India

EPENDYMOMA

Incidence

Ependymoma accounts for approximately 1–3% of adult CNS tumors. In general, most pediatric ependymomas arise intracranially, whereas well over 50% of adult ependymomas arise from the spinal cord. Ependymomas account for less than 10% of tumors arising in the CNS and 25% of primary tumors originating in the spinal cord. Most common spinal cord tumors in adults are intramedullary and account for nearly 60% of cases. In contrast to pediatric patients, supratentorial ependymomas are more frequent amongst adults and can arise in the brain parenchyma from ependymal rests, lateral ventricles and less commonly from third ventricle. Infratentorial sites are the floor or roof of the fourth ventricle or cerebellopontine angle (CPA).[24] The incidence of ependymomas is approximately equal in males and females.

Pathology

Ependymomas, as their name implies, are glial tumors that exhibit ependymal differentiation. Ependymomas arise from ependymal lining of the CNS, including the cerebral ventricles, the central canal of spinal cord and the filum terminale as well as cortical rests.[24] Histopathologically ependymoma are characterized by perivascular pseudorosettes that surround a central vascular space.[24] According to the WHO grading scheme for ependymomas:[1]

- Myxopapillary ependymoma (WHO grade I)
- Subependymoma (WHO grade I)
- Ependymoma (WHO grade II)
  - Cellular
  - Papillary
  - Clear cell
- Anaplastic ependymoma (WHO grade III)

Presentation

The most common intracranial symptoms are severe headache, vomiting that is related to increased intracranial pressure from either mass effect or obstructive hydrocephalus. Spinal cord tumor is generally associated with an insidiously worsening neurologic deficit effect in the lower extremities and impairment of the sphincter function. Ependymomas have characteristic features on CT scan and MRI that help in differential diagnosis. Intracranial ependymoma are usually enhancing and calcification can be seen in almost 50% of cases. Spread through foramina of Luschka and Magendie may lead to posterior fossa spread. They appear heterogenous on MRI due to calcification, hemorrhage, and necrosis. MRI of the complete spinal axis needs to be done to rule out cerebrospinal fluid (CSF) dissemination, as well as lumbar puncture for CSF cytology is mandatory. Drop metastases are reported in 5% of cases at the time of presentation. T2-weighted MR images are more sensitive because most tumors are hyperintense to the spinal cord on these sequences. On T1-weighted images intramedullary tumors shows slightly hypointense or isointense to the adjacent spinal cord and most of them are enhancing on T1-weighted contrast examinations.[25]

Surgery

Extent of tumor resection is the most consistent factor associated with local control and survival. Second look surgery and reoperation is recommended in those patients with residual disease.[27,28] The impact of histological grade on outcome is controversial, but several large series have confirmed this finding.

Radiotherapy

Gross total resection and negative margins with grade 1 and grade 2 tumors can be kept on close follow-up. Adjuvant RT even in patients with GTR results in improved local control as shown in a retrospective analysis by Rogers et al.[26] 10-year local control rate with and without RT were 50% vs 100%. Long-term follow-up is required as late recurrences are known. Postoperative RT should be given for anaplastic ependymomas, even in cases of GTR. Duration of treatment for less than 50 days was associated with improved 5-year OS of 86% versus 46% and local control was reported to be 71% versus 46%.[29]

Neuraxis dissemination predominantly occurs following local recurrence and rarely as an isolated event.[30] Current recommendation for adult intracranial ependymomas is to deliver involved field radiation using image base treatment planning to a dose of 59.4 Gy.[31] CTV is typically the postoperative tumor bed including residual disease (post-gadolinium MR T1 enhancing lesion) with 1-1.5 cm margin. A further setup margin to CTV as per institutional protocol (Fig. 4) is added. Target volume should respect the anatomic barrier to tumor spread. Craniospinal irradiation (CSI) is indicated in patient with positive CSF cytology and gross spinal metastasis on MRI (Fig. 5). The dose is typically 36-39.6 Gy followed by boost to primary site (59.4 Gy). Myxopapillary and spinal ependymomas are typically treated to an initial large field to cover the tumor bed to 45 Gy followed by boost to residual disease to 50.4-59.4 Gy depending on the location of disease.

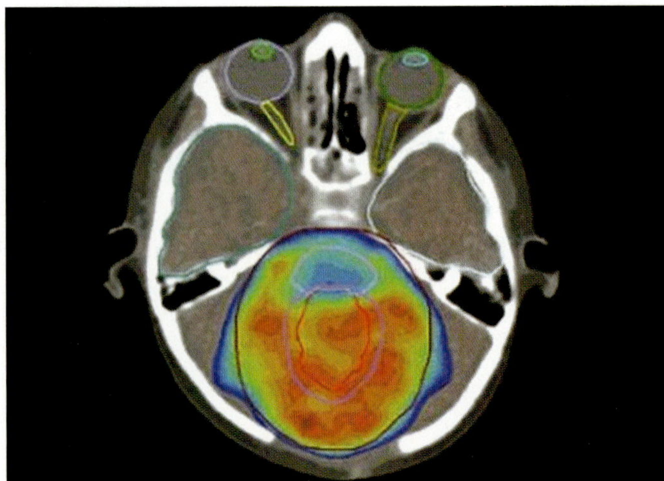

Fig. 4 Target volumes and dose distribution in a posterior fossa ependymoma. GTV: red, PTV45: dark red and PTV 54: (purple)

Courtesy: Dr Tejinder Kataria, Division of Radiation Oncology, Medanta—The Medicity, Haryana, India

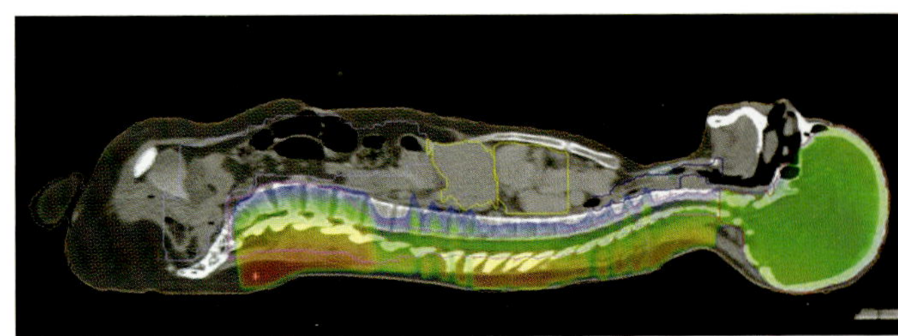

Fig. 5 Craniospinal irradiation in a patient with anaplastic ependymoma

Courtesy: Dr Tejinder Kataria, Division of Radiation Oncology, Medanta—The Medicity, Haryana, India

Chemotherapy

Chemotherapy is reserved for recurrent ependymomas. Response to chemotherapy occurs in only 10-15% of cases. Cisplatin/carboplatin and etoposide are the most active agents. There is no evidence for adjuvant or concurrent chemotherapy in treatment of ependymoma.[32]

Pediatric Ependymomas

Ependymomas account for nearly 8-10% of pediatric CNS tumors. The mean age of diagnosis is 4-6 years, but 25-40% of patients are less than 2 years old.[33] Most common location is posterior fossa. The fourth ventricle is the most common infratentorial site and extension into the subarachnoid space occurs frequently. Both surgery and RT are the main cornerstone of treatment as it is difficult to achieve full resection with surgery due to involvement of lower cranial nerves.

Management

Extent of tumor resection is the most consistent factor associated with local control and survival. 5 years PFS and OS, for those with GTR or STR is approximately 50-75% and 65-85% versus 25-30% and 0-30%. Anaplastic tumors (WHO grade III) fare worse than nonanaplastic tumors but the data on histology is somewhat controversial. In posterior fossa tumors, postoperative RT is the standard of care and in children over 3 years of age due to high rates of local failure if radiation therapy is omitted.[29]

Supratentorial anaplastic ependymoma usually behave worse than posterior fossa ependymomas and will require radiation therapy in postoperative setting. Until recently, it was a standard practice that children under 3 years of age will receive chemotherapy in an effort to delay RT. Duffner et al. showed that RT can be delayed for 1 year with intensive chemotherapy without a decrement in OS.[34] Merchant et al. published their experience from St. Jude's hospital for children 1 year and older with highly conformal involved field RT and showed that the decrement in neurocognitive function over time was minimal.[35] The initial results are preliminary but encouraging and have formed the foundation for the current Children's Oncology Group (COG) phase I protocol looking at immediate postoperative radiation in children as young as 1 year of age and 3 months of chemotherapy with a second look surgery in those with initial STR.[35,36]

Technique/Dose

All pediatric patients must be planned with 3DCRT.[34] Anatomic registration of MRIs (preoperative and postoperative) enables a more precise volume definition. A reference preoperative MRIs and intraoperative notes during the treatment planning are critical. Although current COG protocol prescribes doses to 59.4 Gy at 1.8 Gy/fr, for children over 18 months, the standard dose, off protocol, is between 54 Gy and 55.8 Gy. The dose in COG protocol has been escalated based on St. Jude's experience as local failure is a component in nearly 80% of cases. In very young patients who have been heavily treated with chemotherapy and extirpative surgery, doses as low as 50.4 Gy have been used.

The target volume has evolved over the years from CSI to posterior fossa irradiation to conformal involved field RT for both ependymoma and anaplastic ependymoma. Currently, no evidence that large field RT gives better survival. The GTV includes original tumor bed and resection cavity. Tumors that pushed normal brain aside which has collapsed back into a more normal anatomic position is not considered a part of CTV. The CTV is anatomically defined with a 1 cm margin around GTV. The PTV is not anatomically assigned and is a geometric expansion of 3–5 mm depending on institutional protocol. Care has to be taken to contour and minimize dose to critical structure such as brainstem, bilateral cochlea pituitary gland and hypothalamus.

Choroid Plexus Tumors

Epidemiology

These are rare intraventricular brain tumors, constituting less than 2% of all glial tumors. They are mostly found in the lateral ventricles in children, and in the fourth ventricle in adults. The benign variety is called Choroid Plexus Papilloma (CPP), and the malignant variety is Choroid Plexus Carcinoma (CPC). Atypical choroid plexus papilloma falls intermediate in the continuum of choroid plexus tumors. It is distinguished from the choroid plexus papilloma by increased mitotic activity. Curative surgery is still possible but the probability of recurrence is significantly higher.

Pathology and Biology

Due to CSF overproduction and obstruction of CSF flow, the chief symptom of choroid plexus tumors is hydrocephalus. Dissemination through CSF pathways is common, more so for choroid plexus carcinomas. Histologically, CPPs closely resemble the normal choroid plexus, with a fibrovascular core, covered with modified ependymal cells. Cytokeratin, vimentin, transthretin and S-100 are variably present in both CPPs and CPCs. Ki-67 index for CPPs is around 2%, while that for CPCs is around 13%.[37] CPCs have been reported in association with Li-Fraumeni syndrome with a p53 germline mutation and have a tendency to occur in families with malignant rhabdoid tumor predisposition.

Presentation

They mainly present with signs and symptoms of increased intracranial pressure and hydrocephalus. Intraventricular location on CT/MRI is typical. Neuraxis staging (CSF studies and MRI Spine) is recommended.

Treatment

Surgical resection is the mainstay of treatment. Completely excised CPPs with no evidence of neuraxial dissemination need no further treatment. CPPs with neuraxial dissemination and all CPCs require craniospinal irradiation or adjuvant chemotherapy. 5 years survival for gross totally excised CPPs is 80–95%[38] while that for CPCs is approximately 40 %.[38,39]

Other Neuroepithelial Tumors

Angiocentric glioma: It is mainly a tumor of children and young adults, mean age at surgery being 17 years. Presentation is most commonly as refractory epilepsy. Tumors are mostly located superficially in the frontoparietal cortex or in the temporal/hippocampal area. Although they may extend to the ventricular wall and have features of ependymal differentiation, the predominant clinical symptoms, cortical location, architectural pattern and outcome were considered insufficient to designate, this entity as an ependymoma variant. It behaves as a benign tumor and is amenable to cure by surgical excision alone. It is thus classified as a WHO Grade I tumor.

Neuronal and Mixed Neuronal-Glial Tumors

Ganglioglioma and Anaplastic Ganglioglioma

Ganglioglioma is an "astroglial" form of low grade glioma containing both glial and neuronal elements (other such tumors are pilocytic astrocytoma, pleomorphic xanthoastrocytoma, and subependymal giant cell astrocytoma). It is classified as WHO Grade I or II. Surgery alone is curative.

Radiation therapy is reserved for residual or recurrent cases. Anaplastic ganglioglioma is a higher grade tumour and is better treated with surgery and adjuvant radiation therapy.

Central Neurocytoma and Extraventricular Neurocytoma

Central neurocytoma is a neuronal tumor with pathological features distinct from cerebral neuroblastoma, occurring in young adults, with preferential location in the lateral ventricles in the region of the foramen of Monro and a generally favorable prognosis. Neoplasms occurring in brain parenchyma outside the ventricular system with similar biological behavior and histopathological characteristics are called 'extraventricular neurocytoma'.

MENINGIOMAS

Meningiomas comprise 1–30% of all primary intracranial tumors and are most common in adults in their 4th–6th decades of life and are rare in children.[40] They are extra-axial CNS tumors that originate from the meninges which protect and covers the outer surface of the brain and spinal cord. Most of them (90%) occur in the supratentorial compartment.[41] Reported associated risk factors are past history of ionizing radiation, genetic predisposition like multiple endocrine neoplasia type 1 (MEN1), neurofibromatosis type 2 (NF2) and deletion of chromosome 22, progesterone and estrogen receptors and females with history of breast cancer.

Anatomy

Meningiomas are usually located in cerebral convexity, falx cerebri/parasagittal sinus, sphenoid wing, base of skull, and posterior fossa. Approximately, 90% occur intracranially, and the remaining 10% occur in the spine.

Pathology

Meningiomas arise from the epithelial cells of the arachnoid villi. Microscopically, they have a bland, whorled appearance, with or without psammoma bodies and macroscopically, they are well circumscribed, firm and gray. Histological types are transitional, fibrous, clear cell, chondroid, rhabdoid, and angiomatous. The tumors are graded according to the WHO classification.[1]

World Health Organization Grading of Meningioma

Grade I (Benign meningiomas): Slow-growing tumors with well-defined borders, not invading the adjacent brain parenchyma, and with low mitotic index (90% of all meningiomas).

Grade II (Atypical meningiomas): Mitotic index > 4 mitosis per 10 high-power field (HPF), 5–7% of all meningiomas. Variant of chondroid and clear cell are included.

Grade III (Malignant meningiomas): These tumors have the highest mitotic index (> 20 per 10 HPF) and form 1–3% of all meningiomas. Papillary and rhabdoid variants are considered malignant meningiomas.

Diagnosis

Benign meningiomas are usually asymptomatic and often discovered as incidental findings on a head CT or brain magnetic resonance images. For other variants, signs and symptoms depend on their location of origin. On CT scan, they appear as well-circumscribed extra-axial space occupying lesions, and with homogenous contrast enhancement. On MRI, they are isointense on T1-weighted sequence and isointense to hyperintense on T2 with homogenous contrast enhancement. Dural tail of enhancement is due to the migration of cells along dura is characteristic but is not pathognomonic. Malignant meningiomas are aggressive in nature, and are prone to recur after surgery.

Treatment

Treatment of choice is surgical resection and GTR is attempted as definitive treatment for all benign meningiomas (Table 4). With STR, recurrence rate is higher and outcomes are poorer. They are highly vascular and selected cases are considered for angiography and embolization. Unresectable cases or cases with anticipated high-risk of morbidity with aggressive resection, surgeons must weigh the risks of surgical morbidity of a GTR against the risk of local recurrence with incomplete resection.

Table 4 Simpson grading of surgical resection and corresponding recurrence rates[42]

Simpson grade	*Extent of resection*	*Recurrence rate (%)*
I	Complete tumor resection and removal of dural attachments and abnormal bone	9%
II	Complete tumor resection and coagulation of dural attachment	19%
III	Complete tumor resection without removal or coagulation or dural attachment or extradural extensions	29%
IV	Partial tumor resection	40%
V	Decompression with or without biopsy	NA

Surgical Resection

Approximately, one-third are unresectable or incompletely resected due to large size or due to location (skull base, cavernous sinus, CPA). Surgical resection involves resection of tumor, any involved dura mater, soft tissue or bone. Most of the tumors in the cerebral convexity or parasagittal falx region will have GTR, whereas tumors in the clivus, cavernous sinus, sella, sphenoid ridge, posterior fossa and CPA carry a higher risk of morbidity if GTR is attempted. It is often difficult to achieve GTR for grade II and III tumors because of involvement of dura mater or brain invasion.

Radiation Therapy

Adjuvant RT is recommended after STR of benign meningioma and for all atypical or malignant variant. As a definitive treatment, radiation therapy is indicated for unresectable or recurrent tumors and optic nerve sheath meningiomas (ONSMs).[43]

Maximal safe surgical resection is the primary treatment for benign meningioma. They recur locally and the local recurrence rate after surgery alone for benign type is approximately 20–25% at 10 years with complete surgical resection and 60% with STR. Adjuvant radiation has resulted in improved local control and PFS rates for cases with STR.[44,45] Atypical and malignant meningiomas are relatively more aggressive and they recur more frequently after complete or incomplete resections. Adjuvant radiation is indicated in all these cases after GTR or STR.[46-48] For unresectable meningiomas or if a patient refuses or cannot undergo surgery, external-beam radiation can be used for definitive treatment. Recurrent tumors after surgery may be treated with definitive or adjuvant radiation. The prognosis for both unresectable and recurrent tumors is relatively less favorable. ONSMs, constitute 1–2% of all meningiomas, are typically treated with radiation, which may retain or improve vision (Figs 6A to D).[49,50]

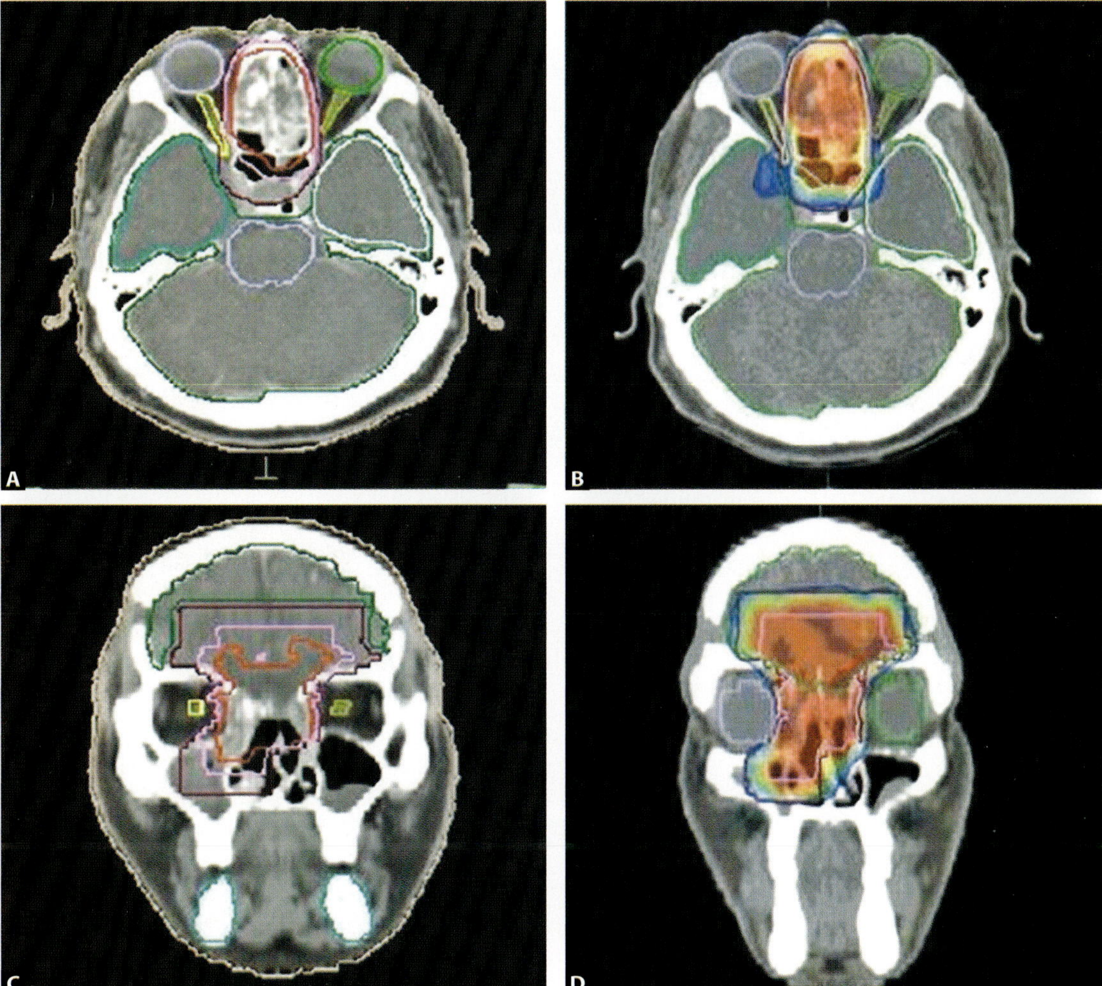

Figs 6A to D Target volumes and dose distribution in grade 2 meningioma after subtotal resection

Courtesy: Dr Tejinder Kataria, Division of Radiation Oncology, Medanta—The Medicity, Haryana, India

Target Volume Delineation (RTOG 0539)

Gross tumor volume

CT simulation is done in supine position with proper head immobilization and fused with a diagnostic T1-weighted MRI for better target delineation. The GTV for benign histologies (WHO Grade I) includes the postoperative residual tumor only and for atypical and malignant meningioma (i.e. WHO grade II and III), GTV should include enhancement plus the entire tumor bed on the preoperative MRI.[51] The "dural tail" or edema component are not included within the GTV.[53]

Clinical target volume

Grade 1 with STR/grade 2 with GTR/recurrent grade 1: CTV54 is GTV plus a margin of 1.0 cm all around. The CTV54 margin may be reduced to 0.5 cm around natural anatomical barriers to tumor growth such as the skull. PTV54 is an additional margin of 5.0 mm around the CTV 54.

Grade 2 meningioma with STR/recurrent grade 2/grade 3: CTV54 is GTV with a margin of 2.0 cm all around. CTV60 is GTV with a margin of 1.0 cm. CTV54 margin is reduced to 1 cm (thus corresponding to the PTV60) around natural barriers to tumor growth such as the skull and the PTV margin is 5.0 mm.

For stereotactic radiosurgery (SRS), the contrast-enhancing tumor (GTV) is treated without any margin.

Treatment planning technique

Intensity-modulated radiation therapy is the preferred technique to minimize toxicities to various critical structures including the optic pathway, eyes, brain stem, and normal brain parenchyma. If 3DCRT technique is used, goals can be better achieved by using multiple non-coplanar beams.

Dose and treatment delivery

Recommended doses and organ at risk constraints (Table 5):

- Grade 1 with STR/grade 2 with GTR/recurrent grade 1: 54 Gy in 30 fractions
- Grade 2 with STR/recurrent grade 2/grade 3: 60 Gy in 30 fractions
- Optic nerve sheath meningioma: 50–54 Gy in 25–30 fractions.[52]
- Stereotactic radiosurgery: 15–20 Gy for meningiomas not close to critical structures 12–20 Gy in 1 fraction and 12 Gy for tumors close to critical structures such as the brain stem.[49-51]

Toxicities

Common acute toxicities associated with radiation for meningioma may be fatigue, focal alopecia, and skin erythema. Rare toxicities include encephalomalacia, cerebrovascular events, cranial neuropathies, cerebral or brainstem necrosis, second malignancies and edema. Irradiation for ONSM carries a risk of cataracts, eye dryness, orbital pain, visual defects or pituitary dysfunction.

Follow-up

Routine follow-up is important after definitive treatment because of the risk of local recurrence. MRI of the brain should be performed every 3–4 months for the first 2 years, every 6 months for the next 3 years, then annually.

G Lymphomas and Hematopoietic Neoplasms

Malignant Lymphomas

Epidemiology: Primary CNS lymphomas (PCNSL) comprise <3% of primary intracranial malignancies. Immunodeficiency, either congenital or acquired (organ transplant or HIV disease), is the only known risk factor for the development of primary CNS lymphoma. Immunocompromised individuals present with this disease at a younger age (3rd to 4th decade) than immunocompetent individuals (6th to 7th decade).

Pathology: Most PCNSL are B-cell lymphomas of intermediate or high grade. It is essential to prove the absence of a systemic lymphomatous process to label the disease as a primary CNS lymphoma. Imaging appearance on MRI is of intensely enhancing, solitary or multiple periventricular masses in the cerebral hemispheres, or sometimes in the meninges, vitreous or retina. CSF involvement is common. Primary intraocular lymphoma is associated with the subsequent development of CNS lymphoma in up to 80% of patients.

Presentation: The symptoms and signs of CNS lymphoma are those of any intracranial mass lesion. An open or stereotactic

Table 5 Recommended dose constraints[51]

Organ at risk	*Dose (Gy)*	*End point*	*Rate (%)*
Brainstem	D_{max} < 54 (1–10 cc < 59)	Permanent neuropathy	< 5%
Optic nerve/chiasm	D_{max} < 55	Optic neuropathy	< 3%
Optic nerves/chiasm	D_{max} 55–60	Optic neuropathy	3–7%
Retina	D_{max} < 50	Blindness	< 1%
Cochlea	Mean dose < 45	Sensorineural hearing loss	< 30%

biopsy helps attain tissue diagnosis and to rule out other primary or metastatic tumors. Immunohistochemical analysis determines B- versus T-cell type. Staging investigations include an ophthalmologic assessment to rule out ocular involvement, CSF cytology, complete blood count, Epstein-Barr virus, and HIV serology. Systemic staging (CT of chest and abdomen, bone marrow biopsy) should be performed if systemic symptoms are present (weight loss, night sweats, fever).

Treatment: Surgical excision is not warranted. Tissue diagnosis is obtained by means of a stereotactic biopsy. It is prudent to avoid giving corticosteroids prior to obtaining tissue sample as the disease often responds remarkably to steroids, and may lead to difficulty in tissue diagnosis later. Mainstay of treatment is whole brain radiation therapy to doses of 40–45 Gy in non-immunocompromised patients, along with systemic chemotherapy. High dose methotrexate, Cytosine Arabinoside, cyclophosphamide, doxorubicin, and vincristine are some chemotherapy agents effective in treating PCNSL. In patients with ocular involvement, the whole eye should be treated to 30–40 Gy, with shielding of the anterior chamber and lacrimal apparatus after this dose. CSI has been advocated for patients with documented CSF involvement. However, intrathecal chemotherapy may be equally efficacious and less toxic, with less impact on bone marrow reserve. The combination of radiation and chemotherapy may be superior to radiation alone; 5-year survival rates are 22%–40% compared with 3%–26% with radiotherapy alone.

Germ Cell Tumors

Epidemiology: CNS Germ cell tumors are rare tumors of adults and children, with a male preponderance.

Pathology: These tumors are broadly classified as Germinomatous and Non-germinomatous germ cell tumors. Germinoma, like its extra-CNS counterpart, seminoma, is highly radio- and chemo-sensitive. Nongerminomatous germ cell tumors (including embryonal carcinoma, yolk sac tumor, choriocarcinoma, and teratoma) are less sensitive to therapy. Mixed germ cell tumors exhibit both germinomatous and non-germinomatous components. All germ cell tumors have propensity for neuraxial dissemination.

Presentation: These are often midline tumors and may present with obstructive symptoms, and signs of raised intracranial pressure. MRI brain with contrast and neuraxial staging (CSF studies and MRI spine) is recommended. Serum and CSF alpha-fetoprotein and beta-human chorionic gonadotropin (β-hCG) are important for diagnostic and staging purpose, and to decide about line of management.

Treatment: For disseminated disease, chemotherapy agents may be tried initially, which include carboplatin/etoposide combination or ifosfamide/etoposide combination. In the event of favorable response, this is followed by craniospinal irradiation up to 24–36 Gy, and focal boost up to 45–54 Gy, using a 1 cm CTV. Those with a partial response may be considered for second line chemotherapy or surgery. For localized disease, whole ventricle irradiation to 24–30 Gy, followed by boost up to 45–50 Gy should be sufficient.[54]

REFERENCES

1. Louis DN, Ohgaki H, Wiestler OD, (Eds). et al. WHO Classification of Tumours of the Central Nervous System. Lyon: IARC; 2007.
2. Pan E, Prados MD. Familial Tumors Syndromes of the Central Nervous system. In: Kufe DW, Pollock RE, Weichselbaum RR, Bast RC, Gansler TS, Holland JF, Frei E (Eds). Holland-Frei Cancer Medicine, 6th edn. Hamilton: BC Decker; 2003.
3. Gupta K, Salunke P. Molecular markers of glioma: an update on recent progress and perspectives. J Cancer Res Clin Oncol. 2012;138(12):1971-81.
4. Claus EB, Horlacher A, Hsu L, Schwartz RB, Dello-Iacono D, Talos F, et al. Survival rates in patients with low-grade glioma.
5. Berger MS, Deliganis AV, Dobbins J, et al. The effect of extent of resection on recurrence in patients with low grade cerebral hemisphere gliomas. Cancer. 1994;74(6):1784-91.
6. Pignatti F, van den Bent M, Curran D, Debruyne C, Sylvester R, Therasse P, et al. Prognostic factors for survival in adult patients with cerebral low-grade glioma. J Clin Oncol. 2002; 20(8):2076-84.
7. Karim AB, Maat B, Hatlevoll R, Menten J, Rutten EH, Thomas DG, et al. A randomized trial on dose-response in radiation therapy of low-grade cerebral glioma: European Organization for Research and Treatment of Cancer (EORTC) Study 22844. Int J Radiat Oncol Biol Phys. 1996;36(3):549-56.
8. Shaw EG, Wang M, Coons SW, Brachman DG, Buckner JC, Stelzer KJ, et al. Randomized trial of radiation therapy plus procarbazine, lomustine, and vincristine chemotherapy for supratentorial adult low-grade glioma: Initial results of RTOG 9802. J Clin Oncol. 2012:30(25):3065-70.
9. Weller M, Felsberg J, Hartmann C, Berger H, Steinbach JP, Schramm J, et al. Molecular predictors of progression-free and overall survival in patients with newly diagnosed glioblastoma: a prospective translational study of the German Glioma Network. J Clin Oncol. 2009;27(34):5742-50.
10. Curran WJ, Scott CB, Horton J, Nelson JS, Weinstein AS, Fischbach AJ, et al. Recursive partitioning analysis of prognostic factors in three radiation therapy oncology group malignant glioma trials. J Natl Cancer Inst. 1993;85(9):704-10.
11. Stupp R, Hegi ME, Mason WP, van den Bent MJ, Taphoorn MJ, Janzer RC, et al. Effects of radiotherapy with concomitant and adjuvant temozolomide versus radiotherapy alone on survival in glioblastoma in a randomized phase III study: 5-year analysis of the EORTC-NCIC trial. Lancet Oncol. 2009;10(5):459-66.

12. Amundson EW, McGirt MJ, Olivi A. A contralateral, transfrontal, extraventricular approach to stereotactic brainstem biopsy procedures. Technical note. J Neurosurg. 2005;102:565-7.
13. Cairncross G, Berkey B, Shaw E, et al. Intergroup Radiation Therapy Oncology Group Trial 9402, Phase III trial of chemotherapy plus radiotherapy compared with radiotherapy alone for pure and mixed anaplastic oligodendroglioma: Intergroup Radiation Therapy Oncology Group trial 9402. J Clin Oncol. 2006;24(18):2707-14.
14. Albert FK, Forsting M, Sartor K, et al. Early postoperative magnetic resonance imaging after resection of malignant glioma: objective evaluation of residual tumour and it influence on regrowth and prognosis. Neurosurgery. 1994;34(1):45-60.
15. McGirt MJ, Chaichana KL, Gathinji M. Independent association of extent of resection with survival in patients with malignant brain astrocytoma. J Neurosurg. 2009;110(1):156-62.
16. Stummer W, Pichlmeier U, Meinel T, Wiestler OD, Zanella F, Reulen HJ. Fluorescence guided surgery with 5-aminolevulinic acid for resection of malignant glioma: a randomized controlled multicenter phase III trial. Lancet Oncol. 2006;7(5):392-401.
17. Engelhard HH. The role of interstitial BCNU chemotherapy in the treatment of malignant glioma. Surg Neurol. 2000; 53(5):458-64.
18. Walker MD, Alexander E, Hunt WE, MacCarty CS, Mahaley MS, Mealey J, et al. Evaluation of BCNU and/or radiotherapy in the treatment of anaplastic gliomas. A cooperative clinical trial. J Neurosurg. 1978;49(3):333-43.
19. Tofts PS, Kermode AG. Measurement of the blood-brain barrier permeability and leakage space using dynamic MR imaging. 1. Fundamental concepts. Magn Reson Med. 1991;17(2):357-67.
20. Perry J, Zuraw L. For the Neuro-Oncology Disease Site Group. Adjuvant systemic chemotherapy, following surgery and external beam radiotherapy, for adults with newly diagnosed malignant glioma: a clinical practice guideline. Evidence-based series 9-2. Section 1. Toronto: Cancer Care Ontario; March 2004, updated May 2006.
21. Muacevic A, Kreth FW. Quality-adjusted survival after tumor resection and/or radiation therapy for elderly patients with glioblastoma multiforme. J Neurol. 2003;250(5):561-8.
22. Phillips C, Guiney M, Smith J, Hughes P, Narayan K, Quong G. A randomized trial comparing 35 Gy in ten fractions with 60 Gy in 30 fractions of cerebral irradiation for glioblastoma multiforme and older patients with anaplastic astrocytoma. Radiother Oncol. 2003;68(1):23-6.
23. Wallner KE, Sheline GE, Pitts LH, Wara WM, Davis RL, Boldrey EB. Efficacy of irradiation for incompletely excised acoustic neurilemomas. J Neurosurg. 1987;67(6):858-63.
24. Kleihues P, Cavenee WK (Eds). WHO Classification of Tumors Pathology and Genetics of Tumours of Nervous System. Lyon: IARC Press; 2000.
25. Macdonald J. Advances in imaging techniques in neuroendocrine tumors: miscellaneous papers of interest. Curr Opin Oncol. 1990;2(1):117-8.
26. Rogers L, Pueschel J, Spetzler R, Shapiro W, Coons S, Thomas T, et al. Is gross-total resection sufficient treatment for posterior fossa ependymomas? J Neurosurg. 2005;102(4):629-36.
27. Paulino AC, Wen BC, Buatti JM, Hussey DH, Zhen WK, Mayr NA, et al. Intracranial ependymomas: an analysis of prognostic factors and patterns of failure. Am J Clin Oncol. 2002; 25(2):117-22.
28. Shaw EG, Evans RG, Scheithauer BW, et al. Postoperative radiotherapy of intracranial ependymoma in pediatric and adult patients. Int J Radiat Oncol Biol Phys. 1987;13(10):1457-62.
29. Merchant TE, Jenkins JJ, Burger PC, Sanford RA, Sherwood SH, Jones-Wallace D, et al. Influence of tumor grade on time to progression after irradiation for localized ependymoma in children. Int J Radiat Oncol Biol Phys. 2002;53(1):52-7.
30. Mansur DB, Perry A, Rajaram V, Michalski JM, Park TS, Leonard JR, et al. Postoperative radiation therapy for grade II and III intracranial ependymoma. Int J Radiat Oncol Biol Phys. 2005;61(2):387-91.
31. Taylor RE. Review of radiotherapy dose and volume for intracranial ependymoma. Pediatr Blood Cancer. 2004; 42(5):457-60.
32. Merchant TE, Fouladi M. Ependymoma: new therapeutic approaches including radiation and chemotherapy. J Neurooncol. 2005;75(3):287-99.
33. Merchant TE. Current management of childhood ependymoma. Oncology (Williston Park). 2002;16(5):629-42, 644; discussion 645-6, 648.
34. Duffner PK, Horowitz ME, Krischer JP, Friedman HS, Burger PC, Cohen ME, et al. Postoperative chemotherapy and delayed radiation in children less than three years of age with malignant brain tumors. N Engl J Med. 1993;328(24):1725-31.
35. Merchant TE, Mulhern RK, Krasin MJ, Kun LE, Williams T, Li C, et al. Preliminary results from a phase II trial of conformal radiation therapy and evaluation of radiation-related CNS effects for pediatric patients with localized ependymoma. J Clin Oncol. 2004;22(15):3156-62.
36. Merchant TE, Li C, Xiong X, Kun LE, Boop FA, Sanford RA. Conformal radiotherapy after surgery for paediatric ependymoma: a prospective study. Lancet Oncol. 2009;10(3):258-66.
37. Rickert CH, Paulus W. Tumours of the choroid plexus. Micros Res Tech 52:104,2001.
38. Krishnan S, Brown PD, Scheithauer BW, et al. Choroid Plexus papillomas: a single institution experience. J Neuro-oncol 68: 49,2004.
39. Wolff JE, Sajedi M, Brant R, et al. Choroid plexus tumours. Br J Cancer 87:1086,2002.
40. Longstreth WT, Dennis LK, McGuire VM, et al. Epidemiology of intracranial meningioma. Cancer. 1993;72(3):639-48.
41. Bondy M, Ligon BL. Epidemiology and etiology of intracranial meningiomas: a review. J Neurooncol. 1996;29(3):197-205.
42. Simpson D. The recurrence of intracranial meningiomas after surgical treatment. J Neurol Neurosurg Psychiatry. 1957:20(1):22-39.
43. Glaholm J, Bloom HJ, Crow JH. The role of radiotherapy in the management of intracranial meningiomas: the Royal Marsden Hospital experience with 186 patients. Int J Radiat Oncol Biol Phys. 1990;18(4):755-61.

44. Soyuer S, Chang EL, Selek U, Shi W, Maor MH, DeMonte F. Radiotherapy after surgery for benign cerebral meningioma. Radiat Oncol. 2004:71(1):85-90.
45. Goldsmith BJ, Wara WM, Wilson CB, et al. Postoperative irradiation for subtotally resected meningiomas. A retrospective analysis of 140 patients treated from 1967 to 1990. J Neurosurg. 1994;80(2):195-201.
46. Condra KS, Buatti JM, Mendenhall WM, Friedman WA, Marcus RB Jr, Rhoton AL. Benign meningiomas: primary treatment selection affects survival. Int J Radiat Oncol Biol Phys. 1997:39(2):427-36.
47. Glaholm J, Bloom HJ, Crow JH. The role of radiotherapy in the management of intracranial meningiomas: the Royal Marsden Hospital experience with 186 patients. Int J Radiat Oncol Biol Phys. 1990:18(4):755-61.
48. Taylor BW, Marcus RB, Friedman WA, et al. The meningioma controversy: postoperative radiation therapy. Int J Radiat Oncol Biol Phys. 1988;15(2):299-304.
49. Lo SL, Chang EL, Suh JH. Recent advances in therapeutic radiation: an overview. In: Lee JH (Ed). Meningiomas—Diagnosis, Treatment and Outcomes. Berlin Heidelberg New York: Springer; 2008. pp. 253-8.
50. Simon SL, Tinnel B, Suh JH. Conventional radiation for meningiomas. In: Lee JH (Ed). Meningiomas—Diagnosis, Treatment and Outcomes. Berlin Heidelberg New York: Springer; 2008. pp. 259-65.
51. Lawrence YR, Li XA, el Naqa I, Hahn CA, Marks LB, Merchant TE, et al. Radiation dose-volume effects in the brain. Int J Radiat Oncol Biol Phys. 2010;76(3 Suppl):S20-7.
52. Lo SL, Chao S, Suh JH. 3D Conformal RT. In: Jeremic B, Pitz S (Eds). Optic Nerve Sheath Meningioma. Berlin Heidelberg New York: Springer; 2008. pp. 85-94.
53. Miralbell R, Linggood RM, de la Monte S, Convery K, Munzenrider JE, Mirimanoff RO. The role of radiotherapy in the treatment of subtotally resected benign meningiomas. J Neurooncol. 1992;13(2):157-64.
54. Shirato H, Aoyama H, Ikeda J, ET AL. Impact of margin for target volume in low-dose involved field radiotherapy after induction chemotherapy for intracranial germinoma. Int J Radiat Oncol Biol Phys 60:214-217, 2004.

10 CHAPTER

Surgical Management of Head and Neck Cancer

Ajay Kumar Dewan, Abhinav Dewan

"Decisions are more important than incisions."

INTRODUCTION

Worldwide there were 6,86,328 new cases of head and neck cancers diagnosed and 3,75,665 deaths reported in year 2012.[1] Incidence is more than twice (ratio 2:1 to 4:1) in men than in women.[2] Oral cavity cancer is the most common type of head and neck cancer with 240,000 cases diagnosed every year. Oral cancer has the highest incidence in Western Europe, India, South Africa and Australia.[3] Cancer of the tongue and buccal mucosa are quite common in India, mostly attributable to local customs of chewing *pan* and betel leaf with tobacco.[4] Smokeless tobacco and areca nut chewing have important therapeutic implications.

There is little good quality evidence to help define the optimal treatment of each tumor subsite. A large number of nonrandomized single center case series report the local control, survival and morbidity rates associated with both surgical resection and radiotherapy (RT), but this evidence is not of sufficient quality to support a clear recommendation regarding the best modality for treating the primary tumor in each subsite. Surgery may be the treatment of choice if the primary tumor can be excised with an appropriate margin of normal tissue without resulting in major functional compromise given the lack of good quality evidence. The choice of definitive local therapy must take into account the following factors:

- Likely functional outcome of treatment
- Resectability of tumor
- Performance status and associated comorbidities
- Patient's preference.

PRINCIPLES OF SURGICAL TREATMENT

The aim of treatment is to maximize locoregional control and survival with minimal resulting functional damage. The most important functions that must be considered when planning treatment are swallowing, respiration and speech.[5]

Cancers of head and neck should be managed by a multidisciplinary team. The team should include a radiation oncologist, head and neck cancer surgeon, pathologist, medical oncologist, dental surgeon (prosthodontist), reconstructive and plastic surgeon, speech and swallowing therapist, dietician, physiotherapist, counselor and head and neck specialist nurse if available. Treatment plans should be formulated by the multidisciplinary team in consultation with the patient. As part of this process, dental, speech and nutritional assessments are essential.

- Whenever possible, surgery for a primary head and neck cancer should preserve organ function.
- Whenever necessary, resection should be followed by reconstruction using the most appropriate techniques.
- Nonsurgical treatment like RT with or without chemotherapy (CT) should be offered to patients if survival rates are comparable with that of surgical resection.
- Salvage surgery must be available if an organ preservation approach is to be pursued.
- Following resection; adjuvant RT and CT should be considered wherever indicated.[5]

The main aim of surgery is to excise the area of malignancy ensuring that a margin of normal tissue surrounding the tumor is also removed and that radical excision is performed with curative intent. Access to the hidden recesses of head and neck is essential to excise the tumor and perform surgical reconstruction. Various approaches to tumors include open/conventional; minimally invasive approaches incorporating endoscopes or robotic arms. There are no randomized controlled trials (RCTs) comparing different resection techniques in the tumor subsites. If an inadequate initial excision has been performed or tumor has been excised with positive margins, re-resection should be considered.

In early stage head and neck cancer, surgery is preferred over RT as a single modality in:

- Young patients due to high incidence of second primary cancer.
- In presence of submucous fibrosis.
- Lesions involving or close to bone/mandible.
- Sites where surgery is not morbid (cosmetically and functionally).

Criteria of Unresectability

Primary Disease

- Adequate surgical access is not achievable.
- Extensive infratemporal fossa/skull base involvement.
- *Extensive soft tissue disease:* Satellite nodules/Brawny induration.

Nodal Disease

- Clinically fixed nodes.
- Infiltration of internal/common carotid artery.
- Extensive infiltration of prevertebral muscles/skull base.

SURGERY OF PRIMARY LESION

Lip: Surgical treatment for early lesion (0.5–1.5 cm) uses a V- or W-shaped excision, depending on the size of the defect, which facilitates cosmetic primary closure. If the vermilion is diffusely involved with little or no involvement of the muscle, a vermilionectomy may be performed and the mucosa from the labial vestibule of the oral cavity advanced to cover the defect.[6]

Floor of mouth: Small lesions (≤0.5 cm in size) may be excised transorally with a 1 cm margin with primary closure or a skin graft. If the submandibular duct is involved, the submandibular gland and duct are removed in continuity. Rim resection of the mandible in continuity with excision of the primary lesion preserves the arch and may be combined with postoperative RT.[6] Periosteal invasion is often an indication for this procedure. Partial segmental mandibulectomy with resection of the floor of the mouth is done through a lip-splitting incision or by using a visor flap. The primary lesion and neck specimen are removed in continuity. An osteomyocutaneous flap is usually used to repair the defect. For lesions of the anterior floor of mouth, a full-thickness resection of the anterior mandible (arch) may be required.[6]

Oral tongue: For early lesions (T1 or T2), partial glossectomy and primary closure is performed. Advanced (≥T3) deeply infiltrative lesions are managed by partial or total glossectomy followed by adjuvant treatment.[6] RT failure is managed by surgery. Surgical failure occasionally is salvaged by re-resection.

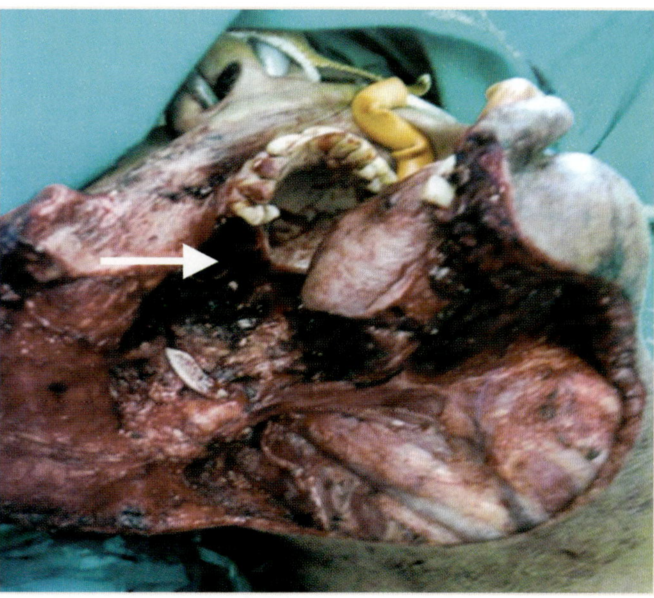

Fig. 1 Composite resection of buccal mucosa with infratemporal fossa clearance (arrow depicting the infratemporal fossa)

Buccal mucosa: Lesions that invade the mandible or maxilla require resection of the bone alongwith the soft tissues. A myocutaneous flap repairs full-thickness defect of the cheek (Fig. 1).

Alveolus: For discrete T1-T2 carcinomas with minimal cortical bone invasion, at least 1 cm of the inferior border of the mandible is preserved, thereby maintaining its biomechanical integrity. For lesions with transcortical bone invasion into the medullary space, a segment of the mandible is removed in continuity with the tumor. Massive anterior lesion may necessitate removal of the mandible from angle to angle; tumors that invade the mandible posterior to the angle may require condylar resection. Reconstruction is ideally accomplished with a revascularized osteomyocutaneous flap.[6] Salvage procedures frequently are not attempted because of the advanced nature of the recurrence and the low chance of cure.

Oropharynx: The occasional patient with a low volume T1 or early T2 cancer may be suitable for transoral laser excision or robotic surgery (Fig. 2) in combination with a neck dissection. Historically the surgical approach requires an incision that splits the lip and mandibulotomy, which permits lateral rotation of the mandible. Suprahyoid, transhyoid, and infrahyoid approaches also can be used to resect small lesions. After the tumor has been removed, the mandibular edges are reapproximated and stabilized with a titanium plate. Only one lingual artery may be sacrificed.[7] Removal of a large tumor may require simultaneous removal of part or the entire larynx. Radiotherapy treatment failures are treated

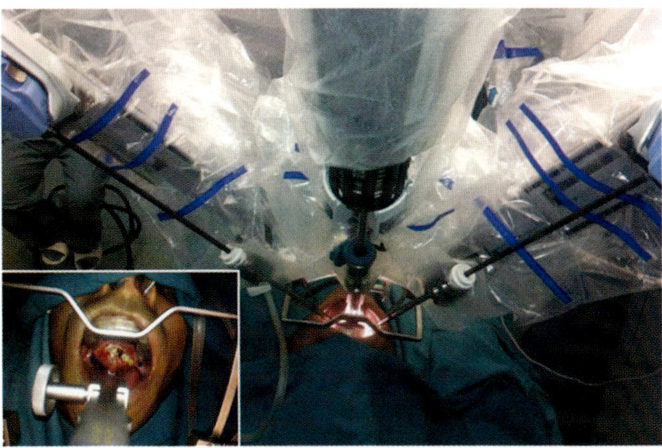

Fig. 2 Transoral robotic surgery (TORS) for oropharyngeal cancer

surgically; salvage is infrequent. Surgical treatment failures are rarely salvaged.

Larynx: For early vocal cord lesion (T1, T2), RT is the treatment of choice with surgery reserved for salvage of RT failure. Open partial laryngectomy also produces comparable cure rates for selected T1 or T2 vocal cord lesions. Endoscopic transoral laser resection is increasingly being used nowadays.[6] Open partial laryngectomy or total laryngectomy may be used as a salvage operation after RT failure. Verrucous carcinomas are treated with transoral laser resection or open partial laryngectomy. Cordectomy is used for well-defined lesions of the middle third of the vocal cord. Hemilaryngectomy or partial laryngectomy allows removal of limited cord lesion with voice preservation. In supraglottic laryngectomy, the arytenoids and true vocal cords are preserved. If one of the arytenoids is sacrificed, the vocal cord is fixed in the midline to prevent aspiration.

The last surgical alternative is total laryngectomy with or without a neck dissection. The entire larynx is removed, the pharynx is reconstituted, and a permanent tracheostoma is created. There are several options to accomplish voice rehabilitation after total laryngectomy. Prosthetic devices (e.g. the Blom-Singer voice prosthesis) have been developed for insertion into a tracheoesophageal fistula which permits the patients to speak without aspiration.[6]

Hypopharynx: For posterior pharyngeal wall, if the lesion is high on the posterior wall, a transoral approach can be used. Lower lesions can be accessed via a transhyoid approach, a lateral pharyngotomy, or a midline mandibulolabial glossectomy. More recently, transoral laser microsurgical resection has been employed to reduce the morbidity.[6]

Pyriform sinus: Partial laryngopharyngectomy removes the false cords, epiglottis, aryepiglottic fold, and pyriform sinus; one arytenoid may be removed when necessary. The vocal cords are preserved. Total laryngopharyngectomy removes the larynx and varying amounts of pharyngeal wall.[6] Advanced lesions require excision of nearly the entire circumference of pharynx. The continuity of pharynx is re-established by primary closure after a partial pharyngectomy or reconstruction with a pectoralis major myocutaneous flap or radial forearm free flap. If the lesion extends into the cervical esophagus, a gastric pull up or jejunal free flap may be necessary.

Nasopharynx: The treatment of nasopharyngeal cancer is RT based because complete surgical resection is usually not feasible. Neck dissection is used less often in the management of neck disease because of the relatively high success rate with RT or chemoradiation.

Nasal cavity and paranasal sinuses: Surgery alone is preferred for the occasional very small lesion of nose. Excision of lesions in the nasal vestibule usually involves removal of cartilage as well as skin. If the alar cartilage has been sacrificed, either a composite graft consisting of skin and cartilage from the ear or a nasolabial flap can be used to repair the defect. If the entire external nose is resected, a prosthesis is used.[6]

Surgery for maxillary sinus carcinoma depends on which walls are involved. If the floor of the orbit is free of disease, then the eye and orbital rim may be left undisturbed. If, however, there is involvement through the orbital floor, then a maxillectomy with resection of the floor with or without an orbital exenteration must be performed. A split-thickness skin graft is used to line the cavity, and a removable dental prosthesis is then used to fill the resulting deformity in the palate. An interim prosthesis is constructed prior to surgery so it can be placed at the time of operation and act as a stent. The permanent prosthesis is constructed about 6 months after the operation.[6] Localized lesions of ethmoids require ethmoidectomy with or without the resection of ipsilateral maxilla and/or orbit. Extensive lesions require a craniofacial procedure. Minimally invasive surgical approach circumvents the need for craniotomy.

Temporal bone tumors: Excision is satisfactory for small lesions that can be removed without damage to normal structures. Stereotactic radiosurgery is an option for early lesions. Early lesions of the tympanic cavity can be managed successfully by excision without loss of hearing or vestibular function. For the glomus jugulare tumors, surgery is reserved for RT failure, in which case a radical mastoidectomy or a subtotal temporal bone resection would be required.[6] Some surgeons advocate a skull base approach.

Parotid tumor: Ideally, 1 cm circumferential cuff of "normal" parotid tissue should be resected along with the tumor. However, close margins of less than 1 mm are frequently encountered as most parotid gland tumors lie close to branches of the facial nerve (Fig. 3). In such cases, completely encapsulated tumors can frequently be resected

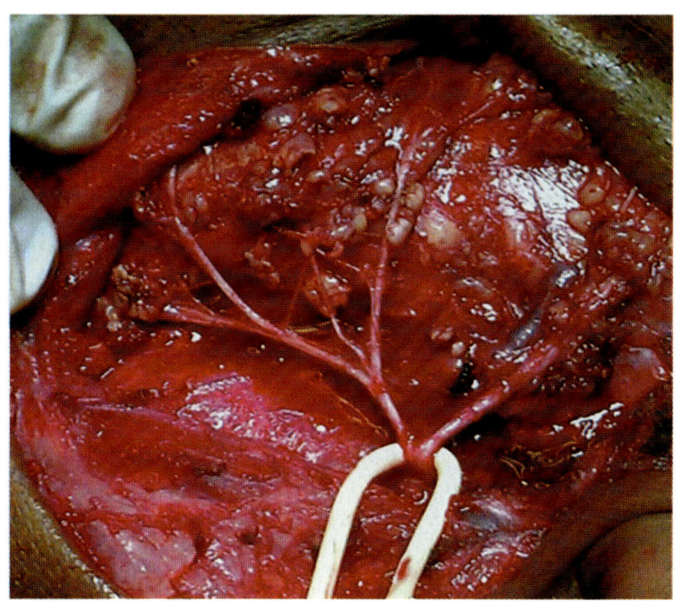

Fig. 3 Branches of facial nerve in total parotidectomy

with confidence. On the other hand, facial nerve passing through the tumor or when there is gross extracapsular extension in the parotid gland, the adequacy of resection is determined by frozen sections. The nerve is dissected free from the underlying deep lobe and the deep lobe and tumor are removed. The mandible may be divided to gain access to the retromandibular portion of the deep lobe. A partial mandibulectomy is required when the mandible is invaded by the tumor. A radical parotidectomy implies removal of the entire parotid, the facial nerve, and other involved tissues such as skin, bone or muscle.[6]

Salvage surgery: A meta-analysis of retrospective case series reported the weighted average of 5-year survival following salvage surgery for recurrent previously irradiated laryngeal, hypopharyngeal and oral cancers as 39% in 1,080 patients from 28 different institutions.[8] Disease-free survival following salvage surgery is not influenced by the modality (surgery or RT) used to treat the original tumor.[8] Following salvage surgery for head and neck cancer, the total complication rates vary from 39% to 53% (39–53%) with an operative mortality of 3.2–5.2%.[7,8] An increased rate of postoperative complications is seen with increasing stage of recurrent cancer.[7] Even the quality of life following salvage surgery correlates with the stage and not with the site of recurrence.[8]

Salvage surgery should be considered in any patient with a resectable locoregional recurrence of oral cavity, oropharynx, or hypopharyngeal cancer following previous radiation or surgery. Salvage surgery should be performed by an experienced team in centers with adequate facilities for medical support, reconstruction and rehabilitation.

Palliative surgery: Aim of palliative surgery is to debulk tumor mass, reduce symptoms like pain, bleeding and dyspnea associated with tumor growth. These procedures include tracheostomy, external carotid artery ligation, laser debulking, percutaneous endoscopic gastrostomy (PEG) and nerve blocks, etc. Appropriate surgical procedure should be considered for palliation of particular symptoms taking local expertise into consideration.[5]

Reconstruction: Extensive resection of soft tissue, bone and cartilage may leave a major physical defect that may not be repaired by primary closure.[5] Reconstruction aims to repair any physical deficit and restore or minimize functional deficit that would arise from the loss of resected tissue. Reconstruction techniques are diverse and vary by anatomical region. Free flap transfer is safe and reliable technique for reconstruction in head and neck cancer defects and is particularly useful for oral cavity and hypopharynx.[9-16] There is evidence that the free jejunal transfer is effective in swallowing but is poor for speech rehabilitation following hypopharyngeal resection.[17] Pectoralis major myocutaneous flap is suitable for elderly and frail patients.[18] Choice of reconstructive technique should be made on an individual basis for each patient, according to the tumor location, comorbidities and patient's and surgeon's preferences.

SURGICAL TREATMENT OF NECK

Neck dissection removes both soft tissues and neck nodes. A number of dissections have been described.[19,20]

- *Comprehensive neck dissection:*
  - *Radical neck dissection (RND):* All ipsilateral nodes from level I to V along with spinal accessory nerve, interior jugular vein and sternocleidomastoid muscle are removed.
  - *Modified neck dissection (MND):* As RND with preservation of one or more nonlymphatic structures.
- *Selective neck dissection:* One or more of lymphatic groups normally removed in RND are preserved. Nodes removed are based on the pattern of metastasis which are predictable of each site of the disease.[5]
- *Extended neck dissection:* Additional lymph node groups or nonlymphatic structures are removed.

MANAGEMENT OF N_0 NECK

Clinical and radiological examinations are unable to detect microscopic disease in lymph nodes. A study of computer-assisted decision analysis, using data from retrospective series has suggested that prophylactic treatment of neck is required if the risk of occult nodal metastasis is more than 20%.[21] Not adequately powered RCTs compare prophylactic treatment of N_0 neck with observation and therapeutic neck dissection.

There is a body of evidence from retrospective studies suggesting that in patients who do not have prophylactic therapy of the clinically N_0 neck, there is often a low salvage rate for disease recurrence.[22-28] A large retrospective series comparing elective neck dissection and prophylactic radiation of neck in patients with oral cavity, oropharyngeal and laryngeal cancer reported no statistically significant difference in disease control at 5 years.[29]

Patients with clinically N_0 neck, with more than 20% risk of occult nodal metastasis, should be offered prophylactic treatment of neck, either by appropriate selective neck or MND or by external beam RT.[5]

CLINICALLY NODE POSITIVE NECK

When there is clinical or imaging evidence of disease in neck nodes, active treatment is required. There is no RCT that clearly defines the best treatment for patients with clinically positive neck node. If the involved neck node is fixed and unresectable, RT or chemoradiation may be the only therapeutic option. MND or RND result in equivalent rates of disease control in N_1 neck when performed in appropriately selected cases.[30-36]

There is increased risk of local recurrence following neck dissection if histological examination reveals node of more than 3 cm or two or more histologically positive nodes.[37] Postoperative radiation or chemoradiation reduces the risk of recurrence in these situations. In patients where the primary tumor is small and nodal disease is resectable, neck dissection may be performed before treating both the primary and neck with radiation or chemoradiation. In patients with clinically N_2 or N_3 disease, there is poor correlation between clinical and pathological response following chemoradiotherapy.[38] Even if clinical and radiological complete response has been achieved after chemoradiation, more than 30% patients with N_2/N_3 neck may have pathological evidence of residual disease on histological examination of neck dissection specimen.[38-40] MND following chemoradiation irrespective of the response to treatment confers a disease free and overall survival advantage to patient with N_2 and N_3 neck, but not N_1 disease.[38]

CONSERVATION OF ORGAN VERSUS PRESERVATION OF ORGANS

Nonsurgical approaches to laryngeal preservation in carcinoma larynx include either radiation alone or chemoradiation. These nonsurgical approaches are often referred to as "organ preservation" strategies. Currently, a broad spectrum of surgical procedures is available for preserving the larynx in the setting of laryngeal carcinoma. This is called "conservation surgery". After conservation surgery, the patient should be able to speak and eat without a permanent tracheostomy at the point when no local recurrence is expected. The conservation surgery options include cordectomy, supraglottic partial laryngectomy and vertical partial laryngectomy.

Surgical margins: The main aim of surgery is to remove the primary tumor completely with negative margins. Internationally, it is generally accepted to achieve a 1 cm margin of normal tissue around the tumor at the time of resection. Margins shrink after formalin fixation and pathological processing by 30–50%. This means that in order to obtain 5 mm of pathologically clear margin, an in situ margin of resection of atleast 8–10 mm needs to be taken.[41] Clear margin means no tumor around 5 mm of index tumor and close margin means tumor within 5 mm of surgical margin. When surgery fails to remove the tumor completely, this can be corrected surgically in two ways. Either frozen sections are used or re-excision is done at same time or redo surgery is performed if final pathology report is positive for margins. If it is not feasible, then chemoradiation is given for close/positive margins.

COMPLICATIONS IN HEAD AND NECK SURGERY

Head and neck surgery has the potential of many complications due to presence of a large number of major vessels and nerves.[42] These complications can arise due to airway compromise, vascular injury and infections. Carefully performed surgery can prevent many complications. Complications can be classified as intraoperative and postoperative (early and delayed). Complications related to different subsites (excluding thyroid surgery) are as follows:

- Neck dissection (Table 1)
- Oral surgery
  - Orocutaneous fistula
  - Flap dehiscence
  - Wound sepsis
  - Skin flap necrosis
- Laryngectomy
  - Pharyngocutaneous fistula
  - Vascular blowout especially in salvage surgery after radical RT
- Parotidectomy
  - Facial nerve paresis/palsy
  - Frey's syndrome

Table 1 Intraoperative neurovascular complications

Nerve injury	*Vascular injury*
Marginal mandibular nerve	Internal jugular vein
Spinal accessory nerve	Facial artery
Phrenic nerve	Transverse cervical artery
Vagus nerve	

- Flap complication
  - Flap necrosis and leaks
- Others
  - Thoracic duct injury
  - Airway obstruction in immediate postoperative period
  - Osteomyelitis
  - Reactionary/secondary hemorrhage
  - Cerebrospinal fluid (CSF) leaks
  - Pulmonary and cardiac problems.

Many of the complications are preventable. Meticulous attention to details and thorough check after completion of the procedure will ensure optimal results.

Although early stage head and neck cancers have high cure rates, up to 70% of head and neck cancer patients present with advanced disease. Cure rates decrease in locally advanced cases, whose probability of cure is inversely related to tumor size and even more so to the extent of regional node involvement. For cancers of oropharynx the survival has improved in last 2 decades. It is known that head and neck cancers associated with HPV are more sensitive to chemotherapy and radiation. Additionally, young patients are more likely to have HPV-related tumors which may help explain the reason for the greater improvement in survival in younger patients.

CONCLUSION

Most of the head and neck cancers need multimodality treatment and an interdisciplinary approach. The aim of surgery with curative intent in head and neck cancer is complete microscopic surgical excision. There should be no compromise in the extent of resection, when the morbidity is not materially affected by a more radical approach with appropriate reconstruction. For any head and neck surgeon, it is not only important to know how to operate, but also when and when not to operate.

REFERENCES

1. Ferlay J, Soerjomataram I, Ervik M, et al: Globocan 2012 v1.0, Cancer incidence and mortality Worldwide: IARC Cancer Base No. 11. Lyon, France: International Agency for research on Cancer; 2013.
2. American Cancer Society. Cancer Facts and Figures 2007. [online] Available from www.cancer.org/downloads/STT/CancerFacts& FiguresTM.pdf. [Accessed April, 2015].
3. Ferlay J, Bray F, Pisani P, Parkin DM. Globocan 2002: Cancer Incidence, Mortality and Prevalence Worldwide. IARC Cancer Base No. 5, version 2.0. Lyon: IARC Press; 2004.
4. Thomas G, Hashibe M, Jacob BJ, Ramadas K, Mathew B, Sankaranarayanan R, et al. Risk factors for multiple oral premalignant lesions. Int J Cancer. 2001;107(2):285-91.
5. Scottish Intercollegiate Guidelines Network (SIGN). Diagnosis and management of head and neck cancer. A national clinical guideline. SIGN publication No. 90. Edinburgh, Scotland: Scottish Intercollegiate Guidelines Network (SIGN); 2006.
6. DeVita VT, Lawrence TS, Rosenberg SA, DePinho RA, Weinberg RA (Eds). DeVita, Hellman, and Rosenberg's Cancer: Principles & Practice of Oncology, 9th edition. Philadelphia, PA: Lippincott Williams & Wilkins; 2011.
7. Agra IM, Carvalho Al, Pontes E, Campos OD, Ulbrich FS, Magrin J, et al. Postoperative complications after en bloc salvage surgery for head and neck cancer. Arch Otolaryngol Head Neck Surg. 2003;129(12):1317-21.
8. Goodwin WJ. Salvage surgery for patients with recurrent squamous cell carcinoma of the upper aerodigestive tract: when do the ends justify the means? Laryngoscope. 2000; 110(3):1-18.
9. Chiarini L, De Santis G, Bedogni A, et al. Lining the mouth floor with prelaminated fascio-mucosal free flaps: clinical experience. Microsurgery. 2002;22(5):177-86.
10. Azizzadeh B, Yafai S, Rawnsley JD, Abemayor E, Sercarz JA, Calcaterra TC, et al. Radial forearm free flap pharyngoesophageal reconstruction. Laryngoscope. 2001;111(5):807-10.
11. Jol JK, Quak JJ, De Bree R, et al. Larynx preservation surgery for advanced posterior pharyngeal wall carcinoma with free flap reconstruction: a critical appraisal. Oral Oncol. 2003;39(6):552-8.
12. Disa JJ, Pusic AL, Hidalgo DA, et al. Microvascular reconstruction of the hypopharynx: defect classification, treatment algorithm, and functional outcome based on 165 consecutive cases. Plast Reconstr Surg. 2003;111(2):652-60; discussion 61-3.
13. Genden EM, Kaufman MR, Katz B, et al. Tubed gastro-omental free flap for pharyngoesophageal reconstruction. Arch Otolaryngol Head Neck Surg. 2001;127(7):847-53.
14. Villaret DB, Futran NA. The indications and outcomes in the use of osteocutaneous radial forearm free flap. Head Neck. 2003;25(6):475-81.
15. Hayden RE, Deschler DG. Lateral thigh free flap for head and neck reconstruction. Laryngoscope. 1999;109(9):1490-4.
16. Makitie AA, Beasley NJ, Neligan PC, Lipa J, Gullane PJ, Gilbert RW. Head and neck reconstruction with anterolateral thigh flap. Otolaryngol Head Neck Surg. 2003;129(5):547-55.
17. Julieron M, Germain MA, Schwaab G, Marandas P, Bourgain JL, Wibault P, et al. Reconstruction with free jejunal autograft after circumferential pharyngolaryngectomy: eighty-three cases. Ann Otol Rhinol Laryngol. 1998;107(7):581-7.
18. Castelli ML, Pecorari G, Succo G, Bena A, Andreis M, Sartoris A. Pectoralis major myocutaneous flap: analysis of complications in difficult patients. Eur Arch Otorhinolaryngol. 2001;258(10):542-5.
19. Royal College of Pathologists. Standards and Datasets for Reporting Cancers: Datasets for Histopathology Reports on Head and Neck Carcinomas and Salivary Neoplasms, 2nd Edition. London: The Royal College of Pathologists; 2005.
20. Robbins KT, Clayman G, Levine PA, Medina J, Sessions R, Shaha A, et al. Neck dissection classification update: revisions

proposed by the American Head and Neck Society and the American Academy of Otolaryngology-Head and Neck Surgery. Arch Otolaryngol Head Neck Surg. 2002;128(7): 751-8.
21. Weiss MH, Harrison LB, Isaacs RS. Use of decision analysis in planning a management strategy for the stage N0 neck. Arch Otolaryngol Head Neck Surg. 1994;120(7):699-702.
22. McGuirt WF, Johnson JT, Myers EN, et al. Floor of mouth carcinoma. The management of the clinically negative neck. Arch Otolaryngol Head Neck Surg. 1995;121(3):278-82.
23. Fakih AR, Rao R, Borges A, et al. Elective versus therapeutic neck dissection in early carcinoma of the oral tongue. Am J Surg. 1989;158(4):309-13.
24. Van den Brekel MW, Castelijns JA, Snow GB. Diagnostic evaluation of the neck. Otolaryngol Clin North Am. 1998;31(4):601-20.
25. Ho CM, Lam KH, Wei WI, et al. Treatment of neck nodes in oral cancer. Surg Oncol. 1992;1(1):73-8.
26. Lydiatt DD, Robbins KT, Byers RM, et al. Treatment of stage I and II oral tongue cancer. Head Neck. 1993;15(4):308-12.
27. Grandi C, Mingardo M, Guzzo M, Licitra L, Podrecca S, Molinari R. Salvage surgery of cervical recurrences after neck dissection or radiotherapy. Head Neck. 1993;15(4):292-5.
28. Vandenbrouck C, Sancho-Garnier H, Chassagne D, Saravane D, Cachin Y, Micheau C. Elective versus therapeutic radical neck dissection in epidermoid carcinoma of the oral cavity: results of a randomized clinical trial. Cancer. 1980;46(2):386-90.
29. Chow JM, Levin BC, Krivit JS, et al. Radiotherapy or surgery for subclinical cervical node metastases. Arch Otolaryngol Head Neck Surg. 1989;115(8):981-4.
30. Molinari R, Cantu G, Chiesa F, et al. Retrospective comparison of conservative and radical neck dissection in laryngeal cancer. Ann Otol Rhinol Laryngol. 1980;89(6):578-81.
31. Jesse RH, Ballantyne AJ, Larson D. Radical or modified neck dissection: a therapeutic dilemma. Am J Surg. 1978; 136(4):516-9.
32. Lingeman RE, Helmus C, Stephens R, et al. Neck dissection: radical or conservative. Ann Otol Rhinol Laryngol. 1977;86(6): 737-44.
33. Brandenburg JH, Lee CY. The eleventh nerve in radical neck surgery. Laryngoscope. 1981;91(11):1851-9.
34. Andersen PE, Shah JJ, Cambronero E, et al. The role of comprehensive neck dissection with preservation of the spinal accessory nerve in the clinically positive neck. Am J Surg. 1994;168(5):499-502.
35. Bocca E, Pignataro O. A conservation technique in radical neck dissection. Ann Otol Rhinol Laryngol. 1967;76(5):975-87.
36. Chu W, Strawitz JG. Results in suprahyoid, modified radical, and standard radical neck dissections for metastatic squamous cell carcinoma: recurrence and survival. Am J Surg. 1978;136(4): 512-5.
37. Vikram B, Strong EW, Shah JP, et al. Failure in the neck following multimodality treatment for advanced head and neck cancer. Head Neck Surg. 1984;6(3):724-9.
38. Brizel DM, Prosnitz RG, Hunter S, Fisher SR, Clough RL, Downey MA, et al. Necessity for adjuvant neck dissection in setting of concurrent chemoradiation for advanced head-and-neck cancer. Int J Radiat Oncol Biol Phys. 2004;58(5):1418-23.
39. Frank DK, Hu KS, Culliney BE, Persky MS, Nussbaum M, Schantz SP, et al. Planned neck dissection after concomitant radiochemotherapy for advanced head and neck cancer. Laryngoscope. 2005;115(6):1015-20.
40. Wang SJ, Wang MB, Yip H, et al. Combined radiotherapy with planned neck dissection for small head and neck cancers with advanced cervical metastases. Laryngoscope. 2000;110(11):1794-7.
41. Johnson RE, Sigman JD, Funk GF, et al. Quantification of surgical margin shrinkage in the oral cavity. Head Neck. 1997;19(4):281-6.
42. Pai PS. Complications in head and neck surgery. Otorhinolaryngology Clinics: An International Journal. 2010; 2(1):61-7.

11

CHAPTER

Radiation in Treatment of Head and Neck Cancer

Tejinder Kataria, Ashu Abhishek

INTRODUCTION

Conventional radiation planning for head and neck cancers defined placement of radiation fields and shaping the beams based on the bony anatomy acquired by simulator diagnostic quality X-ray or through fluoroscopic imaging on a 2D simulator. The advances in 1980s, on the imaging front, with advent of computed tomography (CT) and magnetic resonance imaging (MRI) have given a new dimension to image-based three-dimensional radiation treatment planning (3D RTP). Simultaneous introduction of advanced treatment planning systems and multileaf collimators (MLCs) in the linear accelerators in 1990s gave a powerful way to visualize and deliver the dose clouds.

THREE-DIMENSIONAL CONFORMAL THERAPY

The newer technologies have changed the implementation of external beam radiation therapy techniques, allowing the conformation of high-dose region closely to the tumor-target volume and reducing the volume of normal tissues receiving a high dose. This form of external beam radiation was given the name of three-dimensional conformal radiation therapy (3D CRT).[1-3] Three-dimensional planning and delivery is not an add-on to the conventional way of treatment, it is a new way of treatment. It is a new way of approaching the three-dimensional tumor with the addition of image-based visualization, use of an increased member of beams that may be angled and/or shaped to conform to a planning target volume (PTV).[4] This may include use of conventional beam modifiers like wedges, compensating filters or with MLCs.

The 3D CRT has been succeeded by its more advanced form since the late 1990s by intensity-modulated radiotherapy (IMRT). IMRT can achieve a higher degree of conformity by modeling the radiation beam intensity (fluence) throughout each shaped beam.[5,6]

INTENSITY-MODULATED RADIOTHERAPY

Intensity-modulated radiotherapy includes the use of radiation fields where intensity varies across the field, depending upon the thickness of the target and critical tissues in their path. The technical advancement of computer-controlled MLCs and 'inverse-planning optimization' algorithms helped the onset of IMRT utilization in clinical radiotherapy. A computerized optimization program determines the intensity of beam required to satisfy a specified set of dose distributions. Beamlets of varying intensity are created by moving the leaves in a MLC assembly through the beam during gantry rotation around the patient.[6] IMRT delivery with an MLC linear accelerator can be in the form of:

- *Dynamic mode:* With the leaves sweeping across the target, at each gantry position while the beam is on, with their speed being the determinant of radiation fluence.
- *Static, segmental or step and shoot mode:* Here each field consists of multiple segments with different intensities and the MLC shapes up after the gantry stops at its given angle of delivery.
- *Intensity-modulated arc therapy (IMAT):* Here the gantry angle, MLC position and radiation dose rate are continuously changing throughout an arc. IMAT, volumetric-modulated arc therapy (VMAT) and rapid arc are the clinically available modes at present.

The complexity of IMRT plans cannot be achieved by forward planning available with the 3D-CRT process, i.e. by beam shaping alone. The anatomy of neck is complex and many radiation-sensitive structures lie in close vicinity to the target/s. These include the major salivary glands, minor salivary glands within the oral cavity, mandible, pharyngeal musculature, brachial plexus, inner and middle ears, the temporomandibular joints, temporal lobes of brain, optic pathways, brain stem and spinal cord. Head and neck cancers are more eminently suited to IMRT planning as the organ motion is limited and patient set-up uncertainties can be minimized with immobilization.

IMAGE-GUIDED RADIOTHERAPY

The goal of dose escalation and increased tumor control can be achieved further, by an increase in the geometric precision. Rigid immobilization and set-up aids are in use to reduce the systematic and random components of set-up errors and organ motion. The availability of in-room imaging has made it possible to provide additional information acquired immediately before or during the course of treatment. Conventional treatment techniques do not distinguish between target volumes, normal tissue volumes, geometric uncertainties and penumbral width in the design of a treatment portal. The wide fields around the tumor accommodate all these uncertainties and do not need daily correction. For 3D CRT and IMRT or the volume-based planning and delivery, there is an inherent risk that the geometric uncertainty in daily treatment may not be covered. There are devices that aid in reduction of random or systematic set-up errors through in-room imaging and can be used for on-line or off-line correction. Such a corrected treatment delivery has been named as image-guided radiotherapy (IGRT). The in-room devices used for IGRT are:

- Electronic portal imaging device (EPID)[7]
- K-V cone beam CT[8,9]
- M-V cone beam CT[10]
- Cyberknife[11]
- Tomotherapy[12]
- CT on rails[13]
- BAT ultrasonography[14]
- Infrared light emitting diodes.[15]

Patient Selection for Intensity-modulated Radiotherapy

Intensity-modulated radiotherapy planning is a labor-intensive process for head and neck cancers. The maximum benefit is achieved for the patients with paranasal sinus cancers where the targets are close to optic pathways, nasopharynx and oropharynx cancers that mandate a large field, covering major salivary glands and are have proximity to spinal cord and brain stem besides optic chiasma and temporal lobes. Patients with laryngeal cancers not involving nodes and tumors that need irradiation of ipsilateral neck alone may not benefit with IMRT.

Immobilization

Head and neck immobilization is performed with thermoplastic mask over the patient's head, face and neck extending to cover both the shoulder joints and the sternal angle. The mask is prepared with the patient is supine position, both hand by the side of the body and lying on a flat table top that bears graduations identical to the linear accelerator treatment table top. For treatment plans designed with 3D treatment planning tools, the portals are shaped to the target in the beam's eye-view (BEV) with a small margin. In IMRT, the high-dose region is shaped to conform to the geometry of the target with a rapid fall-off around the target in all three dimensions. Such radiation delivery techniques are sensitive to set-up accuracy and thus require adequate and effective immobilization. Clinical studies have shown an increase in recurrence rates for stage III laryngeal cancers if the tumor dose delivery is changed by 5%.[16] In another study, inadequate tumor coverage was responsible for reducing the slope of dose-response curve to approximately zero in nasopharyngeal cancers.[17] Besides immobilizing the patient and reducing set-up uncertainty, such a device can reduce the daily set-up time, stabilize the relationship of external fiducial markers to internal structures and make the patient less apprehensive.

Concept of Volumes and Margins

The International Commission on Radiation Units and Measurements (ICRU) has recommended definition of terms and concepts for volumes and margins in radiotherapy.[4,18]

- *Gross tumor volume (GTV):* The clinically and or radiologically demonstrable tumor volume.
- *Clinical target volume (CTV):* The volume that includes GTV and the subclinical disease, i.e. volumes containing suspected tumor infiltration or spread.
- *Planning target volume (PTV):* Includes the CTV with margins to account for geometric uncertainties. The final plan requires a 5–7 mm margin around the PTV from the beam edge to account for the penumbra of the beam.
- *Treatment volume:* This is the volume enclosed by the prescribed isodose surface, specified by the radiation oncologist, to achieve the goal of treatment and this volume is larger than PTV.
- *Irradiation volume:* The volume of tissue that receives a dose considered significant with respect to tissue tolerance, viz. tissue in the exit region of nonopposed beam or within the penumbra of individual beams.
- *Planning organ at risk volume (PRV):* It is a margin around the organ at risk.

Target Localization and Treatment Planning

The aim of target localization is to fix the relationship between the radiation beam and the target. The target is generally deep seated and may not be directly visible or palpable, hence external fiducials are applied during the simulation and data acquisition to reproduce alignment of the target to the beam. For conformal and intensity-modulated treatments, data acquisition is done after preparation of an immobilization device, in head and neck cancers. A CT, MRI and/or PET-CT imaging are done to identify the tumor-target and the anatomy in proximity. The patient is taken on a CT or CT-simulator and the external fiducials placed over the immobilization device are aligned with moving room lasers and/or the CT-lasers. The CT images are taken at 1–3 mm slice thickness depending upon the proximity of critical organs, viz. optic chiasma. At our center, we take CT scans from the top of vertex to T4 (thoracic) vertebra. An MRI can be taken at the same consult or diagnostic MRI images can be fused with the CT-images to delineate the soft tissue extensions or intracranial involvement. Bone and cartilage destruction is better appreciated on CT-scans. An MRI gives a better soft tissue delineation and is useful to ascertain dural breach and intracranial extension. PET-CT has been found to be useful in cancers of nasopharynx and oropharynx for identification of equivocal lymph node involvement and intracranial extension in cases of nasopharyngeal cancers. The CT-images, MRI images and PET-CT images are transferred to a treatment planning or contouring computer through a dedicated IP address, PACS or through a data-holding device (CD).

A consult with a radiologist, MR or nuclear medicine specialist is sought at the time of contouring at our center for difficult cases. The present day contouring tools include good fusion capabilities for all three modalities; however, treatment planning is always done on CT-images, as the electron density is not available in MRI and PET imaging. After contouring the various target volumes and organs at risk the dose prescription for each target and dose constraints for OARs are given by the radiation oncologist and DICOM (Digital Imaging and Communications in Medicine) structure sets are sent to the treatment-planning system (TPS) for the physicist to start the treatment planning process.

Selection and Delineation of Target

Earlier 3D CRT and at present IMRT has given a potential to improve tumor control by reducing the limitation for tumor dose delivery due to proximity of critical organs. For head and neck cancers, another benefit has been the elimination of need for posterior neck electron fields that were used for the conventional planning. IMRT is more feasible in head and neck cancers due to absence of organ motion during treatment.

A potential pitfall of IMRT or conformal plan development is failure to select and delineate the targets accurately. Before expanding on the site-wise delineation of target volumes, it is prudent to revisit patterns of spread in head and neck cancers.

Patterns of Spread

The tumor spread in head and neck cancers includes: (a) contiguous, (b) lymphatic, (c) perineural, and (d) hematogenous dissemination. The site of origin and histopathology determine the pattern of cancer spread. For IMRT planning the hematogenous spread is not important as these tumors are locoregional in a vast majority of cases.

Target Definition in Head and Neck Cancers

The GTVs include primary tumor and the lymph nodes with apparent or suspected metastases. The primary tumor (GTVp) is defined with clinical, radiologic and histopathology details. Lymph node GTVs include nodes that are grossly enlarged, positive on biopsy and/or have radiologic criteria of involvement, i.e. diameter more than 1 cm, smaller nodes with spherical rather than ellipsoidal shape, nodes containing in homogeneities with necrotic centers and cluster of three or more nodes.[19] The clinical target volume around the primary tumor contains the microscopic and subclinical tumor extension. Secondary lymphatic CTVs include nodal areas at risk of metastatic disease without involvement.

Primary Tumor Clinical Target Volume Delineation

The CTV margins in each case include tumor site, size, stage, differentiation, morphology and histopathology if the patient is an operated case.[20] Site-wise recommendations are as follows:

Oral Cavity Cancers

Floor of mouth: The CTV encompasses the muscles of floor of mouth including genioglossus, geniohyoid bilaterally, sublingual and submandibular gland ipsilaterally (or bilaterally, if a midline tumor) the medial alveolus ridge and root of tongue muscles.

Oral tongue: CTV includes the extrinsic, intrinsic muscles of the tongue, floor of mouth, glossotonsillar sulcus, anterior tonsillar pillar and the base of tongue (Fig. 1A).

High-risk CTV includes at risk anatomical regions in proximity to the primary lesion (extrinsic, intrinsic muscles of the tongue, floor of mouth glossotonsillar sulcus, anterior tonsillar pillar and the base of tongue with involved neck nodal regions, if any) and low-risk CTV includes neck nodal regions (level 1–4) not included in high-risk CTV. Level 1A and ipsilateral level 1B are usually covered by the CTV for primary. Nodal CTV includes bilateral level 2–4 (for N0) or additional level 5 on the side with N+ disease.

Buccal mucosa: The CTV includes the upper and lower buccal gingival sulci, infratemporal fossa and submandibular gland. Anteriorly, it extends to include the commissure of lip and posteriorly the retromolar trigone (Fig. 1B).

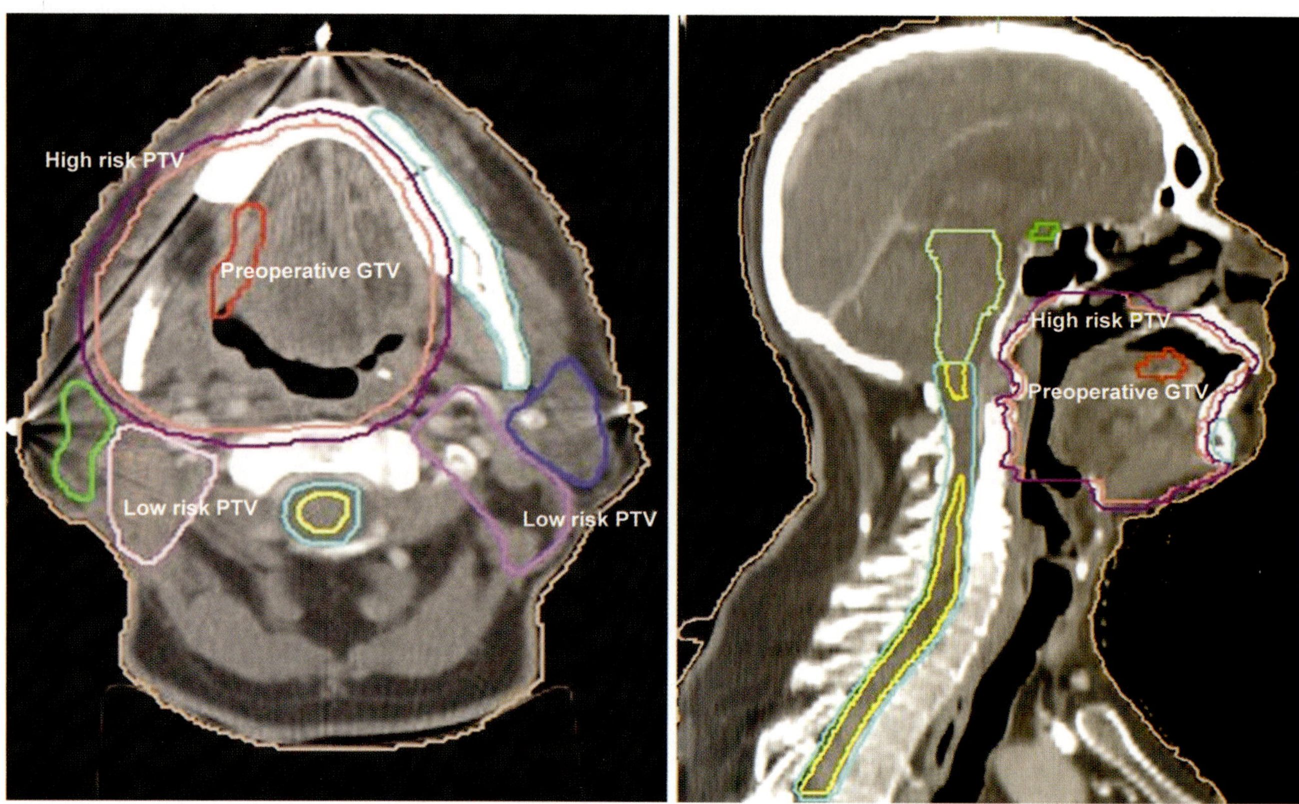

Fig. 1A Axial and sagittal planning CT sections showing target delineation for primary and neck nodes in a postoperative case of carcinoma oral tongue

Abbreviations: PTV, planning target volume; GTV, gross tumor volume
Courtesy: Dr Tejinder Kataria, Division of Radiation oncology, Medanta—The Medicity, Haryana, India

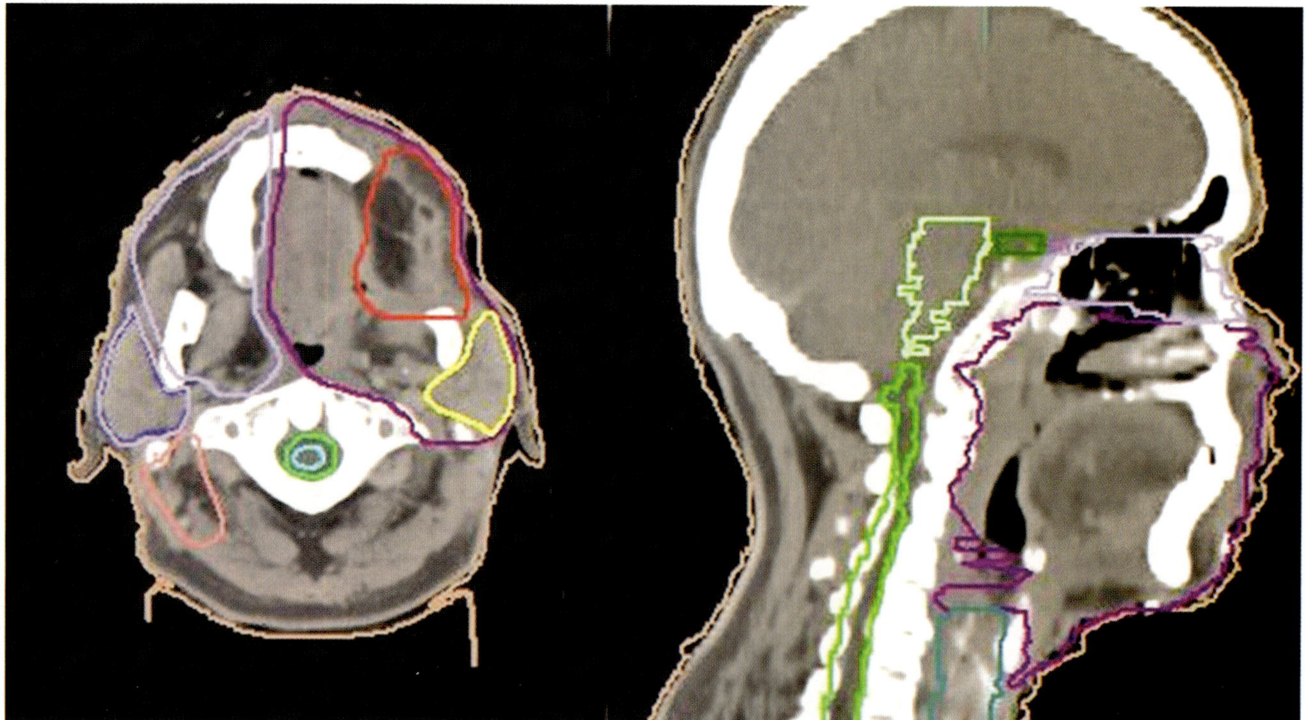

Fig. 1B Planning CT sections showing target volume coverage in carcinoma buccal mucosa.
Courtesy: Dr Tejinder Kataria, Division of Radiation Oncology, Medanta—The Medicity, Haryana, India

Cancers of the Oropharynx

Cancer tonsil: The CTV includes the palate, base of tongue and adjacent buccal mucosa with the involvement of posterior tonsillar pillars, CTV extends to include the pharyngoepiglottic fold. Ipsilateral medial mandible, pterygoid muscles, parapharyngeal space and adjacent nasopharynx are included in advanced cases (Fig. 2A).

Cancer base of tongue: CTV includes the whole of base of tongue, at least 2 cm of oral tongue beyond the GTV and vallecula. Suprahyoid epiglottic larynx is included in case of extension to vallecula (Fig. 2B).

Pharyngeal wall cancers: In pharyngeal wall cancers, skip lesions and longitudinal mucosal spread are known to coexist besides the visible gross tumor. The CTV includes the cranial extension through the nasopharynx and caudal extension through hypopharynx including parapharyngeal space.

Cancer of the soft palate: It includes the entire soft palate, superior extension of tonsillar pillars, tonsillar fossa and pterygopalatine fossa. Adjacent nasopharynx and pterygoid muscles are included in advanced tumors. An assessment with MRI can help distinguish involvement of skull base in case of tumors extending to pterygopalatine fossa. The sphenoid sinus and skull-base foramina are included in the CTV with pterygopalatine fossa involvement for adenoid cystic carcinoma and high-grade acinic cell carcinomas. In case of tumor extension to pterygomaxillary fissure, the course of maxillary nerve through cavernous sinus to the fifth nerve ganglion in Meckel's cave is included due to risk of perineural spread.

Cancer Larynx

In early stages, parallel-opposed portals give the best coverage and are encouraged. For advanced cancers, preoperative or postoperative radiation with or without chemotherapy is encouraged. The CTV includes the entire larynx, pyriform sinuses, vallecula, paraglottic, pre-epiglottic spaces and entire thyroid cartilage in advanced cases. The tracheostomy site is included when a tracheostomy has been performed (Fig. 3).

Hypopharyngeal Cancer

The CTV includes the parapharyngeal tissues from skull base to 2 cm below the cricoid to cover the submucosal longitudinal spread for pyriform sinus cancers, ipsilateral hemilarynx and posterior pharyngeal wall. Ipsilateral thyroid lobe is included for cancers with lateral extension for pyriform fossa tumors.

Nasopharyngeal Cancer

The CTV includes the skull base, superior parapharyngeal space, pterygoid plates and pterygoid muscles. The sphenoid and cavernous sinuses are included in the skull base besides foramen

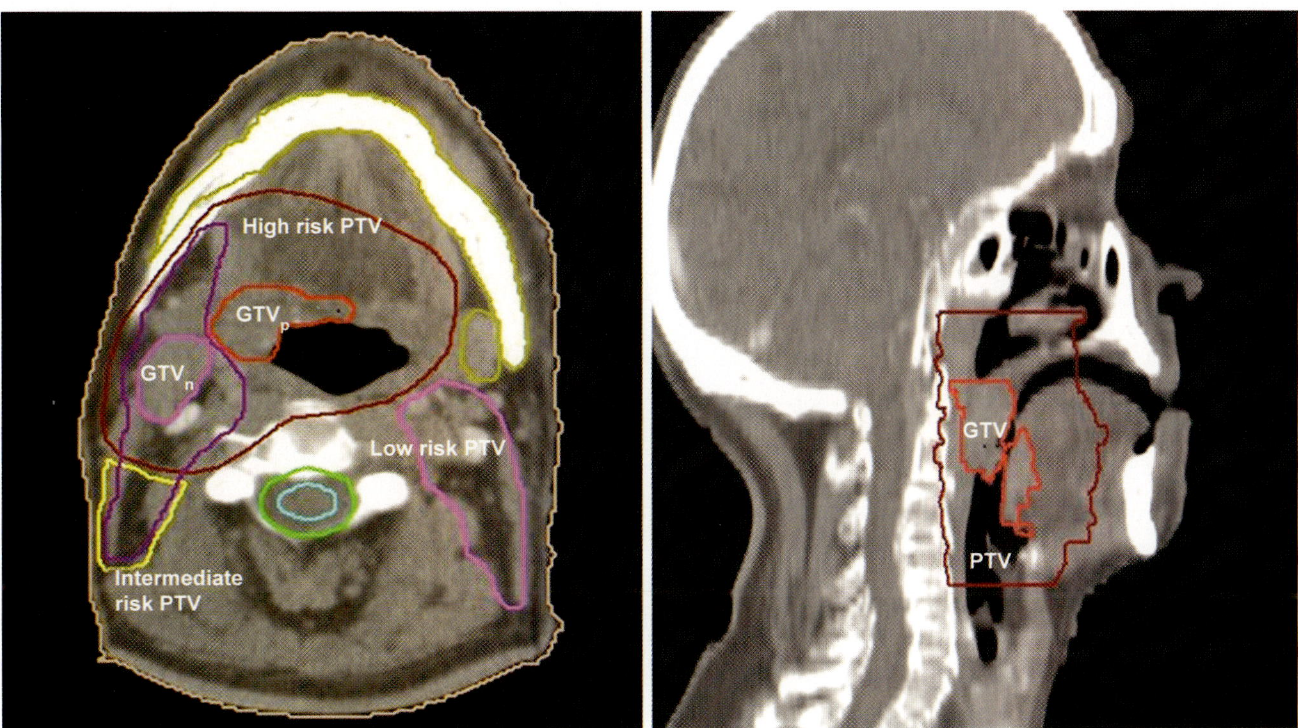

Fig. 2A Axial and sagittal planning CT sections in a case of carcinoma right tonsil

Abbreviations: PTV, planning target volume; GTVp, primary gross tumor volume; GTVn, gross tumor volume for lymph nodes; GTV, gross tumor volume

Courtesy: Dr Tejinder Kataria, Division of Radiation Oncology, Medanta—The Medicity, Haryana, India

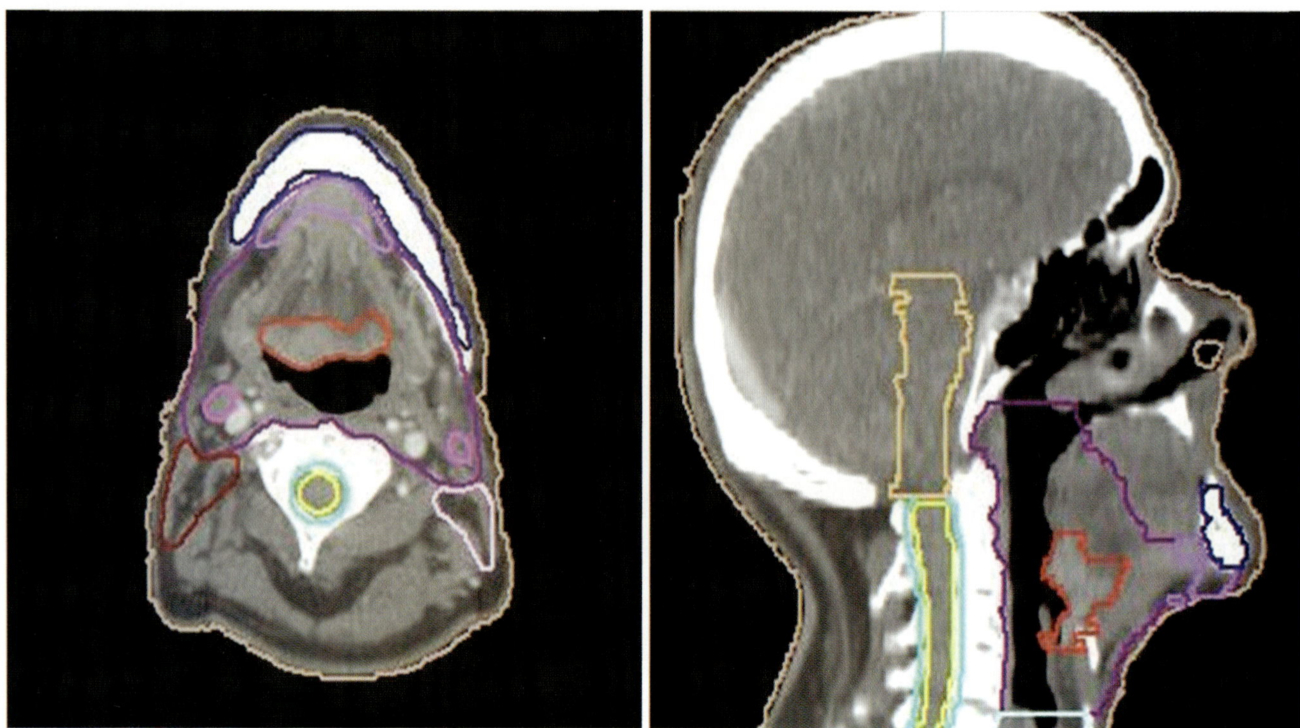

Fig. 2B Axial and sagittal sections of planning contrast-enhanced computed tomography showing target volume coverage in carcinoma base of tongue

Courtesy: Dr Tejinder Kataria, Division of Radiation Oncology, Medanta—The Medicity, Haryana, India

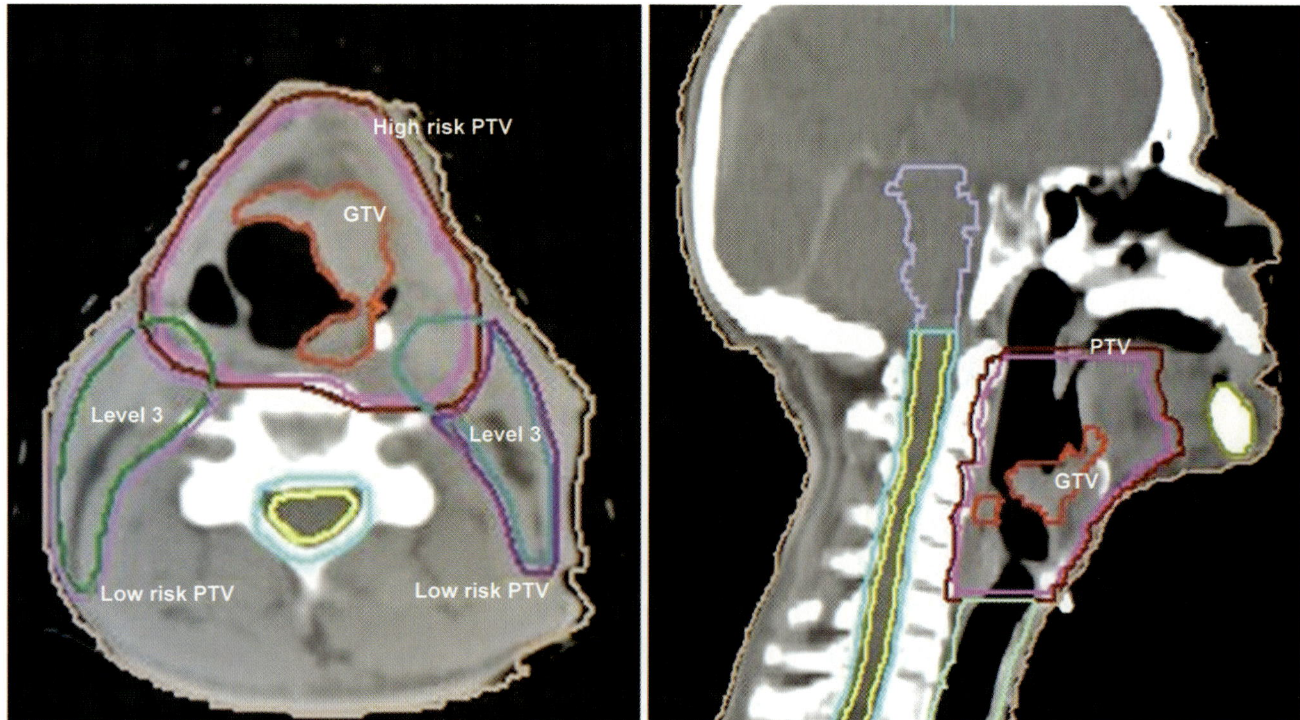

Fig. 3 Planning CT sections in a case of carcinoma larynx

Abbreviations: PTV, planning target volume; GTV, gross tumor volume

Courtesy: Dr Tejinder Kataria, Division of Radiation Oncology, Medanta—The Medicity, Haryana, India

ovale, carotid canal and foramen spinosum. Retropharyngeal nodes are covered up to the hyoid bone and parapharyngeal space included to reach the mid tonsil level. Posteriorly the clivus, the posterior one-third of maxillary sinuses anteriorly, posterior ethmoid sinus and the posterior one-third of nasal cavity form the anterior extension of the CTV. Pituitary fossa, optic chiasma and optic nerves need to be included in base of skull involvement by tumor. The dose to latter should be limited to 45–54 Gy at conventional fractionation (Fig. 4).

Cancers of the Paranasal Sinuses

Maxillary and ethmoid cancers are commonly encountered sites amongst the paranasal sinus tumors. CTV for maxillary cancers includes palate, alveolar ridge, nasopharynx and nasal cavity. Medial orbit needs to be encompassed for ethmoid and medial maxillary tumors. Superior extension includes the sphenoid sinus, foramen rotundum and posterior extension includes pterygopalatine and infratemporal fossa. In cases of neural involvement on MRI, the CTV should cover the cavernous sinus. Anterior cranial fossa is covered in tumors with intracranial involvement and cribriform plate with a part of frontal lobe are included in ethmoid sinus and nasal cavity involvement.

Lymph Node Delineation

The pattern of cervical lymph node metastases has been established from studies published by Memorial Sloan Kettering, Brazilian Head and Neck Study Group, recommendations of imaging classification of cervical lymph nodes proposed by Som et al. and critically reviewed by Robbins et al.[21-26] The incidence of skip metastases in 270 patients from M.D. Anderson Cancer Center from 1970 to 1990 was reported to be 12% by Byers et al.[27]

Tentative guidelines for treatment of neck nodes are recommended below; however, the final decision needs to be taken in multidisciplinary meeting for complex cases. For N0 patients with squamous cell carcinoma of head and neck, viz. oral cavity, nasopharynx, orophrynx, hypopharynx and larynx except for T1 glottic laryngeal primary, elective treatment of neck is recommended.[28,29]

- Levels I–IV should be treated for oral cavity cancers and levels II–IV for oropharyngeal, hypopharyngeal and laryngeal tumors.
- Levels II–V, junctional nodes at the junction of level II and spinal accessory chain and retropharyngeal nodes for nasopharyngeal tumors should be treated bilaterally (Figs 5A to E).

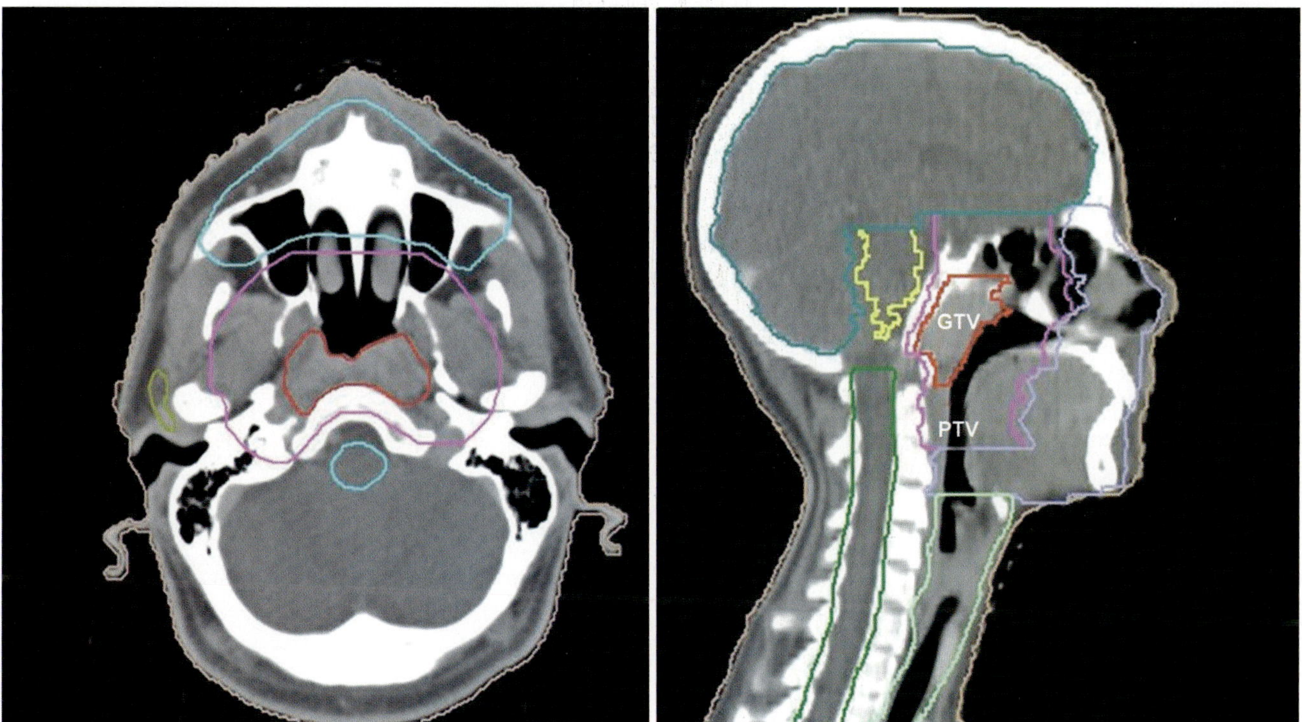

Fig. 4 Axial and sagittal CT sections showing target volumes for carcinoma nasopharynx

Abbreviations: GTV, gross tumor volume; PTV, planning target volume
Courtesy: Dr Tejinder Kataria, Division of Radiation oncology, Medanta—The Medicity, Haryana, India

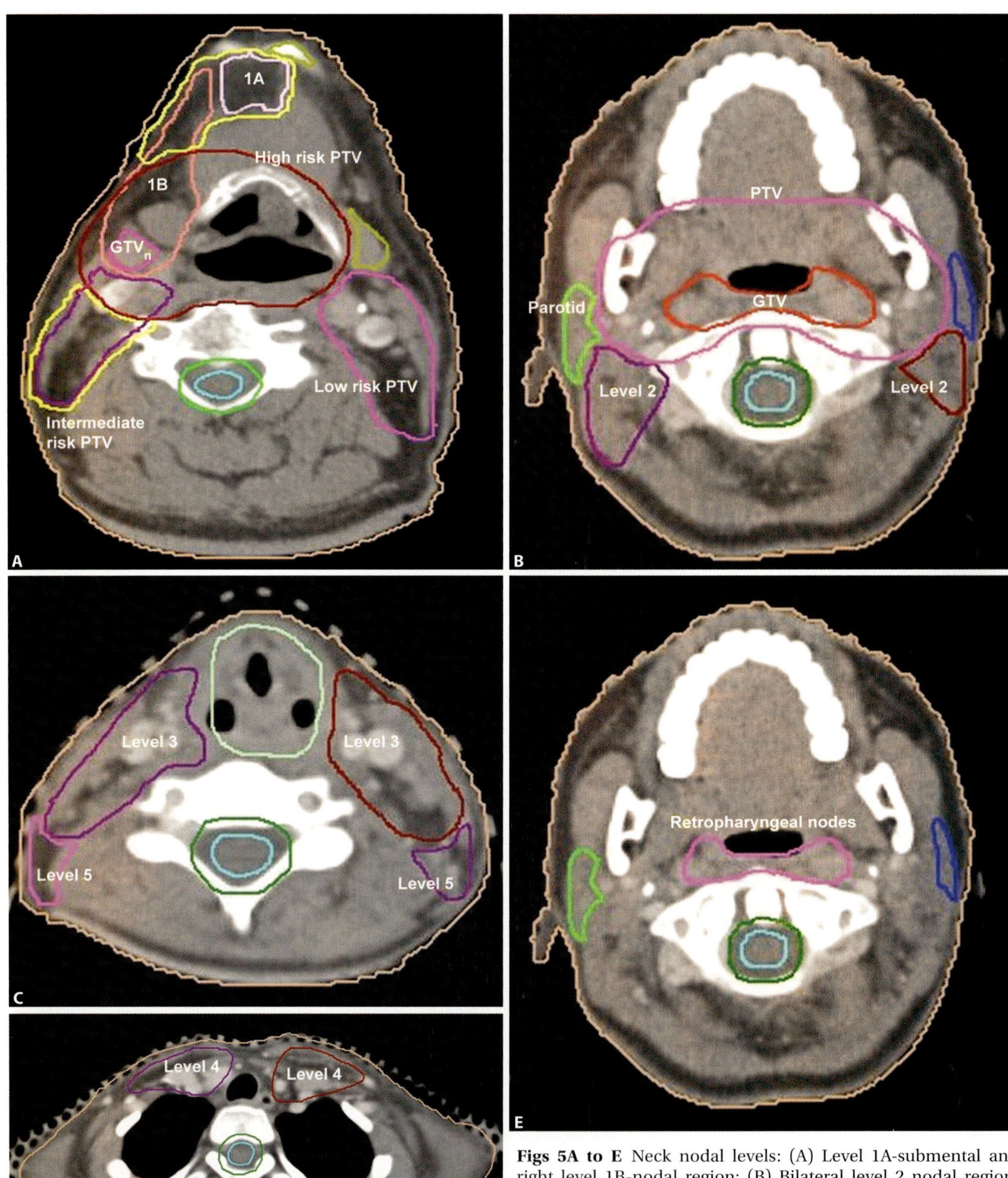

Figs 5A to E Neck nodal levels: (A) Level 1A-submental and right level 1B-nodal region; (B) Bilateral level 2 nodal region; (C) Bilateral level 3 and level 5 nodal regions; (D) Bilateral level 4 nodal regions; (E) Retropharyngeal nodal region

Abbreviations: PTV, planning target volume; GTV, gross tumor volume; GTVn, gross tumor volume for lymph nodes 1A, submental nodes; 1b, submendibular nodes

Courtesy: Dr Tejinder Kataria, Division of Radiation Oncology, Medanta—The Medicity, Haryana, India

- For posterior pharyngeal wall tumors, oropharynx and hypopharynx prophylactic treatment of retropharyngeal nodes is recommended.
- For subglottic tumors with subglottic and transglottic extension or hypopharynx extending to esophagus, level VI nodes need to be covered in treatment fields.

The treatment portals need to be defined for each primary site depending upon N1–N3 status, number of lymph nodes and extracapsular spread.[30,31]

The nodal stations have been defined in literature with appropriate guidelines available for delineation of these regions.[23,32,33]

We have treated about 1,000 cases of head and neck cancers since 2002, starting with IMRT, beginning with physical intensity-modulated compensators from February 2002 to April 2004 (N=74), graduating to MLC-based intensity modulation since 2004–2007 at RGCI (N=334), implementing IGRT (KV-cone beam CT) at Artemis Health Institute, from January 2008 to September 2009 (N=100) and Medanta Cancer Institute at Medanta-the Medicity, February 2010 till date (N = 500). The most common histology seen in our cases has been a squamous cell histology followed by, adenoid cystic carcinomas, mucoepidermoid carcinomas, non-Hodgkin's lymphomas and acinic cell tumors. We introduced the VMAT in 2010 and after the learning curve of this new technology, we have adopted it for more than 95% of our treatments for head and neck cancers.

Image-guided Radiotherapy in Head and Neck Cancer

Image guidance is a standard tool that aids in verification and delivery of precise high-dose radiation to the sites where radiotherapy has a role. Image verification and delivery helps in irradiating the desired site to the planned dose with precision by reducing the errors induced due to set-up uncertainties. It has a vital role to play in sites like head and neck where major vital organs are densely packed in a small space. Although internal motion may not be of much concern in these sites, the margin of error is very low due to close approximation of the structures to each other. They are also of importance in cases of reirradiation where each millimeter of normal tissue may count and sparing of which may increase the therapeutic ratio to a large extent.

By image guidance, although the radiotherapy planning remains the same, the mode of delivery changes wherein, daily intra- or interfraction movement is recorded and necessary adjustments made to deliver the planned dose as approximately as possible, by reducing the modifiable errors like difference in daily set-up positions.

In image guidance, reference images generated from the initial planning images are used over which acquired images during daily treatment set-up are overlaid and then matched to assess the set-up uncertainties. Both the translational and rotational errors are recorded and as per departmental policies and equipments available, these may be used for couch correction to maintain precision up to 1 mm in daily set-up and treatment delivery.

Set-up Uncertainties and Planning Target Volume Margins in Head and Neck Cancers

Planning target volume as defined by ICRU, 62 aids in taking care of the variation in actual dose delivery to the planned target volumes, due to various reasons, set-up uncertainties being one of them.[33] Institutional protocols may vary, but as a rule most centers use 5 mm as predefined PTV margins for most of the head and neck cases.

Radiotherapy is an essential component of management in solid tumors, like head and neck cancers and precision in delivery of planned dose has a pivotal role to play in the overall outcomes of treatment. In addition to an understanding of precise and targeted therapies for optimal target coverage with significant sparing of normal tissues, the role of radiotherapy has been redefined in radical and specially organ sparing management protocols for head and neck cancers. Targeted approach is of prime importance in head and neck region, considering densely packed vital structures of functional and cosmetic importance, in a small anatomical area, thus making each millimeter count.

Although strict immobilization is a rule in radiotherapy, even with best of the techniques used, set-up errors are unavoidable and are important considerations in planning the final dose delivery to the target. Like various documented data in past, the authors also have tried to explore the existence and importance of set-up uncertainties in head and neck cancers and validate the PTV margin most commonly used at most centers.[8]

We studied the online set-up uncertainties for 50 cases (37 head and neck and 13 brain) where daily cone beam CT was done as a part of the IGRT delivery. We found mean error in daily set-up as 0.12 ± 0.05 cm in lateral, longitudinal and vertical directions. The recorded systematic errors were 0.07, 0.09 and 0.1 in vertical, lateral and longitudinal directions. Similarly, the random errors recorded were 0.13, 0.11 and 0.15 in all the three directions. Using these data the PTV margins calculated were 0.23 cm, 0.25 cm and 0.31 cm (Strooms') and 0.26 cm, 0.30 cm and 0.36 cm (van Herks') in anteroposterior, mediolateral and superoinferior directions, respectively. The authors thus validated the use of 5 mm isotropic expansion of site-specific CTVs for the final PTV in an individual head and neck case, ensuring more than 90% population coverage for 95% prescribed dose (van Herks') or 99% CTV coverage by 95% prescribed dose (Strooms').[34,35]

Calculated PTV margins may actually vary in every institution and also in any particular case depending on the set-up used, treatment techniques applied, individual variations, etc. The basic idea is to understand the factors responsible for these errors estimate the minimum PTV margin required and then formulate a standard PTV protocol for a set of cases at one center. Centers not equipped with estimation of daily set-up errors may adhere as closely to the dictum of strict immobilization and use the most commonly used PTV margin of 5 mm with safety, till further validation of margin reduction in special settings are formulated. Centers using IGRT as a part of treatment in selected cases, have added confidence to a more precise delivery of the planned dose, when they use the above margin. These centers may use the same 5 mm margins, considering the residual errors left even after correction, else, plan for margin reduction using appropriate tools for image guidance and set-up error avoidance and correction, and validating the same in clinical settings. Till that time, universal 5 mm PTV margins in all head and neck cancers remains a valid choice. Optimal studies may in future help us to understand and aim at further margin reduction using appropriate tools for adequate targeted therapy (Figs 6A and B).

BRACHYTHERAPY IN HEAD AND NECK CANCER

Introduction

Brachytherapy, an age-old yet ever evolving technique of radiotherapy derived its nomenclature from Greek word brachys, which is used to depict short distance. It is also popularly known as internal radiotherapy, curietherapy, endocurietherapy or sealed-source radiotherapy. It is popularly used to deliver radiation close to mucosal or target surfaces and is said to deliver radiation inside out.[36-37]

It was in year 1901, when Pierre Curie and Henri Danlos thought of a radioactive source that could be used for treatment after insertion inside a tumor.[38,39] Alongwith Alexander Graham Bell, there were studies that reported significant reduction of tumor after such procedures.[39]

Following an initial peak in interest of using brachytherapy, there was a gradual decline, especially in Europe and the USA due to problems related to postprocedure radiation exposure reported after manual application of sources in clinics.[39,40]

With reports of these risks, remote after loading techniques were developed that allows the radiation to be delivered from a shielded safe, reducing the operator and patient exposure.[38] Aided with more technological advances in the field of imaging, radiation planning and more sophisticated delivery system, brachytherapy has been made much more safe and effective treatment in today's world.

Perspective in Head and Neck Cancer

Brachytherapy is a therapeutic modality that may provide a significant improvement in the therapeutic ratio when appropriately applied, and hence, is an appealing treatment strategy for the head and neck cancer management.[41] The benefits of achieving a good locoregional control with minimal treatment related functional deficits and improved quality of life, makes brachytherapy an important treatment tool for head and neck cancers. Moreover, due to possible risks of second primaries and locoregional recurrences needing reirradiation, availability of brachytherapy implants is particularly appealing in selected cases.[42] The scope in head and neck cancer management could be:

- For early stage lesions with low risk of nodal disease, brachytherapy can be used for definitive or as local treatment in adjuvant setting, postsurgery.
- As local boost, postexternal-beam radiation therapy (EBRT) for head and neck cancers.
- For reirradiation in recurrent or second primary occurring within a previously irradiated region.

Basic Principles

Patient Selection

Appropriate patient selection is the key to success of effective brachytherapy. The selected patients must be able to comply with their baseline self-care needs along with care of the tracheostomy, nasogastric tubes, etc. as required.[41]

Risk-benefit Assessment

Assessment of location, size and extent status of oral/dental hygiene is important in patients being considered for brachytherapy, especially in regard to the risk of mandibular osteoradionecrosis. Dental evaluation is also of importance in such cases.[42]

Permanent vs Temporary Implants

Decision for technique is important, based on its appropriateness for planning and preparation. Due to easy maneuverability and accurate positioning, temporary implants are preferred over permanent implants. Risk of radiation exposure is also negligible as compared to permanent implants. Procedure involves using a nylon catheter that serves as guiding wire for the after loading low-dose rate (LDR) sources. This allows optimal dosimetry and optimization. Reduced treatment time, ability to treat less hypoxic tumor bed early in postoperative period, reduced effect of hypoxia and exploitation of cell cycle specific radiosensitization are other benefits of the temporary implants. Due to differences in repair potentials of tumor and normal tissues, the risk of late normal complications are thus decreased. Good source handling and strict radiation precautions are mandatory for departments dealing with brachytherapy sources.

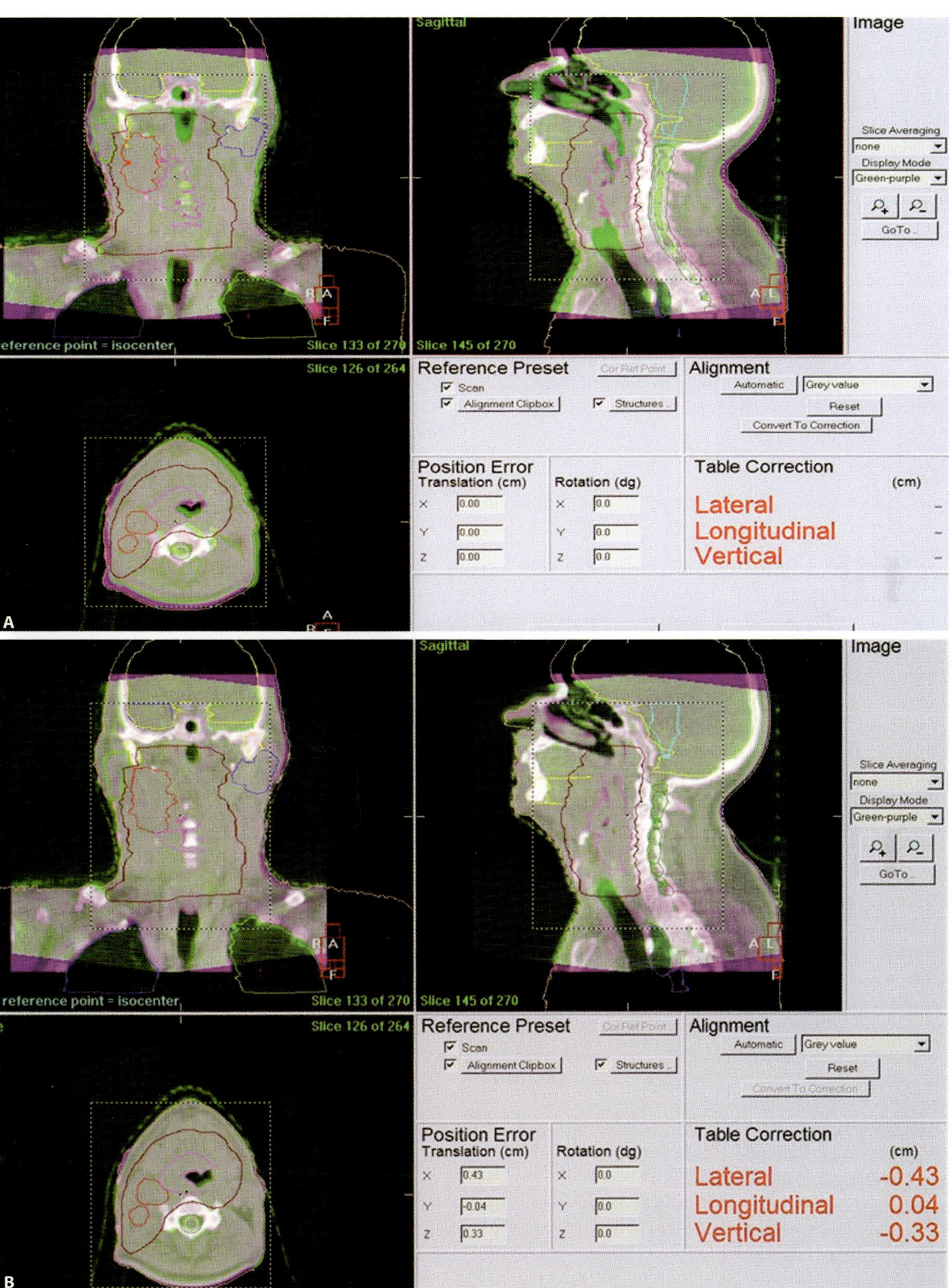

Figs 6A and B Image-guided radiotherapy-XVI (X-ray volume imaging,-Kilovoltage-Cone Beam CT). (A) Carcinoma oropharynx-before correction; (B) Carcinoma oropharynx-after correction

Courtesy: Dr Tejinder Kataria, Division of Radiation Oncology, Medanta—The Medicity, Haryana, India

Alternatively, high-dose rate (HDR) sources with computer-guided remote after loading significantly reduce the radiation exposure risks and required precautions. Fractionated radiotherapy is delivered with a single iridium-192 source fixed to the end of a guidewire that may be variably stepped along the length of each catheter. High-dose rate implants have greater flexibility in conforming the implant dosimetry to the target volume and yield a relatively more homogeneous dose distribution, compared to that of LDR implants. Moreover, as the delivery of the radiation occurs over a shorter time, it is less subject to the effects of organ movement. This precise geometric sparing may yield a lower complication rate. However, concerns remain regarding the risk of increased late complications from the higher dose rate of radiation.[43] This has prompted studies to define optimal fractionation schedules to reduce this risk.

Indications

The general indications for brachytherapy in head and neck cancer management are:

- Accessible lesions
- Small (preferable < 3 cm) tumors
- Lesions away from bone
- No nodal status
- Superficial lesions.

The application of brachytherapy among different subsites of head and neck region will be discussed here.

Nasopharynx

Recurrent disease remains the main indication for brachytherapy implant, which has shown sustained local control rates of 20–60% in many reported series. The variability is generally due to differences in reirradiation dose and extent of the recurrence.[44,45] Most experience has been with LDR implants.

In selected series treating disease confined to the nasopharynx mucosa amenable to either an intracavitary or interstitial implants, sustained local control rates of 50–60% have been realized. The use of interstitial iodine-125 implants may be particularly useful for discrete lesions located in the posterior or superior nasopharynx.[46] However, late radiation-related complications, including soft-tissue and bone necrosis, fistula formation, trismus and neurologic complications such as radiation myelitis and temporal lobe necrosis has been reported in literature.

The published reports of HDR brachytherapy experience are with favorable outcome and acceptable toxicities. Ng et al. in 2005, reported their work on 38 patients with EBRT/HDR brachytherapy boost delivered via customized catheters in a noninvasive, accurate and reproducible method under direct fiberoptic visualization. The procedure was well tolerated without any incidents of soft tissue or bone necrosis and with minimal decrease of oral aperture. Median follow-up time was 47 months (range, 2–84 months); 35 patients had at least 1 year of follow-up. The 5-year actuarial rate of local control, disease-free survival and overall survival were 96.0%, 81.4% and 92.7%, respectively.[47]

The recent report of brachytherapy boost in locally advanced nasopharyngeal carcinoma from International Atomic Energy Agency (IAEA) randomized trial evaluated in both LDR and HDR setting. The trial evaluated, brachytherapy boost by either LDR–11 Gy or HDR–3 fractions of 3.0 Gy brachytherapy.[48] The EBRT doses given were 70 Gy to the primary tumor and positive lymph nodes and 46 Gy to the negative neck. They concluded that addition of a brachytherapy boost to external beam radiotherapy and chemotherapy did not improve outcome in locoregionally advanced nasopharyngeal carcinoma.[49]

Soft Palate and Tonsil

Older series reported their experience with brachytherapy implants at these sites, typically administered as a boost (20–30 Gy) following EBRT (45–50 Gy) due to the risk of lymph node metastases.[50-52] This is particularly relevant for posterior tonsillar pillar lesions requiring treatment of the retropharyngeal lymph nodes. Most experience has been with temporary interstitial LDR implants using iridium-192. When combined with EBRT, brachytherapy produces local control rates of 85% or greater for T1 and T2 lesions and 65– 70% for selected T3 lesions.

Pernot and colleagues at the Centre Alexis Vautrin recently updated their series of 361 patients treated from 1977 to 1991, with 343 patients receiving EBRT (50 Gy) followed by an implant (20–30 Gy) using the Paris system.[15] The 5- and 10-year local control rates were 80% and 74% respectively.

The long-term outcome of HDR brachytherapy in oropharyngeal carcinoma has been reported from National Institute of Oncology, Hungary and they evaluated 60 patients (mean age, 57 years; range, 36–78 years) with T1–T4 and N0–3 carcinoma of base of tongue. Fifty-six patients (93%) had advanced (Stage III-IV) disease. HDR brachytherapy boost (mean dose, 17 Gy; range, 12–30 Gy) was delivered after 50–70 Gy (mean 62 Gy) locoregional external beam irradiation. The conclusion was external beam irradiation combined with interstitial HDR brachytherapy boost results in good local tumor control with an acceptable rate of late side effects in patients with base of the tongue carcinoma.[53]

The effectiveness of brachytherapy boost and stereotactic boost was also compared among 250 consecutive patients with T1-2N0-3 oropharyngeal carcinoma with 46-Gy of IMRT followed by boost using brachytherapy (BT) or stereotactic body radiotherapy. The results suggested comparable outcome, toxicity and QoL-scores were achieved with both modalities.[54]

Table 1 Characteristics of literatures investigating low-dose rate (LDR) vs high-dose rate (HDR) for oral cancer

Author	*Year*	*Anatomy*	*LDR patients*	*LDR implant*	*LDR dose (Gy)*	*HDR patients*	*HDR implant*	*HDR dose (Gy)*
Ghadjar et al.[56]	2011	Lip	70	^{192}Ir	60	33	^{192}Ir	36
Averra et al.[57]	2010	Lip	100	^{192}Ir	60–70	21	^{192}Ir	45–50
Umeda et al.[58]	2005	Tongue	78	^{226}Rd/ ^{137}Cs	61	26	^{192}Ir	59
Kakimoto et al.[59]	2003	Tongue	61	^{192}Ir	69	14	^{192}Ir	49
Inoue et al.[60]	2001	Tongue	26	^{192}Ir	70	25	^{192}Ir	60
Inoue et al.[61]	1997	Floor of mouth	41	^{198}Au	72	16	^{192}Ir	53

Oral Cavity Cancers

Brachytherapy has been used alone or in combination with EBRT, demonstrating local control efficacy. The historical experience over 600 patients from the Curie Institute researchers reported local control rates of 86%, 78% and 71% for T1, T2 and T3 lesions, respectively.[55] Early T1 and T2 lesions were treated with temporary interstitial LDR iridium-192 implants alone, delivering 70 Gy in 6–9 days. Larger T2 and T3 lesions were treated with EBRT (50–55 Gy) followed by an implant (20–30 Gy).[56]

A recently published meta-analysis compared the efficacy and safety of HDR and LDR brachytherapy in treating early-stage oral cancer.[57] They did a systematic search of MEDLINE, EMBASE and Cochrane Library databases. A total six trials, consisting of one RCT and five trials with control were analyzed and of those eligible trials, 607 patients treated with LDR (n= 447) or HDR (n =160) were taken into account. Four studies compared LDR versus HDR brachytherapy alone, while two others combined adjuvant routine radiotherapy. The pertinent results being elaborated in Table 1.

The authors concluded that the results of HDR brachytherapy were a competent alternative to LDR brachytherapy for early-stage oral cancer. The potential advantages of HDR brachytherapy being:[62]

- Accurate calculations made possible by complete fixation of the guide tubes.
- Parallel source arrangement with sophisticated technique.
- Homogeneous dose distribution due to stepping source optimization.
- Better patient care in normal wards without medical staff radiation exposure, administration on an outpatient basis in several cases.
- No shifting of seeds within the tissues.

There are detailed guidelines regarding all the steps involved in head and neck cancer brachytherapy formulated by GEC-ESTRO group, which are beyond the scope of present discussion.[63]

CONCLUSION

A brachytherapy implant may be used in the management of head and neck squamous cell carcinoma for several tumor sites including the tonsil and soft palate, base of tongue and lip. The use of an implant in the lip, oral tongue, and base of tongue has the advantage of being a functional organ-preserving treatment strategy. In specific circumstances, it may be used as an alternative to surgery for selected cancers of the floor of the mouth.

REFERENCES

1. In: Meyer JL, Purdy JA (Eds). 3-D Conformal Radiotherapy: A new Era in the Irradiation of Cancer. Frontiers of Radiation Therapy and Oncology. Basel, Switzerland: Karger Publishing Co.; 1996(2).
2. Goitein M, Abrams M, Rowell D, Pollari H, et al. Multidimensional treatment planning: II. Neam's eye view, back projection and projection through CT-sections. Int. J. Radit. Oncol Biol Phys. 1983;9:789-97.
3. In: Purdy JA, Emami B (Eds). 3-D Radiation Treatment Planning and Conformal Therapy. Medison, Wisconsin: Medical Physics Publishing; 1995. p. 465.
4. ICRU. ICRU report No. 50: prescribing, recording and reporting photon beam therapy. Washington, D.C.: International Commission on Radiation Units and Measurements; 1993.
5. In: Sternick ES (Ed). The Theory and Practice of Intensity Modulated Radiation Therapy. Madison, WI: Advanced Medical Publishing, 1997.
6. Webb S. Intensity Modulated Radiation Therapy. London: IOP Publishing Ltd; 2001.
7. Lebesque JV, Remeijer P, Van Riel V, Vos P, de Boer JCJ, Visser AG, et al. Clinical evaluation of set-up verification and correction protocols: results of multicentre studies of Dutch Co-operative EPID Group, proceedings of the 5th international workshop on electronic portal imaging, Phoenix, AZ; 1998.
8. Kataria T, Abhishek A, Chadha P, et al. Set-up uncertainties: online correction with X-ray volume imaging. J Cancer Res Ther. 2011;7(1):40-6.

9. Jaffrat DA, Drake DG, Moreay M, et al. Radiographic and tomographic localization of bone and soft-tissue targets on a clinical accelerator. Int J Radiat Oncol Biol Phys. 1999;45(3):773-89.
10. Hansan EK, Larson DA, Aubin M, Chen J, Descovich M, Gillis AM, et al. Image-guided radiotherapy using megavoltage cone-beam computed tomography for treatment of paraspinous tumors in presence of orthopedic hardware. Int J Radiat Oncol Biol Phys. 2006;66(2):323-36.
11. Gibbs IC, Kamnerdsupaphon P, Ryu MR, Dodd R, Kiernan M, Chang SD, et al. Image-guided robotic radiosurgery for spiral metastases. Radiother Oncol. 2007;82:185-90.
12. Kaiser A, Schultheiss TE, Wong JYC, Smith DD, Han C, Vora NL, et al. Pitch, roll and yaw variations in patient positioning. Int J Radiat Oncol Biol Phys. 2006;66(3):949-55.
13. Uematsir M, Shioda A, Suda A, et al. Intrafractional tumor position stability during computed tomography (CT)-guided frameless stereotactic radiation therapy for lung or liver cancers with a fusion of CT and linear accelerator (FOCAL) unit. Int J Radiat Oncol Biol Phys. 2000;48(2):443-8.
14. Lattanzi J, McNeeley S, Pinover W, Horwitz E, Das I, Schultheiss TE, et al. A comparison of daily CT localization to a daily ultrasound-based system in prostate cancer. Int J Radiat Oncol Biol Phys. 1999;43:719-25.
15. Meeks SL, Bova FJ, Wagner TH, Buatti JM, Friedman WA, Foote KD. Image localization for frameless stereotactic radiotherapy. Int J Radiat Oncol Biol Phys. 2000;46:1291-9.
16. Stewart JG, Jackson AW. The steepness of the dose response curve both for tumor cure and normal tissue injury. Laryngoscope. 1975;85:1107-11.
17. Marks JE, Bedwinek JM, Lee F, et al. Dose-response analysis for nasopharyngeal carcinoma: an historical perspective. Cancer. 1982;50:1042-50.
18. van den Brekel MW1, Stel HV, Castelijns JA, Nauta JJ, van der Waal I, Valk J, et al. Cervical lymph node metastasis: assessment of radiologic criteria. Radiology. 1990;177(2):379-84.
19. Kataria T. Newer technology in radiation therapy for oral cancer. Journal of International Medical Services Academy. 2003;16(1).
20. Shah JP. Patterns of cervical lymph node metastasis from squamous cell carcinomas of upper aerodigestive tract. Am J Surg. 1990;160:405-9.
21. Brazilian Head and Neck Cancer Study Group. Results of a prospective trial on elective modified radical classical versus supraomohyoid neck dissection in the management of oral squamous cell carcinoma. Am J Surg. 1998;176:422-7.
22. Som PM, Curtin HD, Mancuso AA. A imaging-based classification for the cervical nodes designed as an adjunct to recent clinically based nodal classifications. Arch Otolaryngol Head Neck Surg. 1999;125:388-96.
23. Robbins KT. Classification of neck dissection: current concepts and future consideration. Otolaryngol Clin North Am. 1998;31:639-55.
24. Robbins KT. Integrating radiological criteria into the calcification of cervical lymph node disease. Arch Otolaryngol Head Neck Surg. 1999;125:385-7.
25. Andersen PE, Shah JP, Cambronero E, et al. The role of comprehensive neck dissection with preservation of the spiral accessory nerve in the clinically positive neck. Am J surg. 1994;168:499-502.
26. Byers RM, Weber RS, Andrews T, McGill D, Kare R, Wolf P. Frequency and therapeutic implications of "skip metastases" in the neck from squamous cell carcinoma of oral tongue. Head Neck. 1997;19:14-9.
27. Clayman GL, Frank DK. Selective neck dissection of anatomically appropriate levels is as efficacious as modified radical neck dissection for elective treatment of the clinically negative neck in patients with squamous cell carcinoma of the upper respiratory and digestive tracts. Arch Otolaryngol Head Neck Surg. 1998;124:348-52.
28. Spiro JD, Spiro RH, Shah JP, Sessions RB, Strong EW. Critical assessment of supraomohyoid neck dissection. Am J Surg. 1988;156:286-9.
29. Cole I, Hughes L. The relationship of cervical node metastases to primary sites of carcinoma of upper aerodigestive tract: a pathological study. Aust NZ J Surg. 1997;67:860-5.
30. Gregoire V, Coche E, Cosnard G, et al. Selective and delineation of lymph node target volumes in head and neck conformal radiotherapy. Proposal for standardizing terminology and procedure based on surgical experience. Radiother Oncol. 2000;56:135-50.
31. Nowak PJ, Wijers OB, Lagerwaard FJ, et al. A three-dimensional CT-based target definition for elective irradiation of neck. Int J Radiat Oncol Biol Phys. 1999;45:33-9.
32. Robbins KT. Integrating radiological criteria into the classification of cervical lymph node disease. Arch Otolaryngol Head Neck Surg. 1999;125:385-7.
33. International Commission on Radiation Units and Measurements (ICRU) report no. 62: "Prescribing, recording and reporting photon beam therapy (supplement to ICRU report 50)." Bethesda, MD: ICRU; 1999.
34. Van Herk M, Remeijer P, Rasch C, et al. The probability of correct target dosage: dose-population histograms for deriving treatment margins in radiotherapy. Int J Radiat Oncol Biol Phys. 2000;47:1121-35.
35. Stroom JC, de Boer HC, Huizenga H, et al. Inclusion of geometrical uncertainties in radiotherapy treatment planning by means of coverage probability. Int J Radiat Oncol Biol Phys. 1999;43:905-19.
36. In: Alain G, Richard P, Jean-Jacques M, et al. (Eds). The GEC ESTRO Handbook of Brachytherapy. Leuven, Belgium: European Society for Therapeutic Radiology and Oncology; 2002. ISBN 978-90-804532-6-5.
37. Gupta VK. Brachytherapy—past, present and future. J Med Phys. 1995;20:31-8.
38. Nag S. A brief history of brachytherapy. Retrieved 25 September, 2009.
39. Aronowitz, J. The "Golden Age" of prostate brachytherapy: a cautionary tale. Brachytherapy. 2008;7:55-9.
40. Quon H, Harrison LB. Brachytherapy in the treatment of head and neck cancer. Oncology. 2002;16:1379-95.
41. Mazeron JJ, Gerbaulet A, Simon JM, et al. How to optimize therapeutic ratio in brachytherapy of head and neck squamous cell carcinoma? Acta Oncol. 1998;37:583-91.
42. Pernot M, Luporsi E, Hoffstetter S, Peiffert D, Aletti P, Marchal C, et al. Complications following definitive irradiation for

cancers of the oral cavity and the oropharynx (in a series of 1134 patients). Int J Radiat Oncol Biol Phys. 1997;37:577-85.
43. Lau HY, Hay JH, Flores AD, et al. Seven fractions of twice daily high dose-rate brachytherapy for node-negative carcinoma of the mobile tongue results in loss of therapeutic ratio. Radiother Oncol. 1996;39:15-8.
44. Pryzant RM, Wendt CD, Delclos L, et al. Re-treatment of nasopharyngeal carcinoma in 53 patients. Int J Radiat Oncol Biol Phys. 1992;22:941-7.
45. Kwong DL, Wei WI, Cheng AC, Choy DT, Lo AT, Wu PM, et al. Long term results of radioactive gold grain implantation for the treatment of persistent and recurrent nasopharyngeal carcinoma. Cancer. 2001;91:1105-13.
46. Harrison LB, Sessions RB, Fass DE, Armstrong JG, Hunt M, Spiro RH. Nasopharyngeal brachytherapy with access via a transpalatal flap. Am J Surg. 1992;164:173-5.
47. Ng T, Richards GM, Emery RS, Ho G, Yung R, Cheng A, et al. Customized conformal high-dose-rate brachytherapy boost for limited-volume nasopharyngeal cancer. Int J Radiat Oncol Biol Phys. 2005;61:754-61.
48. Rosenblatt E, Abdel-Wahab M, El-Gantiry M, Elattar I, Bourque JM, Afiane M, et al. Brachytherapy boost in loco-regionally advanced nasopharyngeal carcinoma: a prospective randomized trial of the International Atomic Energy Agency. Radiat Oncol. 2014;9:67.
49. Esche BA, Haie CM, Gerbaulet AP, Eschwege F, Richard JM, Chassagne D. Interstitial and external radiotherapy in carcinoma of the soft palate and uvula. Int J Radiat Oncol Biol Phys. 1988;15:619-25.
50. Pernot M, Malissard L, Hoffstetter S, Luporsi E, Aletti P, Peiffert D, et al. Influence of tumoral, radiobiological, and general factors on local control and survival of a series of 361 tumors of the velotonsillar area treated by exclusive irradiation (external beam irradiation+brachytherapy or brachytherapy alone). Int J Radiat Oncol Biol Phys.1994;30:1051-7.
51. Hoffstetter S, Marchal C, Peiffert D, Luporsi E, Lapeyre M, Pernot M, et al. Treatment duration as a prognostic factor for local control and survival in epidermoid carcinomas of the tonsillar region treated by combined external beam irradiation and brachytherapy. Radiother Oncol. 1997;45:141-8.
52. Takácsi-Nagy Z, Oberna F, Koltai P, Hitre E, Major T, Fodor J, et al. Long-term outcomes with high-dose-rate brachytherapy for the management of base of tongue cancer. Brachytherapy. 2013;12(6):535-41.
53. Al-Mamgani A, Van Rooij P, Sewnaik A, Mehilal R, Tans L, Verduijn GM, et al. Brachytherapy or stereotactic body radiotherapy boost for early-stage oropharyngeal cancer: comparable outcomes of two different approaches. Oral Oncol. 2013;49(10):1018-24.
54. Decroix Y, Ghossein NA. Experience of the Curie Institute in treatment of cancer of the mobile tongue: I. Treatment policies and result. Cancer.1981;47:496-502.
55. Liu Z, Huang S, Zhang D. High dose rate versus low dose rate brachytherapy for oral cancer—a meta-analysis of clinical trials. PLoS One. 2013;8(6):e65423.
56. Ghadjar P, Bojaxhiu B, Simcock M, Terribilini D, Isaak B, Gut P, et al. Treatment of lip cancer using high dose-rate or low dose-rate brachytherapy. Int J Radiat Oncol Biol Phys. 2012;83(4):1205-12.
57. Ayerra AQ, Mena EP, Fabregas JP, et al. HDR and LDR brachytherapy in the treatment of lip cancer: the experience of the Catalan Institute of Oncology. J Contemp Brachyther. 2010;2(1):9-13.
58. Umeda M, Komatsubara H, Ojima Y, Minamikawa T, Shibuya Y, Yokoo S, et al. A comparison of brachytherapy and surgery for the treatment of stage I-II squamous cell carcinoma of the tongue. Int J Oral Maxillofac Surg. 2005;34(7):739-44.
59. Kakimoto N, Inoue T, Inoue T, Murakami S, Furukawa S, Yoshida K, et al. Results of low- and high-dose-rate interstitial brachytherapy for T3 mobile tongue cancer. Radiother Oncol. 2003;68(2):123-8.
60. Inoue T, Inoue T, Yoshida K, Yoshioka Y, Shimamoto S, Tanaka E, et al. Phase III trial of high- vs. low-dose-rate interstitial radiotherapy for early mobile tongue cancer. Int J Radiat Oncol Biol Phys. 2001;51(1):171-5.
61. Inoue T, Inoue T, Yamazaki H, Koizumi M, Kagawa K, Yoshida K, et al. High dose rate versus low dose rate interstitial radiotherapy for carcinoma of the floor of mouth. Int J Radiat Oncol Biol Phys. 1998;41(1):53-8.
62. Yamazaki H, Yoshida K, Yoshioka Y, Shimizutani K, Furukawa S, Koizumi M, et al. High dose rate brachytherapy for oral cancer. J Radiat Res. 2013;54(1):1-17.
63. Mazeron JJ, Ardiet JM, Haide-Meder C, Kovacs G, Levendag P, Peiffert D, et al. GEC-ESTRO recommendations for brachytherapy for head and neck squamous cell carcinomas. Radiother Oncol. 2009;91:150-6.

12

CHAPTER

Principles of Breast Cancer Surgery

Kanchan Kaur, Hemant Singhal

INTRODUCTION

The role of surgery in the treatment of breast cancer has seen a dramatic change over the past century, from that of the only chance for cure to becoming one weapon in a range of treatment options. Since the first radical mastectomy by Halsted in 1891, surgery remained the mainstay of breast cancer treatment. The evolution of radiation therapy and then the development of chemotherapy with the discovery of alkylating agents and hormonal manipulation, it soon became apparent that cancer could be treated using more than one modality.

The management of patients with breast cancer now involves more than one specialist. Management decisions are made within a multidisciplinary team including surgeons, medical and radiation oncologists, radiologists, pathologists and specialists in palliative care. Increasingly, specialist breast nurses are also intimately involved in coordinating this multidisciplinary activity. Breast cancer care therefore cuts across the traditional specialties, and the development of multidisciplinary team provides a more efficient and complete service for patients. The breast surgeon may be called upon to assist with diagnosis, assessment of tumor staging and removal of tumor. A further aspect of breast practice is in screening to detect malignancy before it has caused symptoms, or the identification of patients at high-risk of developing breast cancer.

DIAGNOSIS AND STAGING

The diagnosis of breast cancer is achieved through triple assessment (Fig. 1). The first step of triple assessment is clinical examination, which allows the clinician to assess the symptoms and signs. Based on this, the second step is breast imaging, which includes mammogram, ultrasonography (USG) and if indicated, an MRI.[1,2] This allows proper local staging prior to the institution of treatment. In appropriate patients, systemic imaging like a PET CT scan may be required to ascertain metastasis. Once the number and size of the lesions is established in the breast, the third step in the assessment process is to obtain tissue diagnosis through a biopsy.

The mainstay of preoperative diagnosis is a biopsy. A biopsy is "to procure enough neoplastic tissue to establish an accurate diagnosis without jeopardizing local tumor control or the patient". Biopsies for diagnosis can be done with fine-needle aspiration, core-needle biopsy or incisional or excisional biopsy.[3,4]

Fine-needle Aspiration

Fine-needle aspirations obtain cell suspensions suitable for cytology or flow cytometry. This technique can be helpful in aspirating a breast lump, or an axillary lymph node. The advantages of fine-needle aspiration include the lack of a scar, lack of need for anesthetic, good patient tolerance of the procedure and rapid reporting of the cytology results. However, breast cancer cytology cannot distinguish between invasive and noninvasive cancers. Because of the possibility of false-positive results, cytology is not considered sufficient for proceeding with a major surgical resection such as a mastectomy.

A fine-needle aspiration can be done when the determination of atypical or malignant cells will help in

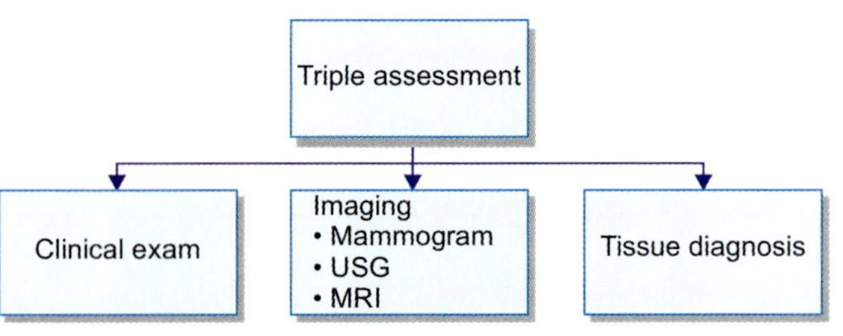

Fig. 1 Triple assessment

diagnosis or treatment, such as documenting whether a lesion is recurrent cancer in a patient with a known history of the disease.

Core-needle Biopsy

Core-needle biopsies can be done percutaneously by palpating a mass or lymph node or by radiologic guidance. A core biopsy yields tissue architecture, including the diagnosis of malignancy, whether a tumor is noninvasive or invasive, and determination of tumor grade, lymphovascular invasion, estrogen receptor status, progesterone receptor status and Her-2/neu gene amplification. Advantages include the ability to do the biopsy with image guidance under local anesthesia, minimal scarring and improved patient tolerance of the procedure.

A core-needle biopsy can allow planning for either neoadjuvant therapy or for extent of surgical resection. For example, a core-needle biopsy of a large breast mass can allow neoadjuvant chemotherapy for a breast malignancy and possibly downstage the patient to being a breast conservation candidate. Thus, it is usually the procedure of choice for making a pathologic diagnosis.

Incisional Biopsy

Incisional biopsies are usually done when a needle biopsy is technically not feasible. For cutaneous lesions like suspected Paget's disease of the nipple, an incisional biopsy will sample all layers of skin including the subcutaneous fat. This procedure can be performed under local anesthesia.

Excisional Biopsy

An excisional biopsy can be cosmetically unacceptable and obligate a mastectomy. Excisional biopsy implies the removal of the entire breast lesion or lump. Disadvantages include the resultant scar, the need for anesthetic, and the potential need for re-excision for margins. It is important to orientate excisional biopsy specimens in three dimensions for the pathologist to determine margins if surgical re-excision is needed. Care should be taken, when biopsying more than one lesion of the same patient. In this setting, precise labeling of each biopsy specimen in separate containers is needed in the event that only one of the biopsied lesions is malignant to correctly identify the area to be further treated.

PLANNING OF BREAST CANCER SURGERY

Proper preoperative planning is essential to the success of breast cancer surgery. This is even more important in the current context of breast and axilla conserving procedures. The surgeon has to plan the appropriate surgery based on clinical and imaging findings. The axillary surgical procedure is independent of the procedure being planned for the breast. Where preoperative assessment indicates axillary nodal involvement, an axillary clearance is performed. However, in patients where axillary nodes do not appear to be involved, a sentinel node biopsy is performed.

The surgical options available for a patient of breast cancer are:

- *Breast conserving surgery (BCS)*
  - Wide local excision
  - Wire-guided or imaging-guided wide local excision (for impalpable lesions).
- *Mastectomy*
  - Radical mastectomy (Halsted's), first performed in 1882, involves removal of entire breast, axillary nodes, pectoralis major and pectoralis minor muscle.
  - Simple mastectomy
  - Modified radical mastectomy, removal of entire breast along with axillary contents (fat, fascia and nodes), sparing pectoralis major muscle.
  - Skin and nipple sparing mastectomy
  - Skin sparing mastectomy.

Reconstruction should be offered to all patients undergoing a mastectomy. This can be done in the primary or delayed setting.

BREAST CONSERVING SURGERY

The safety of breast conservation in a patient diagnosed with breast cancer has been proven in six randomized trials (Table 1).[5-10] In the appropriately selected patient, mastectomy can be avoided.

The three main criteria for deciding upon a breast conserving operation are:

1. Oncological safety
2. Preserving cosmesis
3. Patient choice and counseling.

Oncological Safety

It is imperative to be certain that the breast can be saved in a diagnosed case of breast cancer. The following factors help decide suitability:

- *Size of the tumor:* There is no fixed criterion on the exact size of the tumor, which is suitable for BCS. It is the ratio of the size of the tumor to the size of the breast, which helps guide the decision process. Generally speaking, breast conservation is feasible if negative margins can be achieved while preserving cosmesis. The borderline limit may range from 2 cm for small sized breasts to 5 cm for larger breasts. In patients who have larger tumors, two options are available:
  - *Neoadjuvant chemotherapy*: Upfront chemotherapy affords the possibility of breast conservation. This allows to shrink large tumors to a size whereby a wide local excision can be performed.[11,12]

Table 1 Prospective randomized trials comparing mastectomy and breast conserving surgery

Trial	*N*	*Follow-up*	*05 (5%)—Mastectomy*	*OS(%)—BCS + RT*
NSABP B-06	1851	20	47.2%	46.2%
NCl	237	26	44	38
EORTC	903	8	64	66
Danish Breast Cancer Group	793	20	49.1	53.7
Milan	701	20	58.8	58.3
Institute Gustave-Roussy	179	10	80	79

Abbreviations: BCS, breast conserving surgery; RT, radiotherapy; OS, overall surgical; NSABP, National Surgical adjuvant breast

- *Oncoplastic procedures*: The last decade has seen the advent of specialized breast surgical procedures, which involve special techniques aimed at maintaining the breast form after large volume excisions. These procedures combine basic oncological principles with plastic surgical techniques to enhance cosmesis. Particular emphasis is laid on understanding rearrangement techniques based on breast parenchymal flaps. Maintaining nipple position, correcting ptosis and symmetrizing the contralateral breast are the goals of a successful oncoplastic procedure.

- *Number of tumors in the breast:* For patients with multifocal tumors, breast conservation is not a safe option. MRI of breasts is recommended as part of the evaluation for patients either with a higher possibility of multifocal disease (invasive lobular cancer) or with dense breasts where mammogram and USG may miss a second focus (Figs 2A to C).[13,14]

Maintaining cosmesis: As a thumb rule, if more than 20% of breast volume is excised as part of a routine wide local excision, it can lead to breast disfigurement. It is for such patients that oncoplastic procedures are employed. When large volume

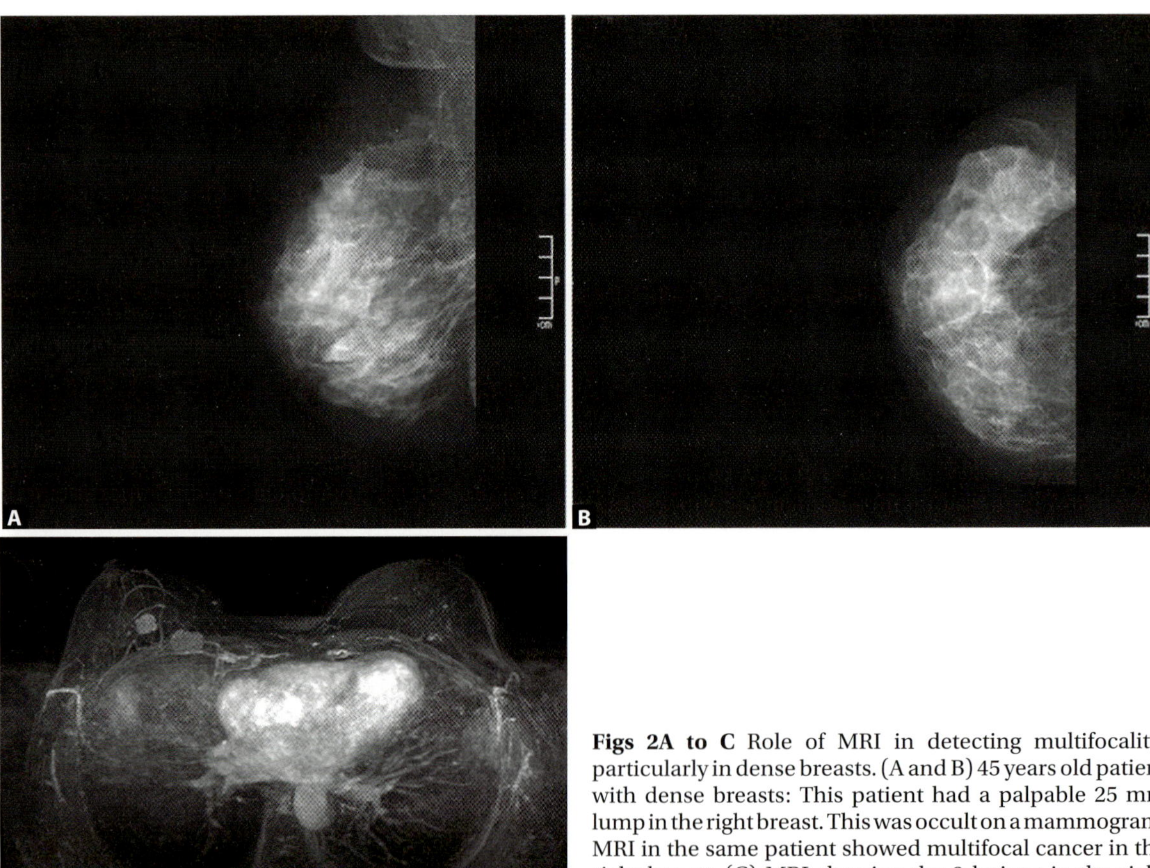

Figs 2A to C Role of MRI in detecting multifocality, particularly in dense breasts. (A and B) 45 years old patient with dense breasts: This patient had a palpable 25 mm lump in the right breast. This was occult on a mammogram. MRI in the same patient showed multifocal cancer in the right breast; (C) MRI showing the 2 lesions in the right breast.

Courtesy: Dr Kanchan Kaur, Consultant, Breast Services, Medanta—The Medicity, Haryana, India

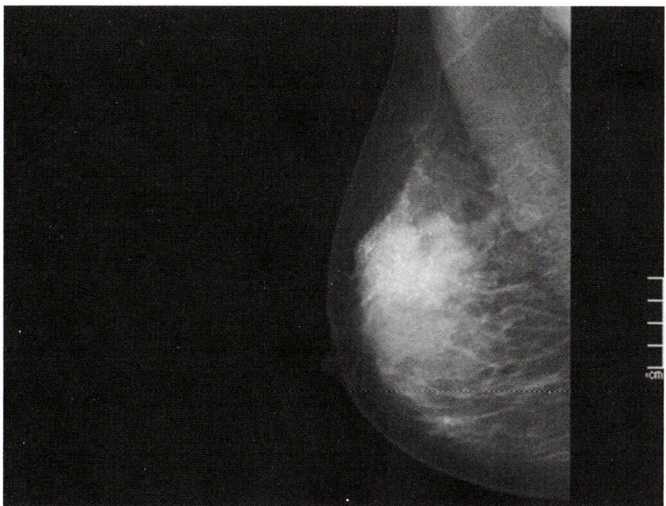

Fig. 3 Extensive malignant microcalcification (not suitable for BCS)

Courtesy: Dr Kanchan Kaur, Consultant, Breast Services, Medanta—The Medicity, Haryana, India

excisions are performed, it may become necessary to perform a contralateral symmetrizing procedure.

Patient counseling: Patients who are offered the option of breast conservation must be counseled about the following facts:

- Need for adjuvant radiotherapy
- Possibility of cosmetic asymmetry
- Postradiation sequelae like skin thickening, color change, skin edema.

CONTRAINDICATIONS OF BREAST CONSERVING SURGERY

- Multifocal tumors
- Extensive malignant microcalcification (Fig. 3)
- Inflammatory breast cancer
- Prior chest wall radiation
- Pregnancy (radiation risk).

SURGICAL CONSIDERATIONS IN PLANNING BREAST CONSERVING SURGERY

- Planning the incision
- Margin status
- Planning the repair.

Planning the Incision

Preoperative clinical assessments, coupled with the imaging findings help decide the most suitable incision. Poorly planned incisions lead to unacceptable cosmetic results. Incision placement should anticipate the potential use of oncoplastic techniques in subsequent procedures.

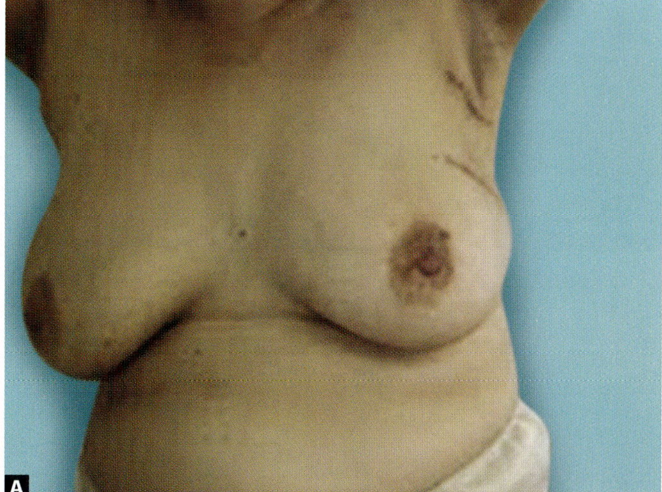

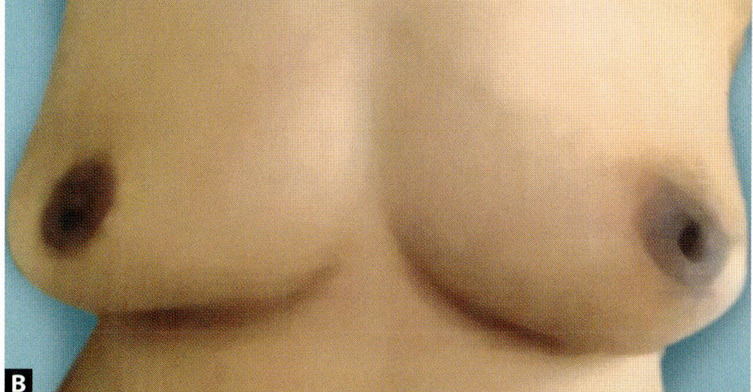

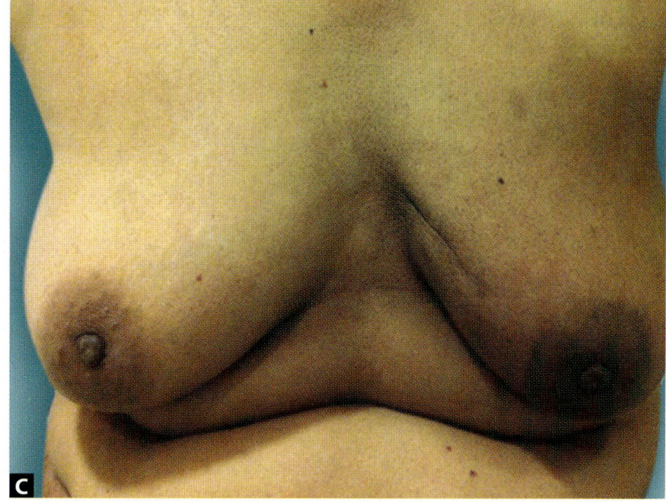

Figs 4A to C Different types of incisions for wide local excision of cancer. (A) Skin crease incision in upper outer quadrant of breast with separate incision for sentinel node biopsy in the axilla; (B) Periareolar incision for left breast lumpectomy; (C) Oblique incision in inner half of the breast for an upper inner quadrant tumor

Courtesy: Dr Kanchan Kaur, Consultant, Breast Services, Medanta—The Medicity, Haryana, India

For palpable tumors, incisions can be:

- Exactly over the tumor (Figs 4A to C)

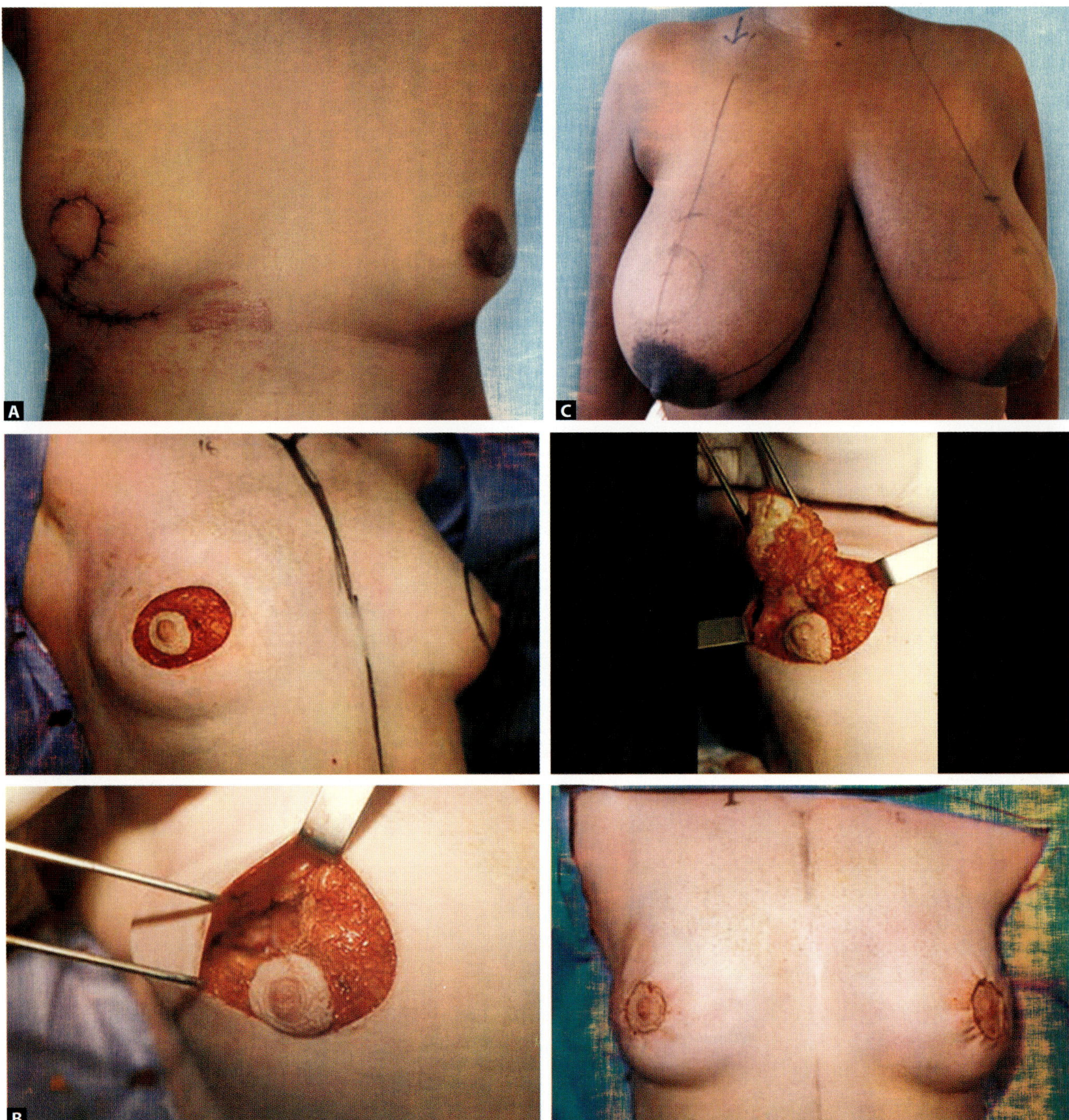

Figs 5A to C Examples of oncoplastic procedures: (A) Grisoti flap for central tumors after excision of nipple areola complex; (B) Round block technique through periareolar incision for a tumor at 12 o' clock position. Contralateral symmetrization procedure performed; (C to F) Reduction mammoplasty (with contralateral symmetrization) with a superomedial pedicle in a patient with two cancers in the lower half of the breast; (C) Preoperative markings

Courtesy: Dr Kanchan Kaur, Consultant, Breast Services, Medanta—The Medicity, Haryana, India

- At a distance from the tumor as part of a planned oncoplastic procedure (Figs 5A to F).

For impalpable tumors, wire placement allows localization and aids excision (Fig. 6). Other less commonly employed techniques are ROLL (radio-guided occult lesion localization) and RSL (radioactive seed localization).[15-17] Specimen X-rays of the excised tissue specimen helps confirm that the lesion has been excised (Figs 7A and B).

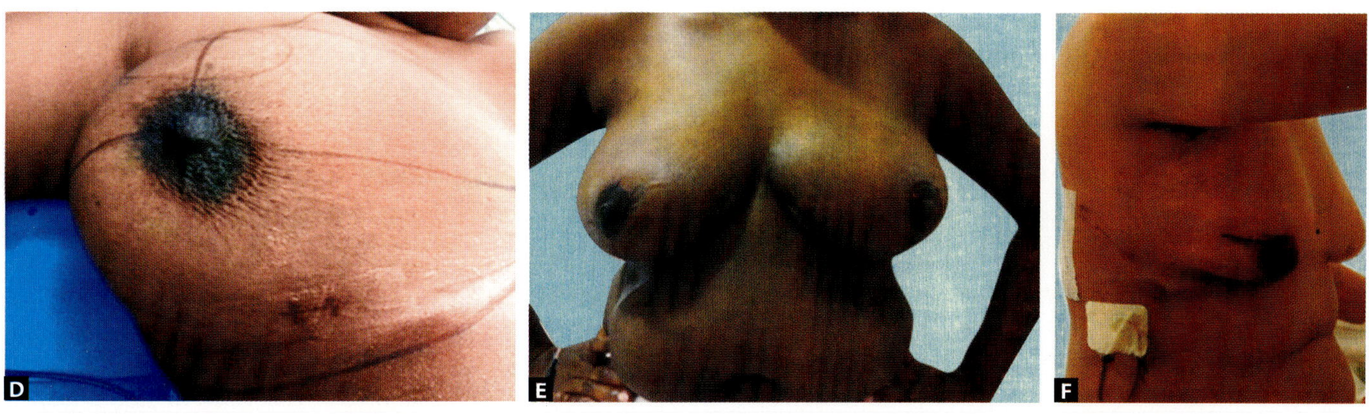

Figs 5D to F (D) Preoperative markings: + signs mark the two tumors; (E) 1 week postoperative. Right axillary drain in place; (F) Skin and nipple sparing mastectomy with primary latissimus dorsi flap reconstruction

Courtesy: Dr Kanchan Kaur, Consultant, Breast Services, Medanta—The Medicity, Haryana, India

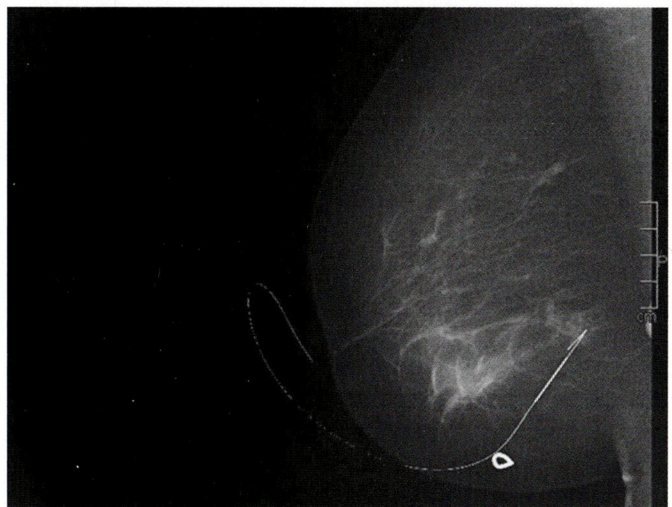

Fig. 6 Wire-guided wide local excision

Courtesy: Dr Kanchan Kaur, Consultant, Breast Services, Medanta—The Medicity, Haryana, India

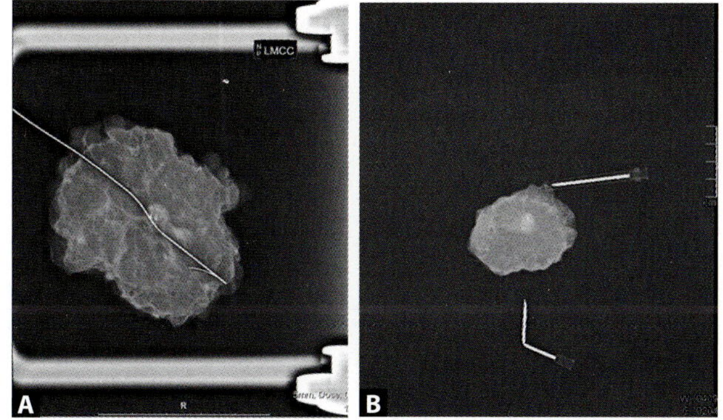

Figs 7A and B (A) Specimen mammograms wire-guided wide excision; (B) Specimen mammogram of wide local excision

Courtesy: Dr Kanchan Kaur, Consultant, Breast Services, Medanta—The Medicity, Haryana, India

Margin Status

Margin status is important to assess adequacy of excision. Intraoperative assessment can be performed by doing an intraoperative USG, specimen X-ray or frozen section of the margins as per surgeon preference. Histopathology gives final confirmation of the margins. Orientation sutures must be placed to guide the pathologist on assessing margins. There has been a long-standing debate over what constitutes an 'adequate margin'. These range from a minimum of 1 mm in some studies to a maximum 10 mm in others. NSABP defines a negative margin as 'no tumor on ink'.[18] A recent meta-analysis found no significant statistical difference between different margin widths and incidence of local recurrence.[19]

Planning the Repair

After an adequate lumpectomy has been performed, the cavity base and margins should be marked with clips. This aids the radiation oncologist while planning cavity boost. It is important to approximate the cavity walls to minimize the dead space. This in turn reduces seroma formation and allows healing. Undermining of the skin and the subglandular space allows easy mobilization of flaps. Care must be taken to avoid excessive mobilization in patients with fatty breasts as this can lead to fat necrosis and poor healing.

SALIENT FEATURES OF BREAST CONSERVING SURGERY

- Ensure proper local staging to confirm safety of BCS
- Proper patient counseling particularly the need for adjuvant radiation must be reinforced
- Individualize the correct lumpectomy/oncoplastic technique best suited to the patient
- Assess the adequacy of lump excision by inking the margins of the specimen and histologic evaluation of the surgical margins

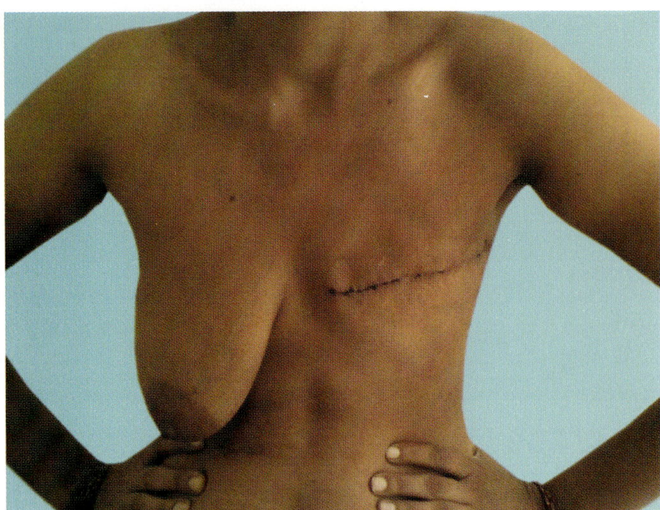

Fig. 8 Simple mastectomy

- Ensure cosmesis
- Use marking clips to mark the excision margins to allow radiotherapy planning.

MASTECTOMY

Mastectomy involves complete removal of the entire breast tissue (Fig. 8). Prior to the advent of the concept of sentinel node biopsy, the procedure of mastectomy invariably involved complete axillary dissection. This procedure is called a modified radical mastectomy (MRM). However, in patients who do not have axillary nodal metastasis (as confirmed by sentinel node biopsy), the axilla is now routinely spared.

Mastectomy may be performed with or without reconstruction. When reconstruction is offered at the same time that the mastectomy is being performed, it is called primary reconstruction. When it is done at a later date it is called delayed reconstruction.

TYPES OF RECONSTRUCTION

- *Autologous:* This entails the use of tissue from another part of the patient's own body to reconstruct the breast. When the continuity of blood supply to the donor site is maintained, the flap is called a pedicle flap. When a new anastomosis is made at the recipient site after completely severing blood supply from the donor site, the flap is called a free flap. Free flaps are at a slightly higher risk of flap necrosis as compared to pedicle flaps.
  Examples of autologous flaps:
  - *Latissimus dorsi (LD flap):* This is a pedicled flap that utilizes the latissimus dorsi muscle. It is the workhorse of most breast reconstructions.
  - *Deep inferior epigastric artery perforator (DIEP) flap:* This is a free flap that utilizes fat from the abdominal wall. It is a free flap based on the deep inferior epigastric artery perforator. Flap complications like necrosis, volume loss are more common.
  - *Transverse rectus abdominis myocutaneous (TRAM) flap:* A TRAM flap utilizes the transverse abdominis muscle. This can be a pedicled or a free flap.
  - *Other steps:* Tissue from gluteal or inner thigh areas can also be used as free flaps for reconstruction.
- *Combined autologous and prosthetic:* The patients own body tissue may not always be sufficient to be able to reconstruct the breast. This is particularly seen in big-breasted women who need larger volumes of tissue to match the normal breast. This extra volume is gained by using external artificial material like silicon prosthesis.
- *Prosthetic:* This form of reconstruction involves using external artificial material to reconstruct the breast mound. An expander is placed in the subpectoral muscle pocket and inflated over a period of weeks with saline, which is injected into a port placed under the skin. Once there is a size match with the contralateral breast, the expander can be exchanged for silicon prosthesis. There are expanders like the Becker's which need not be changed for silicon and can be left in situ once the inflation is complete.

RISK-REDUCING MASTECTOMY

Performing a mastectomy in the absence of a diagnosis of cancer is called risk-reducing mastectomy. It may be unilateral in a patient who is already diagnosed with cancer in one breast, or bilateral in women deemed to be at a high-risk. A prophylactic mastectomy offers the largest absolute breast cancer risk reduction in women with BRCA mutations to the tune of 90–95%.[20,21]

Other potential indications are:

- Atypical hyperplasia or lobular carcinoma *in situ* (LCIS)
- Familial breast cancer
- Age of diagnosis less than 40 years
- History of atypical hyperplasia or LCIS followed by unilateral breast cancer.

SENTINEL NODE BIOPSY

The disease status of the lymph nodes in the armpit axilla is the most important factor that determines the outcome for patients with early stage breast cancer. Accurate assessment of nodes is important for staging, prognosis and guiding treatment selection. A sentinel node biopsy is now considered the gold standard for staging of the axilla.

What is Sentinel Node Biopsy?

It is a procedure, which allows detection of spread of cancer to axillary lymph nodes, without the need for removing all of them, as is usually the case. Breast cancer is believed to spread from the breast to the axillary lymph nodes in a systematic manner. Studies have shown that if the sentinel nodes are not involved with cancer, then a complete axillary dissection can be safely avoided.[22,23]

At the time of preoperative work-up for cancer, the axilla is assessed clinically and by ultrasound. If abnormal lymph nodes are detected, they undergo fine-needle aspiration cytology and if there is proven cancer then the patient does not need a sentinel node biopsy and proceeds to axillary clearance in which all the lymph nodes are removed from the axilla. However, if the preoperative work-up does not identify axillary lymph node involvement, a sentinel lymph node biopsy is planned. This involves testing the sentinel nodes at the time of the primary breast surgery. The results are obtained intraoperatively. If cancer cells are not identified in the glands then nothing further needs to be done. If there is evidence of cancer spread to the sentinel node then a complete axillary dissection is performed at the same time.

What are the Benefits of Having a Sentinel Node Biopsy?

A sentinel node biopsy avoids an unnecessary axillary clearance in patients who do not have involved lymph nodes. It therefore associated with fewer complications such as infection (cellulitis) of the chest wall and arm, sensory changes, and lymphedema, which may otherwise be associated with an axillary dissection.

How is the Procedure Performed?

The procedure involves injection of two types of dyes into the breast. These travel from the breast to the axillary lymph nodes and help in the identification of the sentinel nodes, which are the first nodes to trap the dyes. One of these is a radioactive dye called Technetium-99. It is injected generally a day prior to the surgery. It imparts radioactivity to the lymph nodes, which are then identified during surgery using a hand-held radiation detector. Another dye, which is injected in the operation theater just prior to surgery is a blue colored dye called patent blue V. This aids visual identification by coloring the nodes blue (Fig. 9).

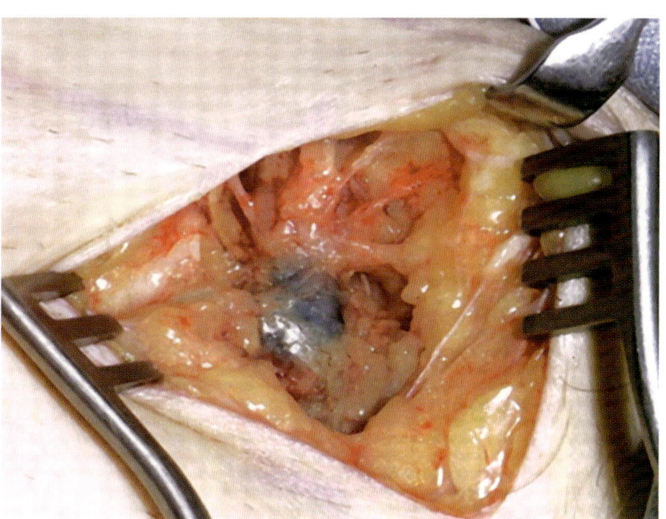

Fig. 9 Blue sentinel node in axilla

Disadvantage of the Procedure

There is a possibility of a false positive or false negative with intraoperative evaluation. The sensitivity of intraoperative analysis has been reported to range from 58% to 76%, depending on tumor characteristics and the method of pathological examination.[24,25]

Axillary Dissection

The axillary lymph nodes represent the most prevalent site of metastasis for breast cancer and represent an important prognostic factor in the staging of the breast cancer patient. For this reason, the removal of the regional lymph nodes is often performed at the time of resection of the primary cancer. Besides staging information, a regional lymphadenectomy provides *regional control* of the cancer.

It is well documented that the removal of these regional lymph nodes can result in long-term survival benefit in approximately 20–40% of individuals depending upon the extent of nodal involvement. Hence, the removal of axillary lymph nodes can be therapeutic.

COMPLICATIONS IN BREAST SURGERY

- *General wound complications:* Wound infections, seroma, hematoma and chronic incisional pain occur in up to 30% cases.
  - *Wound infections:* Staphylococcal organisms are usually implicated in these infections, introduced via skin flora. Obesity, old age, smoking, diabetes mellitus and amount of tissue removed are some of the most consistently identified risk factors for breast wound sepsis.
  - *Seroma:* Seroma occurs at rates ranging from 3% to 85% after breast surgery.
  - *Hematoma:* Such complication continues to occur in 2–10% of cases. Widespread use of electrocautery has largely reduced the incidence of hematoma formation in breast surgery.
  - *Venous thromboembolism (VTE):* There is an 8% and 17% rate of VTE for early and advanced stage breast cancer respectively receiving chemotherapy.
  - *Chronic pain:* Some patients experience chronic incisional pain that can be quite disabling and refractory to standard analgesics. The exact etiology of this syndrome remains obscure, although it is commonly assumed neuropathic in nature.

- *Complication specific to mastectomy procedures—* Incisional dog ears.
- *Complications specific to lumpectomy:*
  - Breast fibrosis
  - Breast lymphedema
  - Breast asymmetry
  - Chronic/recurrent breast cellulitis
  - BCS related angiosarcoma (very rare).
- *Complications related to axillary procedures:*
  - *Upper extremity lymphedema following axillary lymph node dissection:* It is a life-long risk and quite refractory to treatment when it occurs. Lymphedema occurs in 13–27% cases. Risk of lymphedema increases after higher-level axillary dissection compared to less extensive surgery. Other risk factors include obesity, upper limb trauma, infection and regional radiotherapy. Patients can minimize risk of lymphedema by participating in an aggressive and regulated physical therapy program.
  - Stewart-Treves syndrome
  - Winged scapulae after disruption of long thoracic nerve
  - Axillary webs.
- *Complications associated with sentinel lymph node biopsy:*
  - Allergic reactions to blue dye (< 2%): Blue urticaria.

POSTOPERATIVE FOLLOW-UP AND MONITORING

All breast cancer patients, irrespective of the stage at which they were diagnosed, need to have an individualized follow-up routine. The intent of this is early detection of recurrent disease when it is potentially still treatable. A meta-analysis of breast cancer survivors from thirteen studies suggests that the patients detected with asymptomatic recurrence, exhibited superior survival in both the locoregional and contralateral breast cancer recurrence compared to women who presented with symptoms due to recurrent cancer.[26]

National Comprehensive Cancer Network (NCCN) guidelines recommend routine history and physical examination every 4–6 months for the first 5 years after primary therapy and annually thereafter.[27] American Society of Clinical Oncology (ASCO) recommends routine history and physical examination every 3–6 months for first 3 years, every 6–12 months for years 4 and 5, then annually thereafter.[28] Both the NCCN and ASCO do not recommend the use of routine complete blood counts, chemistry panels, tumor markers, bone scans, computed tomography (CT) scans, magnetic resonance imaging (MRI) scans, positron emission computed tomography (PET) scans, or ultrasound examinations in asymptomatic patients without specific clinical examination findings.[27,28]

SUMMARY

The major objective for surgery is to achieve optimal local control. This was well achieved by the Halsted mastectomy, which gave a greater than 90% local control, despite the fact that the overall survival of the patients was not improved. The emergence of multimodal therapy has dramatically affected the surgical approach to many primary cancers, especially when surgical resection of the tumor is combined with radiotherapy. Local control is significantly improved after surgical resection of breast. In fact, the addition of radiation therapy as an adjunctive therapy has allowed for less-radical procedures to be performed with an improvement in the quality of life of patients.

One of the major principles of conservative surgical therapy of the primary tumor is to obtain adequate negative margins around the primary tumor, which could mean different operative approaches depending on the tumor type and its local involvement with adjacent structures.

The overall survival of patients with invasive breast cancer is comparable if treated by mastectomy versus lumpectomy plus adjuvant radiotherapy.[29] This realization has resulted in better cosmesis and quality of life. Adjuvant and neoadjuvant therapies involving chemotherapy, immunotherapy and hormonal therapies have also become standard approaches resulting in improved local control and overall survival.

REFERENCES

1. National Comprehensive Cancer Network (NCCN). NCCN Clinical Practice Guidelines in Oncology: Breast cancer screening and diagnosis, Version 1.2013, http://www.nccn.org.
2. Lee CH, Dershaw DD, Kopans D, et al. Breast Cancer Screening with imaging: Recommendations from the society of breast imagingnand ACR on the use of mammography, breast MRI, breast USG and other technologies for the detection of clinically occult breast cancer. J Am Coll Radiol 2010;7:18-27.
3. Brancato B, Crocetti E, Bianchi S, et al. Accuracy of needle biopsy of breast lesions visible on ultrasound: audit of fine needle versus core needle biopsy in 3233 consecutive samplings with ascertained outcomes. Breast. 2012;21(4):449-54. doi: 10.1016/j.breast.2011.10.008. Epub 2011 Nov 15.
4. Willems SM, van Deurzen CH, van Diest PJ. Diagnosis of breast lesions: fine-needle aspiration cytology or core needle biopsy? A review. J Clin Pathol. 2012;65(4):287-92. doi: 10.1136/jclinpath-2011-200410. Epub 2011 Oct 29.
5. Fisher B1, Anderson S, Bryant J. Twenty-year follow-up of a randomized trial comparing total mastectomy, lumpectomy, and lumpectomy plus irradiation for the treatment of invasive breast cancer. N Engl J Med. 2002;17;347(16):1233-41.
6. Sarrazin D, Lê MG, Arriagada R, et al: Ten-year results of a randomized trial comparing a conservative treatment to mastectomy in early breast cancer. Radiother Oncol 1989; 14:177-84.

7. van Dongen JA, Bartelink H, Fentiman IS, et al: Randomized clinical trial to assess the value of breast-conserving therapy in stage I and II breast cancer, EORTC 10801 Trial. J Natl Cancer Inst Monogr 1992;11:15-8.
8. Blichert-Toft M, Nielsen M, Düring M, et al. Long-term results of breast conserving surgery vs. mastectomy for early stage invasive breast cancer: 20-year follow-up of the Danish randomized DBCG-82TM protocol. Acta Oncol. 2008; 47(4):672-81.
9. Veronesi U, Cascinelli N, Mariani L, et al. Twenty-year follow-up of a randomized study comparing breast-conserving surgery with radical mastectomy for early breast cancer. N Engl J Med. 2002;347(16):1227-32.
10. Simone NL, Dan T, Shih J, et al. Twenty-five year results of the national cancer institute randomized breast conservation trial. Breast Cancer Res Treat. 2012;132(1):197-203.
11. Mieog JSD, van der Hage JA, van de Velde CJH. Neoadjuvant chemotherapy for operable breast cancer. British Journal of Surgery. 2007;94(10):1189-1200.
12. Caudle AS, Kuerer HM. Breast conservation therapy after neoadjuvant chemotherapy: Optimization of a multimodality approach. J Surg Oncol. 2014. doi: 10.1002/jso.23595.
13. Lehman CD, Gatsonis C, Kuhl CK, et al. ACRIN trial 6667. Investigators Group. MRI evaluation of the contralateral breast in women with recently diagnosed breast cnacer. N Engl J Med 2007;356(13):1295-303.
14. http://www.acr.org/~/media/ACR/Documents/PGTS/guidelines/MRI_Breast.pdf
15. Sarlos D, Frey LD, Haueisen H, Landmann G, Kots LA, Schaer G. Radioguided occult lesion localization (ROLL) for treatment and diagnosis of malignant and premalignant breast lesions combined with sentinel node biopsy: A prospective clinical trial with 100 patients. European Journal of Surgical Oncology (EJSO) 2009;35(4):403-8.
16. Richard J., Gray MD, Christopher Salud BA, Keoni Nguyen BS, et al. Randomized Prospective Evaluation of a Novel Technique for Biopsy or Lumpectomy of Nonpalpable Breast Lesions: Radioactive Seed Versus Wire Localization. Annals of Surgical Oncology 2001; 8(9): 711-5.
17. Lovrics PJ, Cornacchi SD, Vora R, et al. Systematic review of radioguided surgery for non-palpable breast cancer. European Journal of Surgical Oncology (EJSO), 2011;37(5)388-97.
18. Fisher E, Anderson S, Tan-Chiu E, et al. Fifteen-year prognostic discriminants for invasive breast carcinoma: National Surgical Adjuvant Breast and Bowel Project Protocol-06. Cancer. 2001; 91:1679-87.
19. Houssami N, Macaskill P, Marinovich ML, et al. The Association of Surgical Margins and Local Recurrence in Women with Early-Stage Invasive Breast Cancer Treated with Breast-Conserving Therapy: A Meta-Analysis.: Ann Surg Oncol 2014;21:717-30.
20. Heemskerk-Gerritsen BAM, Menke-Pluijmers MBE, Jager A. Substantial breast cancer risk reduction and potential survival benefit after bilateral mastectomy when compared with surveillance in healthy BRCA1 and BRCA2 mutation carriers: a prospective analysis Ann Oncol (2013) 24 (8): 2029-35.
21. Timothy R Rebbeck, Tara Friebel, Henry T Lynch, et al. Bilateral prophylactic mastectomy reduces breast cancer risk in BRCA1 and BRCA2 mutation carriers: The PROSE Study Group. JCO 2004;22(6):1055-62.
22. Veronesi U, Paganelli G, Galimberti V, et al. Sentinel-node biopsy to avoid axillary dissection in breast cancer with clinically negative lymph nodes. The Lancet. 1997;349(9069): 1864-7.
23. Robert E Mansel, Lesley Fallowfield, Mark Kissin, et al. Randomized Multicenter Trial of Sentinel Node Biopsy Versus Standard Axillary Treatment in Operable Breast Cancer: The Almanac Trial. Jnci J Natl Cancer Inst. 2006;98(9):599-609.
24. Weiser MR, Montgomery LL, Susnik B, Tan LK, Borgen PI, Cody HS. "Is routine intraoperative frozen-section examination of sentinel lymph nodes in breast cancer worthwhile?" Annals of Surgical Oncology, 2000;7(9):651-5.
25. van de Vrande S, Meijer J, Rijnders A, et al. "The value of intraoperative frozen section examination of sentinel lymph nodes in breast cancer," European Journal of Surgical Oncology; 2009;35(3)276-80. View at Publisher·
26. Lu WL, Jansen L, Post WJ, Bonnema J, Van de Velde JC, De Bock GH. Impact on survival of early detection of isolated breast recurrences after the primary treatment for breast cancer: a meta-analysis. Breast Cancer Res Treat. 2009;114:403-12.
27. NCCN Clinical Practice Guidelines in Oncology (NCCN Guidelines): breast cancer-version 3.2013.
28. Khatcheressian J, Hurley P, Bentug E, Esserman LJ, Grunfeld E, Halberg F. Breast Cancer Follow-Up and Management After Primary Treatment: American Society of Clinical Oncology Clinical Practice Guideline Update. 2013;31:961-5.
29. Clarke M, Collins R, Darby S, et al. Effects of radiotherapy and of differences in the extent of surgery for early breast cancer on local recurrence and 15-year survival: an overview of the randomised trials.Lancet 2005;366(9503):2087-106.

13 CHAPTER

Carcinoma of Breast

Shyam Singh Bisht, Tejinder Kataria, Kushal Narang

NONINVASIVE BREAST CANCER

INTRODUCTION

Noninvasive breast cancer (Stage Tis) includes lobular carcinoma in situ (LCIS), Paget's disease of nipple and ductal carcinoma in situ (DCIS). All three are distinct in clinical presentation, biologic potential and histopathologic characteristics. They currently comprise a larger percentage (20%) of all breast cancer cases because of increased use of mammography. The optimal treatment approach is debatable, although cancer-specific survival for Tis exceeds 95%, regardless of the type of local therapy employed.

LOBULAR CARCINOMA IN SITU

It constitutes areas of abnormal cell growth in the lobules and the milk-producing glands at the end of breast ducts. Initially considered a *direct precursor* to invasive lobular carcinoma, now it is accepted as a *marker of increased risk of invasive carcinoma* (usually ductal > lobular). Invasive cancer develops in approximately *20–25%* of women, with nearly equal risk for both breasts. LCIS has *multicentric distribution* (up to 90% of mastectomy specimens), bilateral involvement (35–59%) and *represents less than 15%* of all noninvasive breast cancer.[1] The majority of women are *premenopausal* at diagnosis with an average age of 45 years. It has not been described in men as they lack lobules.[2]

Lobular carcinoma in situ cells are commonly *estrogen-receptor positive*, the loss of E-cadherin is often observed, while overexpression of c-erbB-2 and p53 is uncommon. Pleomorphic LCIS is an aggressive variant with greater potential for progressing to invasive cancer.[3-5]

Risk Factors

Risk factors for development of LCIS correspond to those identified for invasive carcinoma.

Presentation

It is often detected as an incidental biopsy finding as there are no characteristic clinical or mammographic indicators of LCIS. Rarely, LCIS can be detected with mammographic calcifications.

Magnetic Resonance Imaging as a Screening Tool

In 2009, the National Comprehensive Cancer Network published guidelines reflecting a panel consensus opinion that *annual breast magnetic resonance imaging (MRI) should be considered* in patients with LCIS as it is a marker of increase risk of subsequent development of invasive disease. Studies have revealed a 3.8–4.5% breast cancer detection rate in LCIS, which supporting this consideration.

Management for LCIS

Lobular carcinoma in situ either may be the sole histologic diagnosis or may be associated with another malignancy (DCIS or invasive carcinoma).

If LCIS found with DCIS or invasive disease: Management is as per the dominant malignant histology (DCIS or invasive carcinoma) and LCIS is to be disregarded. In such cases, additional surgery to obtain clear margins for LCIS is not necessary.

If LCIS is the sole histologic diagnosis: (i) Most widely accepted practice is *close observation* with regular physical examination and mammographic surveillance. (ii) *Bilateral prophylactic mastectomy*: Initially, mastectomy was often performed for LCIS. Later, the high frequency of contralateral breast involvement was used to justify contralateral biopsy and even bilateral mastectomy.[6] Now, this approach is employed only for LCIS, which are at highest risk (young age, diffuse high-grade lesion and significant family history). (iii) *Chemoprevention* using tamoxifen or raloxifene.

There is *no role for radiotherapy (RT)* in the management of pure LCIS.

Evidence for the Role of Chemoprevention

NSABP-P1, Level I: This trial randomized healthy patients at high risk of breast cancer to receive placebo versus tamoxifen for 5 years. Among all patients receiving tamoxifen, the relative risk of invasive and noninvasive breast cancer was reduced by 49% and 50%, respectively. Among the 13,388 women enrolled in the study, 826 had LCIS. At a follow-up of 69 months, a 56% reduction in the incidence *of invasive cancer* in the LCIS patient group was observed.[7]

NSABP-P2 (STAR), Level I: STAR trial conducted by the NSABP randomized patients between tamoxifen and raloxifene. They observed both agents to be effective in reducing second cancer events. Results showed that tamoxifen in premenopausal and raloxifene in postmenopausal patients brings about risk reduction in women with LCIS.[8]

PAGET'S DISEASE

The clinical presentation of crusting and eczematous changes of the nipple-areola with an underlying breast cancer was reported by Sir James Paget in 1874. Paget's disease of the nipple is characterized by the presence of Paget's cells located throughout the epidermis. Paget's disease is associated with an underlying malignancy in more than 95% of cases.

Origin

According to the most widely accepted epidermotropic theory, the disease originates from the underlying in situ or invasive disease. This is supported by histologic evidence of intraepithelial extension, immunohistochemical studies and evidence suggesting that the epidermal keratinocytes release a motility factor, heregulin-α, that results in the chemotaxis of Paget's cells, which migrate to the overlying nipple epidermis.

Epidemiology

Paget's disease is rare, representing less than 5% of breast cancer cases and is typically diagnosed in the fifth or sixth decade of life. Synchronous bilateral and male Paget's disease has been reported.

Clinical Presentation

Patients with Paget's disease describe itching and burning of the nipple and areola, with slow progression toward a crusting eczematoid appearance that can extend to the periareolar skin. If neglected, bleeding, pain and ulceration can occur. Alternatively, Paget's disease can be asymptomatic and present as a pathologic finding after incidental surgical removal of the nipple-areolar complex.

Pathology

Malignant cells called Paget's cells are a pathognomonic of the disease. They are found singly or in clusters in the epidermis of the skin of the nipple and the areola and have a large, round appearance under a microscope.

Associated Malignancy

A palpable mass is detected in approximately 50% of patients at diagnosis; in more than 90% of cases, this will be an invasive carcinoma. If no palpable mass is detected, 66–86% will have an underlying DCIS.

Mammographic Findings

Mammographic findings are frequent in the presence of a palpable mass; however, normal mammograms are reported in approximately 50% cases.

Clinical Evaluation

Clinical evaluation includes bilateral breast examination, mammography and biopsy to confirm the diagnosis of Paget's disease and to fully evaluate the extent of the associated malignancy.

Management

The prognosis of Paget's disease *depends on the associated malignancy*. Therefore, local treatment, as well as systemic and regional nodal disease risk management, is directed on the associated disease.

- *Mastectomy:* For many years, mastectomy, with or without axillary lymph node dissection, was regarded as the standard surgery for Paget's disease of the breast.
- *Combined-modality approach:* Breast conserving surgery (BCS) and postoperative whole breast radiotherapy (WBRT) is an appropriate alternative to mastectomy in properly selected patients with underlying noninvasive or invasive carcinoma of limited extent.
  - Breast conserving surgery: Multicentric disease extension should be excluded before BCS. Surgical resection should include the nipple-areolar complex

with microscopically clear margins surrounding both the Paget's disease and the associated malignancy. Management of regional nodes and the risk of systemic disease are dictated by the associated malignancy.
- Whole breast radiotherapy is delivered with standard techniques.

EVIDENCE FOR CONSERVATIVE APPROACH

- The European Organisation for Research and Treatment of Cancer (EORTC) Study 10873 reported a 5-year local recurrence rate of 5.2% for Paget's in patients undergoing complete excision with tumor-free margins of the nipple–areolar complex followed by WBRT. Most of these patients had an underlying DCIS without a palpable mass.[9]
- In a seven-institution collaborative review of 36 patients with Paget's disease without a palpable mass or mammographic density, the actuarial rate of local failure as the only site of first recurrence was 9% at 5 years and 13% at both 10 years and 15 years.[10] Median follow-up was for 9.4 years. The extent of surgical resection varied as patients underwent complete (69%) or partial (25%) excision of the nipple–areolar complex and underlying breast tissue with 6% reported as biopsy only. The final margin status was documented as negative in 56%, positive in 6% and unknown in 39%. All received whole-breast irradiation, and most received an additional boost dose to the tumor bed.

DUCTAL CARCINOMA IN SITU

Ductal carcinoma in situ is a neoplastic process that is confined to the ductal system of the breast and lacks histological evidence of invasion. These cells neither disrupt the basement membrane nor involve the surrounding breast stroma, and lack the ability to metastasize. DCIS is a precursor for invasive ductal carcinoma and exists somewhere along the evolutionary continuum between benign breast tissue and invasive breast carcinoma.

Risk Factors

Risk factors for DCIS are the same as those identified for invasive carcinoma.

Presentation

Before the use of screening mammography, DCIS typically presented as a palpable mass or nipple discharge. An invasive component was commonly found, and pure DCIS was rare. Now, DCIS is mostly (95%) detected as abnormality on mammography with a nonpalpable mass.

Epidemiology

In the US, incidence of DCIS has undergone a tenfold increase in past 20 years. The rate of DCIS detection has been reported to increase from 0.56 per 1,000 mammograms among women aged 40–49 years to 1.07 per 1,000 mammograms among women aged 70–84 years.

Radiology

About 95% of new of DCIS present with mammographic abnormalities, of which microcalcifications are most typical. Calcifications may be amorphous, coarse, fine pleomorphic or fine linear. Linear and segmental calcifications are suspicious and can be associated with DCIS in up to 80% of cases. Linear and branching calcifications frequently are associated with high-grade DCIS and necrosis, whereas fine and granular calcifications are associated with low-grade DCIS. Other findings include noncalcified mammographic abnormalities like asymmetric densities, dominant masses and abnormal galactograms. The extent of the lesion determined mammographically may be used as a guide for excision; however, the size is often underestimated by 1–2 cm when compared with pathologic measurements. Improved MRI imaging acquisition and understanding of non-mass like malignant lesion imaging characteristics has made it a valuable imaging tool for DCIS. MRI has been shown to better establish the extent of DCIS, thus aiding treatment planning.

Pathology and Biology

The diverse histological spectrum of DCIS extends from noncomedo, low-grade DCIS similar in appearance to atypical ductal hyperplasia to comedo, high-grade DCIS. Also, DCIS can extend into lobules, making it difficult to distinguish from LCIS. The five subtypes of DCIS are comedo, solid, cribriform, micropapillary and papillary. Less common subtypes include apocrine, neuroendocrine, signet-cell cystic hypersecretory carcinoma and clinging DCIS.

Pathological features to be documented for DCIS include nuclear grade, presence of necrosis, polarization and architectural pattern(s), margin status, lesion size, extent of microcalcifications and correlation between specimen X-ray and mammographic findings. Knowledge of the anatomy and distribution of DCIS within the mammary ductal tree helps select patients for breast conservation and assure maximal surgical clearance of the lesion while preserving cosmesis. The DCIS growth patterns documented include unicentric (one area only), multicentric (two distinct areas separated by >4 cm), continuous (extension along ductal system without gaps) and discontinuous or multifocal (two or more areas separated by <4 cm).[11] In mammographically detected DCIS, a multicentric growth pattern is rare (<2%) and even with a discontinuous growth pattern, most cases have foci separated by less than 10 mm. Hence, a 1-cm margin of normal tissue around the lesion would lead to complete surgical clearance of histologically evident DCIS in 90% of cases.[11]

Ductal carcinoma in situ has been classified under luminal, basal and erbB2 intrinsic molecular subtypes. The estrogen receptor (ER) is present in 70% of DCIS, expressed more often in low-grade lesions (90%) than high-grade lesions (25%). Approximately 50% of DCIS lesions overexpress HER2/neu, and 25% express p53 tumor suppressor gene. Both molecular markers are noted in less than 20% of low-grade lesions but are present in approximately two-thirds of high-grade lesions. Most features of breast cancer, such as hormone receptor status, level of oncogene expression and histologic grade, are probably determined by the time DCIS evolves, although the lesion may not be a malignant phenotype.

An occult microinvasive tumor (one that does not exceed 0.1 cm in diameter) may be seen with some cases of DCIS. Such cases are classified as *microinvasive breast cancer* and are generally treated according to the guidelines for invasive disease. *Occult microinvasive tumors* are most common in patients with DCIS lesions that are more than 2.5 cm in diameter, those presenting with palpable masses or nipple discharge, and those with high-grade DCIS or comedonecrosis.

Therapy Recommendations for DCIS

General

Patients with a diagnosis of DCIS who have mammographically detected calcifications should have a post-lumpectomy, *pre-RT mammogram* to establish the new baseline, and also to document whether there is any radiographic evidence of residual calcifications.

Treatment options in the management of DCIS include:

- *Lumpectomy with adjuvant RT (Grade A):* The goal of lumpectomy is to remove the tumor with associated microcalcifications in its entirety and achieve negative surgical margins, followed by WBRT.
- Lumpectomy alone followed by observation (Grade B).
- Total mastectomy with/without sentinel lymph node biopsy with/without reconstruction.
- *Indications of total mastectomy are:* (a) multicentric DCIS when there are diffuse malignant calcifications in the breast; (b) lesion is too large to be excised to achieve negative margins with acceptable cosmetic outcome.
- *Adjuvant hormone therapy:* ER is present in about 80% of DCIS lesions and is more common in noncomedo than comedo DCIS. Endocrine therapy reduces local recurrences and prevents new primary in contralateral breast.

Evidence for the Role of Radiotherapy after Lumpectomy

NSAPB B-17 (Level I) is a phase III study that randomized patients between lumpectomy alone (L; 391 patients) and lumpectomy plus 50 Gy RT to whole breast (L + RT; 391 patients).[12] Patients with all subtypes of DCIS benefited from RT. Overall recurrence rate (DCIS + Invasive) at *12 year* follow-up was *32% lumpectomy alone versus 16% lumpectomy plus RT* showing a 50% risk reduction of malignant events. Approximately 50% of the recurrences had in situ histology and the other 50% had invasive recurrences. The limitations of the NSAPB B-17 study are that the margin width was not reported, and data on post-lumpectomy mammograms documenting removal of all radiographic microcalcifications was not routinely performed.

EORTC 108-53: A prospective phase III clinical trial randomized 1,010 patients of DCIS with documented negative margins on lumpectomy to receive 50 Gy RT versus Observation.[13] At a 4-year follow-up, the trial reported the benefit of RT with a lower recurrence rate of 9% among the irradiated patients compared with 16% in the observation group. At 10.5 years median follow-up, the recurrence rate (DCIS + Invasive) was *26% versus 15%* showing a 47% risk reduction.

UK/ANZ trial; follow-up 12.7 years: About 1,030 patients were subjected to a 2 × 2 randomization (RT vs no RT; tamoxifen vs no tamoxifen). The study demonstrated a lower recurrence rate in post-lumpectomy RT arm versus observation alone (21% versus 8%; 68% risk reduction).[14]

Swedish trial: 8 years mean FU: About 1,067 patients were accrued in the study and the results showed an ipsilateral recurrence rate of 29% lumpectomy versus 13% lumpectomy plus RT giving a 60% risk reduction.[15]

In all the above four trials, all subsets benefited from RT, but benefit was more in younger patients.

Evidence for Role of Observation after Lumpectomy

ECOG 5194: In this study, patients with low-risk DCIS were treated with lumpectomy alone. In DCIS with median tumor size of 6 mm and a clear margin width of 5–10 mm, at 5 years, the local recurrence rate was 6.8% compared to 13.7% among those with small high-grade DCIS, suggesting that a select group of patients with DCIS may be observed following lumpectomy.[16]

Observation pitfalls: A study by Wong et al.[17] noted that among a favorable group of patients with grade 1 or 2 DCIS less than 2.5 cm on mammogram and with negative resection margins more than 1 cm, a relatively high local failure rate of 12% at 5 years was observed (*Level IV evidence*).

Evidence for Role of Tamoxifen

NSABP B-24 trial (Level I): It aimed to study the effect of tamoxifen in the prevention of local recurrence or secondary breast cancer in patients treated for DCIS. RT was used for postoperative adjuvant treatment. In this trial, 1,804 women with the diagnosis of DCIS were treated with lumpectomy and RT. This was followed by randomization to placebo (902 women) versus tamoxifen at a dose of 20 mg daily for 5 years (902 women). Resection margins were positive in 16% of the patients. At 7-year follow-up, the ipsilateral breast the recurrence rate decreased from *11% to 8%,* and in the contralateral breast, the reduction in cancer events reduced from *4.9% to 2.3% (53% reduction)*. In a subsequent publication, the response to tamoxifen with respect to the ER status was evaluated. In ER-positive patients, tamoxifen resulted in a 59% reduction of all breast cancer events, whereas in ER-negative patients, only *20% reduction* was observed.[18]

The UK Coordinating Committee on Cancer Research (2003) completed a four-arm randomized trial. About 1,701 patients were randomized after lumpectomy with negative margins to observation versus RT alone versus tamoxifen alone versus tamoxifen and RT. At a median follow-up of 53 months, local relapse rates were *22% (no treatment), 18% (tamoxifen alone), 8% (RT alone), and 6% (RT + Tam)*. Patients receiving any RT had a 6% relapse rate compared to 14% relapse for patients receiving no RT (*UKCCCR, Level I*).[19]

Treatment of Axilla

Pure DCIS does not metastasize to axilla. Studies of axillary dissection in DCIS have found the evidence of 1–2% axillary nodal metastasis due to unrecognized microinvasion. Risk of isolated axillary recurrence with no axillary surgery/RT is less than 0.1%. Thus, routine use of sentinel node biopsy (SNB) is not justified in DCIS. Most investigators advocate selective use of SNB in patients of DCIS at significant risk of having coexistent invasive carcinoma, i.e.

- Patients diagnosed as having DCIS with large vacuum assisted biopsy devices (invasive component seen in 5–18%).
- Diagnosis of DCIS in palpable mass and core biopsy comes as suspicious of microinvasion.
- Performance of mastectomy in DCIS.

Radiation Therapy Dose Fraction Schedule

Whole breast radiotherapy: All the level I data evaluating the efficacy of RT in the management of DCIS used WBRT fields. The dose of RT to whole breast is 45–50 Gy in 1.8–2.0 Gy fractions.

Irradiation of the regional nodal areas is not required because of low risk of nodal metastasis.

BOOST: Although the value of boost has not been formally tested in patients with DCIS, it is generally recommended only in case of microinvasive disease.

EARLY BREAST CANCER

RISK FACTORS

Age

Breast cancer risk increases exponentially up to the age of menopause, and then it slows down. The annual increase in risk of developing breast cancer for women in their late 30s is approximately 0.07% per year, and increases to 0.44% per year for women in their late 70s.

Child Bearing/Parity/Breastfeeding

There is a protective effect of *child bearing* at younger ages on breast cancer risk. For women who had their first childbirth at age more than 35, the risk appears greater than nulliparous women. There is linear relation between relative risk of breast cancer and *age at first birth. Breastfeeding* has protective effect on breast cancer risk.

Ovarian Function (Long Menstrual History; Early Menarche, Late Menopause)

Long menstrual history (early menarche and late menopause) increases breast cancer risk. Early *menopause* (before age 45 years) decreases breast cancer risk.

Exogenous Hormone/Oral Contraceptive Pill

A collaborative meta-analysis from 51 epidemiological studies of over 150,000 women showed an increased relative risk of 1.35 for *current or recent users* of hormonal replacement therapy.[1] A randomized trial of postmenopausal hormone therapy comparing estrogen and progestin with placebo was closed prematurely, demonstrating a 24% increase in breast cancer, coronary heart disease, stroke and pulmonary emboli. A combined use of estrogen and progesterone reportedly increased the relative risk of breast cancer by 8% compared with the risk in nonusers, whereas the use of estrogen alone increased the relative risk only 1%.[2] Such increased risks are associated with *long-term use* of hormonal replacement therapy, and short-term use has not been consistently associated with the same. In post-*hysterectomy patients,* hormone replacement therapy with estrogen alone has a minimal effect on breast cancer risk. The use of *oral contraceptives* has not been consistently shown to increase the risk of breast cancer, although studies demonstrating some amount of risk exist.

Family History/BRCA

For women with a *second-degree relative* (aunt, grandmother) with breast cancer, the risk is about 1.5, and for women with a history in *first-degree relatives* (mother or sister), the risk is 1.7–2.5. About 20%–25% of patients have a positive family history and approximately 10% of women with breast cancer are from families who display an autosomal dominant pattern of breast cancer inheritance.

BRCA1 or BRCA2 mutations are present in less than 1% of the population and account for approximately 5% to 10% of all breast cancer cases. Women carrying these mutations have a lifetime risk of developing breast cancer of up to 70–80%.[3]

The National Comprehensive Cancer Network (NCCN) recommends that genetic testing be offered when:

- The individual has a family history of a known BRCA1/ BRCA2 mutation.
- Personal history of breast cancer plus one of the following:
  - Diagnosed age 45 years or younger
  - Diagnosed age ≤50 years with one or more close blood relatives with breast cancer ≤50 years
  - Two breast primaries when first breast primary occurred before age 50 years
  - Diagnosed at any age, with two or more close blood relatives with breast and/or epithelial ovarian/ fallopian tube/primary peritoneal cancer at any age
  - Close male relative with breast cancer
  - An individual of ethnicity associated with higher mutation frequency (e.g. Ashkenazi Jewish).
- Personal history of epithelial ovarian/fallopian tube/ primary peritoneal cancer.
- Personal history of male breast cancer.

Personal History of Breast Cancer and History of "Benign" Breast Biopsy

Women with a *prior history of invasive breast cancer/DCIS* are at an elevated risk (10–15%) to develop a second contralateral breast cancer. Women with a history of *fibrocystic changes, atypical hyperplasia* (higher risk) have been reported to have an elevated risk of breast cancer.

Radiation Exposure

Risk of radiation-induced cancer of the breast increases approximately linearly with dose and is heavily dependent on age at exposure (early age exposure carries more risk).[4,5]

Body Mass Index, Physical Activity, Diet, Alcohol

Higher *body mass index (BMI)*, especially BMI more than 31 in postmenopausal women, is associated with higher breast cancer risk, because in postmenopausal women, adipose tissue is the primary source of estradiol, whereas in premenopausal women, estradiol is predominantly from the ovaries, so there is little association with BMI and estradiol levels.

Physical activity can have a significant impact on BMI. There is a lower risk of breast cancer among women who are more physically active compared with women who are sedentary.

Diet: A strong link between diet and breast cancer risk have not been clearly established. Although it has been suggested that a high intake of meat, dairy products and fat may increase the risk and fiber, fruits and vegetables and phytoestrogens (soy products) may reduce risk. Daily consumption of four or more *alcohol drinks* a day had a 50% higher breast cancer risk.[6]

Mammographic Density

There is a correlation between higher mammographic breast density and higher breast cancer risk.

Familial Breast Cancer

Approximately 10% of breast cancer patients have familial breast cancer, typically defined as breast cancer showing an autosomal dominant inheritance pattern. Mutations in three important tumor suppressor genes—*p53, BRCA1,* and *BRCA2* are associated with familial breast cancer.

Mutations in p53

The *p53* gene is called the "guardian of the genome" because of its critical role in cellular pathways that recognize and direct a response to DNA injury. The p53 tumor suppressor gene encodes a nuclear phosphoprotein that is important to cell cycle regulation and DNA repair and that also may regulate induction of apoptosis by ionizing radiation. p53 is most frequently mutated in sporadic breast cancer (in 22% cases). Germline mutations in the *p53* gene result in Li-Fraumeni syndrome characterized by an increased risk for a variety of cancers, including childhood sarcomas, gynecologic tumors and breast cancer (most common). The lifetime risk for development of a cancer is estimated to be 90%.

Mutations in BRCA1 and BRCA2

BRCA1 and *BRCA2* are also tumor suppressor genes like p53 and contribute to the stability of the genome. Germline mutations in *BRCA1* and *BRCA2* occur in less than 7% of patients with breast cancer.

BRCA1: Individuals with a germline mutation in *BRCA1* gene have a lifetime breast cancer risk of 65–85%, ovarian cancer (50%) and may also develop colon and prostate cancers.

BRCA2: The lifetime risk of breast cancer for women with germline *BRCA2* mutations is 65–85% but risk of ovarian cancer is much less than BRCA1. BRCA2 is also associated with male breast cancer and pancreatic cancer.

NCCN Recommendations for Individuals with Genetic Mutations (p53, BRCA)

Before the age of 25 years, annual clinical and self-breast examination is recommended. After the age of 25 years, annual mammography or MRI; and semi-annual clinical and self-breast examination are recommended. In addition, annual pelvic examinations with transvaginal sonography, color Doppler examinations of the ovaries, and measurement of serum CA-125 levels are recommended beginning at age 25–35 years. For those women over the age of 35 years, a risk-reducing bilateral salpingo-oophorectomy is recommended, with possible short-term hormone replacement therapy.

Determining an Individual's Risk

Gail et al. have used epidemiologic risk factors to derive a model for predicting an individual's *annual and lifetime risks* of breast cancer.[7] In the Gail model, an individual's annual risk of breast cancer is based on her present age, age at menarche, age at first birth, number of first-degree relatives with breast cancer, number of breast biopsies and history of atypical ductal hyperplasia.

BREAST CANCER PREVENTION STRATEGIES

Tamoxifen/Raloxifene

NSABP-P1: This randomized, placebo-controlled trial was designed to test the efficacy of 5 years of tamoxifen in the prevention of breast cancer. About 13,388 women with a 1.67% or greater predicted risk of developing breast cancer within 5 years (modified Gail model) were enrolled. The results indicated that tamoxifen reduced the rates of invasive and noninvasive breast cancer by 49% and 50%, respectively. The benefit of tamoxifen was seen in all age groups (≤49 years, 50–59 years, ≥6 0 years). In addition, women with a history of atypical ductal hyperplasia had an 86% risk reduction and women with a history of LCIS had a 56% risk reduction. Tamoxifen selectively reduced the incidence of ER-positive tumors; ER-negative tumors developed at an equal rate in the tamoxifen and placebo groups. No evidence was shown of a cardioprotective effect of tamoxifen, but the number of osteoporosis-related fractures was reduced and risk of stage I endometrial cancer (risk ratio of 2.53) increased in the tamoxifen-treated cohort.[8]

NSABP-P2: This trial compared tamoxifen (20 mg OD) to raloxifene (60 mg OD) for 5 years, as a preventative agent in postmenopausal women with breast cancer. Raloxifene was as effective as tamoxifen in reducing the risk of invasive breast cancer. The main benefit of raloxifene was in toxicity. Lesser incidence of uterine cancer and thromboembolic events was observed in raloxifene arm. No differences were found for ischemic heart disease events, or for stroke or osteoporotic fractures.[9]

Prophylactic Surgery

Hartmann et al. analyzed outcomes in women with a family history of breast cancer who underwent bilateral prophylactic mastectomy at the Mayo Clinic between 1960 and 1993.[10] With a median follow-up time of 14 years, only 4 of the 639 treated patients developed breast cancer. According to the Gail model, 37.4 cases of breast cancers would have been expected to develop in this population, so the prophylactic surgery resulted in an 89.5% risk reduction (p <.001).

NATURAL HISTORY

The Halsted model was based on an orderly progression from the breast to the regional lymph nodes and from there to distant metastatic sites.[11] Later, Keynes et al. *suggested alternative hypothesis* that breast cancer is a systemic disease.[12] A third hypothesis put forward by *Hellman* considers breast cancer as a heterogeneous disease with a spectrum extending from a tumor that remains localized throughout its course to one that disseminates systemically.[13]

The growth rate of a tumor in the breast is thought to be constant from the date of origin. Using estimates of doubling time, it would take an average of approximately 5 years for a tumor to reach palpable size. Women with a history of breast cancer have a 10–15% risk of developing a new primary in the contralateral breast.

Axillary Involvement

Higher risk of axillary node involvement exists with a larger tumor size, young age, outer-half tumor location, poor or moderate differentiation, aneuploidy and infiltrating ductal histologic type. *Lower risks of axillary node involvement are seen in* medullary or tubular carcinoma, smaller tumors and medially located tumors. Up to 30–40% of T1/T2 with cN0 may have pathologically involved lymph nodes on dissection.[14] Similarly, clinically node positive, but pathologically negative may be seen in 20–30% cases.[15]

Internal Mammary Nodes

Higher risk of internal mammary node chain (IMC) involvement is seen in larger tumor size, *positive axilla*, medial half and central lesions, and young patient. Patients with positive internal mammary nodes (IMNs) have a significantly worse overall disease-free survival (DFS) than those with negative IMNs.[16]

Clinical failure of the IMNs is extremely rare (<1%), despite the evidence of pathological involvement from these studies.[17,18]

Supraclavicular Spread

Spread to supraclavicular lymph nodes usually follows involvement in the high axillary lymph nodes or IMNs. Three predictive factors for supraclavicular involvement are high histologic grade, more than four positive nodes and axillary level II or III involved nodes.[19] *Clinical failure in the supraclavicular fossa* is relatively rare in patients with early stage breast cancer and is dependent on the degree of axillary involvement. For patients with early breast cancer (EBC) with *no or minimal nodal involvement* (less than three involved axillary nodes), supraclavicular failure is extremely rare (1.3%).[18] For patients with advanced disease or *more than four lymph nodes* involvement, failure rate in supraclavicular nodes, if left untreated, may be as high as 8–20% in the absence of supraclavicular fossa radiation.[20] Radiation to the supraclavicular fossa in these higher risk patient results in high local control rates, with isolated supraclavicular failures occurring in less than 1% of prophylactically treated nodes.

Risk factors for systemic micrometastasis: Larger tumor size (<2, 2–5, >5 cm and pT4) have 25%, 33%, 38% and 60% risk of bone marrow micrometastasis; higher histologic grade, hormone receptor negative tumors also have a higher probability of micrometastasis.[21]

Impact of Local Control on Systemic Metastasis and Breast Cancer Mortality

Studies have identified local control as an independent predictor of systemic metastases, DFS and overall survival (OS).

Against: Fisher et al. in an analysis of patients treated in NSABP B-06, concluded that ipsilateral breast tumor recurrence was a harbinger, but not a cause, of distant metastases. Although local treatment (Surgery + RT) prevented expression of breast relapse, neither lowered the risk of distant metastases, which was determined by a host of prognostic factors.

For: More recent meta-analyses have demonstrated a small but significant impact of local control on systemic metastasis and OS.

- A meta-analysis of randomized trials by Vinh-Hung and Verschraegen comparing BCS without RT to BCS + RT confirms an approximate threefold reduction in local relapse with radiation therapy and an 8.6% improvement in mortality in the radiated cohorts.[22]
- Analysis of the Early Breast Cancer Trialists Collaborative Group (EBCTCG) reveals that RT reduced the 10-year risk of any first recurrence from 35.0% to 19.3% (p < 0.0001) and reduced the 15-year risk of breast cancer death from 25.2% to 21.4% (p < 0.001). In women with pN + disease (n = 1,050), RT reduced the 10-year recurrence risk from 63.7% to 42.5% (p < 0.0001) and the 15-year risk of breast cancer death from 51.3% to 42.8% (p = 0.01). Overall, about one breast cancer death was avoided by year 15 for every four recurrences avoided by year 10.[23]

SCREENING IN BREAST CANCER

X-ray Screening Mammography

Early detection by mammography, followed by appropriate local, regional, and systemic treatment, is associated with reduced breast cancer mortality rates for women 50 years of age and older. Screening mammography in women 40–49 years of age may reduce mortality from breast cancer, and mammographic screening beginning at age 40 years is encouraged in the majority of published guidelines. In a simplified model described by Harris et al., for every 1,000 screening mammograms, 80 women (8%) will be recalled for additional diagnostic imaging, 10 (1%) will require tissue diagnosis, and of those undergoing biopsy only 3 (0.3%) will have a malignancy.[24]

Sensitivity (true positive): 70–90% (i.e. 10–30% false negative).

Specificity (true negative): 80–90%.

Radiation exposure: For women more than 40 years, benefit of screening mammography outweighs the risk. Mean glandular dose of screening mammography is 1–2 mSv per view. (CT thorax 7 mSv, abdominal CT 12 to 20 mSv; whole body environmental radiation dose is 3 mSv per year). It may be estimated that up to 1 breast cancer may be induced per 1,000 women aged 40–80 years, undergoing annual mammogram.

Evidence for Reduction in Mortality by Screening Mammography

Tabár et al.[25] showed that the reduction in mortality rate with screening mammography observed during the service-screening period, adjusted for selection bias, was 48%. In a recent long-term update, there has remained a highly significant reduction in breast cancer mortality in women invited to screening (RR 0.69; 95% CI: 0.56–0.84; p = .001). In contrast, a *Canadian* study revealed that in women aged 50–59 years, the addition of annual mammography screening to physical examination had no effect on breast cancer mortality. The results of the Canadian study may be due to the unbalanced allocation of women with advanced cancers (large tumors, four or more positive nodes) to the screened group, the poor quality of the mammography in the trial, and insufficient sample size.[26,27]

Screening in Women under Age 50 Years

Although the majority of studies clearly support the impact of screening mammography on mortality in women over 50 years of age, data on screening younger women are more conflicting.

No benefit: Frisell, et al. found no benefit of screening mammography in age group 40–49 in *Stockholm mammographic trial:* The relative risk of breast cancer death in screened versus non-screened women was 1.08 (95% CI, 0.54 to 2.17).[28]

Benefit in less than 50 years: Screening *trial in United Kingdom* involving 45,841 women aged 45–64 years at 16 years follow-up found a 35% decrease in mortality rate in mammographically screened women for all cohorts aged 45–64 years at entry. There was no evidence of decreased benefit in women aged 45–49 years at initial screening.[29] In a *Swedish* study evaluating women in the 40–49-year age group, Hellquist et al. reported 803 breast cancer deaths in a screening study group compared with 1,238 deaths in a control group after 16 years of follow-up. The estimated relative risk for women screened in this younger population was 0.74 (95% CI, 0.66 to 0.83), concluding that screening mammography reduced the breast cancer mortality rate in this younger population.[30]

Screening Mammography Guidelines

Standard risk women: The National Cancer Institute, American Cancer Society, and the American College of Radiology recommend a baseline mammogram at the age of 35 years (30 years in high-risk groups). Repeat examinations should be carried out every 2 years beginning at 40 years of age. In women older than 50 years, mammograms should be performed annually (Fig. 1).

High-risk women: Annual screening may be started at an earlier age (before 40 years). These women include those with a personal history of breast cancer, those who have had therapeutic radiation to the breast area especially for Hodgkin lymphoma, *BRCA*-positive women, women with a family history of a first-degree relative with breast cancer at a young age, and women with a biopsy diagnosis of LCIS or atypical ductal hyperplasia.

Digital versus Screen Film Mammography

Advantages of digital mammography include no film processing and faster image acquisition. Results of a large-scale American College of Radiology Imaging Network (ACRIN) trial of 49,000 women revealed that digital mammography was at least as good as screen film mammography but was superior in younger women and women with dense breasts.[31]

Magnetic Resonance Imaging Screening

Magnetic resonance imaging (Fig. 2) is unlikely to replace mammography for screening of the general population. Although MRI has not yet been shown to impact mortality, its sensitivity over mammography in high-risk population has been demonstrated. In a landmark study by Kriege et al., 1,909 eligible women (cumulative lifetime risk of breast cancer of 15% or more) at high risk for familial breast cancer were screened with an annual MRI and mammography.[32] The

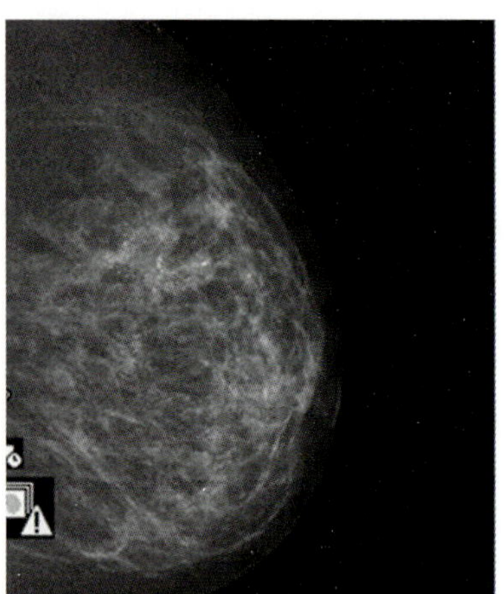

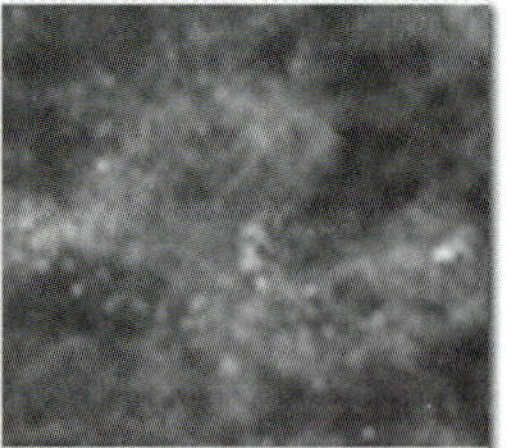

Fig. 1 X-ray mammography with microcalcifications

Courtesy: Dr Shyam Bisht, Associate Consultant, Division of Radiation Oncology, Medanta—The Medicity, Haryana, India

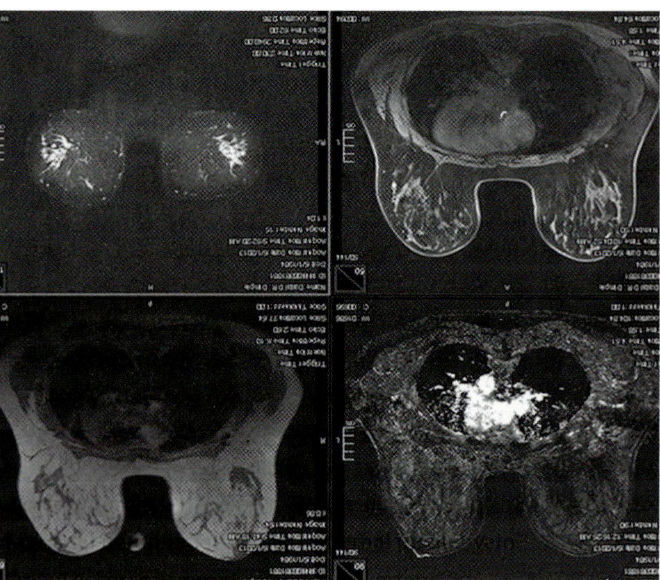

Fig. 2 Magnetic resonance mammography in prone position

Courtesy: Dr Shyam Bisht, Associate Consultant, Division of Radiation Oncology, Medanta—The Medicity, Haryana, India

sensitivity of clinical breast examination, mammography and MRI for detecting invasive breast cancer was 17.9%, 33.3% and 79.5%, respectively and the specificity was 98.1%, 95.0% and 89.8%, respectively. The overall discriminating capacity of MRI was significantly better than that of mammography ($p < .05$).

PROGNOSTIC AND PREDICTIVE FACTORS

Prognostic Marker

It provides information about patient's overall cancer outcome (likely course of cancer disease), regardless of therapy. The factors that determine or correlate with the natural history of the disease, in the absence of intervening adjuvant systemic therapy and which are therefore reflective of the inherent aggressiveness of the cancer are termed *prognostic markers*. Prognostic markers include nodal status, tumor size, pathologic subtypes, demographic characteristics and other molecular biomarkers involved in tumor metastases and disease progression. Generally, prognostic markers can be used to help determine a need to further systemic therapy, but not to discriminate relative benefits of particular therapies.

Predictive Marker

It provides information about the effect of therapeutic intervention (identify patients who are most likely to respond to a given therapy). Conversely, *predictive markers* are those associated with response or lack of response to a particular therapy. The most notable example of a predictive marker is the ER, which predicts for response to hormonal therapies in the adjuvant, neoadjuvant and metastatic settings.

In addition, some factors may share both *prognostic* and *predictive* properties. ER expression is a weak prognostic factor for favorable outcome and a strong predictive factor for benefit from hormonal therapy. Expression of the growth factor receptor cerbB2 (ERBB2, formerly HER-2/*neu*), is a *prognostic* factor associated with poorer clinical outcome and its amplification is also predictive of response to trastuzumab and possibly *predictive* of a better response to anthracyclines or poorer response to hormonal agents as tamoxifen.

Prognostic Factors for Survival and Metastasis

At present, the standard prognostic and predictive factors in primary breast cancers in clinical practice are as follows:

- Tumor size
- Axillary lymph node status, including micrometastasis (Nmic)
- Histologic subtype
- Nuclear or histologic grade
- Proliferation indices, including mitotic index
- Estrogen and progesterone receptor (PR) status (mainly as predictive markers of response to hormonal therapies)
- ERBB2 amplification or overexpression (mainly as a predictive marker of response to trastuzumab and possibly as predictive of benefit from anthracyclines)
- Multiparameter-based markers (mainly as prognostic indicator of recurrence risk).

Prognostic factors for local relapse after mastectomy differ substantially from prognostic factors for local relapse after lumpectomy and radiation.[33]

The College of American Pathologists presented a Consensus Statement in 1999 summarizing prognostic factors in breast cancer. Factors were category I if they were proven to be of prognostic importance and useful in clinical patient management. These included tumor size, lymph node status, micrometastasis, histologic grade, mitotic count and hormonal receptor status. Category II factors had been extensively studied biologically and clinically, but their importance remains to be validated in studies. These included HER-2/neu expression, p53 mutations, lymphovascular invasion and DNA ploidy. Category III included all other factors not sufficiently studied to demonstrate their prognostic value, like tumor angiogenesis, EGFR, transforming growth factor, Bcl-2, and cathepsin D overexpression.[34]

Tumor Size

After nodal status, tumor size is one of the most consistent and powerful prognostic factor for distant relapse, DFS and OS especially in node-negative patients. Tumor size also correlates strongly with the presence and number of involved axillary lymph nodes. In a study with an over 20-year follow-up, Rosen et al. reported a recurrence-free survival rate of 88% for tumors less than 1 cm, 72% for tumors 1.1–3 cm, and 59% for tumors 3.1–5 cm.[35] In an analysis of 826 women with node-negative breast cancer treated by mastectomy, Quiet et al. reported a 20-year DFS of 79% for patients with tumors less than 2 cm, compared to 64% with tumors more than 2 cm.[36]

Axillary Nodal Status

Of all prognostic factors, nodal status continues to be the strongest predictor of DFS and OS and is the primary factor that governs breast cancer staging. NSABP trials treated primarily with local and regional therapy alone revealed 5-year survival rates of 82.8% for node-negative group, 73% for 1–3 positive nodes group, 45.7% for 4–12 positive nodes and 28.4% for more than 13 positive nodes.

Tumor Type

The tubular, mucinous and medullary subtypes have a more favorable prognosis, compared to invasive ductal. Invasive lobular tumors appear to have a prognosis similar to invasive ductal tumors. Poor prognostic categories include metaplastic, undifferentiated and other rarer subtypes.

Tumor Grade

Grade has been shown to be of independent prognostic significance.

The Scarff-Bloom-Richardson classification system utilizes mitotic index, differentiation and pleomorphism, each with scores of 1–3. Scores of 3–5 are well differentiated, 6–7 moderately differentiated and 8–9 poorly differentiated.

Elston and Ellis of the Nottingham group refined this methodology. The revised technique involves evaluation of three morphological features: the percentage of tubule formation, the degree of nuclear pleomorphism and an accurate mitotic count using a defined field area.

Estrogen and progesterone hormonal receptors in tumor cells: Patients with hormonal receptors positivity have a significantly higher survival rate. Tumors that express both ER and PR have the greatest benefit from hormonal therapy, but those containing only ER or PR still have significant responses. Two types of estrogen receptors (ERs), ER-β and ER-α, have now been identified. PR also exists in two forms, PR-albha and PR-beta.

Lymphatic and vascular invasion (LVI) in the peritumoral region is of prognostic significance.

Proliferative Indices (S-Phase/Thymidine Labeling Index)

Proliferative rate of a tumor has been shown to correlate with distant metastasis and survival. *Thymidine labeling* represents the fraction of cells in the S-phase of the cell cycle. Thymidine labeling index is a prognostic indicator independent of tumor size, steroid receptors for loco-regional or distant metastases. *S-phase fraction (SPF)*: A higher SPF is associated with a worse tumor grade, absence of steroid receptors, larger tumors and positive axillary lymph nodes. Higher SPF is usually associated with worse DFS and OS rates.

DNA Ploidy Index

DNA ploidy correlates with nuclear grade, with low-grade tumors being diploid and high-grade tumors being aneuploid. Diploid tumors tend to be ER-positive, whereas aneuploid tumors are frequently ER-negative. Diploid tumors tend to have a better prognosis than those with an aneuploid DNA distribution.

HER-2/neu

HER-2/neu proto-oncogene (c-erbB-2) located on chromosome 17 codes for a transmembrane glycoprotein, p185, which has tyrosine kinase activity and is homologous to EGFR. It is amplified or overexpressed in up to 30% of human breast carcinoma. Overexpression of the protein is associated with tumor aggressiveness and decreased DFS in node-positive patients with variable prognostic significance among node-negative patients. HercepTest 3+ cases have worse prognosis, significantly associated with lower ER levels and histologic grade III tumors. More critical than its prognostic significance is the predictive value of Her2/neu status with respect to response to therapy and its value in identifying patients who may benefit from adjuvant targeted therapy directed at the protein.

p53 gene is most frequently mutated in sporadic breast cancer (22% cases). Mutations of p53 were found more often in tumors of younger women, African American women and in tumors lacking ER, PR or both. p53 is an independent prognostic factor for OS and post-relapse survival.

Genetic Profiling

MammaPrint, developed at the Netherlands Cancer Institute, is a 70-gene prognostic signature, which was studied in 295 women and demonstrated a 10-year DFS of 50.6% in 180 poor prognosis signature patients compared to 85.2% in 115 women with a favorable signature. In a validation study, the profiling outperformed classic prognostic criteria, but the magnitude of the prognostic value was not as strong.[37,38]

Oncotype DX: It can be done on paraffin-embedded specimens. A panel of 16 cancer-related genes and five reference genes was employed to compute a recurrence score (0 to 100) and then used to estimate odds of relapse over 10 years. Patients are categorized into low risk (<18 score), intermediate risk (18 to 30), or high risk (31 to 100). The likelihood of distant metastasis is low in those patients with favorable scores treated with tamoxifen alone. These data can be used to determine which patients with ER-positive tumors may avoid chemotherapy.

Age

Young age is a significant prognostic factor for distant metastasis and subsequent DFS, and a predictor of local relapse following BCS. Younger women often present with palpable disease and have larger tumors with a higher percentage of positive nodes, higher proportion of ER-negative and high-grade tumors and lower DFS and breast cancer specific survival.

Obesity/Body Mass Index

Obesity remains a statistically significant prognostic factor. Recurrent disease develops in 32% of obese patients compared with 19% of non-obese women.[39]

Pregnancy

Women with primary childbirth between 20 years and 29 years, experience a significantly reduced risk of death compared with women with primary childbirth before the age of 20 years. The prognosis of the pregnant breast cancer patient is similar to her stage-matched nonpregnant counterparts in most series.[40] There is no strong evidence to suggest that subsequent pregnancy will increase the risk of recurrence.

Tumor Location

There is some evidence that medially located tumors have a poorer prognosis than laterally located tumors, with a twofold risk of relapse and breast cancer death being associated with high-risk medial breast tumors. This may be due to occult spread to IMNs or due to underestimation of axillary lymph node involvement.

Other potentially useful prognostic factors include cathepsin D, vascular endothelial growth factor, epidermal growth factor, Bcl-2, carcinoembryonic antigen, E-cadherin and others. CA 15-3 is a widely used tumor marker in carcinoma of the breast, but its role in the management of patients with early disease is controversial.[41]

MANAGEMENT OF BREAST CANCER

Definition of Risk Categories for Patients with Operated Breast Cancer.[42]

Low Risk

- Node negative and all of the following features:
  - pT2 cm,
  - Grade 1,
  - Absence of peritumoral vascular invasion,
  - HER2/neu gene neither overexpressed nor amplified,
  - Age >35 years.

Intermediate Risk

- Node negative and at least one of the following features:
  - pT >2 cm,
  - Grade 2-3,
  - Presence of peritumoral vascular invasion,
  - HER2/neu gene overexpressed or amplified,
  - Age <35 years.
- Node positive (1–3 involved nodes) and HER2/neu gene neither overexpressed nor amplified.

High-risk

- Node positive (1–3 involved nodes) and HER2/neu gene overexpressed or amplified
- Node positive (4 or more involved nodes).

Mastectomy

Skin-Sparing Mastectomy

Skin-sparing mastectomy is a standard mastectomy, with minimal skin sacrifice at the mastectomy site. This is often performed when immediate reconstruction is planned. It attempts to remove all breast tissue, while preservation of skin provides cosmetic and reconstructive advantages. The procedure is oncologically sound, and patients undergoing skin-sparing mastectomy do not require postmastectomy radiation unless they have risk factors that place them at higher risk (i.e. positive nodes, positive margins, large primary tumors or in case patient has received neoadjuvant chemotherapy (NACT) for down staging a large primary/nodal disease).

Nipple-sparing mastectomy: In this, the nipple and/or nipple areola complex are conserved. This procedure is more controversial and is not routinely employed in cancer patients.

A modified radical mastectomy may be preferable for patients:
- Who wish to avoid radiation,
- In whom lumpectomy is likely to result in suboptimal cosmesis,
- With diffusely positive margins which cannot be cleared with re-excision,
- With diffuse suspicious microcalcifications.

Breast Conservative Treatment

Breast conservative treatment (BCT) usually includes breast conservative surgery (BCS) + axillary management followed by postoperative radiation therapy to whole breast. BCT is the current standard of care for early stage invasive breast cancer. It provides survival equivalent to that of total mastectomy and axillary dissection while preserving the breast. It also enhances the acceptance by women of mammographic screening for early detection of this disease.

Selection of Cases for BCT[43]

- Unicentric primary tumors that are less than 4–5 cm in diameter.
- Larger tumors can undergo NACT for reduction in tumor size, followed by BCT.

Absolute Contraindication of BCT

- Persistently positive diffuse margins, extensive intraductal carcinoma (EIC) after surgery.
- Gross multicentric disease.
- Diffuse malignant appearing microcalcifications.

- History of prior RT to breast.
- Lumpectomy likely to result in unacceptable cosmetic outcome.
- Pregnancy (0–20 weeks) as RT is contraindicated in it. (BCS in 3rd trimester with RT after delivery can be done).

Relative Contraindications of BCT

- Collagen vascular disease.
- Patients with germline mutations that predispose to breast cancer development.
- Patients at higher risk for development of local recurrence.
- High risk of systemic relapse is not a contraindication for BCT but indication for adjuvant systemic treatment.

Breast Conservation Surgery

Various terms have been used to describe the surgical approach, including lumpectomy, wide local excision, BCS, tylectomy, tumorectomy, segmental mastectomy, partial mastectomy, and quadrantectomy. Since cosmesis is a critical reason for performing tumor excision and irradiation instead of mastectomy, wide local excision with microscopically negative margins is preferable to segmental mastectomy or quadrantectomy. Re-excision is indicated when margins are positive or if the biopsy/surgery was performed at an outside hospital and margins of resection were unknown. The rate of positive re-excisions is high (60–90%) if biopsy contains EIC or mammogram detects residual microcalcifications before re-excision. Selected patients with a focally involved margin may be treated with radiation therapy, without re-excision, following lumpectomy with acceptable local control rates.

Surgical Management of Axilla

Clinically Negative Axilla (cN0)

If SNB is positive then complete axillary dissection is needed, else sentinel lymph node dissection (SLND) alone is adequate.

Clinically Positive Axilla (cN+)

Complete axillary lymph node dissection (ALND), including level III, may be performed in patients with clinically positive lymph nodes. A higher incidence of breast and arm edema has been noted with level III axillary node dissection, without any additional benefit. If level I axillary lymph nodes is positive then 25% cases would have had metastases confined to levels II and III. However, only 1.4% of patients show positive level III lymph nodes if levels I and II were negative.[44]

Rates of Axillary Failure

cN0 (clinically no nodes) and no axillary surgery: Approximately 20–40% of patients with carcinoma of the breast and cN0 have pathologic evidence of lymph node metastases. Yet, in patients with stage I or II breast cancer and cN0 if an axillary dissection is not performed, axillary recurrence develops in only approximately 20%. Axillary recurrences after complete axillary dissection range from 1% to 2%.

Sentinel Lymph Node Dissection

Surgical management of axilla has undergone a paradigm change since the concept of lymphatic mapping of the breast was introduced at John Wayne Cancer Institute in 1991. Patients are injected around the tumor with technetium-99 sulfur colloid and vital blue dye, and a hand-held gamma probe is used to identify areas of highest radioisotope uptake in the lymphatic system. The lymph nodes underlying this area (sentinel lymph nodes) are removed.[45,46] The sentinel node procedure is currently an acceptable standard for women with cN0 breast cancer with a high degree of sensitivity and specificity. The overall accuracy of the sentinel node status as reported by Veronesi et al. was 96.9%, the sensitivity 91.2%, and the specificity 100%.[47] Fifty percent of patients with sentinel lymph node metastases have no metastatic disease in nonsentinel lymph nodes on ALND.[49]

SLND in Special Circumstances

SLND after NACT: SLND is technically feasible after NACT. However, the SLN identification rate is decreased in the presence of cN+ at initial clinical examination. The risk of false negative (RFN) findings on SLND performed after NACT is generally higher, especially in the presence of cN+ at initial clinical examination. In such cases a complete clinical axillary response to NACT, combined with a negative SLNB after chemotherapy, is still not enough to warrant exemption of ALND. In patients who are cN0 at initial clinical examination, SLND performed after NACT carries a lower RFN than cN+ patients, although still greater than 5%.[48]

Presence of large tumors: SLND is technically feasible in T3 tumors without adenopathy at clinical examination, with a high SLN identification rate and RFN significantly greater than 5%.

After breast augmentation or reduction mammoplasty: Although some cases of SLND after periareolar or inframammary breast augmentation or reduction have demonstrated the feasibility of this technique, the data is as yet insufficient.

Reoperative sentinel lymph node biopsy in the case of recurrence: Feasibility of the same has not been clearly demonstrated.

SLND is Contraindicated in the Following Cases

- Presence of suspicious palpable axillary lymph nodes
- Ductal carcinoma in situ when mastectomy is not planned, therefore not requiring axillary node assessment

- Inflammatory breast cancer
- Absence of experienced surgeon
- Prior axillary surgery.

SLND is Not Contraindicated in the following Cases

- Ductal carcinoma in situ when a mastectomy is planned
- Multicentric tumors
- Bilateral breast cancer
- Patients aged 65 years or older
- Obese patients
- Male breast cancer patients.

Role of SLND is Less Clear in the following Circumstances

- Presence of internal mammary lymph nodes
- Before preoperative systemic therapy
- T3/T4 tumors
- DCIS (without mastectomy)
- Suspicious palpable axillary nodes
- After preoperative systemic therapy
- Prior diagnostic or excisional breast surgery
- Prior non-oncologic breast surgery
- Pregnancy: For pregnant patients, there are concerns about the safety of blue dye; decisions should be made on a case by case basis.[49]

Trials of Equivalence of SLND to Axillary Dissection in cN0 Axilla

The *ALMANAC (axillary lymphatic mapping against nodal axillary clearance)* trial is a multicenter randomized trial of 1,031 patients randomly assigned to SNB (n = 515) or standard axillary dissection (n = 516) in cN0. The authors concluded that SNB is the treatment of choice for patients who have early stage breast cancer and clinically negative nodes, assuring better quality of life and arm functioning scores.[50]

Veronesi et al. reported a trial of 516 patients with T1 tumors, randomized to either SNB or total axillary dissection. The overall accuracy of the sentinel node status was 96.9%, sensitivity 91.2%, and specificity 100%. Among the 167 patients who did not undergo axillary dissection, after SNB negative, there were no cases of overt axillary metastasis during follow-up.[47]

NSABP-32: David Krag et al. Lancet 2010. No difference in OS, DFS. Improve morbidity in SNB alone arm in patients who did not undergo ALND after negative SNB.[51]

Subset of Patients in which Completion ALND can be omitted after Positive SNB

Although the current standard for patients with a positive sentinel node is to undergo completion axillary dissection, the necessity of this has been questioned in the *ACOSOG Z0011* trial.[52] At a median follow-up time of 6.3 years, there were no statistically significant differences in local recurrence (p = 0.11) or regional recurrence (p = 0.45) between the ALND+ and ALND- groups. All patients in the trial had whole-breast irradiation, but regional nodal irradiation was not allowed. The reason for low regional relapse rates is likely a combination of factors, including a favorable subset of patients with a low likelihood of a high residual axillary burden of disease, use of systemic therapy, and incidental radiation to the residual nodes in level I or II from tangential breast irradiation.

Radiation Therapy to Breast

In 1992, the National Cancer Institute published a monograph that stated that breast conservation treatment is an appropriate method of primary therapy for most women with stage I or II breast cancer and is preferable because it provides survival equivalent to that of total mastectomy and axillary dissection while preserving the breast. Despite the clear evidence of equivalence, some patients will still prefer mastectomy, which remains an acceptable standard of care for all women with operable breast cancers.

Randomized Studies Comparing BCS Plus Radiation Therapy to Mastectomy

Veronesi et al. in *Milan trial* randomized cT1cN0 patients to quadrantectomy and axillary dissection plus irradiation (50 Gy/5 weeks + 10 Gy boost) versus radical mastectomy. Women with positive axillary lymph nodes also received 12 cycles of adjuvant chemotherapy with cyclophosphamide, methotraxate, 5 flouro-uracil (CMF). Actuarial 20-year overall and DFS rates were comparable in the two groups (58%). The incidence of local failure was 2.3% with mastectomy and 8.8% with quadrantectomy and irradiation. There was no difference in the incidence of contralateral breast cancer (10.2% and 8.7%, respectively).[53]

NSABP protocol B-06, less than 4 cm tumors were randomly assigned to total mastectomy or lumpectomy (segmental mastectomy), with or without irradiation (50 Gy with no boost). With a 20-year follow-up, there was no significant difference in survival among patients treated with mastectomy, lumpectomy alone, or lumpectomy combined with irradiation. For the patients treated with lumpectomy alone, the ipsilateral breast relapse rates were approximately 40% if the nodes were negative and 50% if they were positive. For patients treated with lumpectomy and irradiation, the corresponding rates were 10% for all patients and those with negative nodes and 5% for those with positive nodes.[54]

The *Institut Gustave-Roussy* prospective, randomized trial comparing mastectomy with local excision plus irradiation for women with cancers measuring less than or equal to 2 cm showed 15-year DFS rate as 55% for the tumorectomy group and 45% for the mastectomy group (p = .23). The 15-year local recurrence rate was 9% in the conservation surgery and irradiation group and 14% in the mastectomy group.[55]

The *EORTC Breast Cancer Cooperative Group* randomized trial of women with stage I or II breast cancer comparing modified radical mastectomy (420 patients) with breast conservation therapy (448 patients) showed similar actuarial 8-year local tumor control rate was in both arms, 91% in the mastectomy group and 87% in breast-conservation therapy group.[56]

Danish Cooperative Study: High-risk patients (tumor >5 cm, invasion to skin or deep fascia, metastatic axillary lymph nodes) who were treated with breast conservation therapy received radiation therapy to the regional lymph nodes. Those who were treated with mastectomy also received irradiation of the same target volume and all high-risk patients received adjuvant CMF. At 6 years OS rates were 79% and 82%, respectively. There were 12 breast relapses in the former group (3%) and 19 chest wall recurrences in the latter group (4%).[57]

Prognostic Factors for Local Relapse Following BCS Plus Radiation Therapy

Local relapse following BCS and radiation can be governed by a complex array of host, primary tumor, and treatment factors. *Age*: One of the most significant and powerful studies correlating young age with local relapse was the large EORTC boost versus no boost trial.[58] It concluded that young age and breast-conserving therapy are both independent predictors for isolated loco-regional recurrence. Although there is no apparent cut off age where relapse rates significantly change, most of the studies have selected 35 or 40 years of age to demonstrate the differences. Conversely, some older patients more than or equal to 65 years of age with pathologically negative nodes and hormone receptor positive may be treated with wide local excision and adjuvant hormonal therapy alone, omitting the RT, in view of low risk of recurrence.

Margin status: Definition of a negative margin is variable. Some consider no tumor cells seen on the inked margin, as defined by the NSABP, and others consider margins of 1 or 2 mm beyond invasive cancer as negative. Positive margin status has been one of the most consistently reported factors associated with higher local relapse rates. The degree of margin involvement (focal or diffuse) is also important. A focally involved margin, particularly when re-excision is not technically feasible (e.g. focally involved deep margin at the pectoralis fascia) is not a contraindication to BCT. Data on close margins are less consistent. Adjuvant chemotherapy or hormone therapy cannot compensate for the adverse impact of positive margin status.

Effect of systemic therapy on local control: Systemic therapy, in the form of adjuvant tamoxifen or adjuvant chemotherapy, has been clearly shown to impact local control in numerous randomized trials. It is also clearly demonstrated that chemotherapy and tamoxifen are not appropriate substitutes for radiation therapy, but in patients who are treated with radiation therapy, the use of systemic therapy improves local control.

Tumor size: Although tumor size is clearly a strong predictor of systemic relapse and OS, its prognostic value in local relapse has not been consistently reported.

Tumor location: Any specific location is not associated with a higher local relapse rate. Subareolar breast cancer presentation is not a contraindication to breast-conserving therapy in early stage disease although some studies have reported higher local relapse.

Extensive intraductal carcinoma: According to the Harvard definition, EIC means that 25% or more of the primary tumor is intraductal carcinoma, and intraductal carcinoma is seen outside (adjacent to) the infiltrating tumor border. It has been reported that a somewhat higher breast relapse rate in EIC-positive patients was seen only in women younger than 40 years of age. The impact of EIC on local relapse, however, appears to be minimized if negative margins are achieved.

Histology: No higher relapse rates are associated with specific histologic patterns. Literature strongly supports BCT as appropriate therapy for invasive lobular breast cancer. Due to the presumed multicentric nature of lobular carcinomas, several groups have attempted to assess whether these subtypes are more prone to local failure with BCT and found equivalent breast tumor control and survival after BCT in patients with invasive ductal or lobular carcinoma.

Lobular carcinoma in situ as a component of invasive cancers: Presence of LCIS at the margins and the size and presence of multifocal LCIS does not alter the rate of local control. Peritumoral lymphatic infiltration causes poor disease-free and total survival rates, as well as more local recurrences and distant failures.

Nodal status: Although nodal status is the strongest predictor of distant metastasis and OS, effect of nodal status on local control in the conservatively managed breast cancer patient has not been demonstrated. This may be due to the fact that a majority of node-positive patients receive chemotherapy and/or hormonal therapy, which may counteract the effect of any adverse effect on local relapse.

Radiation Therapy Techniques

Conventional Two-dimentional Tangent

Whole breast irradiation is normally delivered with two opposed tangential fields to encompass the breast, often including part of the underlying chest wall and the lower axilla. Beam modifying devices, usually lead wedges, are used to improve dose homogeneity. This technique has been in existence since early 1980s, with little changes until recently (Fig. 3). Increasingly, centers now use computed tomography (CT) to plan radiation therapy, which permits clearer definition of underlying lung and heart and avoidance of these critical structures. CT planning also permits for the correction of underlying lung density and optimization of compensation if necessary.

Usually up to 2–3 cm of underlying lung is included in the tangential portals. Parameters measured from simulator films included the perpendicular distance from the posterior tangential field edge to the posterior part of the anterior chest wall at the center of the field [central lung distance (CLD)], the maximum perpendicular distance from the posterior tangential field edge to the posterior part of the anterior chest wall [maximum lung distance (MLD)], and the length of lung as measured at the posterior tangential field edge on the simulator film. The best predictor of the percentage of ipsilateral lung volume treated by the tangential fields is the CLD. A CLD of 1.5 cm predicted that approximately 6% of the ipsilateral lung would be included in the tangential field, a CLD of 2.5 cm, approximately 16%, and a CLD of 3.5 cm, approximately 26% of the ipsilateral lung.[59]

When the CLD is more than 3 cm, in treatment of the left breast, a significant volume of heart will also be irradiated. Special attention should be paid to minimizing the volume of heart irradiated.

Techniques such as respiratory gating, deep inspiratory breath-hold using Active Breath Coordinator can deliver radiation to breast while minimizing dose to heart (Fig. 4).

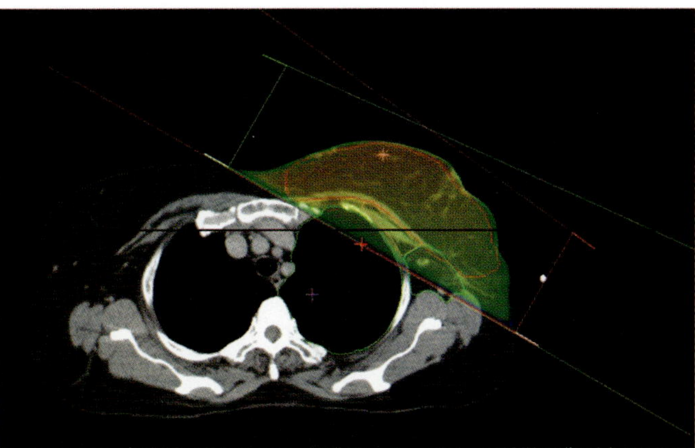

Fig. 3 Relationship of conventional tangents with breast and underlying lung

Courtesy: Dr Tejinder Kataria, Division of Radiation Oncology, Medanta— The Medicity, Haryana, India

Three-dimensional Conformal or Intensity-modulated Radiation Therapy

A number of advances in radiation oncology technologies have significantly improved radiation treatments for breast cancer. CT simulation has replaced fluoroscopic guidance for delineation of treatment fields. Delineating and contouring three-dimensional target volumes and critical normal structures has helped to improve the accuracy of treatment and potentially minimize risks of normal tissue injury. It is important to recognize that the term intensity-modulated radiation therapy (IMRT) has been used in various ways to describe breast cancer treatment. In some studies, IMRT is described as a method of three-dimensional dose compensation without a change in the gantry angles of predesigned tangential fields. In such instances, dose distribution has been improved, but the fields are not more conformal. Accordingly, low dose to other organs is not an

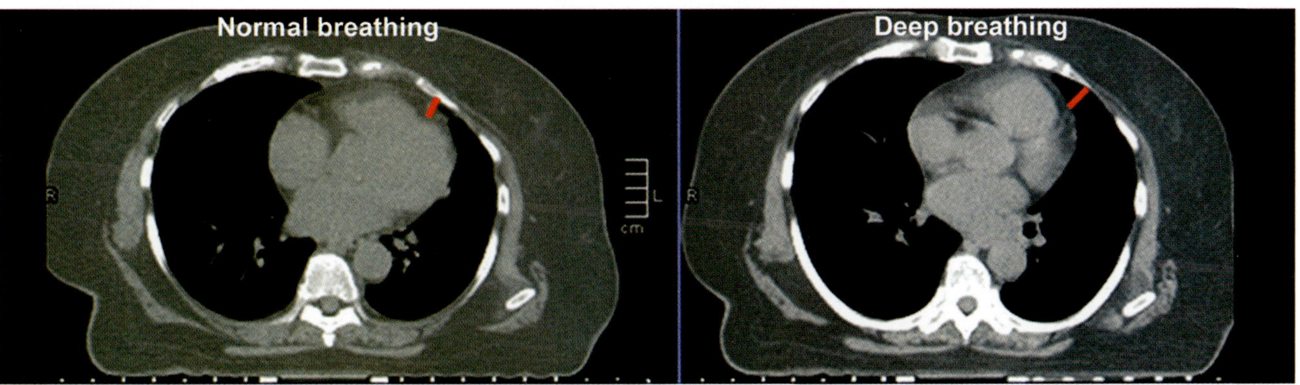

Fig. 4: Relationship of the heart to the radiation fields under free breathing conditions and breath-hold conditions (red line). During deep inspiration breath hold, heart is pushed away and down from chest wall thus sparing the heart

Courtesy: Dr Tejinder Kataria, Division of Radiation Oncology, Medanta—The Medicity, Haryana, India

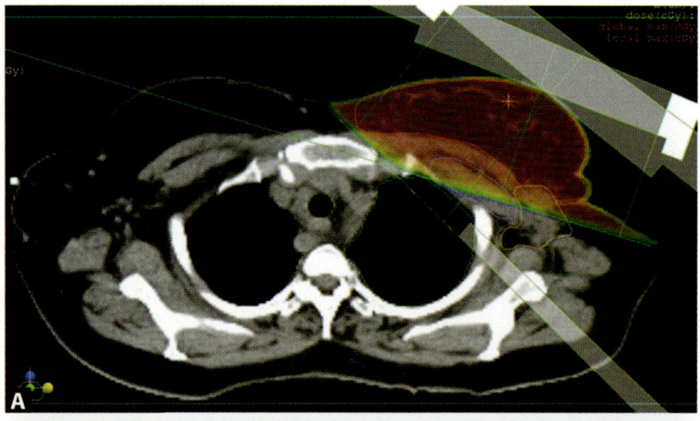

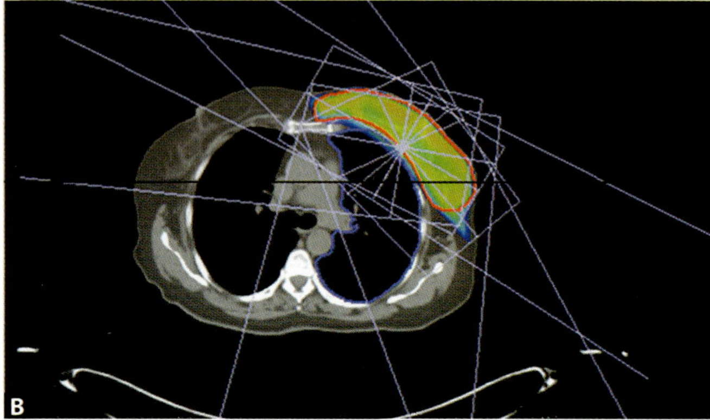

Figs 5A and B Tangent IMRT showing dose distribution has been improved, but the fields are not much conformal; (A) as compared to multibeam IMRT; (B). Increase in the volume of normal tissues that receive low radiation dose increases

Courtesy: Dr Tejinder Kataria, Division of Radiation Oncology, Medanta—The Medicity, Haryana, India

issue. For others, IMRT attempts to improve conformality of the high-dose region by using multiple field angles that increase the volume of normal tissues that receive low radiation dose (Figs 5A and B).

A number of publications have explored the potential advantages of 3D conformal radiation therapy (3D-CRT) or IMRT to treat patients with breast cancer. 3D-CRT involves a reduction in the volume of normal tissues receiving a high dose, with an increase in dose to the target volume that includes the tumor and a limited amount of normal tissue. IMRT can further improve the dose distribution between the target and non-target tissue, but may also increase the volume of tissue exposed to lower doses of radiation.

In a study of 26 patients irradiated to the intact breast with CT scanning-based three-dimensional treatment planning, Muren et al. demonstrated a 50% reduction of the average excess cardiac mortality risk in left-side-treated patients using this technique. Their data showed, without consideration of patient or organ motion, that tangential breast irradiation with less than 1 cm of the heart and less than 2.5 cm of the lung in the treatment volume would lower the anticipated risk for cardiac mortality or pulmonary morbidity to less than 1%.[60]

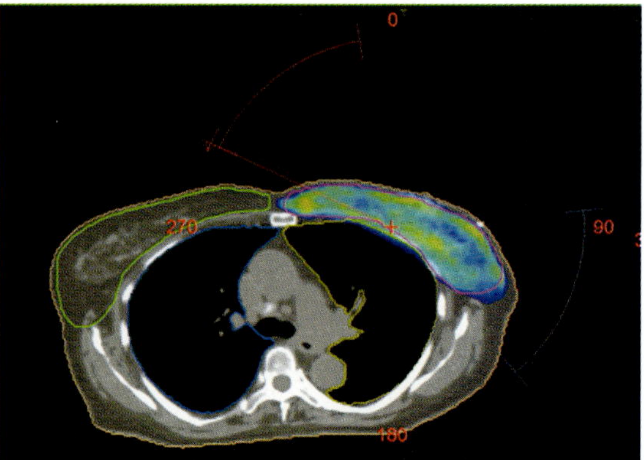

Fig. 6 Volumetric modulated arc therapy with two partial sector arcs

Courtesy: Dr Tejinder Kataria, Division of Radiation Oncology, Medanta—The Medicity, Haryana, India

Cho et al. in a comparison of various techniques in 12 patients with left-sided breast cancer, concluded that the lowest normal tissue complication probability values for heart and lungs were comparable between an oblique electron beam and the IMRT techniques compared with split-beam tangential fields.[61]

Vicini et al. reported on 281 patients treated with whole breast IMRT using multiple static MLC segments. The median volume of breast receiving 105% of the prescribed dose was 11% (range 0–67.6%). The median breast volume receiving 110% of the prescribed dose was 0% (range 0–39%), and the median breast volume receiving 115% of the prescribed dose was also 0%. Only three (1%) experienced grade III toxicity. The cosmetic results at 12 months (95 patients analyzable) were rated as excellent/good in 94 patients (99%). No skin telangiectasia, significant fibrosis, or persistent breast pain was noted. The authors concluded that the use of IMRT with a static MLC technique for tangential whole breast radiation therapy is an efficient method for achieving a uniform and standardized dose throughout the whole breast, and widespread implementation of this technology can be achieved with minimal imposition on clinic resources and time constraints.[62]

In a recently reported trial of patients undergoing breast-conserving therapy, 358 patients undergoing whole breast irradiation were randomized to radiation to the breast with standard wedges or with IMRT. Those randomized to IMRT experienced significantly lower degrees of moist desquamation owing to the improved homogeneity with the IMRT techniques employed.[63] We have implemented the technique of volumetric modulated Arc Therapy (VMAT) at our institute since 2010 with good sparing of the underlying lung and heart (Fig. 6).

Radiation Management of the Regional Lymphatics

The role of radiation therapy in management of the regional lymphatics is influenced by the risk of subclinical microscopic disease in regional nodal basins and patterns of failure. Tangential radiation ports will likely treat most level I nodes and a portion of level II nodes. Reznik et al. analyzed axillary dose-volume data with ST and high tangents. The average doses delivered to levels I, II and III using standard technique were 66%, 44% and 31%, respectively; the dose increasing to 86%, 71% and 73% when the cranial border was raised by 2 cm, reaching up to humeral head (high tangent).[64] In another study, the mean doses delivered to axilla by the three techniques (IMRT, 3D-CRT, ST) were: 78%, 80% and 87% for level I, 70%, 72% and 65% for level II.[65]

pN0 after complete axillary dissection: It is not necessary to irradiate the regional lymphatics if the nodes are pathologically negative and an adequate axillary dissection has been performed.

SNB negative: In patients with a negative sentinel node, it is not necessary to irradiate the regional lymphatics since available studies have demonstrated a low rate of pathologically involved nodes after a negative sentinel node procedure performed by an experienced surgeon.

SNB positive: Current guidelines are to perform completion axillary dissection. If axillary dissection is not done then axillary radiation is required.

Axilla not addressed or positive SNB without completed ALND: Axillary radiation has been shown to result in high rates of regional nodal control.

Indications of Axillary Radiation (I/II)

- N+ with extensive ECE
- SNB positive with no dissection
- Inadequate axillary dissection
- High risk (>10–15% probability of nodal involvement) with no dissection.

Indication of Supraclavicular Fossa/Level III Axilla Radiation

- Clinical N2 or N3 disease
- More than 4 + LN after axillary dissection
- 1–3 + LN with high-risk features (Young age; ECE over 2 mm; extensive LVI; 20% or higher positive nodal ratio)
- SNB positive with no ALND
- High risk (>10–15% probability of nodal involvement) and no dissection.

Indication of IMC Radiation

- Positive axillary nodes with central and medial lesions
- Stage III breast cancer
- Positive SLN in the IM chain
- Positive SLN in axilla with drainage to IM on lymphoscintigraphy.

Axilla RT versus ALND in cN0 but SNB Positive

Patients who have not undergone any axillary staging procedure, or who have a positive sentinel node and did not undergo further axillary staging, axillary radiation has been shown to result in high rates of regional nodal control.[66]

Internal Mammary Node Chain Irradiation

The role of internal mammary nodal irradiation in node-positive breast cancer patients remains a controversial issue. Recently results of NCIC-MA20 trial, EORTC 22922 have come up and they support IMC irradiation in selected group of EBC. In EORTC 22922 phase III trial, after an average follow-up of 10.9 years irradiation of the internal mammary and medial supraclavicular lymph node (IM-MS) chain in stage I to III breast cancer, it was found that patients in the IM-MS treatment group had better OS independent of the number of lymph nodes involved. A total of 382 patients in the IM-MS group died during that period, compared with 429 in the non IM-MS group, and there was no increase in non-breast cancer related mortality in the first group.[67]

Sequencing Chemoradiation in the Conservative Management of Breast Cancer

Most studies evaluating treatment sequencing suggest that a delay in the onset of radiation therapy to permit delivery of chemotherapy does not increase local recurrence rates, contralateral breast cancer, second malignancy or death, provided all modalities are given in a timely fashion.[68,69] Concurrent administration of chemoradiotherapy has been tried, with marginal benefit in terms of reduction of local recurrences in some studies,[70] although with increase in toxicities like subcutaneous fibrosis, telangiectasia, skin pigmentation and breast atrophy.[71]

TECHNICAL ISSUES IN RADIATION MANAGEMENT OF EARLY STAGE BREAST CANCER

Treatment Position

Most patients are treated in the supine position, on breast board, with the arm abducted (90° or greater). Other treatment positions have been used to improve the dosimetry in patients with large, pendulous breasts. A lateral decubitus position has been suggested by investigators at the Institut Curie. Irradiation in the prone position has also been proposed with reduction of dose to the underlying lung and heart and reduction of scattered dose to the contralateral breast.

Treatment Volume

The entire breast and chest wall are included in the irradiated volume. The upper margin of the portals should be placed at the head of the clavicle to include the entire breast. The medial margin, if no internal mammary portal is used, should be at the midline. The lateral-posterior margin should be placed 2 cm beyond all palpable breast tissue, which is usually near the mid-axillary line. The inferior margin is drawn 2–3 cm below the inframammary fold.

In most patients 6 MV is adequate. When separation is more than 22 cm there may be significant dose inhomogeneity in the breast. This problem can be minimized by using higher energy photons (10–18 MV). Bolus should be avoided in conservatively managed patients. Treatment volume should include all the breast parenchymal CT changes as seen in RT planning CT scan.

RTOG has issued consensus definitions of anatomical boundaries for breast cancer contouring atlas http://www.rtog.org/corelab/contouringatlases/breastcanceratlas.aspx.[72]

Doses of Radiation and Fractionation

Whole Breast Dose

With whole breast irradiation, tumor doses of approximately 45–50 Gy are delivered to the entire breast over 5–6 weeks. We use 2 Gy fractions to 50 Gy, since this is the scheme used in the vast majority of randomized trials using whole breast radiation therapy following conservative surgery. Alternative fractionation schemes have been employed: whole breast irradiation of 42.5 Gy in 16 fractions over 22 days. No difference in DFS or OS rates has been detected between above schedules.

Boost to Tumor Site

The need for a boost to the tumor bed following lumpectomy and whole breast radiation remains an area of debate. Most authors report that 65–80% of breast recurrences after conservation surgery and irradiation occur around the primary tumor site. These data provide a strong rationale for a tumor bed boost. Various series suggest that patients treated with higher doses have a greater probability of tumor control.[73,74]

Electron Boosts

An electron energy is selected that covers the target volume depth (usual range is 9–16 MeV electrons), based on review of the physical examination, mammogram, ultrasound, CT, or other imaging used to ascertain the location and depth of the tumor or metallic surgical clips. The 90% prescription isodose line is limited to the chest wall to decrease dose to the lung. The clinical setup for electron boost involves marking the projection of the post-lumpectomy volume on the skin and adding 2–3 cm in all directions.

Radiation Beams

X-ray energies of 4–6 MV are preferred to treat the breast. Photon energies more than 6 MV underdose superficial tissues beneath the skin surface, but higher-energy photons may be helpful in large breasts to decrease the integral breast dose. In these patients, the high-energy photon beam may be degraded to bring the maximum dose to more superficial tissues. It is not necessary to apply bolus as skin is usually not at risk and use of bolus results in impaired cosmetic results. Wedges or compensating filters must be used for a portion of the treatment to achieve a uniform dose distribution in the breast. Although conventional wedges improve dose homogeneity at the central axis of the breast, significant inhomogeneity can occur in the superior and inferior portions of the breast. Currently, with the use of multileaf collimators and more sophisticated treatment planning techniques, optimization of homogeneity throughout the breast can be achieved through the use of a variety of techniques.

ACCELERATED PARTIAL BREAST IRRADIATION

The current standard of care for women with invasive breast cancer remains whole breast irradiation following BCS. In view of long treatment time, accelerated forms of treatment have been developed. The rationale behind this approach is that the majority of breast relapses occur at or near the lumpectomy site. Review of recent clinical and pathologic evidence suggests that the primary target requiring adjuvant treatment following BCS (with negative surgical margins) is likely limited to a 1–2 cm boundary surrounding the lumpectomy cavity, and the same may alone be treated, rather than treating the entire breast in all patients. If it were possible to reduce this target to less than 40% of the whole breast, acceleration of the dose delivery and completion of treatment in less than 5 days becomes more feasible.

The strategy in accelerated RT is of delivering the radiation to a smaller volume of breast tissue around the lumpectomy site, using fewer larger fractions delivered over a shorter time. There are four prevailing techniques and include multicatheter interstitial brachytherapy, balloon catheter brachytherapy, three-dimensional conformal external beam radiotherapy (3D-CRT) and intraoperative RT.

Multicatheter Interstitial Accelerated Partial Breast Irradiation

The accelerated partial breast irradiation (APBI) technique that has been in use the longest and has the most extensive follow-up is the multicatheter interstitial brachytherapy approach.[75] With this technique, after-loading catheters are placed through the breast tissue to surround the lumpectomy cavity. Catheters are generally positioned at 1–1.5-cm intervals to avoid hot and cold spots. These implants generally require 15 to 20 catheters to ensure proper dose coverage. Once the implant geometry is known (through mapping of catheter location), dosimetric planning is completed to determine how to optimally place the radioactive source within the catheters for dose delivery. To date there has only been one prospective phase III trial for which mature results are available to evaluate APBI using primarily interstitial brachytherapy versus whole-breast irradiation (WBI). Polgar et al.[76] reported 5-year results on 258 randomized patients demonstrating similar rates of local recurrence (4.7% and 3.4%; $p = .50$), OS (94.6% vs 91.8%), cancer-specific survival (98.3% vs 96.0%), and DFS (88.3% vs 90.3%) for APBI versus WBI, respectively. After a thorough review of these investigations, it has been suggested that the negative results stem from both a lack of proper patient selection and acceptable dose delivery. Most common fractionation used is 34 Gy in 10 fractions twice a day over 5 days.

MammoSite Radiation Therapy System for Accelerated Partial Breast Irradiation

The MammoSite device consists of a single lumen catheter allowing the passage of high dose rate afterloaded iridium-192 (^{192}Ir) source. The device can be implanted at the time of surgery (open technique) or under ultrasound guidance postoperatively through the same or alternative incision (closed technique). After insertion, the device is filled with radiographic contrast to allow evaluation of placement by CT scan. Device placement is assessed for the adequacy of skin spacing (optimally ≥7 mm) and conformality of the balloon surface to the lumpectomy cavity (>90%). The device is attached to an HDR afterloader for the delivery of 10 fractions of 3.4 Gy each, twice daily for 10 days with a minimum of 6 hours between treatments. Since receiving clearance by the U.S. Food and Drug Administration (FDA) in 2002, MammoSite has become the most widely used form of APBI, implanted in more than 40,000 women by early 2008. Skin spacing 7 mm or more, use of a closed cavity placement technique, use of prophylactic antibiotics, and the use of multiple dwell positions within the device during treatment have been associated with a decreased incidence of acute and late toxicities.

Three-Dimensional Conformal External Beam Radiation Therapy for Accelerated Partial Breast Irradiation

The 3D-CRT technique employs a standard linear accelerator to deliver external beam radiation to a clinical target volume, usually the tumor bed plus a normal breast tissue margin of 10–15 mm, with an additional margin to account for breathing motion and setup uncertainties (generally 10 mm). Three to five beams are typically used to deliver the dose to patients in either the supine or prone position using photons alone or in combination with electrons. Although less studied than catheter techniques, 3D-CRT offers advantages over the latter in being less invasive, greater familiarity of Radiation Oncologists with linear accelerator (LINAC)-based techniques, and consistent and homogenous dose delivery. However, the need for additional margins to account for setup uncertainties can result in increased dose to critical structures, such as the heart, lung and contralateral breast.

Intraoperative Accelerated Partial Breast Irradiation

The University College of London has investigated the use of *low energy x-rays* (maximum energy, 50 kV) delivered by a portable, spherical, radiation-generating device [Targeted Intraoperative Radiotherapy (*TARGIT)*] that is placed into the lumpectomy cavity following tumor resection.[77] A dose of 20 Gy at 1 mm and 6 Gy at 10 mm from the applicator surface is delivered to the cavity. Although the lower energies delivered preclude the need for specially shielded operating rooms, there is concern that such low energies may be inadequate to "sterilize" the target volume of microscopic disease. Initial reports with this technique have reported acceptable cosmetic results, toxicity, and local control rates.

The European Institute of Oncology has used *intraoperative electrons* (generated by a mobile linear accelerator) delivering 21 Gy in one fraction (immediately following quadrantectomy). The breast is surgically manipulated to ensure that all targeted tissue is within the electron field boundaries and nontargeted normal tissue is either outside the electron field or shielded. The Milan group has published on a series of 590 patients using this technique with a median follow-up of 20 months demonstrating a local recurrence rate of 0.5%, with acceptable toxicities.[78] Intraoperative treatment raises some important concerns. The treatment is completed before the availability of the final microscopic margin and axillary nodal status are known, information considered important in patient selection and in the determination of the target extent.

Patient Selection

The Accelerated Partial Breast Irradiation demands the proper selection of patients with an anticipated low risk of harboring in-breast microscopic disease remote from the lumpectomy cavity. In reviewing the literature, requiring negative surgical margins and restricting treatment to patients with smaller tumors are the only two criteria that have been consistently applied within the successful APBI trials.

American Society of Therapeutic Radiology and Oncology (ASTRO) Consensus Statement[79]

- Age ≥60 years
- Infiltrating ductal carcinoma and favorable subtypes
- Less than or equal to 2 cm size
- Lumpectomy achieving microscopically negative margins more than or equal to 2 mm
- Negative axillary lymph nodes
- ER (+) tumors
- No EIC or lymphovascular space invasion (LVSI).

Cautionary Candidates: Any of these Criteria should Invoke Caution and Concern when Considering APBI

- Age 50–59 years
- Lesions 2.1–3.0 cm in size
- Invasive lobular
- Pure DCIS less than or equal to 3cm
- Lumpectomy achieving microscopically negative margins less than 2 mm
- EIC less than 3cm
- Limited/focal LVSI.

Unsuitable Candidates

- Age less than 50 years
- BRCA 1/2 mutation present
- Lesion size more than 3 cm
- Axillary nodes positive
- Extensive LVSI
- EIC more than 3 cm
- Multicentric disease
- Use of neoadjuvant therapy.

FOLLOW-UP OF PATIENTS TREATED WITH BREAST CONSERVATION SURGERY AND IRRADIATION

It is important to closely monitor patients treated with conservation surgery and irradiation because early detection of a local recurrence may allow for another wide local excision or a total mastectomy, without significantly compromising the OS of the patient. Although the optimal interval for follow-up mammography has not been determined, a postradiation bilateral diagnostic mammogram should be obtained within the first year following radiation therapy. A careful history and physical examination are indicated every 3–6 months for 3 years and every 6 months for the following 2 years, and annually thereafter. In patients who underwent breast conservation therapy, a diagnostic mammogram every 6–12 months for the first 2 years and yearly thereafter is sufficient unless the radiologist recommends more frequent examinations. At least yearly evaluation is mandatory even 10 years after therapy because of the possibility of late breast relapses and occasional distant metastases. If there is strong evidence of suspect microcalcifications, masses, or architectural distortions of the breast after conservation surgery and irradiation, a biopsy should be obtained to rule out a recurrence.

Radiographic Findings after Breast Conservation Therapy

Most frequent mammographic findings are parenchymal distortion and fibrosis at the tumor excision site (secondary to surgical scar and irradiation), skin thickening and calcifications, due to fat necrosis, which are coarse and round and have radiolucent centers. Most changes are observed in the first 12 months after therapy, with resolution/stabilization achieved at 12–36 months after completion of therapy. Breast edema is mammographically present in virtually all patients at completion of therapy, with a steady high over 36 months and stabilization by 42 months.

Recurrences commonly contain very suspect patterns of calcification, with linear and pleomorphic forms. The distribution of calcifications is usually clustered. In most of the recurrences, they can be characterized as obviously malignant in majority of cases (77%). Therefore, women without worrisome mammographic patterns need not undergo breast biopsy. If the findings are stable, mammographic follow-up is sufficient. However, a change in number or characteristic pattern warrants a biopsy to rule out recurrent tumor.

Magnetic resonance imaging is increasingly used in the evaluation of patients with equivocal mammographic findings. In suspected cases MRI demonstrates early rise of signal intensity on dynamic T1-weighted, contrast-enhanced images. During the first year after therapy, the diagnostic accuracy is not improved by additional use of contrast-enhanced MRI because of strong and sometimes early and ill-circumscribed enhancement. Later than 12 months after therapy, enhancement decreases significantly and false-positive calls are lesser.

SEQUELAE OF IRRADIATION IN BREAST CANCER

The most frequent complications associated with conservation surgery plus irradiation are arm or breast edema, breast fibrosis, painful mastitis or myositis, pneumonitis, and rib fracture.

Lymphedema/Breast Edema

Arm edema is a common complication of breast cancer therapy that can result in substantial functional impairment and psychological morbidity. Combined axillary dissection and nodal irradiation results in a significantly higher incidence of arm edema compared with either alone.[80]

Preventive measures have not been well studied. Nonpharmacologic treatments, such as massage and exercise, have been shown to be effective therapies for lymphedema, but the effect of pharmacologic interventions remains uncertain. The ALMANAC randomized trial confirms lower morbidity and improved quality of life following SNB compared to axillary dissection. Before the treatment of arm lymphedema after breast carcinoma it is mandatory to differentiate between treatment-associated complications and tumor recurrence in the regional lymphatics. Various treatment regimens to treat lymphedema include the compression pump, arm exercises, compression garments, complex decongestive physiotherapy/complex physical therapy, and manual lymph node drainage.

Skin/breast complications include breast swelling (most frequent) followed by muscle pain (on motion), incision site pain, and general breast discomfort, rib pain, breast discomfort during sexual activity.

Brachial Plexopathy

Brachial plexus dysfunction is a possible complication of regional nodal radiation therapy. In a review of 1,624 patients, Pierce et al. found that brachial plexus sequelae were observed in 1.8% of patients.[81] They also found that the incidence of brachial plexopathy was significantly higher when the axillary dose was more than 50 Gy ($p = .004$). However, dose alone did not determine whether radiation damage would develop in a given patient. Treatment technique (two versus three fields; $p = .0009$) and concomitant chemotherapy were also risk factors. Treatment for radiation brachial plexopathy consists of transdermal electrical nerve stimulation, dorsal column stimulators, neurolysis, and neurolysis with omentoplasty. Physical therapy, tricyclics, antiarrhythmics, anticonvulsants, nonsteroidal anti-inflammatory drugs, and steroids are helpful in therapy of both radiation-induced and metastatic brachial plexopathies. There is no reliable evidence to support hyperbaric oxygen therapy to slow or reverse radiation-induced brachial plexopathy.

Pulmonary Sequelae

Symptomatic pneumonitis is infrequent. This clinical syndrome is noted one to several months after irradiation. Patients present with dry cough (88%), shortness of breath (35%), or fever (53%), and on radiographic studies a pulmonary infiltrate is observed in the irradiated volume. The risk for development of radiation pneumonitis may be related to the volume of lung irradiated. The addition of regional nodal radiation therapy to breast irradiation significantly increases the incidence of symptomatic pneumonitis (1% without and 4% with regional node radiation therapy; $p < .001$). Lingos et al.[82] reported on radiation pneumonitis in a retrospective review of 1,624 patients treated with conservation surgery and irradiation. Overall, pneumonitis developed in 1% of patients. No patient had late or persisting pulmonary symptoms. The incidence of radiation pneumonitis was correlated with the combined use of chemotherapy and a supraclavicular field ($p = .0001$). The effect of tangential field technique on pulmonary function was reported by Lund et al.[83] There was a small but statistically significant decrease in the forced vital capacity and forced expired volume in one second 3 months after irradiation ($p < .05$). These changes normalized within 1 year.

Cardiac Sequelae

The potential for excess cardiac morbidity associated with the use of radiation therapy in breast cancer has been extensively studied. It has been demonstrated, based on data from randomized trials, overview, and meta-analysis, that when using older techniques, excess cardiac mortality from radiation offset some of the benefits that radiation therapy clearly produced with respect to breast cancer mortality. With modern techniques that minimize exposure to the normal cardiac and pulmonary structures, cardiotoxicity have reduced but oncologist should be cautious particularly in the setting of left-sided breast cancers in patients receiving other cardiotoxic therapies, including adriamycin, epirubicin and trastuzumab. Earlier techniques of radiation therapy have clearly been implicated in excess cardiac mortality from large pools of randomized data. In an analysis of over 90,000 Swedish women, comparing left- to right-sided cancers, Darby et al.,[84] from the Oxford group, reported excess ischemic heart disease mortality more than 10 years after initial treatment in the left sided cancer group (HR 1.13, 95% CI, 1.03 to 1.25; $p = .01$). The majority of cardiovascular deaths were from earlier studies using techniques that are no longer used. However, for patients treated after 1980, although the ratio was still 1.11, the confidence intervals were much larger (0.95 to 1.29), so the hazard remains uncertain for the more modern techniques. Cuzick et al.[85] updated cardiac toxicity data from eight randomized trials initiated before 1975 in which RT was the randomized option and surgery was the same for both treatment arms. An initial analysis of these trials demonstrated an increased all-cause mortality rate in 10-year survivors associated with radiation, but in the update this was no longer present. The initial increase mortality in the radiation arms was strongly influenced by the earliest trials, and more recent trials have found a nonsignificant net benefit in overall mortality associated with radiation therapy. However, an excess of cardiac deaths was apparent in both early and more recent trials ($p < .001$), but this was offset by a reduced number of deaths due to breast cancer, especially in more recent trials. Based on this, it is clearly prudent to use techniques that minimize cardiac dose. Although clinical evidence of cardiac morbidity has decreased with modern techniques, care should be taken to exclude heart from the tangential radiation field.

Risk of Stroke with Supraclavicular Radiation

For patients with node-positive disease undergoing supraclavicular radiation, there is a theoretical concern regarding the potential for development of accelerated carotid artery stenosis. Studies have found no significant excess mortality from RT due to stroke. In studies, only age and hypertension are significant predictors of cardiovascular accident/transient ischemic attack.[86]

Contralateral Breast Cancer and Irradiation

Although all patients with a diagnosis of breast cancer are at increased risk for developing contralateral breast cancer, the additional risk contributed by radiation treatment appears to be minimal, particularly when one uses modern techniques and maintains a dose to the contralateral breast that is as low as is reasonably achievable. Although there is some evidence suggesting a slight excess risk in women who are irradiated at a relatively young age (i.e. <45 years at diagnosis), the risk is extremely small and may be related to older techniques, and most experts would agree that the benefit of radiation far outweighs the risk However, the EBCTCG overview analysis does suggest an elevated incidence of contra lateral breast cancer in patients receiving radiation compared to those who did not receive radiation.[87] This overview analysis of all randomized trials comparing radiation to surgery demonstrated an increased relative risk of contralateral breast cancers of 1.18 ($p = .002$). Although the excess risk appears to be driven primarily by older trials using antiquated techniques, these data do demonstrate the potential long-term effects of radiation-related secondary cancers and highlight the need to maintain dose to the contralateral breast as low as possible.

ENDOCRINE THERAPY

Biology of Endocrine Therapy

Endocrine therapy of breast cancer represents the first molecularly targeted therapy for cancer. All endocrine therapies target the ER protein. The PR has not been utilized as a treatment target itself, but its presence indicates a functioning ER pathway because it is an estrogen-induced gene. ER is a nuclear transcription factor. After the binding of estrogen, ER is phosphorylated and its protein conformation is altered. It activates transcription of specific genes important for tumor cell growth and survival. All endocrine therapies target this pathway in one way or another. Selective ER modulators, such as tamoxifen and toremifene, bind ER just like estrogen, but they alter ER conformation in a slightly different way. These drugs demonstrate dual estrogen agonist and antagonist activity depending on the tissue, cell or gene context. Thus, tamoxifen behaves as an estrogen in the endometrium, bone, liver, and even on some genes in the breast, whereas for other genes in the breast, tamoxifen functions as an antagonist to inhibit estrogen-dependent transcription. Ovarian ablation (surgical or medical) and AI lower the level of estrogen, thereby reducing the ligand-induced activation of ER signaling, both genomic and nongenomic. Pure antagonists or ER downregulators (e.g. fulvestrant) bind ER, but have no intrinsic agonist activity. Furthermore, they induce degradation of ER protein.

Adjuvant Therapy with Selective Estrogen Receptor Modulators

Tamoxifen is the most common selective estrogen receptor modulator (SERM) for the treatment of breast cancer. Toremifene, a drug with structural and functional similarities to tamoxifen, is also approved for adjuvant therapy and appears equally effective to tamoxifen, but is much less prescribed. Raloxifene is approved for prevention but not for treatment of breast cancer. These drugs are nonsteroidal compounds that bind to ER and display both estrogen antagonist and estrogen agonist properties. The net result of the binding of tamoxifen to ER is a blockade of cell cycle transit in G1 phase, thereby inhibiting tumor growth. Some evidence suggests that programmed cell death (apoptosis) may also be induced to a slight degree by tamoxifen.

Taking tamoxifen for 5 years prolongs DFS and OS in patients with ER-positive tumors regardless of axillary lymph node status. Equally beneficial effects are seen in premenopausal and postmenopausal women. With AI showing a small DFS benefit over tamoxifen, adjuvant hormonal therapy has shifted more toward the upfront or sequential use of these agents in postmenopausal agents. Tamoxifen should be avoided in women who have medical contraindications, such as a history of thromboembolic disease or blood-clotting disorders. Aromatase inhibitors avoid these problems and may be preferred in these patients. Tamoxifen is certainly an acceptable alternative for women who cannot tolerate or afford an AI, and it is still the endocrine therapy of choice in premenopausal patients.

Aromatase Inhibitors

Upfront Therapy with Aromatase Inhibitors

Upfront therapy with an aromatase inhibitor is beneficial, in terms of DFS, when compared with tamoxifen. It is important to emphasize again that upfront aromatase inhibitors should be used only for women who are verifiably postmenopausal. It should probably be avoided in women with chemotherapy-induced amenorrhea because AI may promote recovery of ovarian function in some of them.

Sequential Adjuvant Therapy with Aromatase Inhibitors Following Tamoxifen

Intergroup Exemestane Study

The Intergroup Exemestane Study (IES) is the largest and most mature switching trial. It tested the concept of whether switching to exemestane after 2–3 years of tamoxifen therapy is more effective than continuing tamoxifen therapy for the remainder of the 5 years of treatment. The primary end point was DFS. The update on this study showed that at a median follow-up of 55.7 months, there were 809 events (354 exemestane, 455 tamoxifen). The hazard ratio was 0.76 (p = .0001) favoring exemestane, and the absolute benefit was 3.3%.[88] Fewer deaths occurred in the exemestane group compared with the tamoxifen group. In addition, switching from tamoxifen to exemestane demonstrated a significant reduction in contralateral breast cancer (HR = 0.56, p = .04).[88]

Combined Analysis of Sequential Trials Using Anastrozole

A combined analysis of the ARNO 95, ABCSG 8, and ITA trials was performed which included more than 4,000 patients.[89] Patients who switched to anastrozole had fewer disease recurrences (92 vs 159) and deaths (66 vs 90) than did those who remained on tamoxifen, resulting in significant improvements in DFS (HR 0.59, p = .0001), event-free survival (HR = 0.55, p <.0001), distant recurrence-free survival (HR = 0.61, p = .002), and OS (HR = 0.71, p = .04), suggesting that postmenopausal women receiving adjuvant tamoxifen should be switched to anastrozole after completing 2–3 years of treatment.

Summary of Sequential Therapy with Aromatase Inhibitors

At the moment it is not clear whether initial treatment with an AI or a few years of tamoxifen followed by an AI is the superior strategy. Some studies suggested that the switching strategy might be only marginally superior for patients whose tumors were ER-positive and PR-positive, whereas initial AI therapy was projected to be significantly better in patients with ER-positive but PR-negative tumors whereas others suggested that initial AI therapy would be superior regardless of the ER or PR status.[90]

Extended Adjuvant Hormonal Therapy

Theoretic reasons support a rationale for prolonged adjuvant hormonal therapy beyond the first 5 years. More prolonged therapy could prevent late recurrences in patients whose breast cancers would otherwise relapse. In addition, tumors resistant to SERM often respond to AI at least in the metastatic setting. On the other hand, side effects and cost of more prolonged therapy are important considerations. Extending tamoxifen, AI, or their sequence beyond 5 years is the subject of several completed and ongoing clinical trials.

Extended Adjuvant Therapy with Tamoxifen

Several trials compared shorter versus longer tamoxifen adjuvant treatment directly. Two large international twin trials (Adjuvant Tamoxifen, Longer Against Shorter [ATLAS] and Adjuvant Tamoxifen: to offer more? [aTTom]) address the issue of very long-term tamoxifen. ATLAS randomized 11,500 women in 38 countries who had completed about 5 years of adjuvant tamoxifen with an additional 5 years of tamoxifen (10 years total) or with stopping therapy. At a mean follow-up of 4.2 years, about 1,500 recurrences were reported, most of them in years 5 through 9. Overall, the recurrence rate was modestly, albeit statistically, significantly lower among those allocated to continue tamoxifen.[91]

Extended Adjuvant Therapy with Aromatase Inhibitors

In the National Cancer Institute of Canada (NCIC)-MA17 trial, more than 5,000 women who had completed 5 years of tamoxifen were randomly assigned to placebo versus letrozole. The study was terminated early after the first interim analysis demonstrated a significant improvement in DFS in the letrozole group, which was confirmed on longer follow-up (HR = 0.58; p < .0001).[92] Another analysis of MA17 that pertains to the issue of duration of an aromatase inhibitor after tamoxifen demonstrated that the hazard ratio in favor of letrozole continued to improve each year throughout the first 4 years of treatment, suggesting that longer treatment might be better.

NSABP B-33, which had a similar design using exemestane, was closed to accrual when the results of MA17 were made public, and patients assigned to placebo were given the option of crossing over to exemestane. At that time, only half of the planned 3,000 patients were enrolled, and more than 40% of patients initially assigned to placebo chose to cross over to receive exemestane. Despite these limitations, a similar trend for improved DFS was observed for the exemestane arm, although it did not reach statistical significance (HR = 0.68, p = .07).[93]

It should be noted that studies of extended adjuvant therapy using tamoxifen or an aromatase inhibitor were performed in patients who received 5 years of initial tamoxifen therapy, a situation that is becoming increasingly less common in postmenopausal women in the era of AI therapy. Additionally, they all demonstrated an impact on DFS but not OS. However, they support the concept of prolonging endocrine therapy beyond 5 years to prevent late recurrences. The type of therapy (tamoxifen, AI, or their sequence) and the optimal duration remain unanswered questions. The NSABP is performing a study of extended adjuvant letrozole following 5 years of upfront AI or sequential therapy, a more modern adjuvant endocrine regimen. Additionally, patients who have completed 5 years of letrozole on the MA17 study are being re-randomized to continue letrozole for 5 more years versus placebo (total 15 years of adjuvant endocrine therapy). Patients on aromatase inhibitors should have serial monitoring of bone mineral density and serum lipids.

Adjuvant Ovarian Ablation

Studies of adjuvant ovarian ablation, either by surgical oophorectomy or by irradiation in premenopausal patients found a significant DFS advantage. Ovarian suppression or ablation (medical or surgical) may be appropriate in selected patients who have a contraindication or do not tolerate tamoxifen. Optimal duration of ovarian suppression (if done medically) is not established, but treating for 3–5 years is reasonable. Combining tamoxifen and ovarian suppression may be utilized in patients at high risk of recurrence. The International Consensus Panel guidelines suggest giving this combination to patients younger than 35 years or to patients with high-risk disease.

Sequencing Tamoxifen and Radiation Therapy in Conservatively Managed Patients

The question of optimal scheduling of hormonal therapy and radiation has been raised due to theoretical concerns that tamoxifen may decrease the radiation sensitivity of tumors. In cell culture studies, tamoxifen causes arrest of breast cancer cells in culture in the relatively radioresistant G_0/G_1 phases of the cell cycle. Although there are conflicting data, suggesting both no effect and increased radiation sensitivity, it is still unclear whether it is reasonable to begin tamoxifen during radiation. In addition, clinical studies have suggested increased pulmonary and breast fibrosis, possibly related to increased concentrations of transforming growth factor with the concurrent use of tamoxifen. Given the lack of definitive data, it appears that either the concurrent or the sequential use of tamoxifen is acceptable in the conservatively managed breast cancer patient.

LOCALLY ADVANCED BREAST CANCER

This term most commonly refers to stage III disease, meaning advanced primary or nodal disease without clinically evident systemic metastases. Patients presenting with such disease are at risk for both loco-regional and distant disease recurrence.[1] Optimal treatment of locally advanced breast cancer requires multidisciplinary management including diagnostic imaging, chemotherapy, appropriate surgery, radiation, and, if indicated, biological and hormonal therapy.

EPIDEMIOLOGY

In the 1980s, the incidence of breast cancer showed an apparent increase partly because of the increase in use of screening mammography.[2] However, the incidence of locally advanced breast cancer decreased as the test helped detect a larger proportion of patients in earlier disease stages, and public education programs prompted women to seek early medical care for a suspected breast lump. Race and ethnicity has a significant bearing on the incidence and prognosis of breast cancer. The primary disease is more commonly advanced, and with positive lymph nodes at presentation in African American women and in cases reported on the Indian subcontinent.[3] Pathologically, the breast cancers in this population are of higher nuclear grade and more frequently have ER-negative disease.[4,5]

NATURAL HISTORY

As cancer grows within the breast, it may infiltrate the dermis or the chest wall. Invasion of Cooper's ligaments may lead to skin retraction. Infiltration or obstruction of the lymphatics may cause edema of the breast, known as *peau d'orange*. In addition, primary tumor growth increases the risk of spread through the lymphatics to involve regional lymph nodes and/or spread hematogenously to involve distant sites such as the liver, lung, bone, and brain.

Most advanced primary tumors are associated with axillary lymph node involvement at the time of diagnosis. The axillary lymph node region is divided into three levels, defined according to their relationship to the pectoralis minor muscle: Level I lymph nodes are inferolateral to the muscle, level II are beneath the muscle, and level III are superomedial to the pectoralis muscle (infraclavicular lymph nodes). The Rotter's nodes (located between the pectoralis minor and pectoralis major muscles), and the supraclavicular and internal mammary lymph nodes may also be involved in locally advanced breast cancer.

The clinical course of locally advanced breast cancer depends on the disease characteristics at presentation and the treatment given. Without treatment, almost all locally advanced breast cancers eventually metastasize to visceral organs and become life threatening. Local disease progression can lead to ulceration of the breast skin, pain, bleeding, and infection. Progression of untreated regional lymphatic disease can cause pain, brachial plexopathy, arm edema, obstruction and thrombosis of the brachial vasculature, and skin ulceration.

Inflammatory breast cancer is characterized by rapid disease onset accompanied with clinical findings of skin erythema, edema (*peau d'orange*), brawny breast induration, warmth and asymmetric enlargement. Typically, extensive lymphovascular invasion by tumor emboli is present that involves the superficial dermal plexus of vessels in the papillary and high reticular dermis.

CLINICAL PRESENTATION

Symptoms and signs for locally advanced breast cancer are most commonly a palpable mass in the breast, local or regional pain, bleeding, paresthesia and paresis. The short history and rapidly progressive course distinguishes Inflammatory Carcinoma from other forms of locally advanced breast cancer.

DIAGNOSTIC WORKUP

For patients with locally advanced breast cancer, the workup should start with a careful history and physical examination. The breast examination should include notation of the breast symmetry as well as careful inspection for involvement or edema of the skin. *Peau d'orange* can be best detected through gentle compression of the dermis between two fingers, which can elicit an increased prominence of the hair follicles and skin thickening compared with the skin overlying the contralateral breast. Fixation of a breast mass to the pectoralis muscle or chest wall should be determined by assessing the mobility of the mass with the pectoralis muscle relaxed and contracted. Regional lymph nodes should be thoroughly evaluated by careful clinical examination with the patient in both supine and sitting positions. Clinical nodal evaluation may be supplemented with ultrasonographic imaging. Investigations required for locally advanced breast cancer include complete blood count and liver function tests, chest radiograph, a USG or CT abdomen, bone scan and incision biopsy for tissue diagnosis and receptor study. MRI Brain is required in case neurologic symptoms are present. Role of FDG-PET is investigational.

Staging

Stage III breast cancer can represent T3 disease (tumors larger than 5.0 cm) with involved lymph nodes, N2 or N3 disease, or T4 disease. This differentiation is of importance as it has implications on patient management. For example, a T4b lesion with skin infiltration requires application of a bolus over the skin during radiation therapy, so as to ensure adequate coverage of the involved skin. Involvement of IMNs, or gross residual disease in axilla post surgery, requires treatment of the same.

GENERAL MANAGEMENT AND TREATMENT RESULTS FOR LOCALLY ADVANCED BREAST CANCER

The aim of treatment of locally advanced disease is to eradicate all disease in the local-regional area and to prevent distant disease recurrence. Use of combined-modality treatments including chemotherapy, surgery, and radiation, and additionally, hormonal therapy for ER/PR-positive and trastuzumab for HER2/neu-positive disease, helps attain this aim.

Locally advanced breast cancer can present as either operable disease or inoperable disease. The current standard of treatment for patients with inoperable breast cancer is to proceed with NACT as the initial therapy. Approximately 80–90% of patients with advanced breast cancer show partial or complete clinical response to NACT,[6,7] and most patients presenting with inoperable breast cancer become candidates for surgery. NACT is recommended if an initial surgical procedure is unlikely to resect all gross disease with achievement of negative surgical margins. Two large randomized trials, namely the NSABP-B18 and EORTC, and a meta-analysis support the fact that NACT before surgery and adjuvant chemotherapy after surgery are equivalent in terms of OS, DFS, risk of death, disease progression, or distant metastases.[6,8-10] However, specific benefits of initiating treatment with each modality exist. Performing surgery first removes the bulk of the disease (and thus the source of distant metastases), reduces the interval between diagnosis and mainstay of treatment, provides complete histopathological extent of disease, provides prognostic information concerning the risk of recurrence after mastectomy and thus, the need for adjuvant treatment. NACT may allow breast conservation in case of favorable disease response, allows in vivo assessment of sensitivity of disease to treatment and permits assessment of pathological disease response, which allows prognostication.

Neoadjuvant hormone therapy has been infrequently used for certain specific indications, namely (i) Lobular breast cancer, in which over 90% of tumors are ER-positive (ii) ER/PR-positive breast cancers with comorbidities precluding chemotherapy use, (iii) Postmenopausal women with locally advanced breast cancer with ER/PR-positive and Her2-neu negative disease.

Breast Conservation Therapy after Neoadjuvant Chemotherapy

An important consideration for performing BCS after NACT concerns the volume of surgical resection. For patients with T3 disease for whom initial BCS would be deforming, only the residual nidus after NACT should be resected. Criteria for carrying out BCS after NACT include resolution of skin edema, favorable clinical response to neoadjuvant treatment, lack of multicentricity, no residual malignant calcifications on postoperative mammogram, and lack of extensive LVSI.[11] In the NSABP-B18 trial,[6] the improvement in breast conservation rates from 60% to 68% for patients treated with NACT showed that 20% of initial mastectomy candidates (8 of 40 patients) could undergo BCS instead. Acceptable outcomes with this approach have been demonstrated in studies from Istituto

Nazionale Tumori, Milan,[12] with 85% of the total 536 patients of predominantly stage II breast cancer undergoing BCS after NACT, with an 8 year rate of ipsilateral breast recurrence rate of 6.8%, and from M.D. Anderson Cancer Centre,[13] with 5 years and 10 years local recurrence rates of 5% and 10%, respectively, despite 72% patients having clinical stage IIB or III disease at presentation.

If the residual after NACT is large in relation to the likely volume of remaining breast tissue, or if the disease is diffuse, multifocal, and scattered throughout the original tumor volume, mastectomy is advisable, because a smaller surgical resection carries the risk of leaving behind gross disease.

For patients with clinical stage T1 or T2 N0 disease who are not interested in breast conservation, a total mastectomy with a SLND may be the treatment of choice. A modified radical mastectomy (removal of the breast plus a level I or II axillary dissection) remains the standard of care for patients with clinically positive lymph nodes or locally advanced disease.

Postmastectomy Radiation Therapy

Mastectomy without radiation offers excellent local-regional control rates for most patients with noninvasive or stage I or IIA disease. In contrast, patients with stage III breast cancer (four or more positive lymph nodes or T3 or T4 primary tumors) have a clinically relevant risk of local-regional recurrence after mastectomy, and thus would benefit from adjuvant radiation. Whether radiation provides a survival advantage for patients with stage II breast cancer and one to three positive lymph nodes, is less clear.

In the analysis by the EBCTCG, based on data from 9,933 patients, postmastectomy radiation therapy reduced the 15-year isolated local-regional recurrence rates for patients with lymph node positive disease from 29% to 8%, which led to a 5% decrease in the 15-year breast cancer mortality rate (60% vs 55%).[14] For patients with lymph node negative disease, a similar proportional reduction in local-regional recurrence was seen, but because the risk of recurrence was much lower, the reduction in the absolute local-regional recurrence risk was much smaller (8% for no-radiation vs 3% radiation).[15] For these patients, this small improvement in local-regional recurrence was not associated with a difference in OS. The addition of systemic therapy to postmastectomy RT leads to an even greater reduction in the risk of any recurrence and the risk of death.

Evidence supporting postmastectomy radiation comes from 15 to 20 years outcome data from three randomized trials that investigated radiation therapy for patients with stage II or III breast cancer. The largest of these studies was the Danish Breast Cancer Cooperative Group 82b trial, which randomly assigned 1,708 premenopausal women with stage II or III breast cancer to receive mastectomy followed by nine cycles of CMF (cyclophosphamide, methotrexate, and fluorouracil) chemotherapy or mastectomy, radiation therapy, and eight cycles of CMF chemotherapy.[16] The loco-regional recurrence rates with and without radiation were 9% versus 32% ($p < 0.0001$), while the survival rates were 45% versus 54% ($p < 0.0001$). The 82c trial had more than 1,300 postmenopausal women randomly assigned to undergo mastectomy and 1 year of tamoxifen versus mastectomy, tamoxifen, and radiation therapy.[17] Here also, the loco-regional recurrence rates were 8% with radiation and 35% without radiation ($p < 0.0001$), and survival rates were 45% with radiation versus 36% without radiation ($p = 0.03$). The British Columbia trial randomly assigned 318 premenopausal women with lymph node-positive disease to undergo mastectomy and CMF chemotherapy with or without postmastectomy radiation therapy.[18] The loco-regional recurrence rates with and without radiation were 13% versus 39% ($p < 0.0001$), the rates of distant metastases were 52% versus 69% ($p = 0.004$) and the survival rates were 47% versus 37% ($p = 0.03$).

However, the risks of recurrence in the Danish and British Columbia trials after mastectomy and chemotherapy were high relative to those reported from large series from the United States and from a European Cooperative Group, which reported the same as between 12% and 15% in the one to three positive lymph nodes cohort.[19-22] Difference in the extent of surgery may account for these discrepancies. In the Danish studies, the local-regional recurrence rate rose relatively consistently by 1% per year between the 10th and 25th follow-up years.[23] Similarly, in the British Columbia randomized trial, approximately 20% of local-regional recurrences in the group that did not receive postmastectomy radiation developed after 10 years of follow-up.[18]

Stage II breast cancer with one to three positive lymph nodes is also heterogeneous with respect to other prognostic factors that affect local-regional recurrence risk. The various cofactors that have been found to increase the risk of local-regional recurrence within this subgroup include age less than 40 years, tumor more than 3–4 cm, ER-negative disease, lymphovascular invasion, tumor grade, and margin status. Even if the risk of local-regional recurrence for most patients with one to three positive lymph nodes is relatively low after a modified radical mastectomy and chemotherapy, radiation could still provide a benefit, but whether this degree of benefit is clinically meaningful with respect to patient survival is unknown.

To summarize, postmastectomy radiation offers a significant benefit for Stage III patients in terms of a 20–40% risk of local-regional recurrence; therefore, it should be recommended for all such patients. It is reasonable to discuss the risks and benefits of radiation for patients with intermediate-risk disease, such as those with pathological stage II breast cancer.

Postmastectomy Radiation Therapy after Neoadjuvant Chemotherapy

In most cases, locally advanced breast cancer is currently treated with NACT as the initial therapeutic approach. NACT changes the extent of pathological disease in 80–90% of cases. The risk of local-regional recurrence for patients given NACT is determined by both the pretreatment clinical stage and the extent of pathologically residual disease after chemotherapy. The same should be taken into account while making a clinical decision to irradiate or not.

The efficacy of postmastectomy radiation therapy for patients treated with NACT was evaluated by Huang et al.[24] Outcomes of 579 patients who received NACT, mastectomy, and radiation therapy as part of different randomized trials were compared with those of 136 patients treated with NACT and mastectomy. Despite the heterogeneous data, with patients with worse disease characteristics more often been treated with radiation therapy, the local-regional recurrence rate was found to be significantly lower in the group treated with postmastectomy radiation therapy than in the group treated with NACT and mastectomy (10-year local-regional recurrence rates were 8% and 22%, respectively; p = 0.001). For patients with clinical stage III disease or extensive disease after chemotherapy, radiation led to significant improvements in local-regional recurrence overall and cause-specific survival rates. Multivariate analyses indicated that radiation was independently associated with a lower risk of local-regional recurrence (hazard ratio for not receiving radiation therapy -7.0; p <0.0001) and a lower risk of breast cancer death (hazard ratio for not receiving radiation therapy -2.03; p <0.0001). Among patients with stage III disease who achieved a PCR, the local-regional recurrence rate for those treated with radiation therapy was 7% versus 33% for those who did not receive radiation therapy (p = 0.040). Radiation use in these patients was also associated with an improvement in survival. The investigators also found that patients with clinical T3N0 disease and those with four or more positive lymph nodes after NACT had high rates of local-regional recurrence.[25] However, the patients with clinical stage II disease who had one to three positive lymph nodes after NACT had a relatively low rate of local-regional recurrence (5-year rate of 8%).

These findings suggest that recommending postmastectomy radiation therapy is reasonable for all patients with clinical T3 or T4 tumors or clinical stage III disease regardless of their response to the chemotherapy regimen. In terms of clinical stage I or II breast cancer, postmastectomy radiation therapy should be recommended for patients with four or more positive lymph nodes after chemotherapy and for the patient in whom the disease progresses and the primary tumor exceeds 5 cm in diameter. But, additional studies are needed to quantify the local-regional recurrence risk for patients who present with T1 or T2 disease and have one to three positive lymph nodes after NACT.

Radiation Treatment Techniques after Mastectomy

Target Definitions

Traditionally, postmastectomy radiation therapy includes treatment to the chest wall and draining lymphatics in the undissected axillary apex/supraclavicular fossa, as the chest wall is the most common site of recurrent disease, and all patients with stage III disease (T3N1, T4, or pathological N2 or N3 disease) have a clinically relevant risk of recurrence in the axillary apex/supraclavicular fossa. For patients who have had a standard ALND (number of lymph nodes recovered more than 10), the 10-year risk of recurrence in this region is only about 3% and not predicted by the extent of axillary disease or extracapsular extension.[26] Hence, an adequately dissected axilla does not constitute the target volume in postmastectomy radiation therapy. IMNs are included in target volume because surgical series have shown that up to 35–50% of patients with clinically advanced disease will have microscopic involvement of lymph nodes within this region.[27,28] Inclusion of the internal mammary lymph nodes also provides a broader coverage of the chest wall, which may prove to be a secondary benefit in avoiding marginal misses. Patients with stage II breast cancer with one to three positive lymph nodes fail predominantly on the chest wall and have a much lower risk of recurrence in the axillary apex/supraclavicular fossa. So, treatment of the chest wall only is advocated in such patients.

Treatment Simulation

Patients should be immobilized with their ipsilateral arm abducted (90–120°) and externally rotated such that the soft tissues of the arm lie cranial to the junction of the tangent and supraclavicular fossa field. Skin folds within the supraclavicular fossa should be avoided. Patients are placed on a 10–15° angle board to flatten the slope of the chest wall in the region of the sternum. Radio-opaque wires are placed on the mastectomy scar. Bolus may be used to treat the skin to therapeutic doses, if indicated. Subsequently, the patient undergoes a treatment planning noncontrast CT scan. Appropriate isocenters and setup points are determined and marked. Targeted areas of interest are then contoured on the CT slices. CT simulation is very useful for precise delineation of target volumes, especially the IMNs, supraclavicular nodes and level III axilla.

Dose Prescription

Initial fields and target volumes should be treated to a total dose of 50 Gy in 25 fractions over 5 weeks. About 3–5 mm bolus over the chest wall should be applied every other day or every day for 2 weeks (20 Gy total dose) to ensure that a brisk radiation dermatitis develops. The chest wall may be further boosted with electron fields (5–10 cm beyond the mastectomy scar and covering the tumor bed location of the original primary) for an additional 10 Gy in five fractions over 1 week beyond the initial 50-Gy course. In addition, all sites of unresected but initially involved adenopathy in the internal mammary, infraclavicular, and supraclavicular regions may be treated with a boost, depending on the status of residual disease present.

Systemic Therapy

Chemotherapy

In the EBCTCG meta-analysis, data from almost 150,000 patients treated on 194 randomized trials that investigated chemotherapy or hormonal therapy was evaluated.[29] The use of chemotherapy was found to reduce the probability of recurrence and the risk of death for both patients with lymph node positive disease and those with lymph node-negative disease. Because patients with positive lymph nodes have a much greater risk of recurrence and death from disease, the absolute percentage who benefit from chemotherapy is greatest in this cohort. Use of multiagent chemotherapy resulted in an improved outcome compared to single-agent chemotherapy. Also, there was a significant benefit in using anthracycline [FAC (fluorouracil, doxorubicin, and cyclophosphamide) or FEC (fluorouracil, epirubicin, and cyclophosphamide)] chemotherapy compared to CMF chemotherapy. The benefits of chemotherapy varied according to patient age, with patients less than 50 achieving a greater proportional reduction in the risk of recurrence (proportional reduction of 36%) than patients 50–69 years old (proportional reduction of 29%). Tamoxifen therapy also provides a significant benefit in reducing recurrence and improving survival for patients with ER-positive disease, with a 31% proportional reduction in the annual risk of breast cancer death rate. Tamoxifen provided a benefit for both younger and older patients with ER-positive or ER-unknown disease, but did not provide a benefit for patients with ER-negative disease. The data indicate that 5 years of tamoxifen therapy provided better outcomes compared to 1–2 years of treatment. For patients with ER-positive or ER-unknown lymph node-negative disease, tamoxifen treatment reduced the 5-year risk from 20.1% (no tamoxifen) to 11% (with tamoxifen). In the lymph node-positive cohort, the risks of recurrence were 40.8% versus 24.7%, respectively. This meta-analysis also found that the benefits of chemotherapy and tamoxifen therapy were additive for patients with ER-positive disease. The estimated cumulative reduction in the risk of mortality from combined anthracycline chemotherapy followed by tamoxifen in young women with ER-positive disease was estimated to be as high as 57%. Recent trials that have shown a benefit for adjuvant taxanes after anthracycline chemotherapy include the CALGB 9344/Intergroup 0148 trial,[30] the NSABP B-28 trial,[31] and the BCIRG 001 trial.[32]

Hormone Therapy

Hormonal therapy is indicated for all patients with ER- or PR-positive disease. Premenopausal women, who continue to have ovarian function after chemotherapy, should receive tamoxifen as the preferred therapy. For postmenopausal women, the use of an aromatase inhibitor is equally appropriate. Aromatase inhibitors have proven to be a significant advance in hormonally responsive breast cancer. Unlike tamoxifen, which directly blocks the ER on tumor cells, aromatase inhibitors provide beneficial effects by decreasing circulating estrogen by inhibiting the conversion of adrenal testosterone-like hormones into estrogen. Accordingly, aromatase inhibitors do not carry some of the same pro-estrogenic effects that have been associated with tamoxifen, such as its potentially beneficial effects against osteoporosis and its potentially harmful effects of stimulating the endometrial lining.

Based on the encouraging results of adjuvant Aromatase Inhibitor trials like ATAC,[33] NCIC MA 17,[34] Intergroup Exemestane Trial[35] and BIG 1-98 trial,[36] there are a number of options for postmenopausal patients, including anastrozole for 5 years, letrozole for 5 years, initial tamoxifen for 2 to 3 years followed by exemestane, or tamoxifen for 5 years followed by 5 years of letrozole.

Targeted Therapy

Trastuzumab for patients with tumors that have gene amplification of the HER2/neu gene is a part of adjuvant therapy for breast cancer patients. A series of randomized prospective trials prove the efficacy of trastuzumab in this setting.[37-40] In all trials, trastuzumab increased the risk for a decrease in cardiac ejection fraction, and it became more fully appreciated that patients who were treated with this agent require careful cardiac supervision. For most of these trials, patients who required radiation received trastuzumab concurrently during radiation treatments. To date, no increase in cardiac events or other serious sequelae have been reported as a consequence of the concurrent use of trastuzumab and radiation.[41]

General Management and Treatment Results for Inflammatory Breast Cancer

Inflammatory breast cancer is considered inoperable at presentation and should be treated initially with NACT (with consideration of trastuzumab if the tumor is HER2/neu-positive). Patients should be carefully monitored for response, and after achievement of the maximal clinical response, patients should be re-evaluated for mastectomy. About 80% of patients with inflammatory breast cancer will achieve a clinical response and their disease will become operable.[42] All patients should receive postmastectomy radiation therapy delivered to the chest wall and the draining lymphatics. Investigators at M.D. Anderson Cancer Center conducted a series of single-group prospective trials for patients with inflammatory breast cancer and found that NACT with FAC followed by local-regional therapy led to a 5-year survival rate of 25%. The addition of taxanes has improved the progression-free and OS of patients with inflammatory disease.[42] Results from this study also confirmed that a complete or partial response to NACT, the use of RT, and the addition of mastectomy to the therapeutic regimen all significantly improved disease-specific survival.[43] After NACT and mastectomy, radiation use can be associated with local-regional control rates of over 80%.[44] An accelerated hyperfractionated radiation delivery schedule in which 51 Gy is delivered to the chest wall, and draining lymphatic fields by giving 1.5 Gy twice a day, and subsequently, the chest wall is boosted to an additional 15 Gy, given in 10 fractions of 1.5 Gy twice daily, as practiced at M.D. Anderson Cancer Centre, helps attain these rates. Efforts at breast conservation in patients with inflammatory carcinoma attaining CR after chemotherapy, have largely been unsuccessful, because of high loco-regional recurrence rates between 30% and 60%.[45,46]

Outcome

Before the era of routine use of systemic treatment, patients with advanced disease were treated with mastectomy, radiation therapy, or both and had 5-year survival rates of only 25% to 45%.[1,47,48] Currently, 5-year survival rates approach 80% for patients with stage IIIA disease and 45% for patients with stage IIIB disease when treated with surgery, radiation therapy, and chemotherapy.[49] With modern treatment strategies that include systemic therapy with taxanes and anthracyclines, appropriate surgical intervention, and local-regional irradiation, 10-year local-regional control rate of 89% has been reported.[24] A reasonable estimate of 10-year survival rates for patients given modern treatments for stage III breast cancer is 40% to 50%.[49]

Historically, less than 5% of patients of inflammatory breast cancer treated with surgery, radiation therapy, or both survived past 5 years, with expected median survival for such patients being less than 15 months. Currently, local control rates for patients treated with chemotherapy, mastectomy, and postmastectomy radiation now approach 70–80%, and 5-year survival rates are 30–40%.[50,51]

Prognosis of advanced breast cancer may vary according to the disease biology. An elderly lady with a hormone receptor positive disease, with an indolent course over many years may have a markedly different outcome than a young lady with hormone negative cancer with a rapidly progressive course. Stage migration resulting from difference in sensitivities of diagnostic tests may also create an apparent difference in the analyzed outcome.

Recurrent Breast Cancer

Development of a local-regional recurrence after primary treatment of an invasive breast cancer signifies a grave event. All patients with local-regional recurrence should have a biopsy for histopathological confirmation and for re-evaluation of hormone receptor and HER2/neu status, along with complete disease restaging to rule out metastatic disease.

For recurrence in the breast after Breast Conservation Therapy, mastectomy remains the standard salvage treatment as most such patients will have been previously treated with breast irradiation and therefore would not be candidates for a breast-conserving approach. Patients with recurrence in the breast are also at risk of axillary metastases. Patients who initially underwent sentinel lymph node surgery should have an ALND at the time of recurrence. The use of systemic therapy after breast recurrence needs to be decided on an individual basis according to the risk of metastatic disease, the previous systemic treatments used, and hormone receptor status. Generally, patients with an interval to development of recurrence of less than 2 years have a worse outcome than those who develop recurrent disease many years after treatment, partly because early breast recurrences are believed to develop from repopulation of persistent microscopic disease, whereas most late breast recurrences represent a new primary tumor. New primary tumors are generally associated with one of the following: Location in the breast remote from the original tumor bed site, a change in histology, or a change from aneuploid to diploid status.

Patients with recurrent disease after initial mastectomy have a worse prognosis than those with recurrent disease after initial breast conservation therapy. In the Danish trial, the 5-year rate of distant metastatic disease development after an isolated local-regional recurrence was 73%, and the rate was no different for those in whom disease recurred after mastectomy only versus those with recurrent disease after mastectomy and radiation.[52] Similarly, in the British Columbia trial, of the 39 patients who developed a local-regional recurrence, 37 eventually developed metastatic disease.[18] Factors of prognostic significance for patients with local-regional recurrence after mastectomy include large initial primary tumor and high number of positive lymph nodes, extracapsular extension, recurrence in the infraclavicular or supraclavicular regions, and a disease-free interval of less than 2 years.[52] In general, patients who present with chest wall recurrence, particularly those who have resectable disease and have not undergone radiation, have a greater probability of disease control and improved outcome. Initial nodal status, time to recurrence, and ability to use radiation to treat the recurrence are independent predictors of outcome for patients with a chest wall recurrence.[53]

Regarding the use of systemic therapy for recurrent disease, as per the M.D. Anderson Cancer Centre experience, for patients with anthracycline-naive disease, the introduction of doxorubicin at the time of recurrence can lead to improved survival and more recently the use of docetaxel also seemed to lead to favorable outcomes for patients who had previously had anthracycline treatment. The 3-year DFS rate for such patients was 58%.[54] Patients with ER-positive disease should receive appropriate second-line endocrine therapy or trastuzumab if the tumor is HER2/neu-positive.

Patients with regional relapse have a less favorable prognosis than patients with intact breast or chest wall recurrences. In general, patients with isolated resectable disease in the low axilla should be treated with axillary dissection, comprehensive radiation to sites not previously treated including the chest wall, and systemic therapy. Most patients with recurrence in the supraclavicular fossa or internal mammary lymph nodes have unresectable disease. If active chemotherapy agents are available, it is reasonable to consider using neoadjuvant systemic treatment and consolidating with radiation at the point of maximal response.

Metastatic Breast Cancer

It is defined by tumor spread beyond the breast, chest wall, and regional lymph nodes. Dissemination can occur through blood and lymphatic vessels and via direct extension through the chest wall. The most common sites for breast cancer metastasis include the bone, lung, liver, lymph nodes, chest wall, and brain. Symptoms are related to the location and extent of the metastatic tumor. The treatment goals in women with advanced breast cancer include prolongation of life, control of tumor burden, reduction in cancer-related symptoms or complications, and maintenance of quality of life and function. Tumor ER, PR, and HER-2 status is critical for all patients, and a detailed assessment of past treatment including timing of therapy as well as patient symptoms and functional assessment is essential. Patients with endocrine-sensitive tumors, particularly those with minimal symptoms and limited visceral involvement, are candidates for initial treatment with endocrine therapy alone. Patients with hormone receptor-negative tumors or those with hormone receptor positive tumors progressing despite the use of endocrine therapy are candidates for chemotherapy. If the tumor is HER-2 positive, then trastuzumab treatment is employed in combination with chemotherapy. Role of RT is mainly limited to palliation for painful bone metastases or prevention of impending bone fractures in weight bearing bones, and palliation for brain metastases causing neurological symptoms. Important prognostic factors for metastatic breast cancer include tumor biology (grade, ER status, *HER-2* status), performance status, cancer-related symptoms, sites of recurrence, number of sites of recurrence, prior adjuvant therapy, disease-free interval, prior therapy for metastatic disease, and response/duration of treatment with prior therapy for metastatic disease.

REFERENCES

Noninvasive Breast Cancer

1. Haagensen CD, Bodian C, Haagensen DE. Lobular Neoplasia (Lobular Carcinoma In Situ). Breast Carcinoma: Risk and Detection. Philadelphia, PA: WB Saunders; 1981. 238-92.
2. Frykberg ER, Bland KI. In situ breast carcinoma. Adv Surg. 1993;26:29-72.
3. Fisher ER, Redmond C, Fisher B, Bass G. Pathologic findings from the National Surgical Adjuvant Breast and Bowel Projects (NSABP). Prognostic discriminants for 8-year survival for node-negative invasive breast cancer patients. Cancer. 1990;65(9 Suppl):2121-8.
4. Schnitt SJ, Morrow M. Lobular carcinoma in situ: current concepts and controversies. Semin Diagn Pathol. 1999;16:209-23.
5. Acs G, Lawton TJ, Rebbeck TR, LiVolsi VA, Zhang PJ. Differential expression of E-cadherin in lobular and ductal neoplasms of the breast and its biologic and diagnostic implications. Am J Clin Pathol. 2001;115:85-98.
6. Andersen JA. Lobular carcinoma in situ of the breast—an approach to rational treatment. Cancer. 1977;39:2597-02
7. Fisher B, Costantino J, Wickerham DL, Redmond CK, Kavanah M, Cronin WM, et al. Tamoxifen for prevention of breast cancer: report of the National Surgical Adjuvant Breast and Bowel Project P-1 study. J Natl Cancer Inst. 1998;90:1371-88.
8. Vogel VG, Costantino JP, Wickerham DL, Cronin WM, Cecchini RS, Atkins JN, et al. Effects of Tamoxifen vs Raloxifene on the Risk of Developing Invasive Breast Cancer and Other Disease Outcomes: The NSABP Study of Tamoxifen and Raloxifene (STAR) P-2 Trial. JAMA. 2006;295:2727-41.
9. Bijker N, Rutgers EJT, Duchateau L, Peterse JL, Julien JP, Cataliotti L, et al. Breast-conserving therapy for Paget disease of the nipple: a prospective European Organization for Research and Treatment of Cancer study of 61 patients. Cancer. 2001;91:472-7.
10. Marshall JK, Griffith KA, Haffty BG, Solin LJ, Vicini FA, McCormick B, et al. Conservative management of Paget disease of the breast with radiotherapy. Cancer. 2003;97:2142-9.
11. Faverly DRG, Burgers L, Bult P, Holland R. Three dimensional imaging of mammary ductal carcinoma in situ; clinical implications. Semin Diagn Pathol. 1994;11:193-8.
12. Fisher B, Dignam J, Wolmark N, Mamounas E, Costantino J, Poller W, et al. Lumpectomy and radiation therapy for the treatment of intraductal breast cancer: Findings from National Surgical Adjuvant Breast and Bowel Project B-17. J Clin Oncol. 1998;16:441-52.
13. Julien JP, Bijker N, Fentiman IS, Peterse JL, Delledonne V, Rouanet P, et al. Radiotherapy in breast-conserving treatment for ductal carcinoma in situ: First results of the EORTC randomised phase III trial 10853. EORTC Breast Cancer

Cooperative Group and EORTC Radiotherapy Group. Lancet. 2000;355:528-33.
14. Cuzick J, Sestak I, Pinder SE, Ellis IO, Hackshaw A, Bundred N, et al. Beneficial effects of tamoxifen for woman with DCIS: Long-term results from the UK/ANZ DCIS trial in women with locally excised DCIS. Cancer Res. 2009;69:34.
15. Emdin SO, Granstrand B, Ringberg A, Sandelin K, Arnesson LG, Nordgren H, et al. SweDCIS: radiotherapy after sector resection for ductal carcinoma in situ of the breast. Results of a randomised trial in a population offered mammography screening. Acta Oncol. 2006;45(5):536-43.
16. Hughes LL, Wang M, Page DL, Gray R, Solin LJ, Davidson NE, et al. Local Excision Alone Without Irradiation for Ductal Carcinoma In Situ of the Breast: A Trial of the Eastern Cooperative Oncology Group. J Clin Oncol. 2009;27(32):5319-24.
17. Wong JS, Kaelin CM, Troyan SL, Gadd MA, Gelman R, Lester SC, et al. Prospective study of wide excision alone for ductal carcinoma in situ of the breast. J Clin Oncol. 2006;24(7):1031-6.
18. Allred DC, Anderson SJ, Paik S, Wickerham DL, Nagtegaal ID, Swain SM, et al Adjuvant tamoxifen reduces subsequent breast cancer in women with estrogen receptor-positive ductal carcinoma in situ: a study based on NSABP protocol B-24. J Clin Oncol. 2012;30(12):1268-73.
19. UK Coordinating Committee on Cancer Research (UKCCCR) Ductal Carcinoma in situ (DCIS) Working Party on behalf of DCIS trialists in the UK, Australia, and New Zealand. Radiotherapy and tamoxifen in women with completely excised ductal carcinoma in situ of the breast in the UK, Australia, and New Zealand: randomised controlled trial. Lancet. 2003;362:95-102.

Early Breast Cancer

1. Breast cancer and hormone replacement therapy: collaborative reanalysis of data from 51 epidemiological studies of 52,705 women with breast cancer and 108,411 women without breast cancer. Collaborative Group on Hormonal Factors in Breast Cancer. Lancet 1997;350:1047-59.
2. Rossouw JE, Anderson GL, Prentice RL, et al. Risks and benefits of estrogen plus progestin in healthy postmenopausal women: principal results From the Women's Health Initiative randomized controlled trial. JAMA. 2002;288:321-33.
3. Robson ME, Boyd J, Borgen PI, Cody HS 3rd. Hereditary breast cancer. Curr Probl Surg. 2001;38:387-480.
4. Land CE, Boice JD Jr., Shore RE, Norman JE, Tokunaga M. Breast cancer risk from low-dose exposures to ionizing radiation: results of parallel analysis of three exposed populations of women. J Natl Cancer Inst. 1980;65:353-76.
5. Land CE. Studies of cancer and radiation dose among atomic bomb survivors. The example of breast cancer. JAMA. 1995;274:402-7.
6. Hamajima N, Hirose K, Tajima K, Rohan T, Calle EE, Heath CW Jr, et al. Alcohol, tobacco and breast cancer--collaborative reanalysis of individual data from 53 epidemiological studies, including 58,515 women with breast cancer and 95,067 women without the disease. Br J Cancer. 2002;87:1234-45.
7. Gail MH, Brinton LA, Byar DP, Corle DK, Green SB, Schairer C, et al. Projecting individualized probabilities of developing breast cancer for white females who are being examined annually. J Natl Cancer Inst. 1989;81:1879-86.
8. Fisher B, Costantino JP, Wickerham DL, Redmond CK, Kavanah M, Cronin WM, et al. Tamoxifen for prevention of breast cancer: report of the National Surgical Adjuvant Breast and Bowel Project P-1 Study. J Natl Cancer Inst. 1998;90: 1371-88.
9. Vogel VG, Costantino JP, Wickerham DL, Cronin WM, Cecchini RS, Atkins JN, et al. Effects of tamoxifen vs raloxifene on the risk of developing invasive breast cancer and other disease outcomes: the NSABP Study of Tamoxifen and Raloxifene (STAR) P-2 trial. JAMA. 2006;295:2727-41.
10. Hartmann LC, Schaid DJ, Woods JE, Crotty TP, Myers JL, Arnold PG, et al. Efficacy of bilateral prophylactic mastectomy in women with a family history of breast cancer. N Engl J Med. 1999;340:77-84.
11. Halsted WS. The results of operations for the cure of cancer of the breast performed at Johns Hopkins Hospital from June 1889 to January 1894. Johns Hopkins Hosp Bull. 1894;4:297.
12. Keynes G. Carcinoma of the breast, the unorthodox view. Proc Cardiff Med Soc. 1954;40.
13. Hellman S. Karnofsky Memorial Lecture. Natural history of small breast cancers. J Clin Oncol. 1994;12:2229-34.
14. Voogd AC, Coebergh JW, Repelaer van Driel OJ, Roumen RM, van Beek MW, Vreugdenhil A, et al. The risk of nodal metastases in breast cancer patients with clinically negative lymph nodes: a population-based analysis. Breast Cancer Res Treat. 2000;62:63-9.
15. Fisher B, Montague E, Redmond C, Deutsch M, Brown GR, Zauber A, et al. Findings from NSABP Protocol No. B-04-comparison of radical mastectomy with alternative treatments for primary breast cancer. I. Radiation compliance and its relation to treatment outcome. Cancer. 1980;46:1-13.
16. Veronesi U, Cascinelli N, Bufalino R, Morabito A, Greco M, Galluzzo D, et al. Risk of internal mammary lymph node metastases and its relevance on prognosis of breast cancer patients. Ann Surg. 1983;198(6):681-4.
17. Fowble B, Solin LJ, Schultz DJ, Goodman RL. Frequency, sites of relapse, and outcome of regional node failures following conservative surgery and radiation for early breast cancer. Int J Radiat Oncol Biol Phys. 1989;17:703-10.
18. Galper S, Recht A, Silver B, Manola J, Gelman R, Schnitt SJ, et al. Factors associated with regional nodal failure in patients with early stage breast cancer with 0-3 positive axillary nodes following tangential irradiation alone. Int J Radiat Oncol Biol Phys. 1999;45:1157-66.
19. Chen SC, Chen MF, Hwang TL, Chao TC, Lo YF, Hsueh S, et al. Prediction of supraclavicular lymph node metastasis in breast carcinoma. Int J Radiat Oncol Biol Phys. 2002;52(3):614-9.
20. Strom EA, Woodward WA, Katz A, Buchholz TA, Perkins GH, Jhingran A, et al. Clinical investigation: regional nodal failure patterns in breast cancer patients treated with mastectomy without radiotherapy. Int J Radiat Oncol Biol Phys. 2005;63(5):1508-13.

21. Braun S, Vogl FD, Naume B, Janni W, Osborne MP, Coombes RC, et al. A pooled analysis of bone marrow micrometastasis in breast cancer. N Engl J Med. 2005;353(8):793-802.
22. Vinh-Hung V, Verschraegen C. Breast-conserving surgery with or without radiotherapy: pooled-analysis for risks of ipsilateral breast tumor recurrence and mortality. J Natl Cancer Inst 2004;96:115-121.
23. Clarke M, Collins R, Darby S, Davies C, Elphinstone P, Evans E, et al. Effects of radiotherapy and of differences in the extent of surgery for early breast cancer on local recurrence and 15-year survival: an overview of the randomised trials. Lancet. 2005;366:2087-106.
24. Harris J, Lippman M, Morrow M, et al. Diseases of the breast. Philadelphia: Lippincott Williams & Wilkins, 2004.
25. Tabar L, Vitak B, Chen HH, Yen MF, Duffy SW, Smith RA. et al. Beyond randomized controlled trials: organized mammographic screening substantially reduces breast carcinoma mortality. Cancer. 2001;91:1724-31.
26. Kopans DB, Feig SA. The Canadian National Breast Screening Study: a critical review. AJR Am J Roentgenol. 1993;161:755-60.
27. Miller AB, To T, Baines CJ, Wall C. Canadian National Breast Screening Study-2: 13-year results of a randomized trial in women aged 50-59 years. J Natl Cancer Inst. 2000;92:1490-9.
28. Frisell J, Lidbrink E. The Stockholm Mammographic Screening Trial: risks and benefits in age group 40-49 years. J Natl Cancer Inst Monogr. 1997:49-51.
29. UK Trial Group. 16-year mortality from breast cancer in the UK trial of early detection of breast cancer. Lancet. 1999;353: 1909-14.
30. Hellquist BN, Duffy SW, Abdsaleh S, Björneld L, Bordás P, Tabár L, et al. Effectiveness of population-based service screening with mammography for women ages 40 to 49 years: evaluation of the Swedish Mammography Screening in Young Women (SCRY) cohort. Cancer. 2011;117(4):714-22.
31. Hendrick RE, Cole EB, Pisano ED, Acharyya S, Marques H, Cohen MA, et al. Accuracy of soft-copy digital mammography versus that of screen-film mammography according to digital manufacturer: ACRIN DMIST retrospective multireader study. Radiology. 2008;247(1):38-48.
32. Kriege M, Brekelmans CT, Boetes C, Besnard PE, Zonderland HM, Obdeijn IM, et al. Efficacy of MRI and mammography for breast-cancer screening in women with a familial or genetic predisposition. N Engl J Med. 2004;351:427-37.
33. Veronesi U, Marubini E, Del Vecchio M, Manzari A, Andreola S, Greco M, et al. Local recurrences and distant metastases after conservative breast cancer treatments: partly independent events. J Natl Cancer Inst. 1995;87:19-27.
34. Fitzgibbons PL, Page DL, Weaver D, Thor AD, Allred DC, Clark GM, et al. Prognostic factors in breast cancer. College of American Pathologists Consensus Statement 1999. Arch Pathol Lab Med. 2000;124:966-78.
35. Rosen PR, Groshen S, Saigo PE, Kinne DW, Hellman S. A long-term follow-up study of survival in stage I (T1N0M0) and stage II (T1N1M0) breast carcinoma. J Clin Oncol. 1989;7:355-66.
36. Quiet CA, Ferguson DJ, Weichselbaum RR, Hellman S. Natural history of node-negative breast cancer: a study of 826 patients with long-term follow-up. J Clin Oncol. 1995;13:1144-51.
37. Buyse M, Loi S, van't Veer L, Viale G, Delorenzi M, Glas AM, et al. Validation and clinical utility of a 70-gene prognostic signature for women with node-negative breast cancer. J Natl Cancer Inst. 2006;98:1183-92.
38. van de Vijver MJ, He YD, van't Veer LJ, Dai H, Hart AA, Voskuil DW, et al. A gene-expression signature as a predictor of survival in breast cancer. N Engl J Med. 2002;347:1999-2009.
39. Senie RT, Rosen PP, Rhodes P, Lesser ML, Kinne DW. Obesity at diagnosis of breast carcinoma influences duration of disease-free survival. Ann Intern Med. 1992;116:26-32.
40. Psyrri A, Burtness B. Pregnancy-associated breast cancer. Cancer J. 2005;11:83-95.
41. O'Hanlon DM, Kerin MJ, Kent PJ, Skehill R, Maher D, Grimes H, et al. A prospective evaluation of CA15-3 in stage I carcinoma of the breast. J Am Coll Surg. 1995;180:210-2.
42. Goldhirsch A, Glick JH, Gelber RD, Coates AS, Thürlimann B, Senn HJ, et al. Meeting highlights: international expert consensus on the primary therapy of early breast cancer 2005. Ann Oncol. 2005;16:1569-83.
43. Veronesi U. NIH consensus meeting on early breast cancer. Eur J Cancer. 1990;26:843-4.
44. Pigott J, Nichols R, Maddox WA, Balch CM. Metastases to the upper levels of the axillary nodes in carcinoma of the breast and its implications for nodal sampling procedures. Surg Gynecol Obstet. 1984;158:255-9.
45. Clarke D, Khonji NI, Mansel RE. Sentinel node biopsy in breast cancer: ALMANAC trial. World J Surg. 2001;25:819-22.
46. Krag DN, Harlow S, Weaver D, Ashikaga T. Radiolabeled sentinel node biopsy: collaborative trial with the National Cancer Institute. World J Surg. 2001;25:823-8.
47. Veronesi U, Paganelli G, Viale G, Luini A, Zurrida S, Galimberti V, et al. A randomized comparison of sentinel-node biopsy with routine axillary dissection in breast cancer. N Engl J Med. 2003;349:546-53.
48. Weir L, Worsley D, Bernstein V. The value of FDG positron emission tomography in the management of patients with breast cancer. Breast J. 2005;11(3):204-9.
49. Gropper AB, Calvillo KZ, Dominici L, Troyan S, Rhei E, Economy KE, et al. Sentinel lymph node biopsy in pregnant women with breast cancer. Ann Surg Oncol. 2014;21(8):2506-11.
50. Mansel RE, Fallowfield L, Kissin M, Goyal A, Newcombe RG, Dixon JM, et al. Randomized multicenter trial of sentinel node biopsy versus standard axillary treatment in operable breast cancer: the ALMANAC Trial. J Natl Cancer Inst. 2006;98:599-609.
51. Krag DN, Julian TB, Harlow SP, Weaver DL, Ashikaga T, Bryant J, et al. NSABP-32: Phase III, randomized trial comparing axillary resection with sentinel lymph node dissection: a description of the trial. Ann Surg Oncol. 2004;11:208S-10S.
52. Delpech Y1, Bricou A, Lousquy R, Hudry D, Jankowski C, Willecocq C, et al. The exportability of the ACOSOG Z0011 criteria for omitting axillary lymph node dissection after positive sentinel lymph node biopsy findings: a multicenter study. Ann Surg Oncol. 2013;20(8):2556-61.
53. Veronesi U, Cascinelli N, Mariani L, Greco M, Saccozzi R, Luini A, et al. Twenty-year follow-up of a randomized study comparing breast-conserving surgery with radical mastectomy for early breast cancer. N Engl J Med. 2002;347:1227-32.

54. Fisher B, Anderson S, Bryant J, Margolese RG, Deutsch M, Fisher ER, et al. Twenty-year follow-up of a randomized trial comparing total mastectomy, lumpectomy, and lumpectomy plus irradiation for the treatment of invasive breast cancer. N Engl J Med. 2002;347:1233-41.
55. Sarrazin D, Le MG, Arriagada R, Contesso G, Fontaine F, Spielmann M, et al. Ten-year results of a randomized trial comparing a conservative treatment to mastectomy in early breast cancer. Radiother Oncol. 1989;14:177-84.
56. van Dongen JA, Bartelink H, Fentiman IS, Lerut T, Mignolet F, Olthuis G, et al. Randomized clinical trial to assess the value of breast-conserving therapy in stage I and II breast cancer, EORTC 10801 trial. J Natl Cancer Inst Monogr. 1992;(11):15-8.
57. Blichert-Toft M, Rose C, Andersen JA, Overgaard M, Axelsson CK, Andersen KW, et al. Danish randomized trial comparing breast conservation therapy with mastectomy: six years of life-table analysis. Danish Breast Cancer Cooperative Group. J Natl Cancer Inst Monogr. 1992;(11):19-25.
58. de Bock GH, van der Hage JA, Putter H, Bonnema J, Bartelink H, van de Velde CJ. Isolated loco-regional recurrence of breast cancer is more common in young patients and following breast conserving therapy: long-term results of European Organisation for Research and Treatment of Cancer studies. Eur J Cancer. 2006;42:351-6.
59. Bornstein BA, Cheng CW, Rhodes LM, Rashid H, Stomper PC, Siddon RL, et al. Can simulation measurements be used to predict the irradiated lung volume in the tangential fields in patients treated for breast cancer? Int J Radiat Oncol Biol Phys. 1990;18:181-7.
60. Muren LP, Maurstad G, Hafslund R, Anker G, Dahl O. Cardiac and pulmonary doses and complication probabilities in standard and conformal tangential irradiation in conservative management of breast cancer. Radiother Oncol. 2002;62: 173-83.
61. Cho BC, Hurkmans CW, Damen EM, Zijp LJ, Mijnheer BJ. Intensity modulated versus non-intensity modulated radiotherapy in the treatment of the left breast and upper internal mammary lymph node chain: a comparative planning study. Radiother Oncol. 2002;62:127-36.
62. Vicini FA, Sharpe M, Kestin L, Martinez A, Mitchell CK, Wallace MF, et al. Optimizing breast cancer treatment efficacy with intensity-modulated radiotherapy. Int J Radiat Oncol Biol Phys. 2002;54:1336-44.
63. Pignol J, Olivotto I, Rakovitch E, et al. Proceedings of the 48th Annual Meeting of the American Society for Therapeutic Radiology and Oncology, 48th Annual Meeting of the American Society for Therapeutic Radiology and Oncology. Int J Radiat Oncol Biol Phys. 2006;66(3):A1-A84, S1-S752.
64. Reznik J, Cicchetti MG, Degaspe B, Fitzgerald TJ. Analysis of axillary coverage during tangential radiation therapy to the breast. Int J Radiat Oncol Biol Phys. 2005;61:163e8.
65. Kataria T, Bisht SS, Gupta D, Goyal S, Jassal K, Abhishek A, et al. Incidental radiation to axilla in early breast cancer treated with intensity modulated tangents and comparison with conventional and 3D conformal tangents. Breast. 2013; 22 (6):1125-9.
66. Recht A. Should irradiation replace dissection for patients with breast cancer with clinically negative axillary lymph nodes? J Surg Oncol. 1999;72:184-92.
67. Poortmans PSH, Kirkove C, Budach V, Maingon P, Valli MC, Collette S, et al. Irradiation of the internal mammary and medial supraclavicular lymph nodes in stage I to III breast cancer: 10 years results of the EORTC radiation oncology and breast cancer groups phase III trial 22922/10925. EJC 2013;47(Suppl 2).
68. Recht A. Integration of systemic therapy and radiation therapy for patients with early stage breast cancer treated with conservative surgery. Clin Breast Cancer. 2003;4:104-13.
69. Bellon JR, Come SE, Gelman RS, Henderson IC, Shulman LN, Silver BJ, et al. Sequencing of chemotherapy and radiation therapy in early-stage breast cancer: updated results of a prospective randomized trial. J Clin Oncol. 2005;23:1934-40.
70. Rouesse J, de la Lande B, Bertheault-Cvitkovic F, Serin D, Graïc Y, Combe M, et al. A phase III randomized trial comparing adjuvant concomitant chemoradiotherapy versus standard adjuvant chemotherapy followed by radiotherapy in operable node-positive breast cancer: final results. Int J Radiat Oncol Biol Phys. 2006;64:1072-80.
71. Toledano A, Garaud P, Serin D, Fourquet A, Bosset JF, Breteau N, et al. Concurrent administration of adjuvant chemotherapy and radiotherapy after breast-conservative surgery enhances late toxicities: long-term results of the ARCOSEIN multicenter randomized study. Int J Radiat Oncol Biol Phys. 2006;65(2):324-32.
72. The Radiation Therapy Oncology Group. (2015). Breast Cancer Atlas. [Online] Available from http://www.rtog.org/corelab/contouringatlases/breastcanceratlas.aspx [Access on April 2015].
73. Romestaing P, Lehingue Y, Carrie C, Coquard R, Montbarbon X, Ardiet JM, et al. Role of a 10-Gy boost in the conservative treatment of early breast cancer: results of a randomized clinical trial in Lyon, France. J Clin Oncol. 1997;15:963-8.
74. Bartelink H, Horiot JC, Poortmans P, Struikmans H, Van den Bogaert W, Barillot I, et al. Recurrence rates after treatment of breast cancer with standard radiotherapy with or without additional radiation. N Engl J Med. 2001;345:1378-7.
75. Polgar C, Major T, Fodor J, Németh G, Orosz Z, Sulyok Z, et al. High-dose-rate brachytherapy alone versus whole breast radiotherapy with or without tumor bed boost after breast-conserving surgery: Seven-year results of a comparative study. Int J Radiat Oncol Biol Phys. 2004;60:1173-81.
76. Polgar C, Fodor J, Major T, Németh G, Lövey K, Orosz Z, et al. Breast-conserving treatment with partial or whole breast irradiation for low-risk invasive breast carcinoma: 5-year results of a randomized trial. Int J Radiat Oncol Biol Phys. 2007;69(3):694-702.
77. Vaidya JS, Tobias JS, Baum M, Massarut S, Wenz F, Hilaris B, et al. Intraoperative radiotherapy for breast cancer. Lancet Oncol. 2004;5:165-73.
78. Veronesi U, Orecchia R, Luini A, Galimberti V, Gatti G, Intra M, et al. Full-dose intraoperative radiotherapy with electrons during breast-conserving surgery: experience with 590 cases. Ann Surg. 2005;242:101-6.

79. Smith Bd, Arthur DW, Buchholz TA, Haffty BG, Hahn CA, Hardenbergh PH, et al. Accelerated partial breast irradiation consensus statement from the American Society of Therapeutic Radiology and Oncology. Int J Radiat Oncol Biol Phys. 2009;;74(4):987-1001.
80. Dewar JA, Sarrazin D, Benhamou E, Petit JY, Benhamou S, Arriagada R, et al. Management of the axilla in conservatively treated breast cancer: 592 patients treated at Institut Gustave-Roussy. Int J Radiat Oncol Biol Phys. 1987;13:475-81.
81. Pierce SM, Recht A, Lingos TI, Abner A, Vicini F, Silver B, et al. Long-term radiation complications following conservative surgery (CS) and radiation therapy (RT) in patients with early stage breast cancer. Int J Radiat Oncol Biol Phys. 1992;23: 915-23.
82. Lingos TI, Recht A, Vicini F, et al. Radiation pneumonitis in breast cancer patients treated with conservative surgery and radiation therapy. Int J Radiat Oncol Biol Phys. 1991;21:355-360.
83. Lund MB, Myhre KI, Melsom H, Johansen B. The effect on pulmonary function of tangential field technique in radiotherapy for carcinoma of the breast. Br J Radiol. 1991;64:520-3.
84. Darby SC, McGale P, Taylor CW, Peto R. Long-term mortality from heart disease and lung cancer after radiotherapy for early breast cancer: prospective cohort study of about 300,000 women in US SEER cancer registries. Lancet Oncol. 2005;6: 557-65.
85. Cuzick J, Stewart H, Peto R, Baum M, Fisher B, Host H, et al. Overview of randomized trials of postoperative adjuvant radiotherapy in breast cancer. Cancer Treat Rep. 1987;71: 15-29.
86. Jagsi R, Griffith KA, Koelling T, Roberts R, Pierce LJ. Stroke rates and risk factors in patients treated with radiation therapy for early-stage breast cancer. J Clin Oncol. 2006;24:2779-85.
87. Clarke M, Collins R, Darby S, Davies C, Elphinstone P, Evans E, et al. Effects of radiotherapy and of differences in the extent of surgery for early breast cancer on local recurrence and 15-year survival: an overview of the randomised trials. Lancet. 2005;366:2087-106.
88. Coombes RC, Kilburn LS, Snowdon CF, Paridaens R, Coleman RE, Jones SE, et al. Survival and safety of exemestane versus tamoxifen after 2-3 years' tamoxifen treatment (Intergroup Exemestane Study): a randomised controlled trial. Lancet. 2007;369(9561):559-70.
89. Jonat W, Gnant M, Boccardo F, Kaufmann M, Rubagotti A, Zuna I, et al. Effectiveness of switching from adjuvant tamoxifen to anastrozole in postmenopausal women with hormone-sensitive early-stage breast cancer: a meta-analysis. Lancet Oncol. 2006;7(12):991-6.
90. Coates AS, Keshaviah A, Thürlimann B, Mouridsen H, Mauriac L, Forbes JF, et al. Five years of letrozole compared with tamoxifen as initial adjuvant therapy for postmenopausal women with endocrine-responsive early breast cancer: update of study BIG 1-98. J Clin Oncol. 2007;25(5):486-92.
91. Peto R, Davies C. On Behalf of the ATLAS Collaboration. ATLAS (Adjuvant Tamoxifen, Longer Against Shorter): international randomized trial of 10 versus 5 years of adjuvant tamoxifen among 11,500 women preliminary results. In San Antonio Breast Cancer Symposium. San Antonio, 2007.
92. Goss PE, Ingle JN, Martino S, Robert NJ, Muss HB, Piccart MJ, et al. A randomized trial of LET in postmenopausal women after five years of tamoxifen therapy for early-stage breast cancer. N Engl J Med. 2003;349:1793-802.
93. Mamounas EP, Jeong J-H, Wickerham DL, Smith RE, Ganz PA, Land SR, et al. Benefit from exemestane as extended adjuvant therapy following five years of adjuvant tamoxifen : Intent-to-treat analysis of the National Surgical Adjuvant Breast and Bowel Project B-33 Trial. J Clin Oncol. 2008;26:1965-71.

Locally Advanced Breast Cancer

1. Fracchia AA, Evans JF, Eisenberg BC. Stage III carcinoma of the breast : a detailed analysis. Ann Surg. 1980;192:705.
2. Cancer Facts and Figures 2006. Atlanta, GA: American Cancer Society, 2006;19.
3. Chopra R. The Indian Scene, JCO. 2001;19(18 Suppl):106S-11S.
4. Elledge RM, Clark GH, Chamness GC, Osborne CK. Tumor biologic factors and breast cancer prognosis among white, Hispanic, and black women in the United States. J Natl Cancer Inst. 1994;86:705-12.
5. Li CL, Malone KE, Daling JR. Differences in breast cancer hormone receptor status and histology by race and ethnicity among women 50 years of age and older. Cancer Epidemiol Biomarkers Prev. 2002;11:601-7.
6. Fisher B, Brown A, Mamounas E, Wieand S, Robidoux A, Margolese RG, et al. Effect of preoperative chemotherapy on local-regional disease in women with operable breast cancer: Findings from National Surgical Adjuvant Breast and Bowel Project B-18. J Clin Oncol. 1997;15:2483-93.
7. Kuerer HM, Newman LA, Smith TL, Ames FC, Hunt KK, Dhingra K, et al. Clinical course of breast cancer patients with complete pathologic primary tumor and axillary lymph node response to doxorubicin-based neoadjuvant chemotherapy. J Clin Oncol. 1999;17:460-9.
8. Wolmark N, Wang J, Mamounas E, Bryant J, Fisher B. Preoperative chemotherapy in patients with operable breast cancer: Nine-year results from National Surgical Adjuvant Breast and Bowel Project B-18. Cancer. 2001;30:96-102.
9. Van der Hage JA, Cornelis JH, van de Velde CJ, Tubiana-Hulin M, Vandervelden C, Duchateau L. Preoperative chemotherapy in primary operable breast cancer: Results from the European Organization for Research and Treatment of Cancer trial 10902. J Clin Oncol. 2001;19:4224-37.
10. Mauri D, Pavlidis N, Ioannidis JP. Neoadjuvant versus adjuvant systemic treatment in breast cancer: A meta-analysis. J Natl Cancer Inst. 2005;97:188-94.
11. Singletary SE, McNeese MD, Hortobagyi GN. Feasibility of breast-conservation surgery after induction chemotherapy for locally advanced breast carcinoma. Cancer. 1992;69:2849-52.
12. Bonadonna G, Valagussa P, Brambilla C, Ferrari L, Moliterni A, Terenziani M, et al. Primary chemotherapy in operable breast cancer: Eight-year experience at the Milan Cancer Institute. J Clin Oncol. 1998;16:93-100.

13. Chen AM, Meric-Bernstam F, Hunt KK, Mirza N, Singletary SE, Kuerer HM, et al. Breast-conserving therapy after neoadjuvant chemotherapy: The M.D. Anderson Cancer Center experience. J Clin Oncol. 2004;22:2303-12.
14. Huang EH, Strom EA, Perkins GH, Oh JL, Chen AM, Meric-Bernstam F, et al. Comparison of risk of local-regional recurrence after mastectomy or breast conservation therapy for patients treated with neoadjuvant chemotherapy and radiation stratified according to a prognostic index score. Int J Radiat Oncol Biol Phys. 2006;352-7.
15. Clarke M1, Collins R, Darby S, Davies C, Elphinstone P, Evans E, et al. Effects of radiotherapy and of differences in the extent of surgery for early breast cancer on local recurrence and 15-year survival: An overview of the randomised trials. Lancet. 2005;366:2087-106.
16. Overgaard M, Hansen PS, Overgaard J, Rose C, Andersson M, Bach F, et al. Postoperative radiotherapy in high-risk premenopausal women with breast cancer who receive adjuvant chemotherapy. N Engl J Med. 1997;337:949-55.
17. Overgaard M, Jensen MB, Overgaard J, Hansen PS, Rose C, Andersson M, et al. Randomized trail evaluating postoperative radiotherapy in high risk postmenopausal breast cancer patients given adjuvant tamoxifen: Results from the DBCG 82c trial. Lancet. 1999;353:1641-8.
18. Ragaz J, Olivotto IA, Spinelli JJ, Phillips N, Jackson SM, Wilson KS, et al. Locoregional radiation therapy in patients with high-risk breast cancer receiving adjuvant chemotherapy: 20-year results of the British Columbia randomized trial. J Natl Cancer Inst. 2005;97:116-26.
19. Katz A, Strom EA, Buchholz TA, Theriault R, Singletary SE, McNeese MD. et al. The influence of pathologic tumor characteristics on locoregional recurrence rates following mastectomy. Int J Rad Oncol Biol Phys. 2001;50:735-42.
20. Resch A, Fellner C, Mock U, Handl-Zeller L, Biber E, Seitz W, et al. Locally recurrent breast cancer: Pulse dose rate brachytherapy for repeat irradiation following lumpectomy: a second chance to preserve the breast. Radiology. 2002;225:713-8.
21. Taghian A, Jeong JH, Mamounas E, Anderson S, Bryant J, Deutsch M, et al. Patterns of locoregional failure in patients with operable breast cancer treated by mastectomy and adjuvant chemotherapy with or without tamoxifen and without radiotherapy: Results from five National Surgical Adjuvant Breast and Bowel Project randomized clinical trials. J Clin Oncol. 2004;22:4247-54.
22. Wallgren A, Bonetti M, Gelber RD, Goldhirsch A, Castiglione-Gertsch M, Holmberg SB, et al. Risk factors for locoregional recurrence among breast cancer patients: Results from International Breast Cancer Study Group Trials I through VII. J Clin Oncol. 2003;21:1205-13.
23. Danish Breast Cancer Cooperative Group, Nielsen HM, Overgaard M, Grau C, Jensen AR, et al. Study of failure pattern among high-risk breast cancer patients with or without postmastectomy radiotherapy in addition to adjuvant systemic therapy: Long-term results from the Danish Breast Cancer Cooperative Group DBCG 82 b and c randomized studies. J Clin Oncol. 2006;24:2268-75.
24. Huang EH, Tucker SL, Strom EA, McNeese MD, Kuerer HM, Buzdar AU, et al. Postmastectomy radiation improves local-regional control and survival for selected patients with locally advanced breast cancer treated with neoadjuvant chemotherapy and mastectomy. J Clin Oncol. 2004;22:4691-9.
25. Garg A, Strom EA, McNeese MD, Buzdar AU, Hortobagyi GN, Kuerer HM, et al. T3 disease at presentation or pathologic involvement of four or more lymph nodes predict for local-regional recurrence in stage II breast cancer treated with neoadjuvant chemotherapy and mastectomy without radiation. Int J Rad Oncol Biol Phys. 2004;59:138-45.
26. Strom EA, Woodward WA, Katz A, Buchholz TA, Perkins GH, Jhingran A, et al. Clinical investigation: Regional nodal failure patterns in breast cancer patients treated with mastectomy without radiotherapy. Int J Radiat Oncol Biol Phys. 2005;63:1508-13.
27. Handley RS. Carcinoma of the breast. Ann R Coll Surg Engl. 1975;57:59-66.
28. Urban JA, Marjani MA. Significance of internal mammary lymph node metastases in breast cancer. Am J Roentgenol Radium Ther Nucl Med. 1971;111:130-6.
29. Group EBCTC. Effects of chemotherapy and hormonal therapy for early breast cancer on recurrence and 15-year survival: An overview of the randomised trials. Lancet. 2005;365:1687-717.
30. Henderson IC, Berry DA, Demetri GD, Cirrincione CT, Goldstein LJ, Martino S, et al. Improved outcomes from adding sequential paclitaxel but not from escalating doxorubicin dose in an adjuvant chemotherapy regimen for patients with node-positive primary breast cancer. J Clin Oncol. 2003;21:976-83.
31. Mamounas EP, Bryant J, Lembersky BC, Fehrenbacher L, Sedlacek SM, Fisher B, et al. Paclitaxel following doxorubicin/cyclophosphamide as adjuvant chemotherapy for node-positive breast cancer: Results from NSABP B-28. J Clin Oncol. 2005;23(16):3686-96.
32. Martin M, Peienkowski T, Mackey JR, et al. TAC improves disease free survival and overall survival over FAC in node positive early breast cancer patients, BCIRG 001: 55 months follow-up. Breast Cancer Res Treat. 2003;82:A43 (abstr).
33. Howell A, Cuzick J, Baum M, Buzdar A, Dowsett M, Forbes JF et al. Results of the ATAC (Arimidex, tamoxifen, alone or in combination) trial after completion of 5 years' adjuvant treatment for breast cancer. Lancet. 2005;365:60-2.
34. Goss PE, Ingle JN, Martino S, Robert NJ, Muss HB, Piccart MJ, et al. A randomized trial of letrozole in postmenopausal women after five years of tamoxifen therapy for early-stage breast cancer. N Engl J Med. 2003;349:1793-802.
35. Coombes RC, Hall E, Gibson LJ, Paridaens R, Jassem J, Delozier T, et al. Intergroup exemestane study. A randomized trial of exemestane after two to three years of tamoxifen therapy in postmenopausal women with primary breast cancer. N Engl J Med. 2004;350:1081-92.
36. Thurlimann B, Keshaviah A, Coates AS, Mouridsen H, Mauriac L, Forbes JF, et al. A comparison of letrozole and tamoxifen in postmenopausal women with early breast cancer. N Engl J Med. 2005;353:2747-57.

37. Romond EH, Perez EA, Bryant J, Suman VJ, Geyer CE Jr, Davidson NE, et al. Trastuzumab plus adjuvant chemotherapy for operable HER2-positive breast cancer. N Engl J Med. 2005;353:1673-84.
38. Piccart-Gebhart MJ, Procter M, Leyland-Jones B, Goldhirsch A, Untch M, Smith I, et al. Trastuzumab after adjuvant chemotherapy in HER2-positive breast cancer. N Engl J Med. 2005;353:1659-72.
39. Joensuu H, Kellokumpu-Lehtinen PL, Bono P, Carlini P, Felici A, Cognetti F. et al. Adjuvant docetaxel or vinorelbine with or without trastuzumab for breast cancer. N Engl J Med. 2006;354:809-20.
40. Slamon D, Eiermann W, Robert N, et al. Phase III randomized trial comparing doxorubicin and cyclophosphamide followed by docetaxel (AC T) with doxorubicin and cyclophosphamide followed by docetaxel and trastuzumab (AC TH) with docetaxel, carboplatin and trastuzumab (TCH) in HER2 positive early breast cancer patients: BCIRG 006 study. Breast Cancer Res Treat. 2005;94(Suppl 1):abstr 1.
41. Perez EA, Suman VJ, Davidson NE, Kaufman PA, Martino S, Dakhil SR, et al. Effect of doxorubicin plus cyclophosphamide on left ventricular ejection fraction in patients with breast cancer in the North Central Cancer Treatment Group N9831 Intergroup Adjuvant Trial. J Clin Oncol. 2004;22:3700-4.
42. Cristofanilli M, Gonzalez-Angulo A, Sneige N, Kau SW, Broglio K, Theriault RL, et al. Invasive lobular carcinoma classic type: Response to primary chemotherapy and survival outcomes. J Clin Oncol. 2005;23:41-8.
43. Fleming RY, Asmar L, Buzdar AU, McNeese MD, Ames FC, Ross MI, et al. Effectiveness of mastectomy by response to induction chemotherapy for control in inflammatory breast carcinoma. Ann Surg Oncol. 1997;4:452-61.
44. Liao Z, Strom EA, Buzdar AU, Singletary SE, Hunt K, Allen PK, et al. Locoregional irradiation for inflammatory breast cancer: Effectiveness of dose escalation in decreasing recurrence. Int J Radiat Oncol Biol Phys. 2000;47:1191-200.
45. Swain SM, Lippman ME. Treatment of patients with inflammatory breast cancer. Important Adv Oncol. 1989;129-50.
46. Chevallier B, Asselain B, Kunlin A, Veyret C, Bastit P, Graic Y. Inflammatory breast cancer: Determination of prognostic factors by univariate and multivariate analysis. Cancer 1987;60:897-902.
47. Haagensen CD, Cooley E. Radical mastectomy for mammary carcinoma. Ann Surg. 1969;170:884.
48. Haagensen CD, Stout AP. Carcinoma of the breast: Criteria of inoperability. Ann Surg. 1943;118:859-70.
49. Hortobagyi GN, Singletany EA, Buchholz TA. Locally advanced breast cancer. In: Singletary SE, Robb GL, Hortobagyi GN, (Eds). Advanced Therapy of Breast Disease, 2nd edition. Hammilton, Ontario: B.C. Decker, Inc. 2004. pp 498-508.
50. Fields JN, Perez CA, Kuske RR, Fineberg BB, Bartlett N. Inflammatory carcinoma of the breast: Treatment results on 107 patients. Int J Radiat Oncol Biol Phys. 1989;17:249-55.
51. Krutchik AN, Buzdar AU, Blumenschein GR, Hortobagyi GN, Tashima CK, Gutterman JU, et al. Combined chemoimmunotherapy and radiation therapy of inflammatory breast carcinoma. J Surg Oncol. 1979;11:325-32.
52. Nielsen HM, Overgaard M, Grau C, Jensen AR, Overgaard J. Loco-regional recurrence after mastectomy in high-risk breast cancer: risk and prognosis. An analysis of patients from the DBCG 82 b&c randomization trials. Radiother Oncol. 2006;79:147-55.
53. Chagpar A, Meric-Bernstam F, Hunt KK, Ross MI, Cristofanilli M, Singletary SE, et al. Chest wall recurrence after mastectomy does not always portend a dismal outcome. Ann Surg Oncol. 2003;10:628-34.
54. Hanrahan EO, Broglio KR, Buzdar AU, Theriault RL, Valero V, Cristofanilli M, et al. Combined-modality treatment for isolated recurrences of breast carcinoma: Update on 30 years of experience at the University of Texas M.D. Anderson Cancer Center and assessment of prognostic factors. Cancer. 2005;104:1158-71.

14 CHAPTER

Lung Cancer

Tejinder Kataria, Govardhan HB, Deepak Gupta, Ashu Abhishek

INTRODUCTION

Worldwide, lung cancer is the most common cancer in both incidence and mortality (1.35 million new cases and 1.18 million deaths annually). In the USA, it is the second most commonly diagnosed cancer, with approximately 222,520 new cases diagnosed in 2010, accounting for 105,770 female and 116,750 male patients; lung cancer is responsible for 28% of all cancer-related death each year (~160,000), more than all of breast, colorectal and prostate cancers combined. While the incidence in men has decreased in the past 20 years, the incidence in women has increased; however, it has recently stabilized.[1,2] According to Globocan 2008 data, the incidence of lung cancer amongst males in India is 47/100,000 and 11/100,000 amongst the females. The total number of cases in both sexes is 949,000 and approximately two-third of incident cases, i.e. 633,000 die of lung cancer.[49]

ETIOLOGY

A number of risk factors have been associated with lung cancers:

Lifestyle: Smoking accounts for nearly 90% of cases of lung cancers (98% for small cell). Lifetime risk for developing lung cancer in smokers is 17.2% in males and 11.6% in females. Lung cancers from second-hand smoke exposure increase the relative risk to 1.2–1.3 and accounts for 20,000–30,000 cases annually.[3]

Past medical history: "Scar cancer" has been reported for adenocarcinoma as a radiologically evident tuberculosis (TB) sequel.

Therapeutic radiation: Risks of developing breast and lung cancers are increased in patients exposed to therapeutic radiation for lymphoma during youth.

Radon gas exposure: Radon is a breakdown product of radioactive radium derived from the decay of uranium found in the earth's crust. Radon gas is the second most important risk factor for lung cancer in the USA.

Asbestos exposure: Asbestos exposure has highest risk factor for mesothelioma, and also has synergistic effect to cause lung cancer with smoking. It accounts for 2–3% of lung cancers.

Occupational exposure: Arsenic, bischloromethyl ether, hexavalent chromium, mustard gas, nickel, polycyclic aromatic hydrocarbons, etc. are some of the chemicals linked to development of lung cancers.[3,4]

PATHOLOGY

Lung cancers are broadly categorized as non-small cell lung cancers (NSCLC) and small cell lung cancers (SCLC) lung cancers, accounting for around 85% and 15% of all lung cancers, respectively. The most common histologic subtypes of NSCLC are adenocarcinoma (50%), squamous cell carcinoma (35%), and large cell lung cancer (15%). Subtypes of adenocarcinoma include bronchoalveolar, acinar and papillary; subtypes of large cell lung cancer include giant cell and clear cell carcinomas, both of which carry poor prognosis. Adenocarcinomas are the histologic type least associated with smoking. SCLC (also known oat cell cancer) contains dense neurosecretory granules containing neuroendocrine hormones such as adrenocorticotropic hormone (ACTH) and vasopressin.[5]

The World Health Organization classification of lung cancer is given below:[6]

- Epithelial tumors
  - Benign
    - Papillomas
    - Adenoma

- Dysplasia/carcinoma *in situ*
- Malignant
- Squamous cell carcinoma
  - Spindle cell variant
- Small cell carcinoma
  - Oat cell carcinoma
  - Intermediate cell type
  - Combined oat cell carcinoma
- Adenocarcinoma
  - Acinar
  - Papillary
  - Bronchoalveolar
  - Solid carcinoma with mucin formation
- Large cell carcinoma
  - Giant cell carcinoma
  - Clear cell carcinoma
- Adenosquamous carcinoma
- Carcinoid tumor
- Bronchial gland carcinoma
- Others

• Soft tissue tumors
• Mesothelial tumors
  - Benign
  - Malignant
• Miscellaneous tumors
  - Benign
  - Malignant
• Secondary tumors
• Unclassified tumors
• Tumor-like lesions

Routes of Spread

Local extension, regional spread to the lymphatics, and distant metastasis are the three most common routes of spread in lung cancer.

Local spread: Direct involvement of pleural surfaces, chest wall, ribs, and mediastinal structures can occur causing hemoptysis. Apical tumors can cause superior sulcus syndrome, with involvement of vertebral body, brachial plexus, stellate ganglion (causing Horner's syndrome), subclavian vasculature and superior vena cava (causing SVC syndrome). Direct extension to recurrent laryngeal nerve can cause vocal cord paralysis and hoarseness. Involvement of phrenic nerve causes diaphragmatic paralysis.

Regional lymph node metastasis: First echelon of lymph node drainage includes the hilar and interlobar nodes followed by mediastinal lymph nodes. Mediastinal nodal routes of spread differ between upper and lower lobe tumors.

Distant metastasis: The most common stage at presentation is with distant metastasis (one-third). Most common sites of distant metastasis are contralateral lung, brain, bone, adrenals and liver. Malignant pleural effusion, while strictly not defined as distant metastasis, has poor prognosis and behaves like stage IV disease.

CLINICAL PRESENTATION

Presenting signs and symptoms of lung cancer depend on the location and extent of disease. The symptoms can reflect locoregional spread of disease (either from primary mass or from location of distant metastasis) or systemic manifestation of disease (constitutional symptoms, paraneoplastic syndrome). The three most common presenting sign and symptoms of lung cancer are dyspnea, cough and weight loss. Others are chest pain, hemoptysis, clubbing and bone pain. Headaches, nausea and vomiting, or focal neurologic signs/symptoms may result from brain metastasis.

Locoregional Manifestation of Disease

- *Superior sulcus syndrome*: Invasion of apical structures to cause Horner's syndrome, brachial plexopathy and bone pain
- *Superior vena cava syndrome*: Venous distension of neck and chest wall, cyanosis, facial plethora and upper extremity edema due to mediastinal compression with the primary tumor or nodal disease
- *Nerve plexopathies*: Brachial plexopathy, recurrent laryngeal nerve and phrenic nerve paralysis
- *Pancoast syndrome*: This is observed in superior sulcus tumors. It is characterized by lower brachial plexopathy, Horner's syndrome, and pain in shoulder and ulnar side of arm
- *Horner's syndrome*: This characterized by enophthalmos, ptosis, miosis, ipsilateral sweating loss and hoarseness due to laryngeal nerve invasion
- *Local extension of disease*: Hemoptysis, chest wall pain, rib pain and postobstructive pneumonia.

Systemic Manifestation of Disease

- *Constitutional symptoms*: Fever, weight loss, anorexia, weakness
- *Paraneoplastic disorders (NSCLC)*: Hypercalcemia of malignancy (HCM)
- *Paraneoplastic disorders (SCLC)*: Paraneoplastic syndromes.[7-10]
- Gynecomastia (generally in large cell carcinoma)
- Hypertrophic pulmonary osteoarthropathy (generally in adenocarcinoma)
- Inappropriate antidiuretic hormone secretion is most frequently observed in SCLC.

WORKUP AND STAGING

Complete history, physical examination diagnostic imaging and laboratory tests are necessary for proper diagnosis and staging of lung cancers. The 7th edition of the American Joint Committee on Cancer (AJCC) staging and grouping of lung cancer (both NSCLC and SCLC) is presented below. However, the clinical staging that is commonly used in SCLC is determined by whether the disease can be encompassed within a radiation portal (limited) or not (extensive). Complete history, complete clinical examination, hematology and biochemical tests are a prerequisite to imaging.

Imaging

- Chest X-ray PA and AP view
- CT scan of the thorax and abdomen to study the extent of the disease regionally and to rule out lesions in adrenals and liver. Sensitivity is of a CT scan for lung cancer diagnosis is 64% and specificity is 74%
- FDG-PET (18-fluoro-deoxyglucose positron emission tomography) has been approved by US FDA to workup pulmonary nodules. The size that can be definitely ascertained has a limit set by the PET-crystal size and may vary from 4 mm to 8 mm. Rate of detection of occult metastases by PET-CT range from 6% to 18%. Sensitivity and specificity for staging is 83% and 91%, respectively. Positive predictive value (PPV) is ~80% (false-positive rate ~10–20%) and negative predictive value (NPV) is ~95% (false-negative rate ~5–16%). As the false-positive rate is higher, a positive PET lesion needs to have pathologic confirmation.[11] A PET-CT is shown in Figure 1.
- MRI is more sensitive than CT to detect brain metastasis, and should be done:
  - In patients with advanced disease.
  - For superior sulcus tumors to rule out brachial plexus invasion.
  - For symptomatic patients to rule out cord compression.
  - For all patients diagnosed with small cell lung cancer.
- Bone scan can be done for symptomatic patients. Bone scan is optional if FDG-PET is performed, as FDG-PET is more sensitive for detecting osseous metastasis.

Invasive Procedures

- *Bronchoscopy*: Allows direct visualization and sampling of centrally located tumors. The use of fiberoptic techniques allows visualization and sampling of peripheral lesions.
- *Endobronchial ultrasound* helps visualize extent of invasion in centrally located tumors and mediastinal lymph nodes. Allows sampling of suspicious lymph nodes using fine needle aspiration.[12]
- *Mediastinoscopy*: This is done to evaluate status of enlarged mediastinal lymph nodes seen on CT and/or positive on PET.
- *Chamberlain procedure*: Anterior mediastinotomy.
- *Video assisted thoracoscopic surgery (VATS)*: This is reserved for tumors that remain undiagnosed after bronchoscopy or CT-guided biopsy. VATS plays an important role for confirmation of histology in the presence of a solitary pulmonary nodule (SPN) and for management of malignant pleural effusions.
- *CT-guided biopsy*: This procedure is generally necessary for peripherally located lesions, or at sites of distant disease.

STAGING

AJCC Tumor, Node, Metastasis (TNM) Classification of Lung Cancers (NSCLC and SCLC), 7th Edition[13]

T Staging

T1: Tumor 3 cm or smaller in greatest dimension, is surrounded by lung or visceral pleura, and is without bronchoscopic evidence of invasion more proximal than the lobar bronchus (i.e. not in the main bronchus).

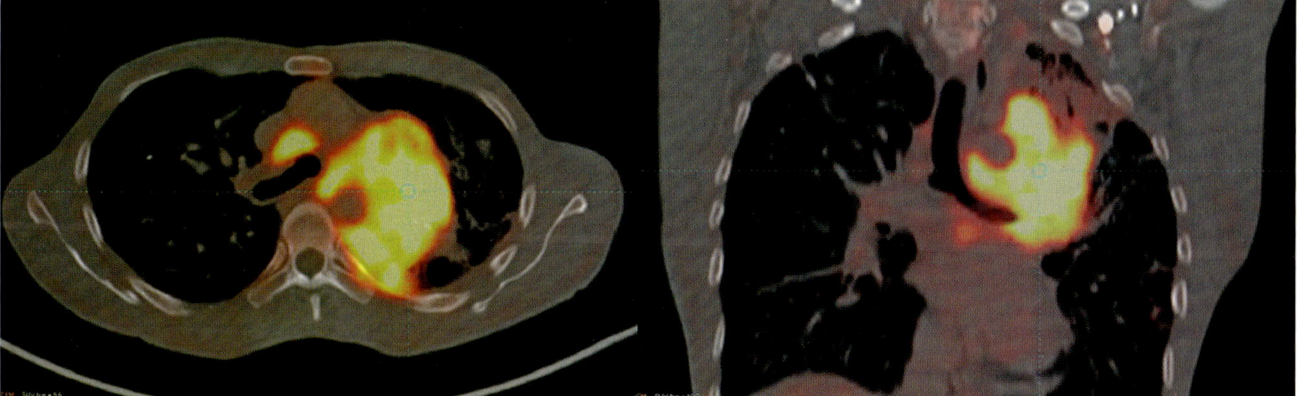

Fig. 1 PET-CT for an upper lobe left sided squamous cell carcinoma with FDG avid central lesion and distal atelectasis

Courtesy: Dr Tejinder Kataria, Division of Radiation Oncology, Medanta—The Medicity, Haryana, India

T1a: Tumor less than or equal to 2 cm.

T1b: Tumor more than 2 cm but smaller or equal to 3 cm.

T2: A tumor with any of the following features of size or extent larger than 3 cm in greatest dimension. Involves the main bronchus and is 2 cm or larger distal to the carina. Invades the visceral pleura. Associated with atelectasis or obstructive pneumonitis that extends to the hilar region but does not involve the entire lung.

T2a: Tumor more than 3–5 cm.

T2b: Tumor more than 5–7 cm.

T3: A tumor more than 7 cm or one that directly invades any of the following: chest wall (including superior sulcus tumors), parietal pleura diaphragm, mediastinal pleura, phrenic nerve, parietal pericardium; or, tumor in the main bronchus less than 2 cm distal to the carina but without involvement of the carina; or, associated atelectasis or obstructive pneumonitis of the entire lung or separate tumor nodules in the same lobe.

T4: A tumor of any size that invades any of the following: mediastinum, heart, great vessels, trachea, recurrent laryngeal nerve, esophagus, vertebral body, carina; or, separate tumor nodules in a different ipsilateral lobe.

N Staging

N0: No regional lymph node metastasis.

N1: Metastasis to ipsilateral peribronchial and/or ipsilateral hilar lymph nodes, and intrapulmonary nodes including involvement by direct extension of the primary tumor.

N2: Metastasis to ipsilateral mediastinal and/or subcarinal lymph node(s).

N3: Metastasis to contralateral mediastinal, contralateral hilar, ipsilateral or contralateral scalene, or supraclavicular lymph node(s).

AJCC Stage Groupings

Stage 0: TisN0M0

Stage IA: T1a-bN0M0

Stage IB: T2aN0M0

Stage IIA: T2bN0M0, T1a-bN1M0, T2aN1M0

Stage IIB: T2bN1M0; T3N0M0

Stage IIIA: T1N2M0; T2N2M0; T3N1M0; T3N2M0; T4N0-1M0

Stage IIIB: Any T, N3M0; T4N2-3, M0

Stage IV: Any T, Any N, M1

PROGNOSIS

Prognostic factors for patients with lung cancer can be divided with regard to patient, tumor and treatment-specific variables. Stanley et al. evaluated 77 prognostic factors in approximately 5,000 patients with inoperable carcinoma of the lung (VA Lung Group Protocols). The three most important prognostic factors affecting survival were patient-specific variables, including performance status (Karnofsky score), stage and weight loss. It is generally believed that epidermoid carcinoma has the best prognosis, followed by adenocarcinoma and undifferentiated large cell carcinoma.[14]

GENERAL MANAGEMENT

Non-Small Cell Carcinoma of Lung

In patients with NSCLC, the most important prognostic factor is tumor stage. Surgery is the treatment of choice for early stage NSCLC, and it is often incorporated for early locally advanced patients as well. Neoadjuvant or adjuvant therapy is recommended for many patients with stage II and III disease. Only about 20% of all patients presenting with lung cancer are suitable candidates for curative surgery. The use of combined-modality therapy including radiation and chemotherapy is recommended for locally advanced stage III disease. Patients with stage IV disease are treated with chemotherapy or palliative radiation therapy (RT) or with supportive therapy alone.

In the past, conventional RT yielded poor outcomes for unresectable early stage patients; however, technologic advances with the advent of stereotactic ablative radiation therapy (SBRT) have contributed to improvements in local control and survival. Locally advanced NSCLC is often managed with concurrent chemotherapy and RT. Postoperative radiotherapy (PORT) is given for patients with positive-margin or pathologic N2 disease. Systemic agents (chemotherapy, targeted agents) are given in the adjuvant setting after surgical resection for stage Ib (tumors > 4 cm) to stage IIIA patients, or for palliation in stage IV patients.

Indications for Surgical Resection

- Treatment of choice for early stage NSCLC (stage I–II).
- May be indicated for early stage IIIA after induction therapies (chemoradiation or chemotherapy) if lobectomy can be performed.
- Lobectomy preferred over wedge resection with mediastinal lymph node dissection.
- Minimum FEV1 necessary for lobectomy more than 1.5 L and for pneumonectomy more than 2.0 L. The marginal %FEV1 is 40% of predicted.
- Generally not indicated for SCLC, although can be considered for small lesions on clinical trial or in the SPN.

Indications for Radiation Therapy

- Definitive treatment for medical inoperable stage I.
- NSCLC using hypofractionated stereotactic body RT.
- Definitive treatment for NSCLC patients unable to tolerate chemotherapy.
- Definitive treatment for locally advanced (stage III) NSCLC and limited-stage SCLC with concurrent chemotherapy.
- Prophylactic cranial irradiation in all stages of SCLC after response to primary treatment.
- Postoperative radiation after surgical resection with pathologic N2 disease, T4 disease except for separate nodules in the same lobe, close/positive surgical margins, gross residual disease.
- Palliation for pain, bleeding, SVC syndrome, brain metastasis, cord compression.

Techniques of Radiation Therapy

- External beam radiation with 3D-CRT, IMRT or stereotactic body RT.
- Proton beam therapy is a promising modality for the management of thoracic malignancies.
- Intraoperative HDR used after wedge resection may improve local control rates.
- *Endobronchial brachytherapy*: Palliation of endobronchial disease recurrent after EBRT, palliation of endobronchial disease from metastatic disease and boost treatment after initial course of definitive EBRT for primary cancer with endobronchial component.

Treatment of NSCLC (Stages I–II, IIIA) Operable Lung Cancers

Surgical resection with lobectomy is preferred, based on a randomized trial. LCSG 921 was a randomized study comparing an anatomic lobectomy versus limited (wedge or segmental) resection for peripheral T1 pulmonary carcinomas. The locoregional recurrence rate for limited resection was three times greater than for lobectomy, 17% versus 6.4%. However, the report did not differentiate true local recurrences from regional nodal metastases.[15]

Stereotactic Body Radiation Therapy

The development of three-dimensional conformal radiotherapy (3DCRT) and stereotactic body radiation therapy (SBRT) allows precise targeting and delivery of radiotherapy. SBRT for lung cancer uses elements of 3DCRT and also incorporates a variety of systems for taking tumor motion into consideration and decreasing setup uncertainty using image-guided radiotherapy techniques. These systems allow reduction of treatment volumes, facilitating hypofractionation with markedly increased daily doses and a significantly reduced overall treatment time. Image-guided SBRT with delivery of biological equivalent dose (BED) more than 100 Gy is feasible and safe in the treatment of peripherally located inoperable stage I and selective II NSCLC. The 3–5 years local control and overall survival rates seem to be much better than those for conventional radiotherapy, and the toxicity is minimal. Timmerman et al. reported 3 years primary tumor control rate was 97.6% [95% confidence interval (CI), 84.3–99.7%] with a SBRT dose of 54 Gy in 3 fractions.[47] Particularly for stage Ia (T1N0M0) disease, SBRT achieved results comparable to those for surgical resection. SBRT is becoming the standard treatment for inoperable stage I NSCLC. To take tumor motion into consideration, image-guided SBRT is required and crucial. The optimal dose regimen remains unclear, but BED higher than 100 Gy seems to be needed. We need to balance the potential improvement of tumor control and treatment-related toxicities.[16]

With the advancement in our experience and technological advances in recent times, Cyberknife, a robot controlled miniaturized radiotherapy tool is one of the best tools of SBRT in lung tumors. With capabilities of real time imaging, coupled with motion management by synchrony software, Cyberknife promises to deliver radiation with pinpoint accuracy to the allocated target (Fig. 2). Cyberknife can be effectively used in treatment of not only early stage medically inoperable lung cancers, but it is also effective in selected oligometastatic lung deposits. Cyberknife SBRT, being an OPD procedure can curtail prolonged treatments and deliver ablative dosages with sub millimeter accuracy in 5–7 fractions (Figs 3A and B). Procedure is safe with minimal acceptable side effects that are self-resolving.

Medically inoperable candidates with T1–T2a (< 5 cm) N0M0 could be amendable for definitive management with stereotactic body radiation (SBRT). Randomized trials comparing surgery with SBRT for resectable patients are underway. Adjuvant chemotherapy is indicated based on multiple randomized trials in stage Ib (> 4 cm) to stage IIIa patients. In a single-institutional, retrospective review by Onishi et al., 277 patients with stage I NSCLC were treated with 18–75 Gy in 1–22 fractions, with median BED = 111 Gy (57–180 Gy), $\alpha/\beta = 10$. The median follow-up is 38 months, and local recurrence related to BED: LC for BED ≥ 100 = 92% and LC for BED < 100 = 57%. The 5 years OS for BED ≥ 100 = 71%; BED < 100 = 30%.[17]

In the RTOG 0236 study, a phase II cooperative trial, patients with T1–3N0 (up to 5 cm) tumors except patients with central lesions (T3 tumors invading mediastinum or those < 2 cm from carina) were selected. Total dose of 60 Gy, i.e. 20 Gy in 3 fractions by SBRT (actual treatment with heterogeneity correction is 18 Gy 3 = 54 Gy) was delivered. Local failure was defined as failure within 1 cm of treated area. A total of 55 patients were evaluable (T1 = 44 patients), with median age = 72 years. The median follow-up of the patient

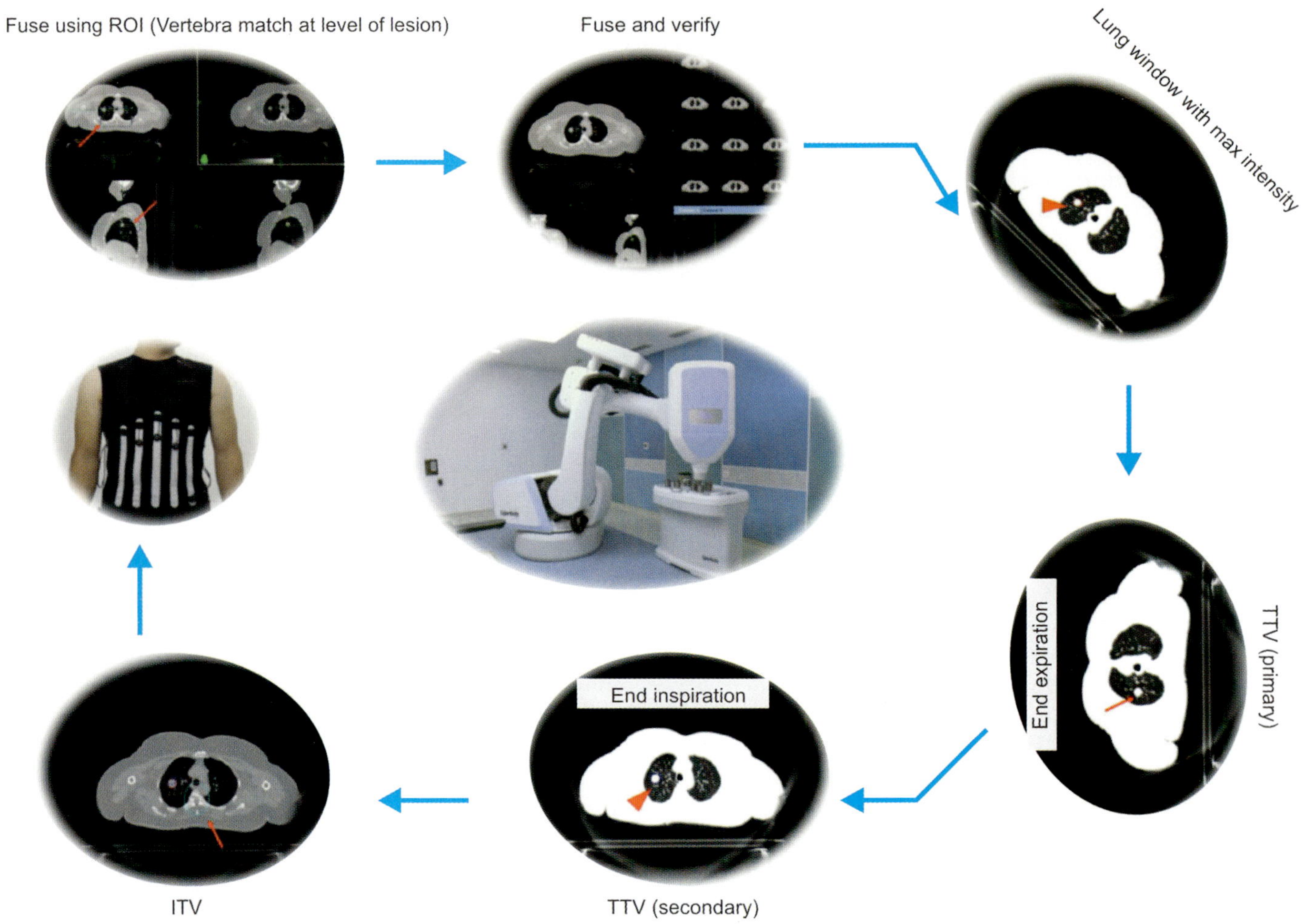

Fuse using ROI (Vertebra match at level of lesion)
Fuse and verify
Lung window with max intensity
TTV (primary)
End expiration
End inspiration
TTV (secondary)
ITV

Fig. 2 Steps of internal target volume generation on cyberknife

Courtesy: Dr Tejinder Kataria, Division of Radiation Oncology, Medanta—The Medicity, Haryana, India

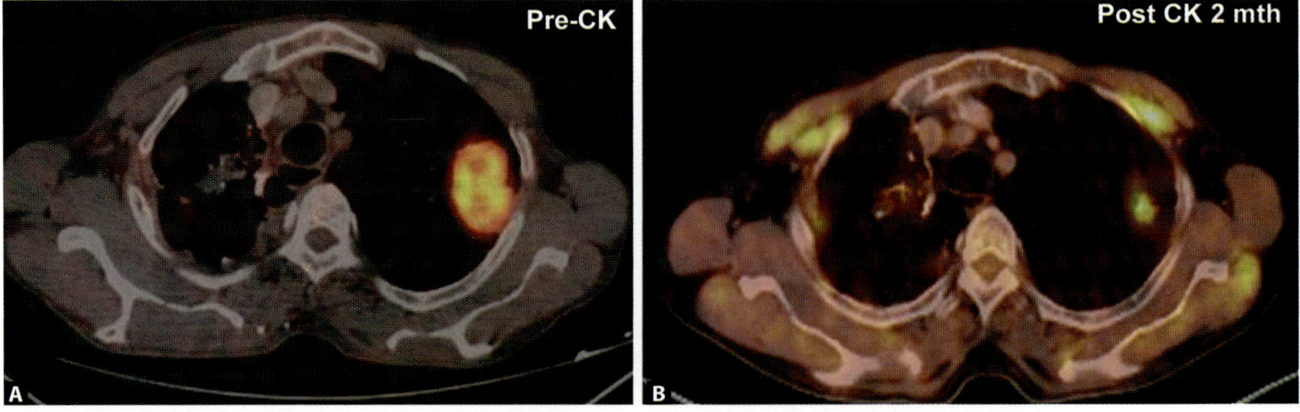

Figs 3A and B Pre- and post-cyberknife treatment PET-CT showing good response to treatment

Courtesy: Dr Tejinder Kataria, Division of Radiation Oncology, Medanta—The Medicity, Haryana, India

was 34 months and 3 years LC = 98%. Three-year Distant Metastasis = 20% median OS = 48 months, 2 years OS = 72%, and 2 years disease free survival (DFS) = 67%.[18]

Stage III non-small cell lung cancer: Approximately, 25–40% of patients with NSCLC have stage III disease. Of these, approximately one-third present with potentially resectable disease, stage IIIA (T1–3 N2, T3 N1). The median survival duration for all patients with stage IIIA (clinical or surgical stage) disease treated with surgical resection is 12 months, and the 5 years survival rate is 9–15%. Within the stage IIIA subset, however, survival rates vary widely.[19]

Preoperative Radiation Therapy

In a prospective randomized multi-institution trial of 478 patients with lung cancer, patients receiving preoperative irradiation (20 Gy in five fractions) followed by surgery were compared with patients receiving surgery alone. There was no difference in the 5 years survival rates among patients with stages I and II disease. However, the survival rates for stage III patients were 49.4% at 3 years and 29.2% at 5 years for the combined-therapy group compared with 28.1% and 15.8%, respectively, for the surgery-alone group.[20]

Preoperative Chemotherapy

Patients with N0 disease usually have a very-high cure rate and are not recommended for neoadjuvant therapy. However, patients with stage II (T1N1 and T2N1) disease, who have lower survival rates (25–50%) after surgical resection, and those with stage III disease, who have a very low survival rate, potentially could benefit from neoadjuvant therapy.[21]

At MD Anderson Cancer Center, 60 patients were randomized to undergo chemotherapy and surgery or surgery alone. Twenty-eight patients received three cycles of cyclophosphamide, etoposide and cisplatin, and then underwent surgery. They were compared with 32 patients treated with surgery alone. The median survival duration was 64 months versus 11 months, favoring neoadjuvant chemotherapy. The 2 years survival rates were 56% in the neoadjuvant group and 15% in the surgery-only group (p = 0.008). In this study, the patients who had positive margins, multiple levels of positive lymph nodes, or extracapsular extension received PORT between 50 Gy and 60 Gy, and only two patients developed local recurrences.[22]

Adjuvant Postoperative Radiation Therapy

In general, PORT is indicated in incomplete resections (close or positive margins) or positive mediastinal metastases (N2). Eradication of local cancer is a prerequisite for cure. As with any other tumor site, if surgical margins are close or positive, PORT is indicated for improvement of local tumor control. The definitions of positive, close and clear surgical margins are rather arbitrary. Generally, if tumor cells are found at the surgical margins (usually inked), these are called positive surgical margins. If less than 0.5 cm of normal tissue is present adjacent to the tumor edge, the surgical margin usually is considered close; more than 1 cm of normal tissue is considered a clear surgical margin. Close or positive bronchial surgical resection margins can occur with peripherally located tumors, often attached to the chest wall, or with centrally located tumors. In these situations, a course of PORT of 50 Gy for potential microscopic disease and 60–66 Gy for a positive-margin in 2 Gy fractions usually is recommended.

Postoperative radiotherapy is currently contraindicated in patients with stage I completely resected disease on the basis of the PORT meta-analysis. The PORT meta-analysis has been widely discussed because of the negative effect of RT on overall survival for all patients examined (stages I–III). Subgroup analysis identified that the decremental effect was statistically limited to patients with stage I disease and was nearly significant for stage II disease. There is a suggestion of benefit with PORT for patients with N2 disease that did not reach statistical significance. There are problems with the nine randomized trials that are included in this meta-analysis, including the inclusion of patients with stage I disease, four of the trials used hypofractionated treatment schedules, and seven of the trials used Cobalt-60. These issues may have contributed significantly to the negative effect of RT on survival for the patients with stages I and II disease.[23]

Postoperative Chemoradiation

The role of adjuvant chemoradiotherapy remains controversial. Keller et al. reported the results of a prospective randomized study designed to determine whether combination chemotherapy with cisplatin/etoposide and thoracic RT was superior to thoracic RT alone for patients with completely resected stage II or IIIa NSCLC.[24] The RTOG recently published the results of a phase II study using paclitaxel and carboplatin concurrently with adjuvant RT. Eighty-eight patients were accrued with stages II and IIIA disease and treated with 50.4 Gy in 28 fractions during 6 weeks with cycles 1 and 2 of chemotherapy. A boost of 10.8 Gy was given for patients with extracapsular extension or T3 lesions. Treatment compliance was good, with 93% completing RT and 86% completing chemotherapy. With a median follow-up of 56.7 months, the median overall survival was 56.3 months with 1-, 2- and 3-year survival rates of 86%, 70%, and 61%, respectively.[25]

Definitive Radiation Therapy

Around 40% of the patients of NSCLC are either medically inoperable or have a locally advanced disease. Definitive RT consists of a minimum dose of 60–75 Gy to the gross disease and 50 Gy to microscopic disease with standard fractionation (1.8 or 2 Gy/fraction). Current RT doses (60 Gy given in single daily fraction of 2 Gy) for patients with unresectable, locally advanced non-small cell carcinoma (stage IIIA and IIIB) were established by RTOG 73-01.[26]

The RTOG recently completed a phase II dose-escalation study (RTOG 93-11). Patients were treated with either radiation alone or radiation following neoadjuvant chemotherapy. Radiotherapy was planned with 3D conformal techniques with target volumes limited to the gross tumor volume (GTV) plus a margin. Because the study was designed to find the maximum tolerated radiation dose, the total volume of normal lung treated dictated the dose. Patients with smaller lung volumes irradiated were treated to higher doses according to the escalation schema. Total doses ranged between 70.9 Gy and 90.3 Gy for the small-volume group and 70.9–77.4 Gy in the larger volume group. The daily fraction size was 2.15 Gy. RTOG 9311 showed that acute toxicity rates were acceptable for the dose up to 90.3 Gy (<15% grade 3 and above pneumonitis, and no esophagitis).[27]

In a phase II hyperfractionated, accelerated RT trial sponsored by the Eastern Cooperative Oncology Group (ECOG 4593), 30 patients were treated with 1.5- to 1.8-Gy fractions three times per day during 16 days, for a total dose of 57.6 Gy. This protocol called for no treatments to be given on weekends. With a minimum follow-up of 19 months, the median survival was 13 months and the 1 year survival rate was 57%. This regimen is being compared with standard radiotherapy (60 Gy during 6–7 weeks) by ECOG in a phase III trial.[28]

A trial from the Netherlands[29] intensified the radiation delivered using a concomitant-boost technique. Thirty-three patients with inoperable NSCLC were treated with 60 Gy in 20 fractions in 25 days. Fifteen patients received 40 Gy in 2-Gy fraction to the primary tumor and a part of the mediastinum, and 18 patients received the same dose to the primary tumor and the whole mediastinum. During each session, a simultaneous boost of 1 Gy was administered to the primary tumor. Moderate acute esophageal toxicity was observed in seven (22%) of 33 patients, and severe late toxicity was seen in one patient (3%). After a mean follow-up of 14 months, 17 patients (52%) had local tumor control, 13 patients (39%) developed a confirmed local recurrence within the treated area, and three patients (9%) had suspected tumor regrowth.

Definitive Chemoradiotherapy

Chemotherapy and RT can be delivered sequentially or concurrently. Conventional radiotherapy alone resulted in a median survival of 10 months and a 5-year survival of 5%. To improve the outcome of treatment, chemotherapy was added to radiotherapy. Multiple phase III trials have demonstrated a survival advantage for the addition of chemotherapy to radiotherapy for NSCLC. The most well-known trial, reported by the CALGB,[30] compared standard radiotherapy of 60 Gy to sequential cisplatin and vinblastine chemotherapy for two cycles followed by 60 Gy. Median and 5-year survivals were superior for the chemoradiation arm (13.8 months vs 9.7 months and 19% vs 7%). These results led the RTOG to conduct a three-arm trial (RTOG 88-08) comparing standard radiotherapy, sequential chemoradiation (CALGB regimen), and 69.6 Gy hyperfractionated radiotherapy.[31] Sequential chemotherapy was statistically superior to both standard radiation and hyperfractionation. Results for the hyperfractionated arm were not statistically different from those for conventional radiation alone.

RTOG 9,410 conducted a three-arm randomized trial to analyze whether the concurrent delivery of cisplatin-based chemotherapy with thoracic radiation therapy (TRT) improves survival compared with the sequential delivery of these therapies for patients with locally advanced, unresected stage II-III NSCLC. The sequential arm included cisplatin (100 mg/m^2) and vinblastine (5 mg/m^2) with 60 Gy of radiotherapy. The concurrent arm used the same chemotherapy with 60 Gy of radiotherapy beginning on day 1 (CON-QD). The third arm employed concurrent cisplatin 50 mg/m^2 with oral etoposide 50 mg with 69.6 Gy in 1.2 Gy twice daily fractions beginning day 1 (CON-BID). For the 595 analyzable patients, the rates of acute grade 3–5 nonhematologic toxicity rates were higher with concurrent than sequential therapy, but late toxicity rates were similar (18–27%). With a minimum and median potential follow-up times of 4.0 and 6.0 years, the median survival and 4-year survivals were 14.6 months and 12% (sequential arm), 17.0 months and 21% (CON-QD radiation therapy), and 15.2 months and 17% (CON-BID RT). The CON-QD RT arm had better survival than the sequential arm ($p = 0.046$). This report demonstrates the long-term survival benefit of the concurrent delivery of cisplatin-based chemotherapy with TRT as compared with the sequential delivery of these therapies. The locoregional failure rates were 50% (sequential arm), 43% (CON-QD), and 34% (CON-BID).[32]

Another trial comparing concurrent versus sequential chemoradiation, reported in 2001 and updated in 2005, also explored the use of consolidation chemotherapy. In this phase III trial from France, 205 patients were assigned to receive two cycles of cisplatin plus vinorelbine followed by 66 Gy of radiation versus cisplatin/etoposide and concurrent radiation to 66 Gy followed by two cycles of consolidation chemotherapy with cisplatin and vinorelbine. Local control rates were improved with the concurrent regimen (40% vs 24%), and the median and 4 years survival times were numerically superior (but not statistically superior) for the concurrent arm

(14.5 vs 16.3 months and 14% vs 21%). However, the incidence of grade 3 esophagitis was significantly higher in the concurrent arm (32% vs 3%), and the toxic death rates were high on both arms (9.5% on the concurrent arm and 5.6% on the sequential arm).[33]

Radiation Treatment Planning and Techniques

Immobilization and Simulation: Patients are placed in the supine position with both arms up and immobilized with a thoracic cast or Vac-LoK bag and T-bar. CT simulation is necessary for conformal treatment planning and contrast enhanced CT scan with 2–3 mm CT slices are required.

Contouring

The GTV should be delineated on the CT images, with guidance from regions of FDG-avidity in PET images. Lymph nodes with short axis larger than 10 mm on CT cr high FDG-avidity on PET images should be included in the gross disease. GTV-P the gross primary disease, and GTV-N gross nodal disease as seen on imaging. The clinical target volume (CTV) was generated by adding 0.6 cm for squamous cell carcinoma and 0.8 cm in adenocarcinoma to GTV in all dimensions. If 4DCT is available, ITV should be generated. An ITV should be generated around CTV. Different techniques can used to overcome tumor motion like active breath holding, generation of ITV using inspiration and expiration CT images, etc. (Fig. 4). A planning target volume (PTV) margin should be given to this volume depending on institutional uncertainties. If patient is treated in free breathing a margin of 1.0 cm radial and 1.5 cm superior inferior should be given to CTV (Fig. 5).

Tumor volume shrinkage during the treatment for lung cancer is well known, replanning during mid-treatment may allow better normal tissue sparing and further improve the therapeutic ratio if GTV decreases by 30% or more[45] (Figs 6A and B).

Curative treatment for NSCLC requires the following dose prescription (Table 1):

- 55 Gy in 20 daily fractions of 2.75 Gy given in 4 weeks, or
- 66 Gy in 33 daily fractions given in 6.5 weeks.

The recommended dose prescription for adjuvant treatment of NSCLC is:

- 50 Gy in 20 daily fractions of 2.5 Gy given in 4 weeks, or
- 60 Gy in 30 daily fractions given in 6 weeks.

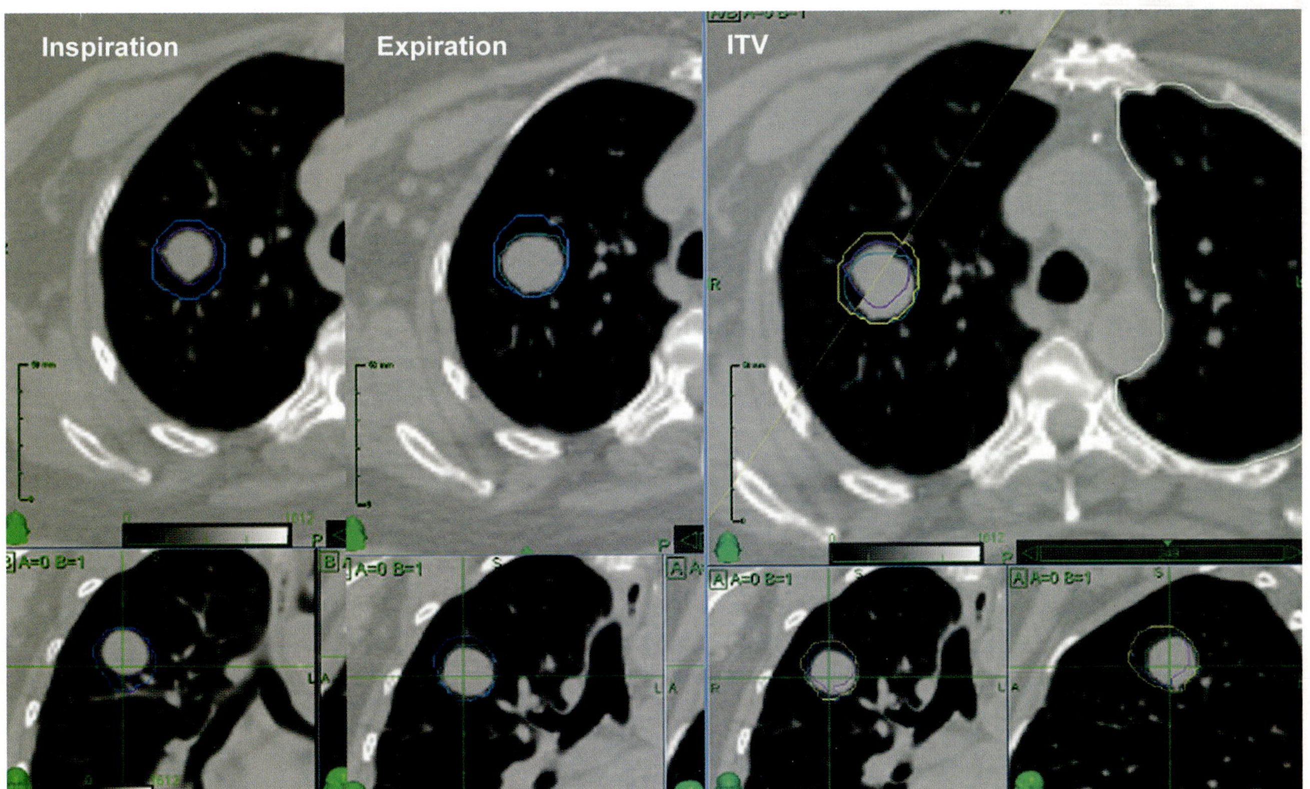

Fig. 4 Internal target volume generation on cyberknife

Courtesy: Dr Tejinder Kataria, Division of Radiation Oncology, Medanta—The Medicity, Haryana, India

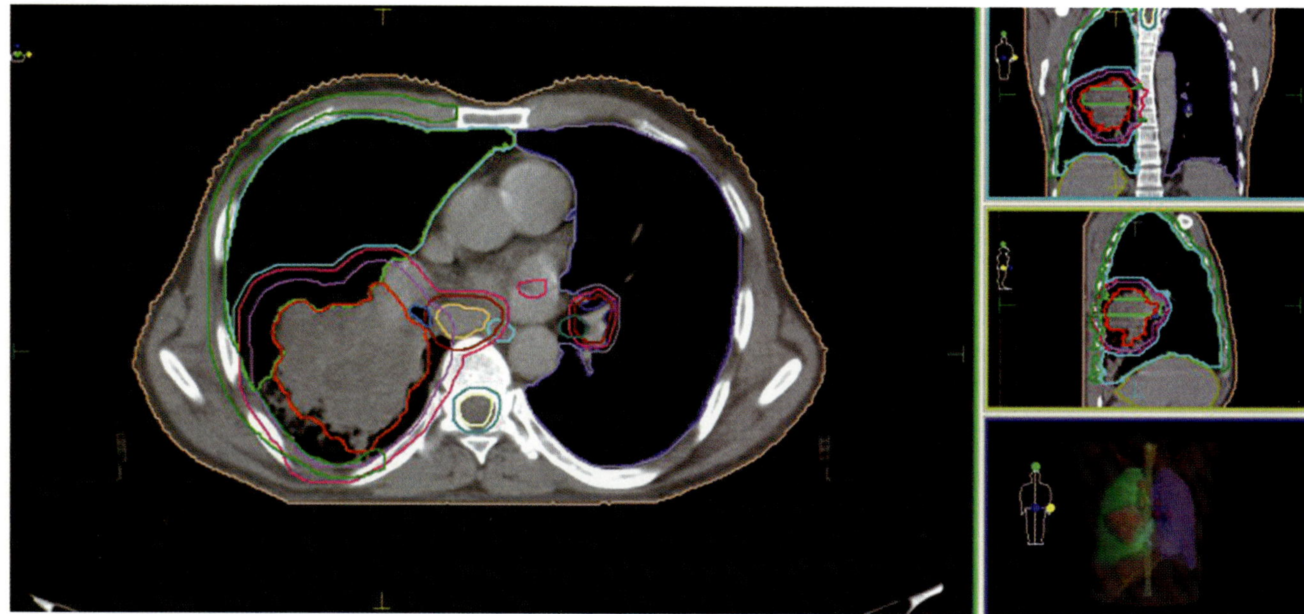

Fig. 5 RT planning CT lobe right sided squamous cell carcinoma lung cT3N1M0

Courtesy: Dr Tejinder Kataria, Division of Radiation Oncology, Medanta—The Medicity, Haryana, India

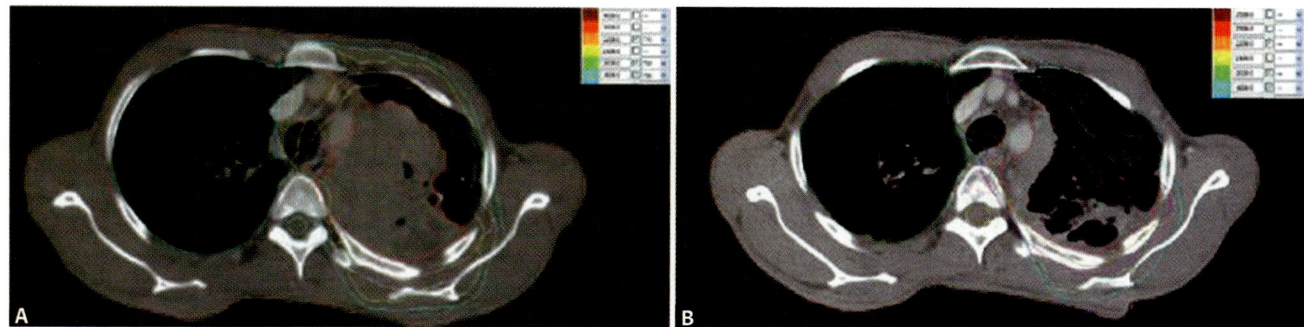

Figs 6A and B RT planning CT for an upper lobe left sided squamous cell carcinoma lung stage III with rescan at 22 fraction

Courtesy: Dr Tejinder Kataria, Division of Radiation Oncology, Medanta—The Medicity, Haryana, India

Table 1 Dose constraint for conventional radiotherapy

Organs at risk	*Doses*
Spinal cord	Maximum < 50 Gy
Lung[66]	V20 < 35%, V5 < 65%, Mean < 20 Gy
Heart[67]	V40 < 80%, V45 < 60G%, V60 < 30%, Mean < 35 Gy
Esophagus[68]	Mean < 34 Gy
Brachial plexus[69]	Maximum < 66 Gy

SBRT Commonly Used Doses

- 25–34 Gy/1 fraction → peripheral, small less than 2 cm tumors, especially more than 1 cm from chest wall
- 45–60 Gy/3 fractions → peripheral tumors more than 1 cm from chest wall
- 48–50 Gy/5 fractions → central or peripheral tumors especially less than 1 cm from chest wall
- 60–70Gy/8–10 fractions → central tumors.

Dose constraints for normal structure for conventional radiotherapy and SBRT were enumerated in Tables 2 and 3.

Stage IV Disease

Around 55% of patients will present with stage IIIB or IV of NSCLC disease that is not amenable to curative treatment. They typically succumb to their disease, with an overall median survival time of 8–10 months. Approximately, one-third of patients with stage IIIB or IV disease are alive at 1 year, and 10–21% of these individuals are alive 2 years after diagnosis. Although these data reflect improvements

Table 2 SBRT dose constraint[65]

		One fraction		*Three fraction*		*Five fraction*		
	Maximum critical volume above threshold	*Threshold dose (Gy)*	*Maximum point dose (Gy)*	*Threshold dose (Gy)*	*Maximum point dose (Gy)*	*Threshold dose (Gy)*	*Maximum point dose (Gy)*	*End point Grade*[3]
Spinal cord	0.35 cc	10	14	18.6 Gy/fx	21.9 (7.3 Gy/fx)	23 (4.6 Gy/fx)	30 (6 Gy/fx)	Myelitis
Spinal cord subvolume 5–6 mm above and below level treated per Ryu	10% of subvolume	10	14	18.6 Gy/fx	21.9 (7.3 Gy/fx)	23 4.6 Gy/fx	30 (6 Gy/fx)	Myelitis
Esophagus	<5 cc	11.9	15.4	17.7 (5.9 Gy/fx)	25.2 (8.4 Gy/fx)	19.5 (3.9 Gy/fx)	35 (7 Gy/fx)	Stenosis/ fistula
Brachial plexus	<3 cc	14	17.5	20.4 (6.8 Gy/fx)	24(8 Gy/fx)	27 (5.4 Gy/fx)	30.5 (6.1 Gy/fx)	Neuropathy
Heart/ pericardium	<15 cc	16	22	24 (8 Gy/fx)	30(10 Gy/fx)	32 (6.4 Gy/fx)	38 (7.6 Gy/fx)	Pericarditis
Great vessels	<10 cc	31	37	39 (13 Gy/fx)	45 (15 Gy/fx)	47 (9.4 Gy/fx)	53 (10.6 Gy/fx)	Aneurysm
Trachea and large bronchus	<4	10.5	20.2	15 (5 Gy/fx)	30 (10 Gy/fx)	16.5 (3.3 Gy/fx)	40 (8 Gy/fx)	Stenosis/ fistula
Bronchus-smaller airways	< 0.5	12.4	13.3	18.9 (6.3 Gy/fx)	23.1 (7.7 Gy/fx)	21 (4.2 Gy/fx)	33 (6.6 Gy/fx)	Stenosis with atelectasis
Rib	<1	22	30	28.8 (9.6 Gy/fx)	36.9 (12.3 Gy/fx)	35 (7 Gy/fx)	43 (8.6 Gy/fx)	Pain or fracture
	<30 cc			30 (10.0 Gy/fx)				
Skin	<10 cc	23	26	30 (10.0 Gy/fx)	33 (11 Gy/fx)	36.5 (7.3 Gy/fx)	39.5 (7.9 Gy/fx)	Ulceration
Lung right and left	1500 cc	7		11.6 (2.9 Gy/fx)		12.5 (2.5 Gy/fx)		Basic lung function, Pneumonitis
	1000 cc	7.4		12.4 (3.1 Gy/fx)		13.5 (2.7 Gy/fx)		Basic lung function, Pneumonitis
Liver	700 cc	9.1		19.2 (4.8 Gy/fx)		21 4.2 Gy/fx)		Basic liver function
Bronchi	4 cc		8.8		30		18	

in the care of patients with advanced lung cancer, treatment remains palliative with the goal of compassionate and effective end-of-life care.

Systemic Chemotherapy

Although systemic chemotherapy is the standard treatment for advanced NSCLC, in some circumstances, the initial treatment can be a local modality to relieve the symptoms. Based on available data from randomized trials, optimal chemotherapy regimens for advanced NSCLC include a platinum drug (cisplatin or carboplatin) and a second drug, such as vinorelbine, gemcitabine, paclitaxel, or docetaxel. Currently, platinum-based combination chemotherapy regimens are preferred for the treatment of advanced NSCLC with good performance status. Patients with an ECOG performance status of 0 or 1 are the best candidates for chemotherapy and can achieve both prolongation of survival and improvement in quality of life. Patients with an ECOG performance status of 2 are at a substantial higher risk of chemotherapy complications and have a significantly poorer prognosis regardless of the use of palliative chemotherapy. Single-agent chemotherapy or regimens with a good tolerance, such as carboplatin and paclitaxel, are advised in performance status 2 patients with advanced NSCLC. Current regimens (particularly those that are carboplatin-based) appear less toxic; however, the overall outcome of patients treated with these newer drug combinations is only marginally better than that reported for patients treated with older regimens.[48]

Newer Agents in NSCLC or Targeted Therapy

Epidermal growth factor receptor (EGFR) is expressed in 40–80% of lung cancers, which makes this an attractive target for molecular intervention in this disease. Gefitinib and erlotinib were the first two agents to target the tyrosine kinase domain of EGFR. Both of these agents have activity in NSCLC.[34]

Initially, it was reported that nearly one-third of patients with NSCLC had overexpression of Her-2/neu.[35] It is becoming increasingly evident that the incidence of Her-2/neu overexpression is perhaps only around 10% in advanced NSCLC. The role of trastuzumab (Herceptin) as a single agent in patients with metastatic NSCLC is currently being studied by the CALGB group (Table 3).

Inhibition of COX-2 has been known to promote apoptosis, to inhibit cell growth and to be synergistic with chemotherapy.[36] Several phase I/II studies are ongoing to assess the role of specific COX-2 inhibitors in combination with chemotherapy and radiotherapy in NSCLC.

Chemotherapy Protocol for Lung Cancer Neoadjuvant and Adjuvant (NCCN 2014)

- *Cisplatin 75 mg/m^2 on day 1 and day 8*: Vinorelbine 25 mg/m^2 day 1, 8, 15, 22 and 28 × 4 cycles.
- *Cisplatin 100 mg/m^2 on day 1*: Vinorelbine 30 mg/m^2 day 1, 8, 15, 22 and 28 × 4 cycles.
- *Cisplatin 75 mg/m^2 IV on day 1*: Docetaxel 75 mg/m^2 IV on day 1 and 21 × 4 cycles.
- *Cisplatin 80 mg/m^2 IV on day 1*: Gemcitabine 1,250 mg/m^2 IV on days 1, 8 and day 21 × 4 cycle.
- *Cisplatin 75 mg/m^2 IV on day 1*: Pemetrexed 500 mg/m^2 day 1 for nonsquamous (without specific histology) every 21 days × 4 days.

If patient unable to tolerate cisplatin, paclitaxel 200 mg/m^2 IV on day 1: Carboplatin AUC 6, on day 1 and day 21 × 4 cycles.

Table 3 Common genetic alteration in lung cancer with available targeted agent

Genetic alteration	*Targeted agent*
EGFR mutation	Erlotinib, gefitinib
ALK mutation	Crizotinib, ceritinib
Her2/neu	Trastuzumab, afatinib
BRAF mutation	Vemurafenib
MET amplification	Crizotinib

Small Cell Lung Cancer

Small cell lung cancer differs from NSCLC in several biologic, clinical and therapeutic aspects. SCLC has a larger growth fraction, grows more rapidly, and more often has disseminated disease at diagnosis. The disease is characterized by large central tumors, and very few patients are asymptomatic at diagnosis. SCLC has a response rate of 60–80% to initial combination chemotherapy, but despite such high response rates, the overall long-term (5 years) survival is less than 10%.

Staging

The TNM staging system is typically not used in patients with SCLC because surgical resection is rarely considered once the diagnosis is established, but most lung cancer clinical trialists would prefer that this system be used.[37,38] SCLC patients are staged according to the two-stage classification originally developed by the Veterans Administration Lung Cancer Study Group, which categorizes patients into limited- or extensive-stage disease (Table 4).

Staging Procedures

The primary objectives of staging procedures are to define the stage of the disease and to evaluate patient's symptoms properly (Box 1). It is appropriate to terminate staging procedures once extensive stage has been established in

Table 4 Definition of limited- and extensive-stage for patients with small cell lung cancer

Stage	*Percent*
Limited Disease confined to one hemithorax with or without ipsilateral or contralateral mediastinal or supraclavicular lymph node metastasis and with or without ipsilateral pleural effusions independent of cytology	30–40%
Extensive: Any disease at sites beyond the definition of limited disease	60–70%

a patient. One possible exception is the evaluation of the brain for metastatic disease.

Box 1 Diagnostic procedures in small cell lung cancer

History and physical examination

Laboratory: Complete blood count, electrolytes, liver function, BUN, creatinine and LDH.

Radiological investigations

- CT scan of the thorax that includes liver and adrenals is necessary in patients with limited-stage disease to plan the radiation fields.
- Brain imaging (MRI with contrast enhancement is preferred).
- Whole body PET scan.

Required in certain patients

- Bone scan
- Bone marrow aspirate and biopsy (rare).

All patients should undergo CT scan evaluation of the chest that includes the adrenals and liver. CT scanning is superior to chest radiographs in evaluating the tumor extent and mediastinal involvement. CT scans are also necessary in patients with limited-stage disease to plan the radiation fields.

Brain is a common site of metastatic disease in SCLC and about 10% of the patients present with intracranial metastases at the first instance. In patients who are being considered for thoracic radiation or surgery, brain imaging should be performed to rule out asymptomatic metastases. MRI with contrast enhancement is more sensitive in detecting brain metastases than are CT scans, particularly with regard to posterior fossa lesions.[39]

Bone marrow is involved in about 20% of patients with SCLC at the time of initial diagnosis. Though bone marrow biopsies were routinely performed for staging SCLC patients in the past, many investigators have reported that a bone marrow examination changes the stage in fewer than 5% of SCLC patients. The general agreement is that a bone marrow examination is not required in patients with normal blood counts.[40] Almost 40% of patients have bone involvement on a radionuclide bone scan at diagnosis, although it is uncommon for bone to be the sole site of metastatic disease. A bone scan is essential in patients deemed to have limited-stage disease, as bone scans can reveal bony metastases in asymptomatic patients.

The role of PET scans in SCLC patients has been reported recently in studies with small numbers of patients. Hauber Schumacher and coworkers[41] reported on the use of PET scans among 26 SCLC patients for initial staging. PET scans upstaged seven patients from limited-stage disease to extensive disease, and all of the sites suspicious for tumor involvement on other staging modalities were also detected on PET scans. In the same study, six patients underwent PET scans after therapy. In one patient, PET scan suggested residual viability in the primary tumor when other staging studies did not detect any residual tumor. Another prospective trial studied the effect of FDG-PET on the staging of 102 patients with NSCLC (? SCLC) and found that the sensitivity, specificity, NPV and PPV of FDG-PET alone for the detection of mediastinal metastases were 91%, 86%, 95%, and 74%, respectively, as compared with CT scan alone, which had a sensitivity of 75% and a specificity of 66%.[42]

Paraneoplastic Syndromes

Paraneoplastic syndromes are more common in SCLC than in NSCLC. Many of the paraneoplastic syndromes are mediated by the production of peptide hormones or antibodies. The types of syndromes associated with SCLC are different from the ones observed in NSCLC. Thus, hypertrophic osteoarthropathy and hypercalcemia are uncommon in SCLC, while the syndrome of inappropriate antidiuretic hormone secretion (SIADH), Cushing's syndrome, or neurologic syndromes are by far more common in SCLC than NSCLC.

Approximately, 15% of SCLC patients present with hyponatremia, but only 5% of the patients are symptomatic for this condition. Ectopic production of arginine, vasopressin and atrial natriuretic factor (ANF) production causes hyponatremia and SIADH.[42] In some SCLC patients who do not have evidence of vasopressin production, hyponatremia is a result of ANF production. Cushing's syndrome is clinically apparent in about 5% of SCLC patients. Ectopic production of ACTH precursors is present in many SCLC tumors.

Prognostic Factors

Box 2 shows potential prognostic factors for survival in SCLC.

Box 2 Potential prognostic factors for survival in SCLC[43]

Poor prognostic factors

- Age more than 70 years
- Male gender
- Poor performance status
- Extensive stage
- Elevated LDH
- Multiple metastatic sites.

Albain and colleagues,[44] in an analysis of the Southwest Oncology Group (SWOG) database, found good performance status, age less than 70 years, female gender, white race and normal LDH as significant favorable predictors of survival in patients with limited-stage SCLC. Combined-modality therapy was also a strong predictor of survival. In extensive-stage SCLC, the presence of a single metastatic site and a normal LDH were favorable predictors of survival. Based on these analyses, patients could be classified into four groups with distinct survival outcomes. The best survival occurred in young patients with limited disease without effusion and a normal LDH. The poorest survival occurred in patients with extensive-stage disease and an elevated LDH.

Management

Early stage SCLC is diagnosed in fewer than 5% of SCLC patients. For patients with clinical stage I (T1–2, N0), complete resection with a lobectomy with mediastinal nodal dissection or sampling may be considered. However, mediastinoscopy should be performed to rule out occult nodal disease prior to resection. Postoperative chemotherapy should be considered even if surgical pathology shows no lymph node involvement. For patients with positive lymph node involvement after surgical resection, postoperative chemotherapy and radiotherapy should be considered. PCI should be considered in all cases.

Surgery in Small Cell Lung Cancer

With its propensity for early hematogenous spread, SCLC is a systemic disease that is rarely cured with surgical resection or radiation alone;[45] however, surgical resection followed by chemotherapy is reasonable for a subset of medically operable patients with a peripheral T1 N0 tumor. Phase II trials have demonstrated the feasibility of delivering neoadjuvant or adjuvant chemotherapy in SCLC.[46] However, the only phase III study, which has evaluated surgery after induction therapy in patients with local disease, SCLC failed to demonstrate an improvement in survival with the addition of surgery.[47] Therefore, surgery continues to have only a limited role in the treatment of SCLC.

Chemoradiation

Although early development of distant metastasis is a critical problem, intrathoracic failure becomes more important once distant metastasis is controlled. Two meta-analyses, using different methods, confirmed the value of thoracic irradiation to decrease local recurrence and to improve survival. The study by Warde and Payne,[48] based on results from 11 prospective randomized trials of chemotherapy with or without TRT, showed an absolute increase in overall survival of 5.4% at 2 years and in local control of 25% for patients with limited disease SCLC.

Concurrent Chemoradiation

The potential advantages from concurrent chemotherapy and RT are early use of both modalities, expectation and acceptance of greater toxicity, ability to plan RT more accurately, short overall treatment time (high-dose intensity) and possible sensitization of the tumor. The disadvantages are enhanced normal tissue toxicity (possible dose modification and/or possible treatment breaks) and an inability to assess response to either modality.

Concurrent chemotherapy (cyclophosphamide, doxorubicin, and vincristine) and thoracic radiotherapy was tried at the National Cancer Institute, which successfully treated patients with limited SCLC, although the mortality rate from the treatment was 20%.[49] Because of this high mortality, the use of concurrent TRT and doxorubicin was abandoned. McCracken et al.[50] reported results from a phase II trial of SWOG in which two courses of cisplatin, etoposide and vincristine were given with concurrent RT using one fraction of 1.8 Gy per day, 5 days per week, to a total dose of 45 Gy. Additional chemotherapy with vincristine, methotrexate and etoposide, alternating with doxorubicin and cyclophosphamide for 12 weeks, followed the concurrent therapy. They evaluated 154 patients; with a minimum period of observation of 3 years, the 2 years survival rate was 42% and the 4 years rate was 30%. Updated, this study showed a 5 years survival of 26%.

The National Cancer Institute of Canada clinical trial group[51] studied early versus late TRT in a randomized trial. Three hundred eight patients were randomized to receive early TRT, 40 Gy in 15 fractions during 3 weeks to the primary site with concurrent etoposide and cisplatin at week 3, or to receive late thoracic irradiation at week 15 with the same RT dose and concurrent chemotherapy. After completion of all chemotherapy and TRT, complete responders received PCI, 25 Gy in 10 fractions during 2 weeks. Although complete response rates did not significantly differ between the early and late TRT groups, progression-free survival ($p = 0.036$) and overall survival ($p = 0.008$) were significantly better in the early radiation group. Patients in the late thoracic radiation group had significantly higher rates of brain metastases ($p = 0.006$). This study indicated that the early administration of TRT with concurrent chemotherapy improved survival, possibly by reducing the few last clonogens in the primary.

The Japanese Clinical Oncology Group (JCOG)[52] reported a prospective randomized study for patients with limited SCLC treated by sequential or concurrent chemotherapy; 231 patients younger than 75 years of age with limited SCLC and good performance status were enrolled. Chemotherapy consisted of paclitaxel, 80 mg/m^2 on day 1 and etoposide, 100 mg/m^2 on days 1 through 3 every 3 weeks. RT consisted of 45 Gy twice daily; the concurrent arm started chemotherapy and TRT on day 1 and the sequential arm started TRT after two cycles of chemotherapy. Chemotherapy was given for four cycles. Their data showed significant improvement of survival with concurrent chemoradiotherapy compared with sequential chemotherapy and radiotherapy.

Radiation Therapy Dose and Fractionation

This concept of altered fractionation was tested in an intergroup study that randomized patients to 45 Gy in 25 fractions over 5 weeks or 45 Gy delivered in twice-daily 1.5 Gy fractions over 3 weeks.[53] Patients in both arms received concurrent cisplatin and etoposide. The accelerated radiation arm demonstrated a significant improvement in survival, with 5-year survivals of 26% compared with 16% (p = 0.04) in patients who received conventional fractionation. Intrathoracic failure rate was higher for patients in the conventional fractionation arm (52% vs 36%, p = 0.06). The rate of esophagitis, toxicity not influenced by dose per fraction, was higher in the twice-daily arm (26% vs 11%, p = 0.001).

The other phase III study comparing twice-daily to once-daily radiation was conducted by the North Central Cancer Treatment Group (NCCTG).[54] This trial differed in two major ways from the intergroup study. The RT in both arms was administered starting with the fourth cycle. The other difference was that the patients in the hyperfractionated arm received RT in split course, with a planned 2 weeks break after 24 Gy, while the control arm received the RT without a break. In this study, there was no difference in survival between the twice-daily radiation arm and the control arm of conventional radiation. It is quite likely that the delayed start of the radiation and split-course therapy in the experimental arm lead to negative results.

Most radiation oncologists plan to deliver 60–64 Gy, in single daily fractions of 1.8 Gy to 2.0 Gy in limited-stage SCLC. Currently, it is unclear whether twice-daily radiation to a dose of 45 Gy is superior to conventional fractionation to a dose of 64 Gy. Twice-daily radiation does have practical limitations, such as greater time commitment on the part of the patient. Such considerations have limited the wider use of the twice-daily radiation treatment plans.

Prophylactic Cranial Radiation and Brain Metastases

Brain metastases are a substantial source of morbidity and mortality in patients with SCLC. In earlier studies, the observed rate of brain metastases was 20%. With the introduction of better imaging modalities, rates as high as 50% have been reported at 2–3 years. Chemotherapeutic agents have limited efficacy in preventing brain metastases, as they are unable to cross the blood-brain barrier. This observation led to the proposal of prophylactic cranial irradiation to prevent brain metastases.[55] Early studies of prophylactic cranial radiation (PCI) suggested a reduction in brain metastases, but there did not appear to be a survival benefit. Further, the benefits observed with PCI were limited, in these early studies, to patients who had complete remission after induction therapy.[56]

Prophylactic cranial radiation does appear to be beneficial in patients with SCLC who are in complete remission. In prospective studies, PCI does not appear to increase neurocognitive dysfunction for at least 2 years after PCI. PCI should not be administered concurrently with chemotherapy, as it appears to increase neurocognitive dysfunction. The optimum dose of PCI is unclear, but based on retrospective analyses, a dose of 20–30 Gy at 2.0 Gy/fraction appears to be effective (Fig. 7).

The recommendations for curative dose schedules for SCLC are as follows:

- 40 Gy in 15 daily fractions of 2.67 Gy given in 3 weeks, or
- 64 Gy in 32 daily fractions given in 61/2 weeks, or
- 45 Gy in 30 fractions of 1.5 Gy, treating twice daily, given in 3 weeks.

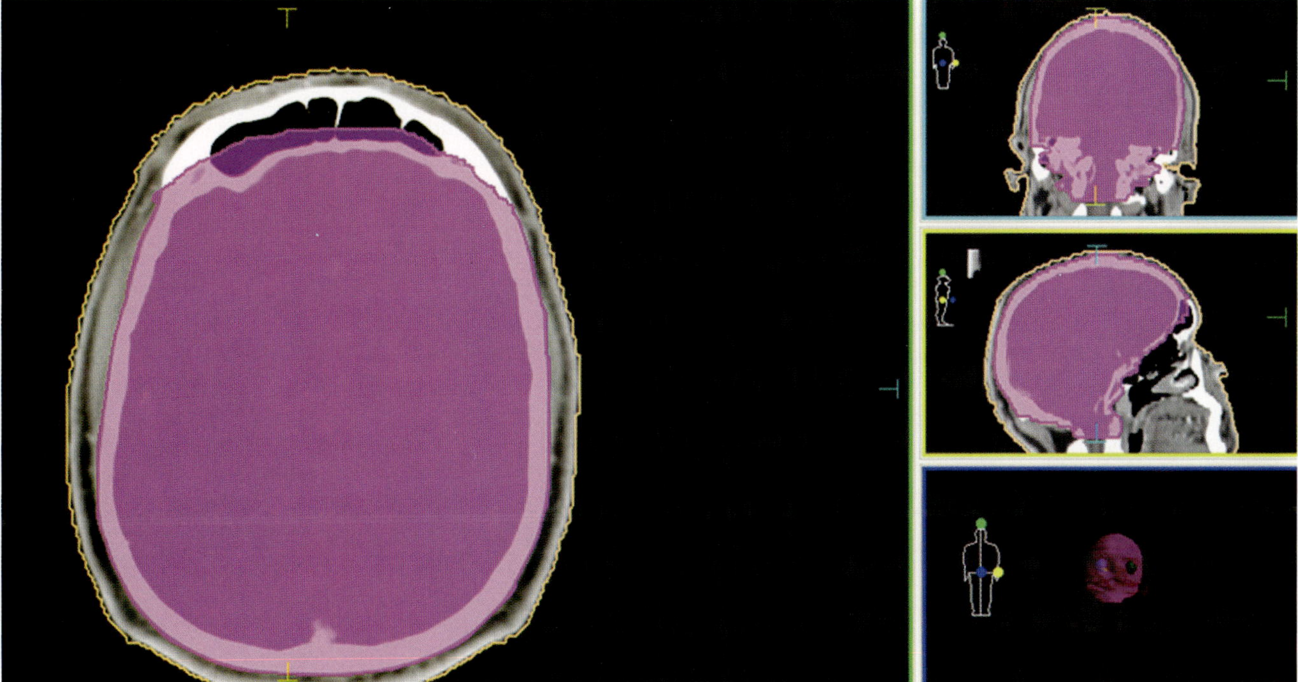

Fig. 7 Target volume for prophylactic cranial irradiation

Courtesy: Dr Tejinder Kataria, Division of Radiation Oncology, Medanta—The Medicity, Haryana, India

Tyrosine Kinase Inhibitors (Targeted Therapy)

Tyrosine kinases (TKs) are enzymes associated with trans-membrane growth receptors. These growth receptors and the associated TKs are overexpressed in many cancers and are involved in cancer cell growth, invasion, angiogenesis and anti-apoptosis. C-kit is a growth receptor that appears to have a role in SCLC proliferation. Some studies have reported C-kit expression in 70% of patients with SCLC, though other studies have found lower expression.[59] Imatinib mesylate inhibits the TK associated with C-kit, and this inhibition has demonstrated therapeutic benefits in gastrointestinal stromal tumors. Imatinib has shown growth inhibition of SCLC cell lines, and this inhibition correlates with inhibition of C-kit TK.[60] A phase II study of imatinib in SCLC patients has been reported. Nineteen patients who were either chemotherapy naive or had sensitive relapse were treated with imatinib; no responses were observed. In retrospective analyses, only four patients had C-kit positive tumor. Other studies are evaluating imatinib in combination with chemotherapy and as maintenance therapy after chemotherapy. Newer drugs that more potently inhibit C-kit are currently undergoing testing. Other TKs, such as C-met, are also being considered as potential targets.[61]

Antibody-based Therapy

In vitro data suggests that peptides such as gastrin releasing peptide can participate in an autocrine growth loop in small cell lung cancer.[62] Thus, targeting such peptides could have therapeutic effect in SCLC. Monoclonal antibody 2A11 was shown to inhibit the binding of gastrin releasing peptide to cellular receptors, with growth inhibition of SCLC in preclinical models.[63] In a phase II study of previously treated patients with SCLC, one of 12 evaluable patients responded completely. Four patients had stable disease. Further testing has been halted due to production issues. Similar antibodies are being evaluated against other targets such as cell surface antigen NKH-1.

Antisense Bcl-2: Bcl-2 is commonly overexpressed in SCLC. Bcl-2 inhibits apoptosis and might contribute to chemotherapy resistance. This is particularly important in refractory or relapsed tumors. Antisense oligonucleotides inhibit the translation of mRNA and thus suppress cellular protein levels. Genasense is a bcl-2 antisense oligonucleotide. Rudin and colleagues[64] treated 12 patients with refractory SCLC with a combination of Genasense and paclitaxel. No objective responses were observed, but 2 of the 12 patients had stable disease. Further evaluation of this agent is ongoing.

Bevacizumab (avastin) is a recombinant monoclonal antibody that blocks vascular endothelial growth factor. On the basis of phase II/III clinical trials, the Eastern Cooperative Oncology Group (ECOG 4599) recommends bevacizumab in combination of paclitaxel and carboplatin as a new treatment for patients with stage IV nonsquamous NSCLC.

Commonly used Chemotherapy Schedules for Lung Cancer

First line

Etoposide	120 mg/m^2 IV on days 1–3 or 120 mg/m^2 PO BID on days 1–3
Cisplatin	60 mg/m^2 IV on day 1
or	
Cisplatin	25 mg/m^2 IV on days 1–3
Etoposide	100 mg/m^2 IV on days 1–3 Repeat cycle every 3 weeks
Carboplatin-based regimens	
Carboplatin	300 mg/m^2 IV on day 1
Etoposide	100 mg/m^2 IV on days 1–3
or	
Carboplatin	100 mg/m^2 IV on days 1–3
Etoposide	120 mg/m^2 IV on days 1–3 Repeat cycle every 4 weeks
Irinotecan plus cisplatin	
Irinotecan	60 mg/m^2 IV on days 1, 8 and 15
Cisplatin	60 mg/m^2 IV on day 1 Repeat cycle every 4 weeks

Note: The optimal duration of treatment for SCLC is 4–6 cycles with interposition of concurrent chemoradiation after the second cycle or upfront for limited-stage disease. The schedules given above are only recommendations and readers are encouraged to review the administration, toxicity and management of toxicity with the chemotherapeutic literature.

The recommended schedules for palliative radiation to bone metastases are:

- 10 Gy in 1 fraction.
- 16 Gy in 2 fractions of 8 Gy a week apart (the dose has been reduced from 17 Gy in 2 fractions to minimize the risk of spinal cord damage if survival is prolonged).

Use of stereotactic body radiation (SBRT) is recommended wherever possible to reduce delays in continuation of chemotherapy.

Prophylactic cranial irradiation: 20–30 Gy in daily fractions of 2 Gy fraction given in 2–3 weeks.

REFERENCES

1. Lu JJ, Brady LW. Decision making in radiation oncology, Berlin: Springer-Verlag Berlin Heidelberg; 2011.
2. Ahmedin J, Ram CT, Taylor M, et al. Cancer statistics 2010. CA Cancer J Clin. 2010;54:8-29.
3. Thun MJ, Henley SJ, Burns D, Jemal A, Shanks TG, Calle EE, et al. Lung cancer death rates in lifelong nonsmokers. J Natl Cancer Inst. 2006;98(10):691-9.
4. Alberg AJ, Samet JM. Epidemiology of lung cancer. Chest 2003;123(1 Suppl):21S.

5. Syrigos Konstantinos N, Nutting Christopher M, Roussos Charalambos I. Tumors of the Chest. New York, Berlin: Springer; 2006. pp 4-13.
6. Brambilla E, Travis WD, Colby TV, et al. The new World Health Organization classification of lung tumours. Eur Respir J. 2001;18:1059-68.
7. Tokuda Y, Maezato K, Stein GH. The causes of hypercalcemia in Okinawan patients: an international comparison. Intern Med. 2007;46(1):23-8.
8. Yang WC, Lin SC, Liu TC, Chen CJ, Yen JH, Ou TT, et al. Clubbed fingers and hypertrophic osteoarthropathy in a patient with squamous cell carcinoma of the lung. Kaohsiung J Med Sci. 2003;19(4):183-7.
9. Müssig K, Horger M, Häring HU, et al. Syndrome of inappropriate antidiuretic hormone secretion and ectopic ACTH production in small cell lung carcinoma. Lung Cancer. 2007;57(1):120-2.
10. Muscolino G, Valente M, Andreani S. Pancoast tumours: clinical assessment and longterm results of combined radiosurgical treatment. Thorax. 1997;52(3):284-6.
11. Gamez C, Rosell R, Fernandez A, Andia E, Arnaiz MD, Cardenal F, et al. PET/CT fusion scan in lung cancer: current recommendations and innovations. J Thorac Oncol. 2006;1(1):74.
12. Fritscher-Ravens A, Bohuslavizki KH, Brandt L, Bobrowski C, Lund C, Knöfel WT, et al. Mediastinal lymph node involvement in potentially resectable lung cancer: comparison of CT, positron emission tomography, and endoscopic ultrasonography with and without fine-needle aspiration. Chest. 2003;123(2):442.
13. AJCC. Lung. In: Edge SB, Byrd DR, Compton CC, Fritz AG, Greene FL, Trotti A, (Eds). AJCC Cancer Staging Manual, 7th edition. New York: Springer; 2010. pp 253-66.
14. Stanley K. Prognostic factors for survival in patients with inoperable lung cancer. J Natl Cancer Inst. 1980;65:25-32.
15. Ginsberg RJ, Rubinstein LV. Randomized trial of lobectomy versus limited resection for T1N0 non-small-cell lung cancer. Lung Cancer Study Group. Ann Thorac Surg. 1995;60:615-22.
16. Onishi H, Kuriyama K, Komiyama T, Tanaka S, Sano N, Marino K, et al. Clinical outcomes of stereotactic radiotherapy for stage I non-small cell lung cancer using a novel irradiation technique: patient self-controlled breath-hold and beam switching using a combination of linear accelerator and CT scanner. Lung Cancer. 2004;45:45-55.
17. Onishi H, Shirato H, Nagata Y, Hiraoka M, Fujino M, Gomi K, et al. Hypofractionated stereotactic radiotherapy (HypoFXSRT) for stage I non-small cell lung cancer: updated results of 257 patients in a Japanese multi-institutional study. J Thorac Oncol. 2007;7:S94-100.
18. Timmerman R, Paulus R, Galvin J, Michalski J, Straube W, Bradley J, et al. Stereotactic body radiation therapy for medically inoperable early stage lung cancer patients: analysis of RTOG 0236. Presented at ASTRO, November, 2009; Chicago.
19. Mountain C, Dresler C. Regional lymph node classification for lung cancer staging. Chest. 1997;111:1718-23.
20. Trakhtenerg A, Kiseleva E, Pitskhelauri V. Preoperative radiotherapy in the combined treatment of lung cancer patients. Neoplasma. 1988;35:459-65.
21. Holmes E. Surgical adjuvant therapy of non-small cell lung cancer. Chest. 1986;89:295-300.
22. Rosell R, Gomez-Codina J, Camps C, Maestre J, Padille J, Canto A, et al. A randomized trial comparing preoperative chemotherapy plus surgery with surgery alone in patients with non-small-cell lung cancer. N Engl J Med. 1994;330:153-8.
23. Port Meta-analysis Trialists Group. Postoperative radiotherapy in nonsmall cell lung cancer: systematic review and meta-analysis of individual patient data from nine randomised clinical trials. Lancet. 1998;352:257-63.
24. Keller S, Adak S, Wagner H, Herskovic A, Komaki R, Brooks BJ, et al. A randomized trial of postoperative adjuvant therapy in patients with completely resected stage II or IIIa non-small-cell lung cancer. N Engl J Med. 2000;343:1217-22.
25. Bradley J, Paulus R, Graham M, Ettinger DS, Johnstone DW, Pilepich MV, et al. Phase II trial of postoperative adjuvant paclitaxel/carboplatin and thoracic radiotherapy in resected stage II and IIIa non-small-cell lung cancer: promising long-term results of the Radiation Therapy Oncology Group RTOG 9705. J Clin Oncol. 2005;23:3480-7.
26. Perez C, Stanley K, Rubin P, Kramer S, Brady L, Perez-Tamayo R, et al. A prospective randomized study of various irradiation doses and fractionation schedules in the treatment of inoperable non oat-cell carcinoma of the lung. Preliminary report by the Radiation Therapy Oncology Group. Cancer. 1980;45:2744-53.
27. Bradley J, Graham M, Winter K, Purdy JA, Komaki R, Roa WH, et al. Toxicity and outcome results of RTOG 9311: a phase I-II dose-escalation study using three-dimensional conformal radiotherapy in patients with inoperable non-small-cell lung carcinoma. Int J Radiat Oncol Biol Phys. 2005;61:318-28.
28. Mehta MP, Tannehill SP, Adak S, Martin L, Petereit DG, Wagner H, et al. Phase II trial of hyperfractionated accelerated radiation therapy for nonresectable non-small-cell lung cancer: results of Eastern Cooperative Oncology Group 4593. J Clin Oncol. 1998;16:3518-23.
29. Schuster-Uitterhoeve A, Hulshof M, Gonzalez G, et al. Feasibility of curative radiotherapy with a concomitant boost technique in 33 patients with non-small cell lung cancer (NSCLC). Radiother Oncol. 1993;28:247-51.
30. Giaccone G, Postmus P, Splinter T, Diaz-Puente M, Van Zandwijk N, Ardizzoni A, et al. Cisplatin/paclitaxel vs cisplatin/teniposide for advanced non-small-cell lung cancer. The EORTC lung cancer cooperative group. The European organization for research and treatment of cancer. Oncology. 1997;11:11-4.
31. Sause W, Kolesar P, Taylor SIV, Johnson D, Livingston R, Komaki R, et al. Final results of phase III trial in regionally advanced unresectable non-small cell lung cancer: Radiation Therapy Oncology Group, Eastern Cooperative Oncology Group, and Southwest Oncology Group. Chest. 2000;117:358-64.
32. Curran W, Scott C, Langer C, et al. Long term benefit is observed in a phase III comparison of sequential vs concurrent chemo-radiation for patients with unresectable NSCLC:RTOG 9410. Proc Am Soc Clin Oncol. 2003;61.
33. Fournel P, Robinet G, Thomas P, Souquet PJ, Léna H, Vergnenégre A, et al. Randomized Phase III trial of

sequential chemoradiotherapy compared with concurrent chemoradiotherapy in locally advanced non-small-cell lung cancer: Groupe Lyon-Saint-Etienne d'Oncologie Thoracique Groupe Francais de Pneumo-Cancerologie NPC 95-01 Study. J Clin Oncol. 2005;23:5910-7.
34. Roman Perex Solar A, Huberman M, Karp D, et al. A phase II trial of the epidermal growth factor receptor (EGFR) tyrosine kinase inhibitor OSI-774, following platinum-based chemotherapy, in patients (pst) with advanced, EGFR-expressing, non-small cell lung cancer (NSCLC). Proc Am Soc Clin Oncol. 2001.
35. Scheurle D, Jahanzeb M, Aronsohn R, et al. HER-2/neu expression in archival non-small cell lung carcinomas using FDA-approved Hercep test. Anticancer Res. 2000;20:2091-6.
36. Stolina M, Sharma S, LIn Y Dohadwala M, Gardner B, Luo J, et al. Specific inhibition of cyclooxygenase 2 restores antitumor reactivity by altering the balance of IL-10 and IL-12 synthesis. J Immunol. 2000;164: 361-70.
37. Mountain C. Revisions in the international system for staging lung cancer. Chest. 1997;111:1710.
38. Zelen M. Keynote address on biostatistics and data retrieval. Cancer Chemother Rep. 1973;4(2):31-42.
39. Davis PC, Hudgins PA, Peterman SB, et al. Diagnosis of cerebral metastases: Double dose delayed CT vs contrast-enhanced MR imaging. Am J Neuroradiol. 1991;12:293.
40. Levitan N, Byrne RE, Bromer RH, Faling LJ, Caslowitz P, Pattern DH, et al. The value of the bone scan and bone marrow biopsy staging small cell lung cancer. Cancer. 1985;56:652.
41. Schumacher T, Brink I, Mix M, Reinhardt M, Herget G, Digel W, et al. FDG-PET imaging for the staging and follow up of small cell lung cancer. Eur J Nucl Med. 2001;28:483.
42. Pieterman R, van Putten J, Meuzelaar J, Mooyaart EL, Vaalburg W, Koeter GH, et al. Preoperative staging of non-small-cell lung cancer with positron-emission tomography. N Engl J Med. 2000;343:254-61.
43. Cerny T, Blair V, Anderson H, et al. Pretreatment prognostic factors and scoring system in 407 small cell lung cancer patients. Int J Cancer. 1987;15:146-9.
44. Albain KS, Crowley JJ, LeBlanc M, et al. Determinants of improved outcome in small cell lung cancer: An analysis of the 2,580-patient Southwest Oncology Group Database. J Clin Oncol. 1990;8:1563-74.
45. Kataria T, Gupta D, Bisht SS, Karthikeyan N, Goyal S, Pushpan L, et al. Adaptive radiotherapy in lung cancer: dosimetric benefits and clinical outcome. Br J Radiol. 2014;87:20130643.
46. Timmerman R, Paulus R, Galvin J, Michalski J, Straube W, Bradley J, et al. Stereotactic body radiation therapy for inoperable early stage lung cancer. JAMA. 2010;303(11):1070-6.
47. Chemotherapy in non-small cell lung cancer: a meta-analysis using updated data on individual patients from 52 randomised clinical trials. Non-small Cell Lung Cancer Collaborative Group. BMJ. 1995;311(7010):899-909.
48. Jimm Grimm, Tamara LaCouture, Raymond Croce, Inhwan Yeo, Yunping Zhu, Jinyu Xue. Dose tolerance limits and dose volume histogram evaluation for stereotactic body radiotherapy. J Appl Clin Med Phys. 2011:12(2);267-92.
49. Behera D. Epidemiology of lung cancer–Global and Indian perspective. JIACM. 2012;13(2):131-7.
50. McCracken JD, Janaki LM, Crowley JJ, et al. Concurrent chemotherapy/radiotherapy for limited small-cell lung carcinoma: a Southwest Oncology Group Study. J Clin Oncol 1990; 8:892-8.
51. Murray N, Coy P, Pater JL, et al. Importance of timing for thoracic irradiation in the combined modality treatment of limited-stage small-cell lung cancer. The National Cancer Institute of Canada Clinical Trials Group. J Clin Oncol 1993; 11:336-44.
52. Goto K, Nishiwaki Y, Takasa M. Final results of a phase III study of concurrent versus sequential thoracic radiotherapy (TRT) in combination with cisplatin (P) and etopside (E) for limited-stage small-cell lung cancer (LD-SCLC): the Japan Clinical Oncology Group (JCOG) study. Proc Am Soc Clin Oncol 1999; 18:468(abstr).
53. Turrisi AT, Kim K, Blum R, et al: Twice-daily compared with once-daily thoracic radiotherapy in limited small-cell lung cancer treated concurrently with cisplatin and etoposide. N Eng J Med 1999; 340:265.
54. Bonner JA, Sloan JA, Shanahan TG, et al. Phase III comparison of twice-daily split-course irradiation versus once-daily irradiation for patients with limited stage small-cell lung carcinoma. J Clin Oncol 1999; 17:2681.
55. Rosen ST, Makuch RW, Lichter AS, et al. Role of prophylactic cranial irradiation in prevention of central nervous system metastases in SCLC: Potential benefit restricted to patients in complete response. Am J Med 1983;74:615.
56. Arriagada R, Le Chevalier T, Borie F, et al: Prophylactic cranial irradiation for patients with small-cell lung cancer in complete remission. J Natl Cancer Inst 1995; 87:183.
57. Michael M, Babic B, Khokha R, et al. Expression and prognostic significance of metalloproteinases and their tissue inhibitors in patients with small-cell lung cancer. J Clin Oncol 1999; 17:1802.
58. Shepherd F, Giaccone G, Debruyne C, et al. Randomized double-blind placebo-controlled trial of marimastat in patients with small cell lung cancer (SCLC) following response to first-line chemotherapy: An NCIC-CTG and EORTC study. Proc Am Soc Clin Oncol 2001; 20:4a.
59. Sekido Y, Obata Y, Ueda R, et al. Preferential expression of c-kit protooncogene transcripts in small cell lung cancer. Cancer Res 1999; 51:2416.
60. Krystal GW, Honsawek S, Litz J, et al: The selective tyrosine kinase inhibitor STI571 inhibits small cell lung cancer growth. Clin Cancer Res 2000; 6:3319.
61. Johnson BE, Fisher B, Fisher T, et al. A phase II study of STI571 (Gleevec) for patients with small cell lung cancer. Proc Am Soc Clin Oncol 2002; 21:293a.
62. Cuttitta F, Carney DC, Mulshine J, et al. Bombesin-like peptides can function as autocrine growth factors in human small-cell lung cancer. Nature 1985; 316:823.
63. Kelley MJ, Linnoila I, Avis IL, et al. Antitumor activity of a monoclonal antibody directed against gastrin-releasing peptide in patients with small cell lung cancer. Chest 1997; 112:256.
64. Rudin C, Otterson GA, George CM, et al. A phase I/II trial of genasense and paclitaxel in chemorefractory small cell lung cancer. Proc Am Soc Clin Oncol 2001; 20:322a.

15

CHAPTER

Carcinoma of Esophagus

Trinanjan Basu, Tejinder Kataria

INTRODUCTION

Esophageal cancer is unique among the gastrointestinal tract malignancies because it embodies two distinct histopathologic types, squamous cell carcinoma and adenocarcinoma. In Western world adenocarcinoma and in developing countries squamous cell carcinoma being the predominant subtype respectively.

India has an age-standardized incidence rate (ASR) of 6.5 per 100,000 male population and 4.2 per 100,000 female population. This translates into approximately 47,000 new cases each year and 42,000 deaths.[1] As per cancer cases projection data, in India by 2020 esophageal cancers will be the second most common gastrointestinal (GI) tract malignancies accounting for about 20% of digestive tract cancers.[2]

ETIOLOGY

The etiological factors related to carcinoma esophagus are described in Table 1.[3-5]

Table 1 Etiological factors related to carcinoma esophagus

Type	*Description*
Patient related	*Lifestyle related:* Smoking is a dose-dependent risk factor and alcohol consumption is an independent risk factor. The majority are squamous cell carcinoma (SCC). Diet rich in vegetables, fruits, fish, and poultry are protective. Typical Western diets low in vitamins and high in red meats are risk factors. Tylosis and Plummer-Vinson syndromes predispose to SCC of the esophagus.
Disease related	*Gastroesophageal reflux disorder and Barrett's esophagitis:* Leading to dysplasia and invasive malignancy. Infectious agents like *Helicobacter pylori* are not known to contribute to esophageal cancers (possibly protective because of atrophic gastritis). Conditions like achalasia, esophageal diverticuli, esophageal webs, and history of squamous cell cancers of the head and neck, due to field cancerization effect.
Environmental exposures	Injury from dye ingestion.

Abbreviations: GERD, gastroesophageal reflux disease; GEJ, gastroesophageal junction.

APPLIED ANATOMY

Three compartments like neck, thorax, and abdomen and are in close association to esophagus. It extends from the cricopharyngeus muscle at the level of the cricoid cartilage to the gastroesophageal (GE) junction. The average length is 25 cm and relative to the incisors, the cervical esophagus spans from 15 cm to 18 cm, the upper thoracic from 18 cm to 24 cm, the midthoracic from 24 cm to 32 cm, and the lower thoracic from 32 cm to 40 cm.

Esophagus has four layers: mucosa with stratified squamous epithelium, submucosa, muscularis propria, and adventitia, but no serosa; hence, it has no barriers to limit locoregional spread. It is drained by a rich network of submucosal lymphatics draining to regional lymph nodes in the cervical, mediastinal, paraesophageal, left gastric, and celiac axis regions. The predominant histological variety is squamous cell carcinoma and adenocarcinoma predominates in the distal esophagus. Adenocarcinomas of the GE junction present a unique challenge as appropriate management of these tumors as either esophageal or gastric cancers has been uncertain. There is Siewert classification which is depending upon demographics, histopathologic variables along with patterns of lymphatic spread and it gives us clarity and is well-established and accepted globally. Type I tumors are adenocarcinomas of the distal esophagus whereas type II and III lesions are classified as gastric cancers (cardia and subcardia). This classification system tailored surgical approach as well as consistency in reporting outcome results after therapeutic interventions.[6]

Lymphatic drainage of the esophagus is important to understanding how the numerous surgical approaches for esophageal cancer have evolved. Tumors of the cervical and upper third of the thoracic esophagus draining into cervical and superior mediastinal lymph nodes whereas middle third of the esophagus tumors draining both cephalad and caudal with lymph nodes at risk being the paratracheal, hilar, subcarinal, periesophageal, and pericardial nodal basins. Lesions in the distal esophagus primarily drain into lower mediastinum and celiac axis region. With this extensive lymphatic network and rich mucosal and submucosal lymphatics inside the wall of the esophagus, skip metastases for upper third lesions have been noted in celiac axis nodal basins. Similarly cervical lymph node metastases have been noted in about 30% of patients with distal esophageal lesions. The basis for extended lymphadenectomy has been derived from this lymphatic spread pattern (Fig. 1).[7,8]

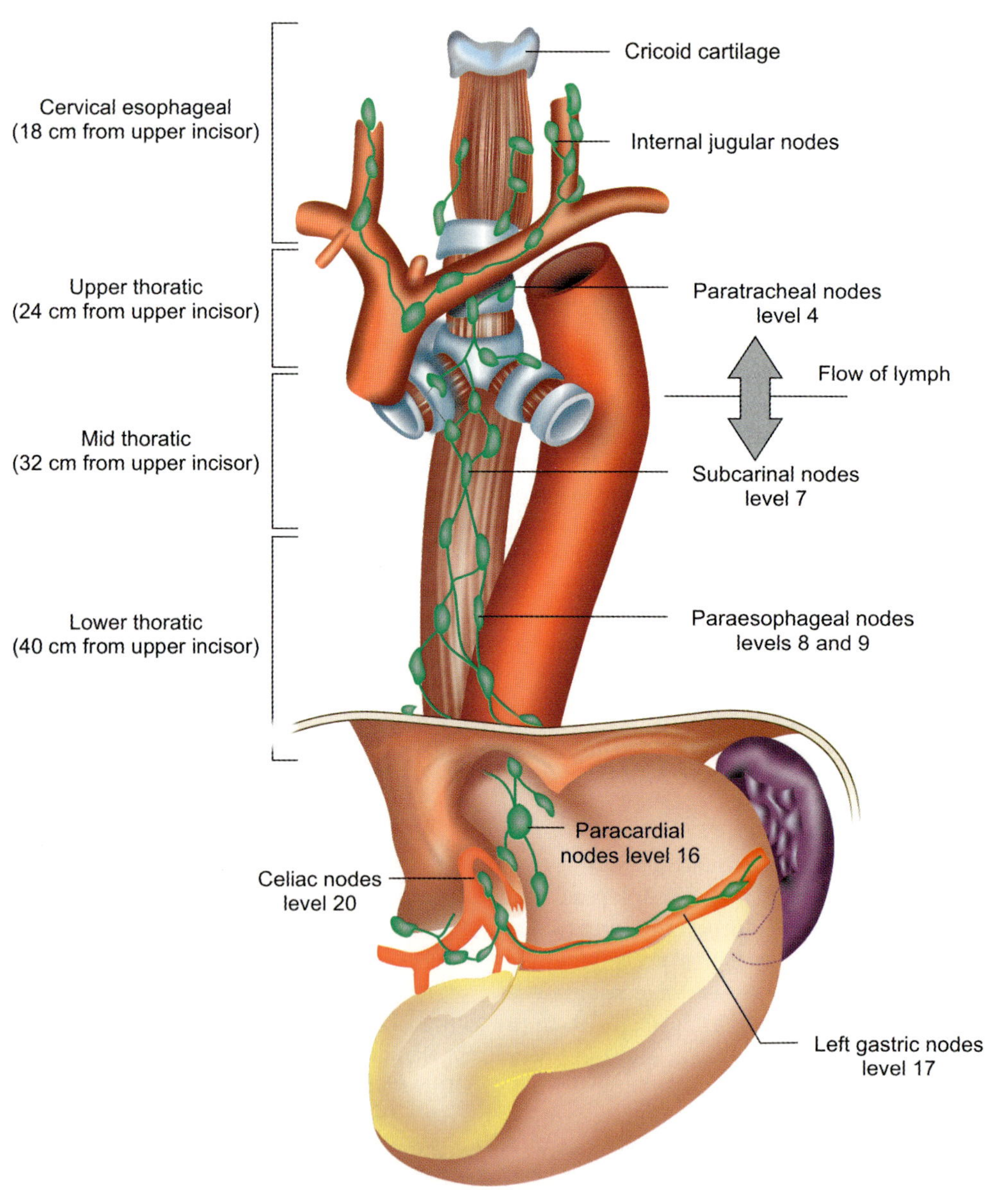

Fig. 1 Anatomical relations of different parts of esophagus

PATTERNS OF SPREAD

The three major routes of spread being local extension, regional (lymphatic), and distant (hematogenous) metastases (Table 2).

DIAGNOSTIC STAGING

Complete history, physical examination, and diagnostic imaging and laboratory tests are required for the proper diagnosis and staging of esophageal cancer. Table 3 summarizes the workup for esophageal cancer.

STAGING

Tumor, node, metastasis (TNM) staging is based on clinical examination and information obtained by imaging: Computed tomography (CT) scan/positron emission tomography-computed tomography (PET-CT) and/or endoscopic ultrasonography (EUS).

Complete history and physical examination regarding the following are important:

- The common symptoms are dysphagia and weight loss. Patients usually describe progressive dysphagia, with difficulty initially to solids and then liquids and in extreme cases to their own saliva as well. In most cases, dysphagia signifies locally advanced disease or distant metastases, or both.
- There is substantial weight loss with dysphagia in approximately 90% of patients with squamous cell carcinoma and mostly arise among lower socioeconomic status. Patients with adenocarcinoma tend to be from middle to upper socioeconomic classes where overweight, history of symptomatic GE reflux and treatment for the above been noted. There is 20% chance of odynophagia accompanying these symptoms.
- Additionally dull retrosternal pain resulting from invasion of mediastinal structures, bone pain secondary to bone metastases, and cough or hoarseness secondary to paratracheal nodal or recurrent laryngeal nerve involvement can also be seen.
- Very rarely pneumonia secondary to tracheoesophageal fistula or exsanguinating hemorrhage due to aortic invasion are also reported.

Table 2 Patterns of spread in carcinoma esophagus

Type	*Description*
Local extension	Lack of serosa permits local extension. Disease can spread locally to invade organs/structures such as the pericardium and heart, trachea, and vertebral bodies.
Regional lymph node metastasis	Paraesophageal lymph node drainage is the first-echelon lymph node. Regional lymph node spread depends on location of the primary disease like below: *Cervical esophagus*: Supraclavicular and cervical nodes. *Thoracic esophagus*: Mediastinal nodal spread is common (paratracheal, subcarinal). *Distal esophagus*: Left gastric and celiac axis nodes.
Distant metastasis	Lung, liver and bone being most common sites and it is much more common in adenocarcinoma.

Table 3 Diagnostic workup in carcinoma esophagus

Type	*Description*
Procedures	*Barium swallow*: Though very basic but can visualize areas of obstruction or fistula. The classic appearance being "Rat tail deformity" with hold-up of barium above growth. Extravasation of barium may indicate fistulous communication. *Esophagogastroduodenoscopy*: Direct visualization of tumor, estimation of distance from incisor teeth an approximate size and aid in diagnostic biopsy. *Endoscopic ultrasound (EUS)*: Assessment for depth of invasion and lymph node involvement. *Fiberoptic bronchoscopy*: For upper and middle thoracic esophagus to rule out tracheal or bronchial involvement.
Imaging studies	*CECT thorax and abdomen*: Accurate assessment of local spread, nodal involvement and to rule our distant metastases. *FDG-PET scan*: Primary disease extent, to rule out metastatic disease and response evaluation after treatment. Can detect occult metastasis in about 15% cases.

DIAGNOSTIC INVESTIGATIONS

- *Barium swallow*: This in most cases is the first investigation among patients presenting with dysphagia. It gives information about:
  - Site
  - Length of lesion
  - Morphology (proliferative/stricturous/ulcerative or combination)
  - Extraesophageal spread (axis deviation, sinuses and fistulation).

However, its clinical utility is questionable as a diagnostic tool as all patients with dysphagia warrant an upper gastrointestinal endoscopy regardless of the barium swallow. More importantly, there is a danger of a "normal" barium swallow missing early esophageal cancers. It does not give any additional information beyond what would be obtained from a good endoscopy.

- *Esophagoscopy*: Fiberoptic esophagoscopy is essential for biopsy or cytology.

STAGING INVESTIGATIONS[9]

- Positron emission tomography-contrast enhanced computed tomography (PET-CECT)
- CECT thorax and abdomen
- Endoscopic ultrasonography
- Fiberoptic bronchoscopy (in selected cases).

CT scan and EUS are complimentary while assessing the lateral extension of disease and lymph node status. EUS scores over CT scan while assessing the depth of tumor invasion, particularly in early stage cancer, and status of regional lymph nodes. However, when there is stricture formation EUS may not always be possible. CT scan is equally accurate in assessment of T3/T4 lesions; abdominal CT scan can additionally screen liver and celiac lymph nodes. Bronchoscopy is an essential investigation for documenting presence or absence of tracheobronchial or esophageal fistulous communication.

Role of EUS[10,11]

- EUS is used for refining locoregional staging and hence should be employed after exclusion of distant metastasis. EUS should be performed by experienced endosonographers.
- Assessment of stenosed tumors should be done using the slim blind tapered probe positioned over a guidewire.[12]
- The use of high frequency EUS catheter probes (20–30 MHz) increases the accuracy for T1 and T2 tumors.[13]
- For T4 stage, EUS had a pooled sensitivity of 92.4% and specificity of 97.4%. With EUS guided fine needle aspiration (FNA), the sensitivity of EUS to diagnose N stage cancer improved from 84.7% to 96.7%, while the specificity of EUS improved from 84.6% to 95.5%.[14]
- Residual inflammation, edema and fibrosis after chemotherapy and radiation makes EUS performance lower for both T and N staging for restaging after neoadjuvant therapy as compared to primary stage evaluation. The T stage accuracy ranges from 27% to 82% and N stage accuracy ranges from 38% to 73%.[15]
- Accuracy of EUS for more than 50% regression in the tumor's maximum transverse cross sectional area after 18 days post-therapy has been used as a marker of response to chemotherapy and chemoradiation and correlates with pathological regression.[16,17]

Role of PET-CECT

Staging

Positron-emission tomography (PET) provides incremental staging information and can lead to management change in a significant number of patients, especially when combined with CT scan (PET-CT).[18] PET can avoid potentially futile thoracotomies by detecting metastatic disease not diagnosed on conventional staging procedures.[19] It should be a part of the diagnostic algorithm in esophageal cancer staging.

Assessment of Response to Treatment and Prognostication

Responders to induction therapy have a significantly improved survival and therapy response can be assessed with 18F-fluorodeoxyglucose (18F-FDG) PET-CT after completion of therapy.[20] Single-center studies investigating response assessment in patients with esophageal cancer have provided promising results. Early metabolic response evaluation is fairly accurate and can possibly guide PET-based treatment algorithms.[21] A prospective validation study confirmed that a decrease in the standard uptake value of 35% or more predicts histologic response and is associated with improved survival and decreased recurrence.[22] Increased rate of detection has been reported with thoracoscopy and laparoscopy for staging but the invasive nature has to be kept in mind.[23]

Functional Evaluation

2D ECHO
PFT + DLCO

A detailed functional evaluation is mandatory for all patients planned for radical treatment (surgery/chemoradio-therapy) and those who have compromised cardiac or pulmonary function. Forced expiratory volume in 1 second (FEV1) and diffusion capacity of the lung for carbon monoxide (DLCO) have been shown to be independent predictors of pulmonary complications after esophagectomy.[24]

Biopsy

Biopsy is required for establishing tissue diagnosis. Analysis of specimens from biopsies combined with cytologic brushings is accurate and reaches up to 100%.[25,26] Targeted biopsy can enhance results with use of chromoendoscopy techniques like indigo carmine, Lugol's solution, methylene blue, and toluidine blue dye as well as they highlight topographic features and epithelial changes and lead to improved diagnostic accuracy.[27,28]

Finally, a study comparing the health care costs and efficacy of staging procedures including CT scan, EUS-FNA, PET, and thoracoscopy-laparoscopy reported that CT plus EUS-FNA was the least expensive and also it offered the most quality-adjusted life-years on average than all the

Table 4 TNM staging for carcinoma of esophagus (7th edition)

Tx	Primary tumor cannot be assessed T1 tumor invades lamina propria, muscularis mucosae, or submucosa
T0	No evidence of primary tumor
Tis	High-grade dysplasia
T1	T1a: Tumor invades lamina propria or muscularis mucosae T1b: Tumor invades submucosa
T2	Tumor invades muscularis propria
T3	Tumor invades adventitia
T4	Tumor invades adjacent structures. T4a: Resectable tumor invading pleura, pericardium, or diaphragm. T4b: Unresectable tumor invading other adjacent structures, such as the aorta, vertebral body, and trachea.
Nx	Regional lymph node(s) cannot be assessed
N0	No regional lymph node metastasis
N1	Metastasis in 1–2 regional lymph nodes
N2	Metastasis in 3–6 regional lymph nodes
N3	Metastasis in 7 or more regional lymph nodes
M0	No distant metastasis
M1	Distant metastasis

other strategies. PET plus EUS-FNA was no doubt effective but at the same time more expensive.[29]

The 7th edition of AJCC TNM staging for esophageal squamous cell carcinoma which came into effect from 2009 is being represented in Table 4.[30]

Histologic Grade (G)

GX grade cannot be assessed—stage grouping as G1.
G1 well differentiated
G2 moderately differentiated
G3 poorly differentiated
G4 undifferentiated—stage grouping as G3 squamous.

The pertinent changes from 6th edition TNM staging:

- A tumor, the epicenter of which is within 5 cm of the esophagogastric junction and also extends into the esophagus is classified and staged according to the *esophageal* scheme.
- M1a designation is no longer recognized and nodes are included in N staging.
- In 6th edition, N staging was site dependent and now it is number of nodes involved.
- T4 is subclassified as T4A (resectable cancer invasion) and T4B (unresectable cancer invasion).
- Histologic grade and tumor location are incorporated.
- Separate stage grouping for adenocarcinoma and squamous carcinoma.

Table 5 Prognostic factors in carcinoma esophagus

Type	*Description*
Disease related	Stage at diagnosis being the most important prognostic factor. Depth of invasion is the most important factor for nodal and distant spread. Tumor volume is also important prognostically. Lymphovascular invasion is a poor prognostic factor.
Patient related	Age of patients per se is not a significant prognostic factor. Performance status may determine the feasibility of definitive therapy for patients with nonmetastatic disease.
Diagnostic or treatment related	Incomplete pathologic response to preoperative therapy (chemotherapy or chemoradiotherapy).

Table 6 Stage-wise prognosis in carcinoma esophagus

Stage	*5-year overall survival*
0	100%
I	50–80%
IIA	30–40%
IIB	10–30%
III	10–15%
IV	0–5%

The staging system for esophageal or esophagogastric junction adenocarcinomas being represented in Table 4.

PROGNOSTIC GROUPS

Prognostic factors in carcinoma esophagus as given in Table 5.

PROGNOSIS OF ESOPHAGEAL CANCER

Table 6 shows stage-wise prognosis in carcinoma esophagus.

PRINCIPLES OF MANAGEMENT

Factors deciding treatment would be:

- Location of the disease.
- Stage of the disease.
- Performance status of the patient.

Key Points in Management

- The preferred treatment of carcinoma of the cervical esophagus is concomitant chemoradiotherapy or radical radiotherapy. In lesions within 5 cm of the cricopharynx, concurrent, radical chemoradiation is the preferred therapeutic strategy to surgery.[31]

- Surgery is the most effective treatment for resectable esophageal cancer in the middle and lower third and esophagogastric junction.[32]
- Early stage lesions can be treated with a single modality—endoscopic mucosal resection[33] (T1mN0)/Surgery (T1/T2, N0)/Surgery (T1/T2, N0).[34]
- Locally advanced disease (T3/T4a/node positive) should receive multimodality treatment. Neoadjuvant chemotherapy or neoadjuvant chemoradiotherapy followed by surgery have superior outcomes to surgery alone. There is insufficient evidence to strongly suggest one of the neoadjuvant treatment strategies.
- Patients with metastatic disease should receive treatment which best palliates their symptoms—palliative radiotherapy/esophageal stenting/palliative chemotherapy.

Prerequisites for Surgery

- Performance status Eastern Cooperative Oncology Group (ECOG) 0,1.
- Adequate cardiopulmonary reserve.
- Potentially resectable lesion on available.

Indications for Surgery

- Early stage disease T1/T2, N0.
- Locally advanced disease T3/T4a, N+ following neoadjuvant treatment.
- Residual disease following chemoradiation if disease is resectable and patient is in good performance status.
- Local recurrence following radical chemoradiation if there is no evidence of distant disease and patient is in good performance status.

Principles of Surgery

- Achieve a longitudinal margin of at least 5 cm proximally[35] and distally[36] from the primary tumor.
- Achieve a free circumferential radial margin.
- No tumor at the cut margin.[37]
- Two field lymphadenectomy should be performed. More extensive lymphadenectomy (three-field/en bloc) may be considered where multiple lymph node fields are involved. However, there is no evidence currently supporting their routine use.
- Minimum lymph node yield of 15 should be achieved to be considered as adequate staging.[38]
- The approach for esophagectomy should be chosen based on location of tumor, ability to achieve negative margins and adequate lymphadenectomy.
- Lesions involving the middle third of the esophagus are best treated by transthoracic total esophagectomy with cervical esophagogastric anastomoses. This approach provides the best access for both resection of the primary and lymphadenectomy.[39]
- Lesions involving the lower third of the esophagus and esophagogastric junction can be resected through different approaches. Transthoracic, transhiatal, left thoracoabdominal and Ivor Lewis are acceptable approaches.[40] A randomized trial comparing transhiatal esophagectomy to transthoracic esophagectomy and lymphadenectomy for adenocarcinoma of the esophagus did not find difference in median overall and disease free survival between the two procedures.[41] However, there was a trend towards superior long-term (5-year) survival, not reaching statistical significance, in favor of transthoracic esophagectomy. The published meta-analysis of over 50 trials (both prospective and retrospective) compared transhiatal to transthoracic esophagectomy did not reveal any difference in the overall survival but the randomized and prospective comparative studies within the meta-analysis showed a significant difference and it favored transthoracic resection.[42]
  The first multicentric randomized trial comparing open versus minimally invasive esophagectomy demonstrated a reduction of almost 30% in pulmonary complications in the minimally invasive group.[43]
  Regarding extent of lymphadenectomy: Three field lymph node dissection (lower cervical, mediastinal and abdominal) is reported to improve survival without significantly increasing procedure related morbidity or mortality.[44] Although, most reported studies are small or have compared results with historical controls. A large nationwide survey from Japan showed benefit with three-field lymphadenectomy.[45]
- *Surgical reconstruction*: Stomach is the preferred conduit for reconstruction,[46] if stomach is unavailable, colon or jejunum may be considered. If stomach is used as conduit, a pyloric drainage procedure should be considered.[47] This has been shown to decrease pulmonary complications, especially aspiration.
- Stapled and handsewn anastomoses have similar leak rates but (end to end anastomosis) staplers have a higher rate of anastomotic strictures.[48]

DEFINITIVE RADIATION AND CHEMORADIATION THERAPY

Key Points

Concurrent chemoradiation is superior to radiation alone (Level IA, Grade A recommendation). Two published [Radiation Therapy Oncology Group (RTOG) and ECOG) randomized trials reported better overall survival with concomitant chemoradiation than radiotherapy alone.[49] However, increasing the dose escalation (50.4 versus 64.8) in concomitant chemoradiotherapy setting did not increase survival (Intergroup trial).[50]

In Cochrane library, meta-analysis of 13 trials combining radiation with chemotherapy was published and reported an absolute reduction in the mortality and local recurrence rate of 7% and 12% respectively in favor of combination therapy, at the cost of increased life- threatening toxicities.[51] Two trials comparing surgery to radiation alone have reported better survival with surgery.[52]

Based on the available evidence, if a patient needs definitive nonsurgical treatment, it should be concomitant chemoradiotherapy, provided performance status is optimal. However, the issues of radiation volumes (margins to the gross tumor, elective nodal irradiation), total doses and optimal concurrent chemotherapy schedule still remain a matter of debate, with most practice being dictated by individual philosophy.

If chemoradiation is used, 5FU with cisplatin has the maximum evidence but due to logistic reasons, taxane with platinum is commonly used.[53,54]

Radiotherapy Technique

Conventional or three-dimensional conformal therapy (3DCRT) is of acceptable standards for radiation therapy. Intensity-modulated radiation therapy (IMRT) with image-guided radiation therapy (IGRT) maybe especially useful for GE junction tumors and for better sparing of organs at risk (OAR). A recently introduced technique of volumetric modulated are therapy (VMAT) was commissioned and implemented, for carcinoma esophagus in 2010 at our hospital and has shown by very good reduction to normal tissues without compromising the dose to the intended target (Fig. 2).

Preoperative Radiotherapy

Single meta-analysis as well as the five published randomized trials comparing preoperative radiation therapy to surgery alone have not shown benefit of preoperative radiation over surgery alone.[55]

Preoperative Concomitant Chemoradiation

There are three major trials and several smaller trials comparing preoperative concomitant chemoradiation to surgery alone. Of these, one trial has shown statistically improved survival with chemoradiation.[56] Meta-analysis of preoperative chemoradiation and surgery to surgery alone (nine trials) has reported improved 3-year survival and reduced locoregional recurrence.[57-60] However, combination treatment is associated with trend towards increased treatment related morbidity and mortality.

A recent randomized controlled trial (CROSS) comparing surgery alone to neoadjuvant chemoradiotherapy followed by surgery showed improved R0 resection, pathological

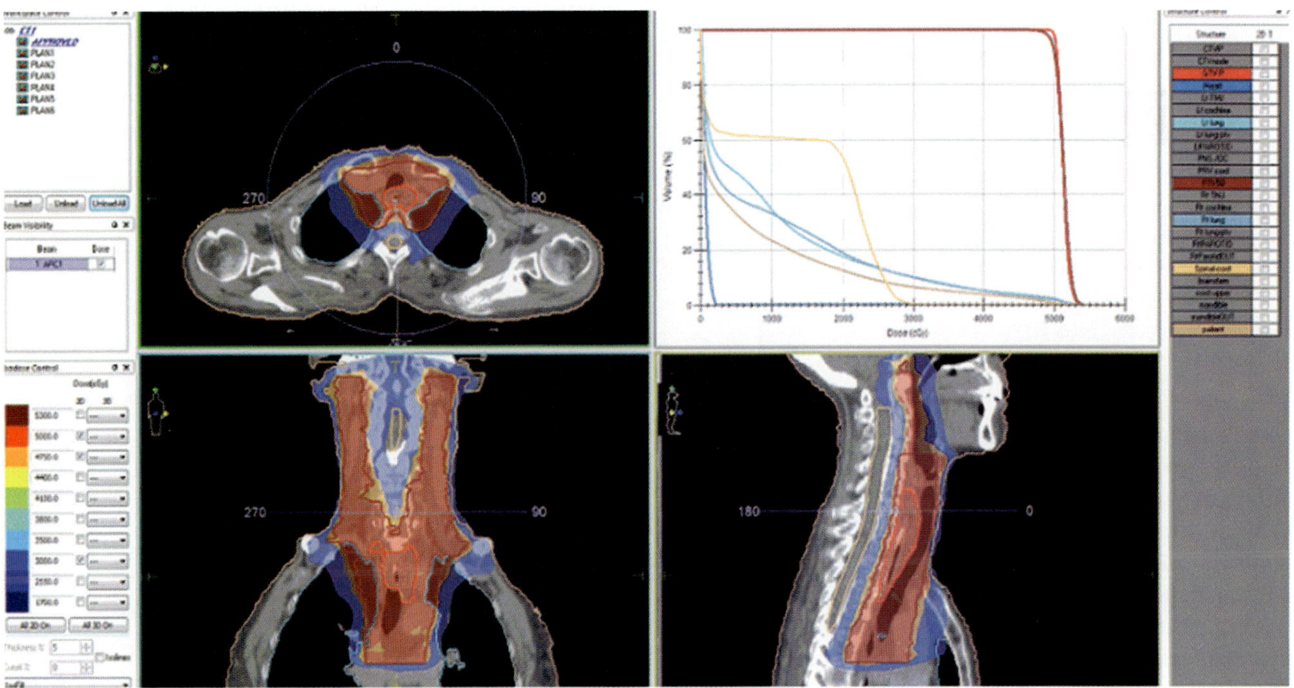

Fig. 2 Volumetric modulated arc therapy (VMAT) plan for mid one-third esophageal cancer with dose-volume histogram (DVH) for important organs at risk (OAR).

Courtesy: Dr. Tejinder Kataria, Division of Radiation Oncology, Medanta—The Medicity, Haryana, India

response and significantly improved survival (49.4 versus 24 months) in the neoadjuvant group, while the postoperative complications and mortality were similar in both groups.[61]

Preoperative Chemotherapy

There are two major and several smaller published trials of preoperative chemotherapy in the management of carcinoma esophagus. The two large trials reported results, which are contradictory. The Intergroup trial, by Kelsen et al. With 440 patients observed no improvement in survival with preoperative combination of cisplatin and fluorouracil among patients with adenocarcinoma or squamous cell carcinoma of the esophagus.[62]

More recently published Medical Research Council (MRC) trial of 802 patients reported improved survival with two cycles of cisplatin and fluorouracil without additional serious events.[63]

The meta-analysis of all trials concluded preoperative chemotherapy plus surgery appears to offer a survival advantage at 3, 4, and 5 years, which is significantly superior to surgery alone for resectable thoracic esophageal cancer irrespective of histologic type.

An updated meta-analysis in 2011 looked at neoadjuvant therapy given to over 4,000 patients with esophageal carcinoma, and found strong evidence for survival benefit with neoadjuvant chemoradiotherapy and neoadjuvant chemotherapy over surgery alone.[64] A clear advantage of neoadjuvant chemoradiotherapy over chemotherapy has not been established.

Among patients with operable gastric or lower esophageal adenocarcinomas, the perioperative regimen of ECF [epirubicin, 5-fluorouracil (5-FU), cisplatin] decreased tumor size and stage and improved progression-free and overall survival as compared to patients who underwent surgery alone.[65] Chemotherapy regimens commonly evaluated in clinical trials are 5-FU/cisplatin and ECF.[66] But due to logistics of administration, taxane and platinum-based chemotherapy is commonly used.[67]

Postoperative Radiotherapy

Three trials have compared surgery and postoperative radiation versus surgery alone. The Chinese trial with 495 patients observed improved 5-year survival among patients with positive lymph nodes and stage III disease. However, the difference in the overall survival between the two groups was statistically nonsignificant.[68]

The meta-analysis of all three trials also reported no benefit of postoperative radiotherapy.[69] Therefore, in the absence of Level I evidence postoperative radiotherapy is indicated only for patients with positive margin and residual disease.

For lower third and GE junction adenocarcinomas with the multiple lymph nodes, positive margins, T3 tumors; adjuvant CTRT maybe considered with the increased incidence of treatment related toxicity.[70]

Postoperative Chemotherapy

Phase III trials of surgery and postoperative chemotherapy have not reported survival benefit over surgery. A Phase III study by Japanese Clinical Oncology Group (JCOG) showed better disease free survival at 5-year with postoperative chemotherapy; however with no difference in the overall survival.[71]

In adenocarcinoma of the cardioesophageal junction (and stomach) postoperative chemoradiotherapy has been shown to improve the median overall survival.[70] Similarly, another randomized trial (MAGIC) showed superior disease free and overall survival with perioperative (three cycles pre and three cycles postoperative) chemotherapy over surgery alone for lower esophageal and GE junction cancers.[72] Thus, in patients with adenocarcinoma of the cardia having good performance status, perioperative chemotherapy or postoperative chemoradiation should be the standard of care.[70,72]

Principles of Radiation Therapy

Radical Radiotherapy

The inclusion criteria are:
- All lesions in upper/mid/lower esophagus.
- Lesion less than 5 cm length (preferred for RT alone).
- Histologically proven esophageal carcinoma.
- Karnofsky performance status (KPS) of more than 60%.
- Metastatic work-up negative (no palpable S/C nodes, bronchoscopy and USG abdomen normal).
  External beam radiotherapy (EBRT) alone.

Dose: 60–64 Gy/30–32 fractions, with reducing fields, conventional fractionation.

Brachytherapy

Whenever feasible, external radiotherapy can be combined with intraluminal radiotherapy (ILRT) as a boost. ILRT is usually avoided with concurrent chemotherapy. ILRT boost: 6 Gy × 2 fractions, high dose rate (HDR), 1 week apart or single fraction 20 Gy low dose rate (LDR).

Palliative Treatment

With acceptable/good performance status,
- Relieving dysphagia by placing esophageal stent alone, preferably self-expanding metallic stent.
- Radiation therapy with intubation if there is significant dysphagia.
- Intraluminal radiotherapy alone.
- Endoscopic laser destruction of tumor.
- Electrocoagulation.
- Palliative radiotherapy.

The intent being quick and good palliation with relief from dysphagia and pain. The inclusion criterias are:

- Lesions in upper/mid/lower esophagus in that order of preference.
- Lesion less than 10 cm long on barium swallow and esophagoscopy.
- Histologically proven cancer.
- Karnofsky performance status of more than 50%.
- Recurrent or metastatic disease.

- Palliative radiation can also be delivered by ILRT alone or in combination with EBRT. Suggested dose per fraction: 8 Gy, in 2 fractions, 1 week apart. No difference in local control or survival between HDR brachytherapy compared with external beam radiation been reported. Various schedules of brachytherapy have been compared and two fractions of 8 Gy are found to be equivalent to three fractions of 6 Gy.[73] Addition of EBRT to ILRT improves the dysphagia free survival.[74]
- *Palliative chemotherapy:* In advanced adenocarcinoma of esophagus palliative chemotherapy improves survival as compared to best supportive care.[75] Targeted therapy with trastuzumab along with chemotherapy in HER-2 positive metastatic gastroesophgeal cancer has improved survival.[76]

When the general condition is poor and patient has limited life expectancy:

- Nasogastric tube placement for feeding.
- Best supportive care.

Treatment of esophageal fistula:

- Esophageal intubation with stent.
- Esophageal and tracheal/bronchial stent placement (double stenting) when possible if the fistula is large or if the tracheal lumen is compromised.

RADIOTHERAPY TECHNICAL DETAILS

Immobilization and Simulation[77]

Patients are placed in the supine position with both arms up and immobilized with a thoracic cast or Vac-LoK bag and T-bar. CT simulation is necessary for conformal treatment planning and contrast enhanced CT scan with 2–3 mm CT slices are required.

Some institution also follow additional oral contrast with barium sulfate emulsion given just before the CT scan for better delineation of target, though we do not follow the same. The cast made in esophageal cancer radiotherapy also varies with the location of primary disease. While thoracic cast subserves in most of the mid to mid-lower esophageal cancers, pure upper 1/3rd lesions actually requires head and neck cast with hands by side position and lower 1/3rd patients will benefit from abdominal cast with hands overhead.

In some institutions four-dimensional (4D)-CT simulation to account for tumor motion and individualizing target volume and margin are applied. Otherwise target volume while contouring should account for motion management.

Target Definition and Delineation

In the era of CT planning and image-guided radiotherapy, margins are defined and contoured on CT scans and respect anatomic boundaries. Gross tumor volume (GTV) is contoured on planning CT scan. The necessary information obtained from clinical examination, endoscopic findings and diagnostic imaging available all are required.

Maximum intensity projection (MIP) imaging (if 4D CT is available) to account for tumor excursion with respiratory motion is helpful.

Gross tumor volume: The primary tumor (GTV-P) and clinically positive lymph nodes (GTV-N) seen on the pretreatment PET scan (SUV > 3), diagnostic CT scan, esophagram or barium swallow, EUS, esophagogastroduodenoscopy (EGD), and/or treatment planning CT (> 1 cm short-axis diameter) will comprise the GTV (Fig. 3).

Clinical target volume (CTV): The CTV is defined to be the GTV-P plus a 0.5–1 cm margin radially and 3–5 cm cranio-caudally, as appropriate to account for microscopic tumor extension. The ipsilateral paratracheal lymph nodes (levels 2 and 4) often comprise part of the CTV. 1 cm margin in all directions on grossly involved LNs (GTV-N). Regional LNs to be covered include periesophageal along entire length of the CTV, celiac axis LNs, peri-gastric LNs along lesser curvature.

Planning target volume (PTV): Includes the CTV plus a total margin of 1.0 cm in all directions. If we do use cone-beam CT (CBCT), then the respective margins on the CTV can be reduced by 0.5 cm, on average.

Dose Constraints for OAR

Normal tissues to be contoured include both lungs, heart, spinal cord, remaining esophagus, kidneys and liver where applicable, breast bilaterally in female patients and HN region OAR for upper one-third esophageal cancers.

All normal tissues assume treatment at 1.8 Gy/Fx (corrected for heterogeneity).

Highest priority = Cord (50 Gy)

Second highest priority = Normal lung (more than 2 cm outside PTV) < 45 Gy and total lung total, defined as the total lung volume minus the CTV (total or the mean lung dose < 20 Gy).

Third highest priority = Kidney (<2/3 total kidney to receive any dose > 20 Gy)

Fourth highest priority = Heart (<1/2 heart to receive any dose > 40 Gy, and the whole heart may receive up to 30 Gy)

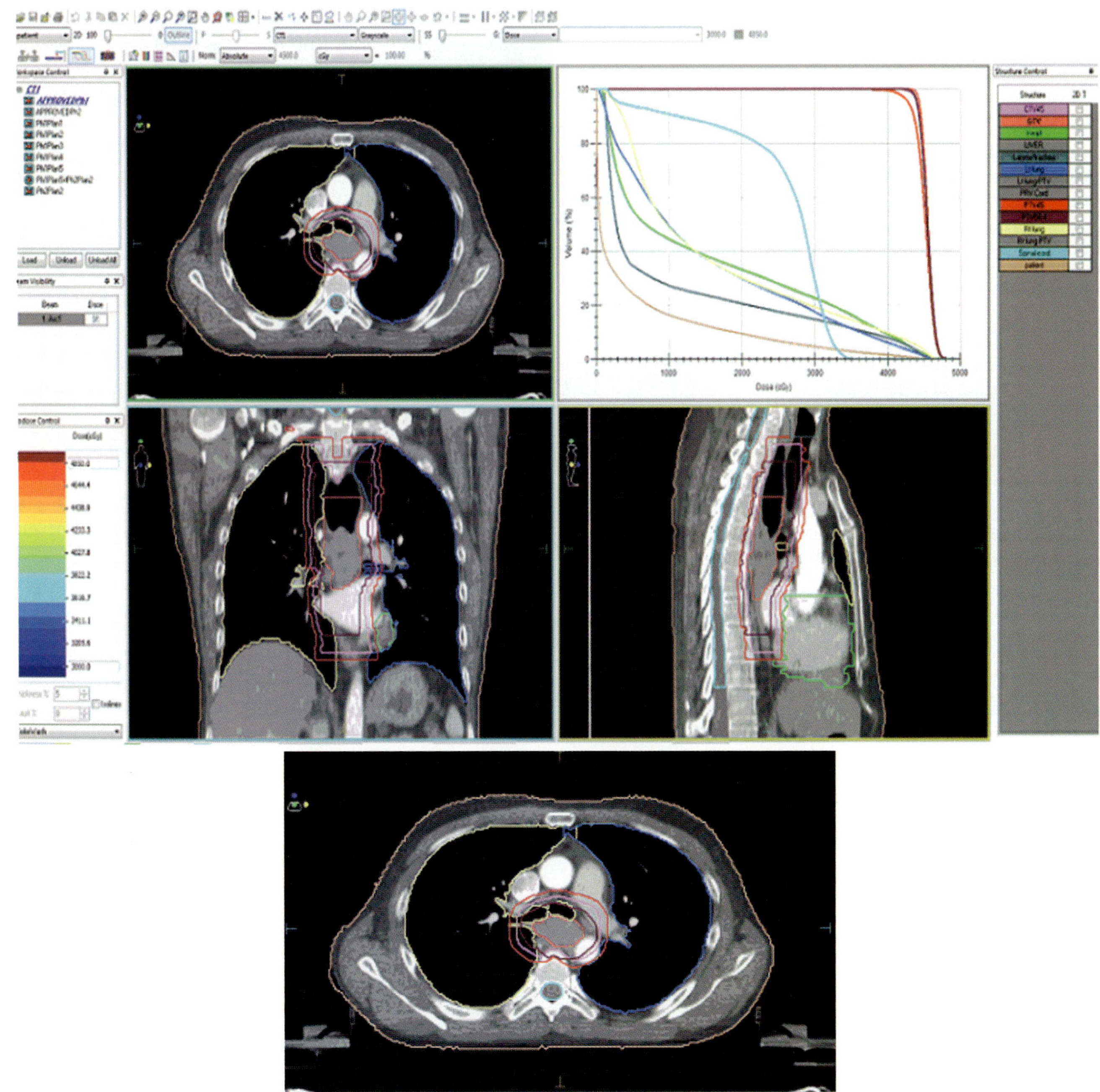

Fig. 3 Phase 1 plan for mid one-third esophageal cancers showing gross tumor volume (GTV) in brick red, CTV in pink and PTV in red.

Courtesy: Dr Tejinder Kataria, Division of Radiation Oncology, Medanta—The Medicity, Haryana, India

Fifth highest priority = Liver (< 1/2 may receive any dose > 30 Gy)

Brachial plexus (< 66 Gy)

Fourth highest priority = Esophagus (mean dose < 36 Gy).

Modern Radiotherapy Techniques[78]

Historically, radiation to the esophagus was delivered with 2D techniques that treated a large volume of normal tissue. Mackley et al.[79] reported that three-dimensional (3D) CT-based radiotherapy planning (3D-CTP) reduces acute esophagitis in patients receiving multimodality therapy for esophageal cancer without compromising clinical outcomes compared with 2D planning. The same study also reported significantly reduced field sizes. When treating esophageal cancers with chemoradiation prior to resection, normal tissue complications are of prime concern. One of the most feared potential late sequelae of intrathoracic irradiation is radiation pneumonitis. Indeed, 3D-CTP provided the ability to evaluate parameters predictive of the side effects.[80] With IMRT, there is not one individual beam of uniform dose as in 3DCRT but rather a series of individual beamlets each programmed to vary the dose intensity across the target or normal tissue interface. This technique can be delivered on a standard linear accelerator or on a tomotherapy unit in which the patient is treated on a machine that resembles a CT scanner, capable of delivering a dose in a 360° rotational fashion.[81,82] However, to avoid underdosing potential disease with a resultant "marginal miss", it becomes more important than ever to optimize delineation of the target volumes and the planned delivery parameters.

With evolving techniques and data supporting them, IMRT or tomotherapy has been established to be efficacious than 3D-CRT.[83-85] Clinical data are now emerging to support the role of IMRT in esophageal cancer. Sridhar et al. have analyzed patients treated by IMRT between 2006 and 2011 with either preoperative or definitive IMRT chemoradiation to 50–60 Gy prescribed to the GTV and 45–50.4 Gy to the CTV concurrently with chemotherapy. IMRT techniques included multifield segmented step and shoot, compensator-based, and volumetric arc therapies. Total 108 patients were analyzed with a median follow-up of 19 months, median OS and disease-free survival (DFS) were 32 and 21.6 months, respectively. A total of 58 patients (53.7%) underwent surgical resection. There was no difference in OS or DFS in patients who underwent surgery compared with patients who were definitively treated without surgery.

Median weight loss was 5.5%, and rates of hospital admissions, feeding tube placement, stent placement, dilation, and radiation pneumonitis were 15.7%, 7.4%, 4.6%, 12%, and 1.9%, respectively. Long-term radiation pneumonitis was observed in 6 (5.6%) patients. The benefits of IMRT over 3D radiation planning are better target conformality and sparing of the surrounding normal tissues.[86]

Another study by Kole et al. showed that IMRT significantly reduced the dose to the heart compared with 3D-CRT. They analyzed 19 patients treated with IMRT and compared 3-field and 4-field 3D CRT plans on those same patients. They showed a significant reduction in mean dose (22.9 versus 28.2 Gy) and V30 (24.8% versus 61.0%; $P < .05$) and a significant improvement in the target conformity with IMRT as measured by the conformality index (ratio of total volume receiving 95% of prescription dose to the PTV receiving 95% of prescription dose), with the mean conformality index reduced from 1.56 to 1.30 using IMRT.[87]

Nguyen et al. analyzed nine patients in a feasibility study to compare lung and heart doses between 3D-CRT and tomotherapy. Mean lung dose (7.4 versus 11.8 Gy; $P = .004$) and heart ventricle dose (12.4 vs 18.3 Gy; $P = .006$) were significantly reduced with tomotherapy.[85] Nicolini et al. compared volumetric modulated arc therapy (VMAT) with multifield IMRT and 3D-CRT plans in patients with esophageal cancer, showing that VMAT and IMRT provided similar target coverage and were superior to 3D-CRT.[88]

Other Technical Issues

Respiratory-associated esophageal tumor motion: Here comes the need of 4D-CT scan for treatment planning.[89-91] Since the intended esophageal target is thus "moving", the question becomes whether a 4D-PET/CT scan that shows the FDG-avid areas in different phases of respiration is a better measure of defining the full physiologic extent of disease and whether this could improve treatment planning. Another option is to place fiducial markers endoscopically in esophageal submucosa to define superior and inferior extent of the disease.[92,93]

Concerns about respiratory-associated tumor motion are particularly important in the setting of GE junction tumors. Multiple investigators have demonstrated increasing radial esophageal motion as the tumor location becomes more distal.[94] Zhao et al.[95] reported that tumors in the left chest may be displaced with cardiac motion. With advanced technology such as IMRT, there is concern that motion may affect the dose distribution. In fact, Kim et al.[96] reported that respiratory motion can reduce the delivered dose by up to 30% in lung tumors that move approximately 1 cm. Motion management strategies should be considered if using IMRT to prevent potential tumor underdosage. Abdominal compression with a device placed to decrease diaphragmatic excursion used daily has been shown to decrease the superior to inferior motion by approximately one-half.[93]

Another strategy involves a solid IMRT approach whereby brass compensators are placed into the pathway of each treatment field to prevent the potential tumor motion mismatch with a static beamlet.[97] Finally, there is also the possibility of incorporating respiratory-gating techniques so that the treatment machine beams "on" only during a specified phase of the breathing cycle.

An additional concern is the variability in day to day stomach motion due to differences in gastric filling with tumors at the GE junction. Bouchard et al.[98] reviewed an analysis of 8 patients who were instructed to fast for 3 hours before daily treatment. The treatment was planned on both a full stomach initial CT scan and an empty stomach initial scan and re-measured with weekly repeated CT scans during treatment. The results showed that the full stomach volumes were a mean of 3.3 (range, 1.7–7.5) times larger than empty stomach volumes. These data emphasize the importance of daily treatment verification when utilizing advanced technologies, a technique termed IGRT. This technique can be incorporated with a daily CT scan on the treatment machine itself, termed a CBCT, which can be fused with the planning CT to ensure that the setup can be reproduced. A daily kilovoltage images of the spine can also be viewed and matched to the initial scan. All of these techniques improve the setup accuracy and may allow for smaller treatment margins to protect additional normal tissue.

Adaptive Radiotherapy for Esophageal Carcinoma: Old Wine in a New Bottle

Radiation treatment planning has evolved considerably since radiotherapy was first used to treat esophageal cancer. With the advent of modern imaging and sophisticated treatment techniques, adapt to tumor response for dose escalation have been tried in many sites of cancer and esophageal cancers are no exception.[99]

But, is it new? Is it something hitherto unknown to the fraternity treating esophageal cancers?

Before CT-based treatment planning, simulation was performed by fluoroscopy and fields were largely designed based on bony landmarks. The traditional techniques for target volumes were:

For phase 1: GTV—Gross disease as evident from clinical-radiological findings taking into considerations for EUS or UGI endoscopic report. The on table barium swallow to ideally delineate GTV on a fluoroscopy was helpful. The CTV is defined as the GTV plus areas at risk for harboring microscopic disease. The CTV is usually the primary tumor GTV, with an additional 4–4.5 cm expansion superior and inferior as well as a 1–1.5 cm radially to include the paraesophageal lymph nodes. In addition, any positive lymph nodes in the GTV should also be included in the CTV volume.[99,100]

With the conventional techniques of radiotherapy with AP-PA portal and simulation based on fluoroscopy the major disadvantage of delivering a radical dose was spinal cord tolerance. The treatment technique was revised in phase 2 around 40 Gy to deliver off-cord and off-heart techniques with 3-field or 3D conformal techniques. To actually reduce the GTV phase 2 CTV expansion was 1–1.5 cm cranio-caudally and 1 cm radially around initial GTV. The PTV in both the phases was 0.5–0.7 cm around CTV depending upon institutional protocol.

Drawbacks of this Approach

- The volume reduction was primarily based on OAR tolerances and not on actual GTV response.
- There is prior assumption of a certain amount of volume reduction after a certain dose level and no actual documentation.
- The margins selected for phase 1 and phase 2 between GTV and CTV was universal and not subjective. Some patients might actually have better response and we tend to over treat in them and those with still persistent disease, we might under treat.

CT-based planning allows for contouring tumor volumes and normal structures and calculating dose to each voxel of a structure. This situation has allowed for more accurate estimation of normal tissue toxicity and dose to the targeted volume. In addition, advances in treatment delivery such as IMRT have allowed more conformal treatment plans with the goal of minimizing toxicity. CBCT or megavoltage CT with tomotherapy allows the ability to perform daily image guidance to ensure that the target volume is in the treatment field and potentially allows margins for setup error to be reduced.

The major leap in the treatment with CT-based adaptive protocol was response based on objective GTV reduction. The evidences, though sparse actually highlight the benefit not only in terms of GTV reduction but also acceptable OAR dose profile. In a recent study with the adaptive RA (RapidArc) plan there was reduced heart D35% and mean dose by 17.35% (p = 0.0011) and 17.16% (p = 0.0012). No significant reduction in spinal cord and liver doses were observed. Normal tissue complication probability (NTCP) for the lung (0.42% versus 0.08%) and heart (1.39% versus 0.090%) was reduced significantly in adaptive plans.[101]

The online imaging system called CBCT which is primarily used for IGRT can however, it can also be employed for an adaptive radiotherapy as Hounsfield unit (HU) values are obtained and can be calibrated for the use in treatment planning.[102] In our Institute it is called Elekta XVI (Elekta Oncology Systems, UK). The application for the same in adaptive radiotherapy has mostly been phantom based and though specifically not meant for esophageal cancers, for thoracic malignancies there was 1.8 ± 1.6% dose difference between CBCT and primary plans.[102]

In conclusion, it is premature to actually recommend adaptive planning for esophageal cancers but the future potential cannot be overlooked. The concept of 2D volume reduction after a certain dose level and implementation of the same in 3D treatment planning reminds us about the concept of "old wine in a new bottle".

REFERENCES

1. Globocan 2008, accessed online at http://globocan.iarc.fr/factsheet.asp on 9th December, 2012.
2. Takiar R, Nadayil D, Nandakumar A. Projections of number of cancer cases in India (2010-2020) by cancer groups. Asian Pac J Cancer Prev. 2010;11(4):1045-9.
3. Jemal A, Bray F, Center MM, Ferlay J, Ward E, Forman D. Global cancer statistics. CA Cancer J Clin. 2011;61(2):69-90.
4. Bosetti C, Levi F, Ferlay J, Garavello W, Lucchini F, Bertuccio P, et al. Trends in oesophageal cancer incidence and mortality in Europe. Int J Cancer. 2008;122(5):1118-29.
5. Cook MB, Chow WH, Devesa SS. Oesophageal cancer incidence in the United States by race, sex, and histologic type, 1977-2005. Br J Cancer. 2009;101(5):855-9.
6. Rüdiger Siewert J, Feith M, Werner M, et al. Adenocarcinoma of the esophagogastric junction. Results of surgical therapy based on anatomic-topographic classification in 1,002 consecutive patients. Ann Surg. 2000;232(3):353-61.
7. Hagen JA, DeMeester SR, Peters JH, et al. Curative resection for esophageal adenocarcinoma: analysis of 100 en bloc esophagectomies. Ann Surg. 2001;234(4):520-30.

8. Altorki NK, Girardi L, Skinner DB. En bloc esophagectomy improves survival for stage III esophageal cancer. J Thorac Cardiovasc Surg. 1997;114(6):948-55.
9. van Vliet EP, Heijenbrok-Kal MH, Hunink MG, et al. Staging investigations for oesophageal cancer: a meta-analysis. Br J Cancer. 2008;12;98(3):547-57.
10. Penman I, Norton S, Harris K. Staging of Oesophago-Gastric Carcinoma by Endoscopic Ultrasonography: Guidance and Minimum Standards; 1e19. 2011, EUS Users Group and the British Society of Gastroenterology (BSG), 2011.
11. Catalano MF, Sivak MV Jr, Bedford RA, Falk GW, van Stolk R, Presa F, et al. Observer variation and reproducibility endoscopic ultrasonography. Gastrointest Endosc. 1995;41(2):115-20.
12. Mallery S, Van Dam J. Increased rate of complete EUS staging of patients with esophageal cancer using the nonoptical, wire-guided echoendoscope. Gastrointest Endosc. 1999; 50(1):53-7.
13. Rosch T, Classen M. staging ESOPHAGEAL CANCER: THE MUNICH EXPERIENCE. In: Van Dam J, Sivak M, (Eds). Gastrointestinal endosonography. Philadelphia: WB Saunders, 1999.
14. Puli SR, Reddy JB, Bechtold ML, et al. Accuracy of endoscopic ultrasound in the diagnosis of distal and celiac axis lymph node metastasis in esophageal cancer: a meta-analysis and systematic review. Dig Dis Sci. 2008;53(9):2405-14.
15. Lightdale CJ, Kulkarni KG. Role of endoscopic ultrasonography in the staging and follow-up of esophageal cancer. J Clin Oncol. 2005;23(20):4483-9.
16. Willis J, Cooper G, Isenberg G, et al. Correlation of EUS measurement with pathologic assessment of neoadjuvant therapy response in esophageal carcinoma. Gastrointest Endosc. 2002;55(6):655-61.
17. Chak A, Canto M, Cooper G, Isenberg G, Willis J, Levitan N, et al. Endosonographic assessment of multimodality therapy predicts survival of esophageal carcinoma patients. Cancer. 2000;88(8):1788-95.
18. Barber TW, Duong CP, Leong T, Bressel M, Drummond EG, Hicks RJ, et al. 18F-FDG PET/CT has a high impact on patient management and provides powerful prognostic stratification in the primary staging of esophageal cancer: a prospective study with mature survival data. J Nucl Med. 2012;53(6):1-8.
19. Meyers BF, Downey RJ, Decker PA, Keenan RJ, Siegel BA, Cerfolio RJ, et al.The utility of positron emission tomography in staging of potentially operable carcinoma of the thoracic esophagus: results of the American College Surgeons Oncology Group Z0060 trial. J Thorac Cardiovasc Surg. 2007;133(3):738-45.
20. Omloo JM, van Heijl M, Hoekstra OS, van Berge Henegouwen MI, van Lanschot JJ, Sloof GW. FDG-PET parameters as prognostic factor in esophageal cancer patients: a review. Ann Surg Oncol. 2011;18(12):3338-52.
21. Lordick F, Ott K, Krause BJ, Weber WA, Becker K, Stein HJ, et al. PET to assess early metabolic response and to guide treatment of adenocarcinoma of the oesophagogastric junction: the MUNICON phase II trial. Lancet Oncol. 2007;8(9):797-805.
22. Ott K, Weber WA, Lordick F, Becker K, Busch R, Herrmann K, et al. Metabolic imaging predicts response, survival, and recurrence in adenocarcinomas of the esophagogastric junction. J Clin Oncol. 2006;24(29):4692-8.
23. de Graaf GW, Ayantunde AA, Parsons SL, et al. The role of staging laparoscopy in oesophagogastric cancers. Eur J Surg Oncol. 2007;33(8):988-92.
24. Ferguson MK, Celauro AD, Prachand V. Prediction of major pulmonary complications after esophagectomy. Ann Thorac Surg. 2011;91(5):1494-500.
25. Cussó X, Monés-Xiol J, Vilardell F. Endoscopic cytology of cancer of the esophagus and cardia: a long-term evaluation. Gastrointest Endosc. 1989;35(4):321-3.
26. Zargar SA, Khuroo MS, Jan GM, et al. Prospective comparison of the value of brushings before and after biopsy in the endoscopic diagnosis of gastroesophageal malignancy. Acta Cytol. 1991;35(5):549-52.
27. Jung M, Kiesslich R. Chromoendoscopy and intravital staining techniques. Baillieres Best Pract Res Clin Gastroenterol. 1999;13(1):11-9.
28. Acosta MM, Boyce HW Jr. Chromoendoscopy--where is it useful? J Clin Gastroenterol. 1998;27(1):13-20.
29. Wallace MB, Nietert PJ, Earle C, Krasna MJ, Hawes RH, Hoffman BJ, et al. An analysis of multiple staging management strategies for carcinoma of the esophagus: computed tomography, endoscopic ultrasound, positron emission tomography, and thoracoscopy/laparoscopy. Ann Thorac Surg. 2002;74(4):1026-32.
30. Rice TW, Rusch VW, Ishwaran H, et al. Worldwide Esophageal Cancer Collaboration. Cancer of the esophagus and esophagogastric junction: data-driven staging for the seventh edition of the American Joint Committee on Cancer/ International Union Against Cancer Cancer Staging Manuals. Cancer. 2010;116(16):3763-73.
31. Tong DK, Law S, Kwong DL, Wei WI, Ng RW, Wong KH. Current management of cervical esophageal cancer. World J Surg. 2011;35(3):600-7.
32. Wright CD. Esophageal cancer surgery in 2005. Minerva Chir. 2005;60(6):431-44.
33. NICE (National Institute for Health and Clinical Excellence). Barrett's Oesophagus Ablative Therapy for the Treatment of Barrett's Oesophagus CG106.1. [online] Available from www.nice.org.uk. [Accessed April 2015]
34. Grotenhuis BA, van Heijl M, Zehetner J, Moons J, Wijnhoven BP, van Berge Henegouwen MI, et al. Surgical management of submucosal esophageal cancer: extended or regional lymphadenectomy? Ann Surg. 2010;252(5):823-30.
35. Law S, Arcilla C, Chu KM, et al. The significance of histologically infiltrated resection margin after esophagectomy for esophageal cancer. Am J Surg. 1998;176(3):286-90.
36. Barbour AP, Rizk NP, Gonen M, Tang L, Bains MS, Rusch VW, et al. Adenocarcinoma of the gastroesophageal junction: influence of esophageal resection margin and operative approach on outcome. Ann Surg. 2007;246(1):1-8.
37. Deeter M, Dorer R, Kuppusamy MK, et al. Assessment of criteria and clinical significance of circumferential resection margins in esophageal cancer. Arch Surg. 2009;144(7):618-24.

38. Veeramachaneni NK, Zoole JB, Decker PA, et al. American College of Surgeons Oncology Group Z0060 Trial. Lymph node analysis in esophageal resection: American College of Surgeons Oncology Group Z0060 trial. Ann Thorac Surg. 2008;86(2):418-21.
39. Cooper JD. Overview of operative techniques. In: Pearson FG, Cooper JD, Deslauriers J (Eds). Esophageal Surgery, 2nd edition. New York: Churchill Livingstone; 2002. p. 793.
40. D'Amico TA. Outcomes after surgery for esophageal cancer. Gastrointest Cancer Res. 2007;1(5):188-96.
41. Hulscher JB, van Sandick JW, de Boer AG, Wijnhoven BP, Tijssen JG, Fockens P, et al. Extended transthoracic resection compared with limited transhiatal resection for adenocarcinoma of the esophagus. N Engl J Med. 2002;347(21):1662-9.
42. Hulscher JB, Tijssen JG, Obertop H, et al. Transthoracic versus transhiatal resection for carcinoma of the esophagus: a meta-analysis. Ann Thorac Surg. 2001;72(1):306-13.
43. Biere SS, van Berge Henegouwen MI, Maas KW, Rosman C, Garcia JR, Gisbertz SS, et al. Minimally invasive versus open oesophagectomy for patients with oesophageal cancer: a multicentre, open-label, randomised controlled trial. Lancet. 2012;379(9829):1887-92.
44. Igaki H, Tachimori Y, Kato H. Improved survival for patients with upper and/or middle mediastinal lymph node metastasis of squamous cell carcinoma of the lower thoracic esophagus treated with 3-field dissection. Ann Surg. 2004;239(4):483-90.
45. Isono K, Sato H, Nakayama K. Results of a nationwide study on the three-field of lymph node dissection in esophageal cancer. Oncology. 1991;48(5):411-20.
46. Davis PA, Law S, Wong J. Colonic interposition after esophagectomy for cancer. Arch Surg. 2003;138(3):303-8.
47. Urschel JD, Blewett CJ, Young JE, et al. Pyloric drainage (pyloroplasty) or no drainage in gastric reconstruction after esophagectomy: a meta-analysis of randomized controlled trials. Dig Surg. 2002;19(3):160-4.
48. Urschel JD, Blewett CJ, Bennett WF, et al. Handsewn or stapled esophagogastric anastomoses after esophagectomy for cancer: meta-analysis of randomized controlled trials. Dis Esophagus. 2001;14(3-4):212-7.
49. Cooper JS, Guo MD, Herskovic A, Macdonald JS, Martenson JA Jr, Al-Sarraf M, et al. Chemoradiotherapy of locally advanced esophageal cancer: long-term follow-up of a prospective randomized trial (RTOG 85-01). Radiation Therapy Oncology Group. JAMA. 1999;281(17):1623-7.
50. Minsky BD, Pajak TF, Ginsberg RJ, Pisansky TM, Martenson J, Komaki R, et al. INT 0123 (Radiation Therapy Oncology Group 94-05) phase III trial of combined-modality therapy for esophageal cancer: high-dose versus standard-dose radiation therapy. J Clin Oncol. 2002;20(5):1167-74.
51. Rebecca Wong, Richard Malthaner. Combined chemotherapy and radiotherapy (without surgery) compared with radiotherapy alone in localized carcinoma of the esophagus (Cochrane Review). The Cochrane Library, Issue 4, 2003.
52. Badwe RA, Sharma V, Bhansali MS, Dinshaw KA, Patil PK, Dalvi N, et al. The quality of swallowing for patients with operable esophageal carcinoma: a randomized trial comparing surgery with radiotherapy. Cancer. 1999;85(4):763-8.
53. Hainsworth JD, Meluch AA, Greco FA. Paclitaxel, carboplatin, and long-term continuous 5-fluorouracil infusion in the treatment of upper aerodigestive malignancies: preliminary results of phase II trial. Semin Oncol. 1997;24(6 Suppl 19):S19-38-S19-42.
54. Kim DW, Blanke CD, Wu H, Shyr Y, Berlin J, Beauchamp RD, et al. Phase II study of preoperative paclitaxel/cisplatin with radiotherapy in locally advanced esophageal cancer. Int J Radiat Oncol Biol Phys. 2007;67(2):397-404.
55. Arnott SJ, Duncan W, Gignoux M, Girling DJ, Hansen HS, Launois B, et al. Preoperative radiotherapy in esophageal carcinoma: a meta-analysis using individual patient data (Oesophageal Cancer Collaborative Group). Int J Radiat Oncol Biol Phys. 1998;41(3):579-83.
56. Walsh TN, Noonan N, Hollywood D, Kelly A, Keeling N, Hennessy TP. A comparison of multimodal therapy and surgery for esophageal adenocarcinoma. N Engl J Med. 1996;335(7):462-7.
57. Urschel JD, Vasan H. A meta-analysis of randomized controlled trials that compared neoadjuvant chemoradiation and surgery to surgery alone for resectable esophageal cancer. Am J Surg. 2003;185(6):538-4.
58. F Fiorica, D Di Bona, F Schepis, Licata A, Shahied L, Venturi A, et al. Preoperative chemoradiotherapy for oesophageal cancer: a systematic review and meta-analysis. Gut. 2004;53(7):925-30.
59. Greer SE, Goodney PP, Sutton JE, et al. Neoadjuvant chemoradiotherapy for esophageal carcinoma: a meta-analysis. Surgery. 2005;137(2):172-7.
60. Gebski V, Burmeister B, Smithers BM, Foo K, Zalcberg J, Simes J, et al. Survival benefits from neoadjuvant chemoradiotherapy or chemotherapy in oesophageal carcinoma: a meta-analysis. Lancet Oncol. 2007;8(3):226-34.
61. van Hagen P, Hulshof MC, van Lanschot JJ, Steyerberg EW, van Berge Henegouwen MI, Wijnhoven BP, et al. Preoperative chemoradiotherapy for esophageal or junctional cancer. N Engl J Med. 2012;366(22):2074-84.
62. Kelsen DP, Winter KA, Gunderson LL, Mortimer J, Estes NC, Haller DG, et al. Long-term results of RTOG trial 8911 (USA Intergroup 113): a random assignment trial comparison of chemotherapy followed by surgery compared with surgery alone for esophageal cancer. J Clin Oncol. 2007;25(24):3719-25.
63. Medical Research Council Oesophageal Cancer Working Group. Surgical resection with or without preoperative chemotherapy in oesophageal cancer: a randomised controlled trial. Lancet. 2002;359(9319):1727-33.
64. Sjoquist KM, Burmeister BH, Smithers BM, Zalcberg JR, Simes RJ, Barbour A, et al. Survival after neoadjuvant chemotherapy or chemoradiotherapy for resectable oesophageal carcinoma: an updated meta-analysis. Lancet Oncol. 2011;12(7):681-92.
65. Cunningham D, Allum WH, Stenning SP, Thompson JN, Van de Velde CJ, Nicolson M, et al. Perioperative chemotherapy versus surgery alone for resectable gastroesophageal cancer. N Engl J Med. 2006;355(1):11-20.
66. Ychou M, Boige V, Pignon JP, Conroy T, Bouché O, Lebreton G, et al. Perioperative chemotherapy compared with surgery alone for resectable gastroesophageal adenocarcinoma: an

FNCLCC and FFCD multicenter phase III trial. J Clin Oncol. 2011;29(13):1715-21.
67. Ferri LE, Ades S, Alcindor T, Chasen M, Marcus V, Hickeson M, et al. Perioperative docetaxel, cisplatin, and 5-fluorouracil (DCF) for locally advanced esophageal and gastric adenocarcinoma: a multicenter phase II trial. Ann Oncol. 2012;23(6):1512-7.
68. Xiao ZF, Yang ZY, Liang J, Miao YJ, Wang M, Yin WB, et al. Value of radiotherapy after radical surgery for esophageal carcinoma: a report of 495 patients. Ann Thorac Surg. 2003;75(2):331-6.
69. Malthaner RA, Wong RK, Rumble RB, et al. Members of the Gastrointestinal Cancer Disease Site Group of Cancer Care Ontario's Program in Evidence-based Care. Neoadjuvant or adjuvant therapy for resectable esophageal cancer: a systematic review and metaanalysis. BMC Med. 2004;2:35.
70. Macdonald JS, Smalley SR, Benedetti J, Hundahl SA, Estes NC, Stemmermann GN, et al. Chemoradiotherapy after surgery compared with surgery alone for adenocarcinoma of the stomach or gastroesophageal junction. N Engl J Med. 2001;345(10):725-30.
71. Ando N, Iizuka T, Ide H, Ishida K, Shinoda M, Nishimaki T, et al. Surgery plus chemotherapy compared with surgery alone for localized squamous cell carcinoma of the thoracic esophagus: a Japan Clinical Oncology Group Study--JCOG9204. J Clin Oncol. 2003;21(24):4592-6.
72. Cunningham D, Allum WH, Stenning SP, Thompson JN, Van de Velde CJ, Nicolson M, et al. Perioperative chemotherapy versus surgery alone for resectable gastroesophageal cancer. N Engl J Med. 2006;355(1):11-20.
73. Sur RK, Levin CV, Donde B, Sharma V, Miszczyk L, Nag S, et al. Prospective randomized trial of HDR brachytherapy as a sole modality in palliation of advanced esophageal carcinoma—an International Atomic Energy Agency Study. Int J Radiat Oncol Biol Phys. 2002;53(1):127-33.
74. Rosenblatt E, Jones G, Sur RK, Donde B, Salvajoli JV, Ghosh-Laskar S, et al. Adding external beam to intra-luminal brachytherapy improves palliation in obstructive squamous cell oesophageal cancer: a prospective multi-centre randomized trial of the International Atomic Energy Agency. Radiother Oncol. 2010;97(3):488-94.
75. Wagner AD, Unverzagt S, Grothe W, Kleber G, Grothey A, Haerting J, et al. Chemotherapy for advanced gastric cancer. Cochrane Database Syst Rev. 2010;(3):CD004064.
76. Bang YJ, Van Cutsem E, Feyereislova A, Chung HC, Shen L, Sawaki A, et al. Trastuzumab in combination with chemotherapy versus chemotherapy alone for treatment of HER2-positive advanced gastric or gastro-oesophageal junction cancer (ToGA): a phase 3, open-label, randomised controlled trial. Lancet. 2010;376(9742):687-97.
77. Lu JJ, Brady LW. Decision making in Radiation Oncology Volume 1 Springer.
78. Shridhar R, Almhanna K, Meredith KL, Biagioli MC, Chuong MD, Cruz A, et al. Radiation therapy and esophageal cancer. Cancer Control. 2013;20(2):97-110.
79. Mackley HB, Adelstein JS, Reddy CA, Adelstein DJ, Rice TW, Saxton JP, et al. Choice of radiotherapy planning modality influences toxicity in the treatment of locally advanced esophageal cancer. J Gastrointest Cancer. 2008;39(1-4):130-7.
80. Martel MK, Sahijdak WM, Ten Haken RK, et al. Fraction size and dose parameters related to the incidence of pericardial effusions. Int J Radiat Oncol Biol Phys. 1998;40(1):155-61.
81. Martin S, Chen JZ, Rashid Dar A, et al. Dosimetric comparison of helical tomotherapy, RapidArc, and a novel IMRT & Arc technique for esophageal carcinoma. Radiother Oncol. 2011;101(3):431-7.
82. Schoenfeld GO, Amdur RJ, Morris CG, Li JG, Hinerman RW, Mendenhall WM. Patterns of failure and toxicity after intensity-modulated radiotherapy for head and neck cancer. Int J Radiat Oncol Biol Phys. 2008;71(2):377-85.
83. Chandra A, Guerrero TM, Liu HH, Tucker SL, Liao Z, Wang X, et al. Feasibility of using intensity-modulated radiotherapy to improve lung sparing in treatment planning for distal esophageal cancer. Radiother Oncol. 2005;77(3):247-53.
84. Chen YJ, Liu A, Han C, Tsai PT, Schultheiss TE, Pezner RD, et al. Helical tomotherapy for radiotherapy in esophageal cancer: a preferred plan with better conformal target coverage and more homogeneous dose distribution. Med Dosim. 2007;32(3):166-71.
85. Nguyen NP, Krafft SP, Vinh-Hung V, Vos P, Almeida F, Jang S, et al. Feasibility of tomotherapy to reduce normal lung and cardiac toxicity for distal esophageal cancer compared to three-dimensional radiotherapy. Radiother Oncol. 2011;101(3):438-42.
86. Shridhar R, Chuong M, Weber J, et al. Outcomes of definitive or preoperative IMRT chemoradiation for esophageal cancer. J Radiat Oncol. 2012:1-8.
87. Kole TP, Aghayere O, Kwah J, et al. Comparison of heart and coronary artery doses associated with intensity-modulated radiotherapy versus three-dimensional conformal radiotherapy for distal esophageal cancer. Int J Radiat Oncol Biol Phys. 2012;83(5):1580-6.
88. Nicolini G, Ghosh-Laskar S, Shrivastava SK, Banerjee S, Chaudhary S, Agarwal JP, et al. Volumetric modulation arc radiotherapy with flattening filter-free beams compared with static gantry IMRT and 3D conformal radiotherapy for advanced esophageal cancer: a feasibility study. Int J Radiat Oncol Biol Phys. 2012;84(2):553-60.
89. Yaremko BP, Guerrero TM, McAleer MF, Bucci MK, Noyola-Martinez J, Nguyen LT, et al. Determination of respiratory motion for distal esophagus cancer using four-dimensional computed tomography. Int J Radiat Oncol Biol Phys. 2008;70(1):145-53.
90. Patel AA, Wolfgang JA, Niemierko A, Hong TS, Yock T, Choi NC. Implications of respiratory motion as measured by four-dimensional computed tomography for radiation treatment planning of esophageal cancer. Int J Radiat Oncol Biol Phys. 2009;74(1):290-6.
91. Cohen RJ, Paskalev K, Litwin S, Price RA Jr, Feigenberg SJ, Konski AA. Esophageal motion during radiotherapy: quantification and margin implications. Dis Esophagus. 2010;23(6):473-9.
92. Fernandez DC, Hoffe SE, Barthel JS, Vignesh S, Klapman JB, Harris C, et al. Stability of endoscopic ultrasound-guided

fiducial marker placement for esophageal cancer target delineation and image-guided radiation therapy. Pract Radiat Oncol. 2013;3(1):32-9.

93. Fernandez DE, Hoffe SE, Dilling TE, et al. Effect of abdominal compression on respiratory motion of esophageal cancer measured with 4D-CT after EUS-guided fiducial marker placement. Int J Radiat Oncol Biol Phys. 2010;78(3):S302.
94. Dieleman EM, Senan S, Vincent A, Lagerwaard FJ, Slotman BJ, van Sörnsen de Koste JR. Four-dimensional computed tomographic analysis of esophageal mobility during normal respiration. Int J Radiat Oncol Biol Phys. 2007;67(3):775-80.
95. Zhao KL, Liao Z, Bucci MK, Komaki R, Cox JD, Yu ZH, et al. Evaluation of respiratory-induced target motion for esophageal tumors at the gastroesophageal junction. Radiother Oncol. 2007;84(3):283-9.
96. Kim S, Bae H, Oh D, et al. Effect of intrafractional organ motion on intensity-modulated radiation therapy dose distribution for lung cancer: a quantitative analysis using free-form deformable registration. Int J Radiat Oncol Biol Phys. 2008;72(1, Supplement):S457.
97. Forster K. The quantification of delivered IMRT doe distributions for mobile targets. Int J Radiat Oncol Biol Phys. 2010;78(3):S754.
98. Bouchard M, McAleer MF, Starkschall G. Impact of gastric filling on radiation dose delivered to gastroesophageal junction tumors. Int J Radiat Oncol Biol Phys. 2010;77(1):292-300.
99. Cooper SL, Russo JK, Chin S. Definitive chemoradiotherapy for esophageal carcinoma. Surg Clin N Am. 2012;92(5): 1213-48.
100. Hawkins MA, Brooks C, Hansen VN, et al. Cone beam computed tomography-derived adaptive radiotherapy for radical treatment of esophageal cancer. Int J Radiat Oncol Biol Phys. 2010;77(2):378-83.
101. Sriram P, Syamkumar SA, Devakumar JS, Prabhakar S, Dhanabalan R, Vivekanandan N. Adaptive volumetric modulated arc treatment planning for esophageal cancers using cone beam computed tomography. Physica Medica: European Journal of Medical Physics. 2012;28:327-32.
102. Srnivasan K, Mohammadi M, Shepherd J. Applications of linac-mounted kilovoltage Cone-beam Computed Tomography in modern radiation therapy: A review. Pol J Radiol. 2014;79:181-93.

16

CHAPTER

Gastric Cancer

Trinanjan Basu, Tejinder Kataria

EPIDEMIOLOGY AND ETIOLOGY

Gastric cancer is the fourth most commonly diagnosed malignancy and the second most common cause of cancer deaths worldwide. It is responsible for about 800,000 deaths globally per year. It is more common in Japan (78 per 100,000 men), Korea, China, other East Asian countries.

As per Indian data gastric malignancies will be the most common type of gastrointestinal (GI) malignancies by 2020.[1] A number of risk factors have been identified for gastric cancer (Table 1). Screening is not performed in most of the world, except in Japan and Korea, where early detection has significantly improved survival.

Table 1 Risk factors for carcinoma stomach

Risk factors	*Description*
Patient related	**Age and gender** Median age at diagnosis: 65 years Before 40 years rare M:F: 1.5:1 **Lifestyle** Smoked and salted food Lack of fruits and vegetables Nitrides and nitrosamines in diet Cigarette smoking Previous radiation exposure **Race** Africans, Asians and Hispanics are at higher risk **Past medical history** *H. pylori* infection associated with 3-6 fold higher risk Autoimmune gastritis, chronic gastritis, pernicious anemia Previous history of gastric polyp **Genetic predisposition** Peutz-Jeghers syndrome Familial adenomatous polyposis and hereditary nonpolyposis colorectal cancer (HNPCC) syndrome [microsatellite instability gene (MSI)] Gene mutations include p53, c-met, k-sam, E-cadherin gene (CDH1), bcl-2, and erb-B2 Slightly increased risk in blood group A

ANATOMY

Stomach begins at the gastroesophageal junction (GEJ) and continues till the pylorus. The left convex border being formed by the greater curvature and the lesser curvature forms the right and concave border. It has four parts, viz. cardia, fundus, body, and antrum. The inner wall has five layers namely mucosa, submucosa, muscularis externa, subserosa, and serosa (Fig. 1). The organ is covered with peritoneum and is closely related to the left lobe of the liver, spleen, left adrenal gland, superior portion of the left kidney, pancreas, transverse colon, and major blood vessels including the celiac axis and superior mesenteric artery.

PATHOLOGY

Adenocarcinoma accounts for more than 90% of all gastric cancers, and will be discussed here.

Adenocarcinomas are further subclassified into *intestinal* versus *diffuse* type (Lauren's classification) (Table 2). Borrmann's classification describes the gross pathologic findings of gastric cancer, and is associated with the aggressiveness of the disease (Table 3).

Routes of Spread

Local extension, regional (lymphatic), and hematogenous metastases are the three major routes of spread in gastric cancer.

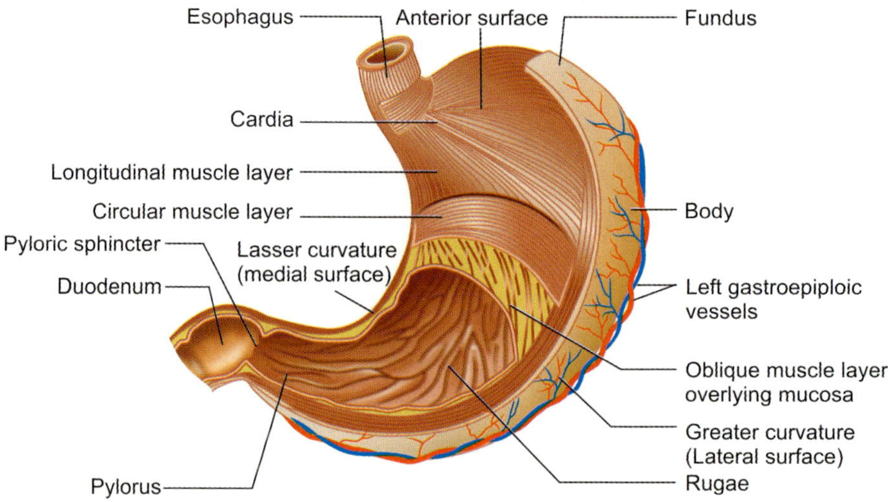

Fig. 1 Anatomy of stomach

Table 2 Lauren's classification

Intestinal type	*Diffuse type*
Occurs in older population	Occurs in younger population
More common in men	More common in women
Occurs usually in body and distal stomach	Occurs usually in the proximal stomach
Associated with *Helicobacter pylori* infection	Associated with hereditary factors
Often preceded by precancerous lesions	Not associated with precancerous lesions
Prone to hepatic metastases	Prone to peritoneal metastases
Associated with a better prognosis	Associated with a poorer prognosis

Table 3 Borrmann's classification

Type	*Description*
I	Polypoid or fungating
II	Ulcerating lesions surrounded by elevated borders
III	Ulcerating lesions with invasion of the gastric wall
IV	Diffusely infiltrating (linitis plastica)
V	Not classifiable

Local Extension

Direct involvement of adjacent structures. The proximal part of greater curvature growth may directly involve the splenic hilum and tail of pancreas, whereas more distal tumors may invade the transverse colon. Proximal cancers may also extend to the diaphragm, spleen, or the left lateral segment of the liver.

Regional Nodal Metastasis

Lymph node (LN) involvement is common and seen in about 80% cases at diagnosis. It also depends on the origin of the primary disease. The lymphatic drainage of the stomach is extensive and LNs have been defined according to their relationship to the stomach and its blood supply.

There are six perigastric LN groups: subpyloric and gastroepiploic along the greater curvature and suprapyloric along the lesser curvature. Proximally are found the right and left pericardial nodes.

The second echelon (extraperigastric) nodes include the common hepatic, left gastric, splenic hilum, and splenic artery lymphatics, which drain into the celiac and periaortic lymphatics. Proximally are the lower esophageal LNs; extensive spread of gastric cancer along the intrathoracic lymph channels may be manifested clinically as LN in the left supraclavicular fossa (Virchow's node) or left axilla (Irish's node).

The different lymph nodal stations anatomically and their radiological identification on contrast enhanced computed tomography (CT) scan being represented in Table 4.

Japanese Classification and its Impact upon Extent of Surgical Resection

Tumors can involve the submucosal lymphatic supply of the stomach becomes extensively and thus other routes of lymphatic drainage may be recruited. Tumor spread to the lymphatics in the hepatoduodenal ligament can extend along the falciform ligament and result in subcutaneous periumbilical tumor deposits known as Sister Mary Joseph's nodes.

Table 4 Japanese Research Society for the Study of Gastric Cancer classification

Station	*Nodes*
1	Right cardial
2	Left cardial
3	Along lesser curvature
4	Along greater curvature
5	Suprapyloric
6	Infrapyloric
7	Along left gastric artery
8	Along common hepatic artery
9	Along celiac axis
10	Along splenic hilum
11	Along splenic artery
12	Hepatoduodenal ligament
13	Postaspect of pancreatic head
14	At the root of mesentery
15	In the mesocolon of transverse colon
16	Para-aortic lymph nodes

The blood supply to the stomach is based on vessels arising from the celiac axis. The right gastric artery, arising from the hepatic artery, and the left gastric artery, arising from the celiac axis directly are along the lesser curvature. Whereas along the greater curvature are the right gastroepiploic artery, which originates from the gastroduodenal artery at the inferior border of the proximal duodenum, and the left gastroepiploic artery, branching from the splenic artery laterally. The short gastric arteries (vasa brevia) arise directly from the splenic artery and make a relatively small contribution to the blood supply to the proximal portion of the stomach. The preservation of any of these vessels in the course of a subtotal gastrectomy for carcinoma is not necessary (nor possible if the operation is performed correctly), and the most proximal few centimeters of remaining stomach are well supplied by collateral flow from the lower segmental esophageal arcade. The rich submucosal blood supply of the stomach is an important factor in its ability to heal rapidly and produce a low-incidence of anastomotic disruption.

The venous supply of the stomach tends to parallel the arterial supply. The venous efflux ultimately passes the portal venous system and is reflected in the fact that the liver is a primary site for distant metastatic spread.

Diagnosis, Staging, and Prognosis

In early stages, stomach cancer is often asymptomatic or causes only nonspecific symptoms. Commonly observed symptoms are abdominal pain, weight loss, anorexia, etc. and detailed in Table 5. The average interval between onset of symptoms and diagnosis is approximately 3 months in 40% of patients and longer than 1 year in approximately 20% of patients.

Table 5 Commonly observed signs and symptoms in gastric cancer

Type	*Description*
General	Usually lack of specific symptoms in the early stage. Indigestion or burning sensation (heartburn) Anorexia Weight loss Lethargy
Locoregional disease	Abdominal pain or discomfort in upper abdomen Nausea or vomiting (secondary to gastric outlet obstruction) Postprandial fullness Diarrhea or constipation Dysphagia Bleeding (hematemesis/melena)
Distant disease	Lymphadenopathy at supraclavicular fossa (*Virchow's node*), is considered distant metastases. *Blumer's shelf* (palpable mass on rectal examination suggests implants to the pelvis. Palpable ovarian mass (*Krukenberg tumor*) suggests ovarian involvement from drop metastasis. Hepatomegaly with disease extension to the liver

Endoscopic ultrasonography (EUS) accuracy for tumor T-classification ranges from 77% to 93% and accuracy for nodal (N) classification is 65% to 90%.

CT scan is accurate for T-classification is 43–70% and sensitivity and specificity for nodal staging range from 65% to 97%, and 49% to 90%. If neoadjuvant chemotherapy, chemoradiation, or surgery is planned staging laparoscopy is used and peritoneal spread being ruled out. Chest CT or X-ray is done to rule out pulmonary metastases. Accuracy of clinical diagnosis approaches 90%. Around 45% of patients have elevated CEA, CA125, CA19-9, and CA72-4 levels (Table 6).

Ideal pathology reporting for gastric cancer should consist of the following:

- Type—subclassify as intestinal or diffuse type as it may have implications on therapy
- Grade
- Depth of tumor invasion
- Vascular invasion
- Status of deep and mucosal margins
- Location of tumor in relationship to the esophagogastric junction (OGJ) (whether tumor crosses OGJ).

Table 6 TNM staging for carcinoma stomach (7th edition)[2]

Stage	*Description*
Primary tumor (T)	
Tx	Primary tumor cannot be assessed
T0	No evidence of primary tumor
Tis	Carcinoma in situ, i.e. intraepithelial tumor without invasion of lamina propria
T1a	Tumor invades lamina propria or muscularis mucosae
T1b	Tumor invading submucosa
T2	Tumor invading muscularis propria
T3	Tumor penetrating subserosal connective tissue without invasion of visceral peritoneum or adjacent structures. T3 tumors also include those extending into the gastrocolic or gastrohepatic ligaments, or into the greater or lesser omentum, without perforation of the visceral peritoneum covering these structures
T4a	Tumor invades serosa (visceral peritoneum)
T4b	Tumor invading adjacent structures like spleen, transverse colon, liver diaphragm, pancreas, abdominal wall, adrenal gland, kidney, small intestine and retroperitoneum.
Regional lymph nodes (N)	
NX	Regional lymph node(s) cannot be assessed
N0	No regional lymph nodal metastasis
N1	Metastasis in 1–2 regional lymph nodes
N2	Metastasis in 3–6 regional lymph nodes
N3	Metastasis in 7 or more regional lymph nodes.
Distant metastases (M)	
M0	No distant metastases
M1	Distant metastases

- Lymph node status and number of LN removed (retrieval of at least 15 LN is recommended to avoid stage migration).
- TRG—assess tumor response to neoadjuvant therapy.
- Human epidermal growth factor receptor 2 (HER 2) testing with immunohistochemistry (IHC) can be considered in all patients with advanced disease.

The most important prognostic factors of gastric cancer include staging at diagnosis (especially the N category), patients' performance status, and treatment modality.

The management of gastric cancer has always been controversial. Different institutions practice different management guidelines and the consensus for the same is also lacking. In Table 7, we briefly highlight the accepted, encouraging and data with inadequate evidence as per management (Table 7).[3] Later on we would elaborate the same.

Current Standard of Therapy

Surgical resection remains the mainstay of treatment. Even after surgical resection the local failure rates being quite high in all the available literature. Local or regional recurrence in the gastric or tumor bed, the anastomosis, or regional LNs occurs in 40–65% of patients after gastric resection with curative intent.[4,5] Only patients with stage IA gastric cancer after curative resection can be kept on follow-up.

Initially people have tried postoperative chemotherapy alone after curative resection of gastric cancer. The results demonstrated no added benefit in survival to surgery alone.[6] The high rate of local recurrence made postoperative radiotherapy as an attractive option in treatment. Four early randomized trials have shown the benefit of 5-fluorouracil-based chemoradiotherapy (CRT) over surgery alone [Gastrointestinal Tumor Study Group (GITSG), 1990, 1982; Klaassen et al. 1985; Moertel et al. 1984]. However, the number of patients in these studies was small (N=62–191) which limits the value of this observation.

In 2001, Mcdonald et al. published their results of more than 500 patients of adenocarcinoma stomach or GEJ treated by curative resection followed by observation or CRT. The median duration of relapse free survival was 30 months in the CRT group and 19 months in the surgery-only group. The 3 years rates of relapse-free survival were 48% in the CRT group and 31% in the surgery-only group. 64% of patients had relapse in the surgery-only group while 43% were in the CRT group (McDonald et al).[8] This study clearly demonstrated the

Table 7 Overview of management options in carcinoma stomach[3]

	Therapy	*Supporting data*
Accepted standard therapy	Postoperative chemotherapy Postoperative chemoradiotherapy Perioperative chemotherapy	Sakuramoto et al. (2007) Macdonald et al. (2001) Kim et al.(2005) Cunningham et al. (2006) Boige and Pignon et al. (2007)
Nonstandard therapy	Preoperative chemotherapy Postoperative combination chemotherapy Hyperthermic intraperitoneal chemotherapy Preoperative radiotherapy Preoperative chemoradiotherapy	Hartgrink et al. (2004) Schuhmacher et al. (2009) Sun etal. (2009) Yan et al. (2007) Florica et al. (2007) Valentini et al. (2009) Ajani et al. (2006)
Modalities with inadequate data	Postoperative radiotherapy Intraoperative radiotherapy	Valentini et al. (2009) Sindelar et al. (1993) Kramling et al(1996) Skoropad et al. (2000)

benefit of adjuvant CRT. With this trial postoperative CRT is currently a standard option in the United States for patients undergoing curative resection of stage Ib–IV gastric cancer who did not receive neoadjuvant therapy.

In a meta-analysis of postoperative CRT, 5-year overall survival is significantly higher with CRT as compared to surgery alone [odds ratio (OR) 0.45, 95% confidence interval (CI) 0.32–0.64]. Although CRT has higher frequency of severe and life-threatening toxicities, overall compliance was 73%. The majority of patients in this analysis are nonetheless derived from the intergroup trial (Fiorica et al. 2007).

Parallel to the development and validation of postoperative CRT the major concern remained the poor performance status postoperatively in these patients. This actually led to the development of neoadjuvant treatment as an attractive option. The main goal of giving neoadjuvant chemotherapy is to treat micrometastatic disease at an early stage and to improve resectability by tumor downsizing and downstaging.

The MRC Adjuvant Gastric Infusional Chemotherapy (MAGIC) trial, randomized 503 patients with advanced (more than submucosal), resectable adenocarcinoma of the stomach, OGJ, or lower esophagus for surgery and perioperative chemotherapy versus surgery alone. Chemotherapy regimen was three preoperative and three postoperative cycles of epirubicin, cisplatin and 5-fluorouracil. R0 resection rates were 66% and 69% for the two groups in favor of the chemotherapy group, and 40% of all resections were D2 LN dissections. About 86% of the patients completed the preoperative chemotherapy schedule, only 55% started postoperative chemotherapy and subsequently 42% completed all the six courses. The major reasons for not starting or finishing postoperative chemotherapy were early progressive disease or death, patient's request and postoperative complications. After a median follow-up of 48 months, 5-year overall survival was significantly higher in the chemotherapy group (36% versus 23%) with no differences according to tumor site. No differences in postoperative morbidity and mortality were observed between the two treatment groups (Cunningham et al. 2006).

A French prospective trial randomized 224 patients with adenocarcinoma of the stomach (25%), the GEJ (64%) or lower esophagus (11%) between chemotherapy plus surgery (N = 113) or surgery alone (N = 111). Chemotherapy regimen included two or three cycles of preoperative 5-fluorouracil and cisplatin and was continued after surgery in case of response to preoperative chemotherapy or stable disease with pN+. Compliance for the preoperative therapy was 87%, whereas 48% of the patients completed the total regimen. After a median follow-up of 5.7 years, 5-year overall and disease-free survival were significantly higher in the chemotherapy group (38% versus 24% and 34% versus 21%) (Boige and Pignon, 2007). Although the final report of this study is still awaited, the results are quite similar to the MAGIC study with better outcomes with perioperative chemotherapy as compared to surgery alone.

The main confusion between perioperative or postoperative treatment regimens has never been studied prospectively until recently Dutch CRITICS trial which had patients receiving three cycles of preoperative ECC (epirubicin, cisplatin and capecitabine), followed by D1+ surgery (D2 dissection without a splenectomy or pancreatectomy). Postoperative therapy consisted of another three cycles of ECC, or CRT with capecitabine and cisplatin without epirubicin (Table 8).

Details of technical consideration in 3D radiotherapy.[7]

Table 8 Current trials in gastric cancer

Trial	*Treatment setting*	*Treatment arm*	*No. of patients required*
CRITICS, Dutch colorectal cancer group	Stage Ib-IV gastric cancer	Perioperative ECC (epirubicin, cisplatin and capecitabine) Versus Preoperative ECC followed by surgery and then adjuvant chemoradiation	788
Magic B, British MRB	Stage Ib-IV resectable adenocarcinoma stomach or Type III GEJ cancers	Perioperative ECC Versus Perioperative ECC and bevacizumab and adjuvant maintenance bevacizumab x 6 cycles	1,100
ARTIST Intergroup CALGB 80101	> D2 resected stage IB-IV gastric cancer. Stage IB-IV resected adenocarcinoma of the stomach or GEJ gastric cancer stage II-IIIB.	Adjuvant CC (cisplatin and capecitabine) Adjuvant CC CRT (chemoradiation) Adjuvant 5FU CRT Adjuvant ECF CRT	490
CLASSIC trial	Stage II-IIIB gastric cancer	D2 resection, adjuvant capecitabine and cisplatin.	1,024

Simulation Considerations

The patient should be in a supine treatment position with arms overhead and should have fasted for 2–3 hours prior to the scan. It is preferable to administer 40–50 mL water per orally just before taking the scans. This helps to distend the remaining stomach and pushes away the intervening small bowels.

During CT simulation, the patient is positioned and straightened and a customized patient immobilization device is used to minimize daily setup variation.

For GEJ tumors, arms are generally placed overhead with knee support underneath the legs for patient comfort. Patients are usually treated in the supine position, although some authors have advocated that patients with mid-esophageal tumor involvement should be simulated in the prone position to maximize distance between the target volumes and spinal cord.[8] The administration of oral contrast medium helps delineate the esophagus and stomach by highlighting the extent of mucosal irregularity. Arterial-phase intravenous contrast medium is generally used to better define mediastinal and abdominal vascular nodal basins, including the celiac axis. Of note, these general principles for CT simulation planning are applicable for intact GEJ tumors as well as in the postoperative setting.

Although relatively little data exist on its use in GEJ tumors, respiratory motion management has been implemented in other disease sites to minimize physiological organ motion and, in turn, target volume movement. The clinical benefit of respiratory motion management still remains a topic of investigation as far as gastric cancers are concerned.

Preoperative or Definitive Therapy

Gross Tumor Volume

After a planning CT is obtained, it is important to determine primary and nodal disease extent for radiation treatment planning purposes. Endoscopy reports as well as various imaging modalities, including barium swallow, CT, positron-emission tomography (PET), and EUS, are useful to determine the gross tumor volume (GTV). Endoscopy remains the best tool both to diagnose and to define primary tumor extent for GEJ tumors. Accurate endoscopic tumor measurement in relation to key anatomic structures (such as distance from the incisors or GEJ) is important to correlate with GTV contours outlined on the planning CT.

In one study from Mayo Clinic, primary tumor (T) staging was correctly identified in only 42% of esophageal cancer patients using CT.[9,10] Additionally, a recent meta-analysis showed that CT sensitivity for detecting regional LN (N) involvement was only 50%.[11]

PET has emerged as an important tool in staging esophageal and GEJ cancer patients, particularly in detecting occult stage IV disease. Flamen et al. prospectively assessed 74 patients with esophageal and GEJ carcinomas and compared staging accuracy of PET and CT. PET demonstrated improved accuracy compared with CT (82% versus 64%) for diagnosing patients with stage IV disease.[11]

In summary, our policy is to use all data derived from swallowing studies, endoscopy, EUS, and PET-CT to define a composite GTV, given the advantages and limitations of each of these modalities.

Clinical Target Volume

An understanding of subclinical disease extent (i.e. clinical target volume or CTV) of the primary tumor is critical for radiotherapy field design. GEJ cancers represent a particular clinical challenge, given the rich submucosal lymphatic network in both the esophagus and stomach. Although not well defined, an approximate 1.5–2 cm radial margin expansion is recommended from the GTV to the CTV.

Dresner et al. evaluated the distribution of LN metastases for 152 patients with resected Siewert type I and II GEJ adenocarcinomas. They found that the frequency of nodal metastases exceeded 30% for the left gastric and paracardial LN basins, regardless of primary tumor location within the GEJ.[12]

Elective LN coverage is largely based on balancing risk of pathologic LN involvement with normal tissue dose constraints and treatment-related morbidity (Table 9). The suggested target volumes as per primary tumor stage and nodal involvement being represented in table originally described by Tepper et al.[13]

Planning Target Volume

The planning target volume is added to the CTV to account for tumor and physiological motion as well as daily setup uncertainty. Intrafraction variations in target location, in large part due to organ motion during the respiratory cycle, or interfraction variability due to stomach filling, can be considerable for GEJ tumors. MD Anderson investigators evaluated tumor motion characteristics for 31 patients with GEJ malignancies using respiratory-gated 4DCT. They demonstrated that 95% of tumors moved 0.75 cm radially and 1.75 cm inferiorly.[16] Other series have also shown GEJ and gastric tumor movement of approximately 1.5 cm superiorly-inferiorly.[17,18]

Postoperative Therapy

Local-regional recurrence rates after surgery alone for lower esophageal cancer are approximately 30–40% after R0 resection[19-21] emphasizing the need for adjunctive therapies.

However, defining an appropriate target volume after resection can be challenging for radiation oncologists.

Clinical Target Volume

Clinical and reoperation series examining recurrence patterns for resected gastric cancer can provide some basic principles for defining the postoperative CTV. In the University of Minnesota reoperation series by Gunderson[22] recurrence rates in the gastric bed, regional LNs, or at the gastric remnant and anastomoses were 55%, 43%, and 27%, respectively. These data can be applied to designing treatment volumes for resected GEJ tumors. Based on the

Table 9 Target volume delineation in gastric cancer[14,15]

Site of primary and TN stage	*Remaining stomach*	*Tumor-bed volume*	*Nodal volume*	*Tolerance organ structures*
GE junction	If allows exclusion of 2/3rd of right kidney	T stage dependent	N stage dependent	Heart, lungs, spinal cord, kidneys, bowel
T2N0 with subserosal invasion	Depends upon surgical-pathological findings Tumors with wide margin (>5 cm) and confirmed negative margin histopathologically, no need to treat remaining stomach	Medial left hemidiaphragm and adjacent body of pancreas	None or perigastric and periesophageal Can exclude if D2 dissection and at least 10–15 nodes being dissected	
T3N0	Depends upon surgical-pathological findings Tumors with wide margin (>5 cm) and confirmed negative margin histopathologically, no need to treat remaining stomach	Medial left hemidiaphragm and adjacent body of pancreas	None or perigastric, periesophageal, mediastinal and celiac. Can exclude if D2 dissection and at least 10–15 nodes being dissected	
T4N0	Preferable	Site of adherence + 5 cm margin and as per T3N0	Nodes related to site of adherence +/- perigastric, periesophageal, mediastinal and celiac	
T1-T2 N+	Preferable	Not indicated for T1, as above for T2 into subserosa	Periesophageal, mediastinal, proximal perigastric, celiac	
T3-T4 N+	Preferable	As for T3, T4N0	As for T1-2N + and T4N0	

recent National Comprehensive Cancer Network guidelines for surgically staged esophageal, GEJ, and gastric cancers, adjuvant chemoradiation is a recommended option for T3/T4 lesions, node-positive tumors, and select T2N0 cancers.

The tumor bed, which can be determined, based on preoperative imaging and/or strategically placed surgical clips, should be included in the CTV. Coverage of the remaining stomach should also be considered, depending on the pathologic T stage (T2 or greater), the presence of adverse tumor histology (such as signet ring), and the surgical margin status, which is 5 cm proximal and distal in optimal cases. However, coverage of the gastric remnant and anastomosis (which is usually transposed to the mid-chest or neck, depending on surgical approach) must be weighed against the morbidity associated with treatment to such a large volume. Pathologically involved LN basins as well as nodal regions deemed at high risk of involvement, including the periesophageal, paracardial, and celiac axis, should be included in treatment volumes for node-positive patients. Coverage of LN basins for node-negative patients depends in part on the extent of LN harvest (Table 1).[23]

Planning Target Volume

The planning target volume expansion in the postoperative setting should be based on the same principles as in the preoperative or definitive setting where there is an intact tumor. However, depending on the site of the anastomosis (i.e. in the upper mediastinum after and Ivor-Lewis esophagectomy), there may not be as much motion relative to an intact primary tumor in the abdomen or at the level of the diaphragm. Motion management can still be used if there is concern about coverage of the nodal regions or mobile anastomosis.

DOSE AND TREATMENT DELIVERY

Conventional fractionation and a total dose of 45–50.4 Gy is recommended for adjuvant radiation therapy with concurrent chemotherapy, using high-energy (6 MV) photons. Positive margins or residual disease can receive boost up to 50.4–54 Gy keeping in mind the tolerances of the surrounding critical organs.

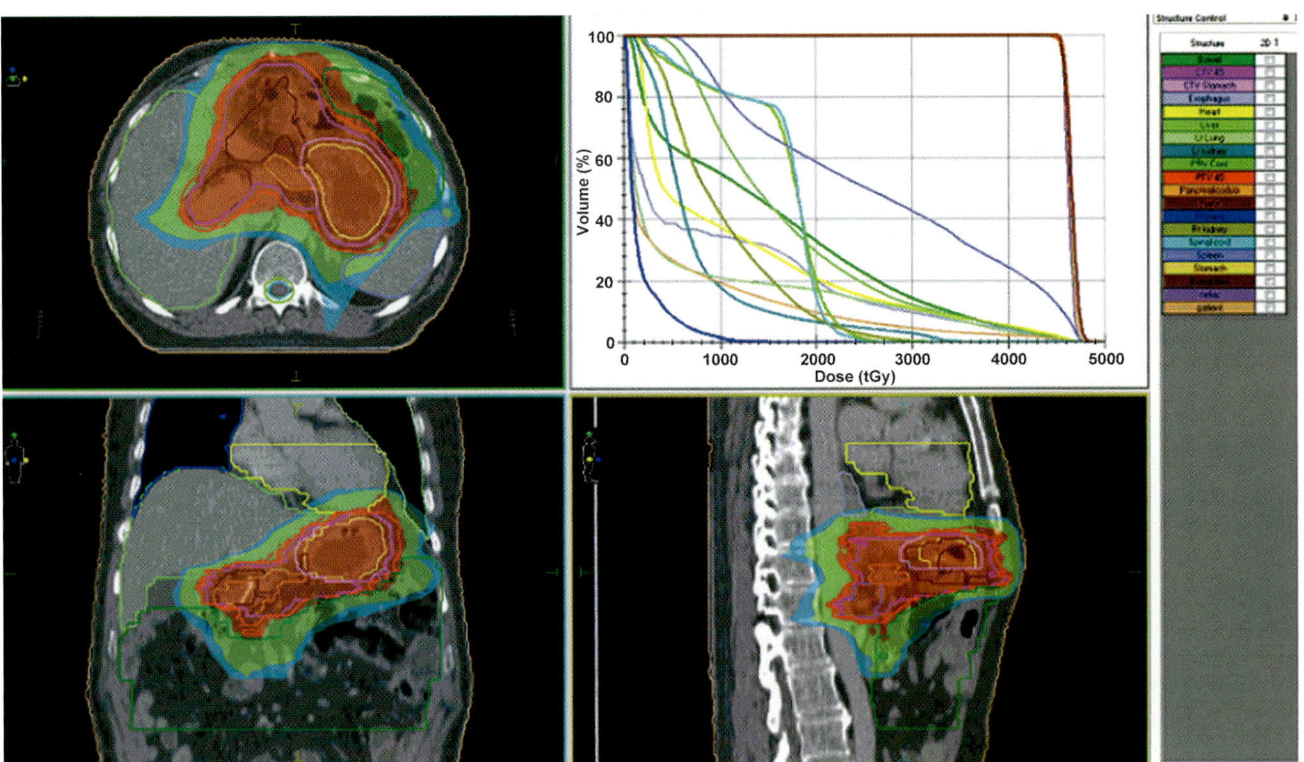

Fig. 2 Dose distribution in intensity-modulated radiotherapy (IMRT) planning in Ca stomach

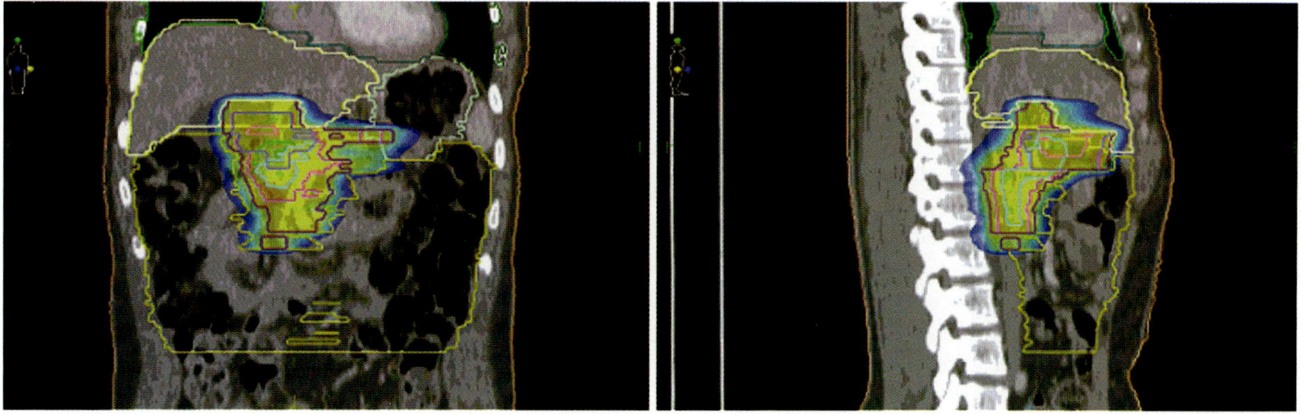

Fig. 3 Coronal and sagittal view of target volume and dose color wash for intensity-modulated radiotherapy (IMRT) plan

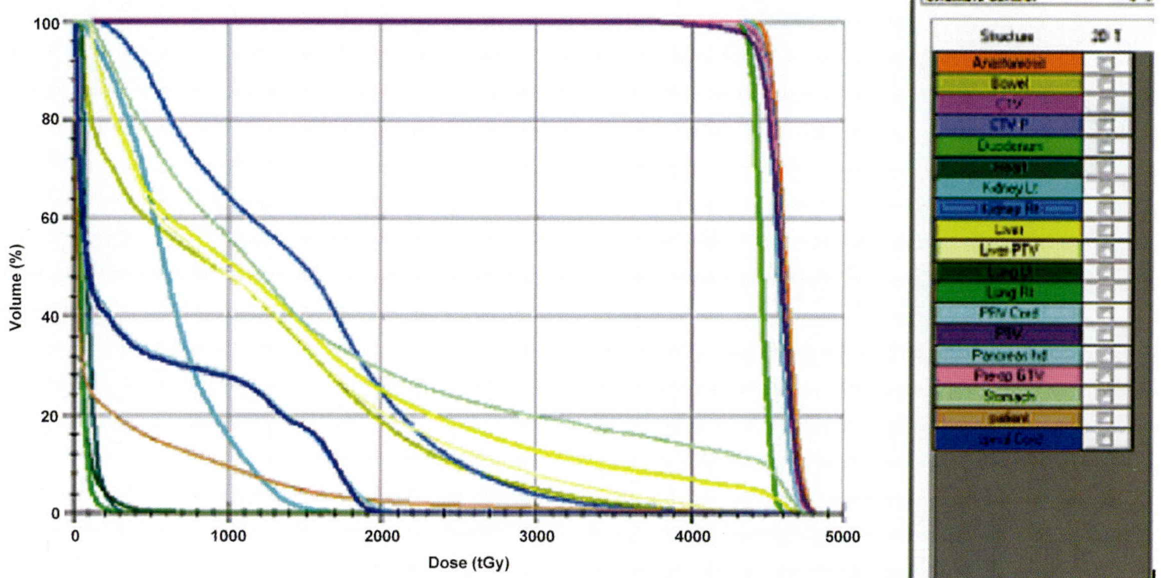

Fig. 4 Dose volume histogram (DVH) for intensity-modulated radiotherapy (IMRT) plan [Purple: PTV, deep blue: Spinal cord, V20 for both kidneys less than 30%, Volume of bowel (yellow) over Dp less than 1 cc]

Role of IMRT in Gastric Cancer

For gastric malignancies intensity-modulated radiation therapy (IMRT) proved to be a better alternative than simple conformal therapy. Initial studies mainly dosimetric clearly highlighted the better sparing of organs at risk, viz. left kidney, bowel, spinal cord (Figs 2 to 4).[14,15]

A comparison of 45 Gy (median dose to target volume) step-and-shoot IMRT versus conventional 8-beam and noncoplanar plans showed best kidney sparing with noncoplanar anteroposterior (AP) and posteroanterior (PA) fields and best liver sparing with IMRT.[24,25] The same group then compared techniques in 15 patients with gastric cancer: 8-field step-and-shoot IMRT, conformal radiation planning, an AP opposed beam arrangement (AP-PA), and intensity-modulated arc therapy or tomotherapy plans using 1- or 2 cm collimation. Step-and-shoot IMRT and tomotherapy were found to improve the target coverage while at the same time reducing the dose to sensitive normal structures. However, the smallest volume of liver was irradiated with the AP-PA technique. IMRT plans were less dependent on individual anatomy. The main problems with IMRT were long treatment time (about 20 minutes) and increased inhomogeneity of dose within the target volume.

Ringash et al.[26] evaluated observer preference for IMRT versus conformal radiation plans. 20 patients who had undergone treatment planning with 5-field conformal plans were replanned with 7- to 9-axial-field IMRT. Two-independent radiation oncologists specializing in GI malignancies reviewed the cumulative dose-volume histograms and organ-dose summaries for each plan.

The IMRT plan was preferred in 17 of 19 cases (89%). In 86% of IMRT plans, the target coverage was improved, while spinal cord, liver, kidney and heart dose was reduced in 74%, 71%, 69% and 69%, respectively. In 4 of the 20 IMRT plans, at least one radiation oncologist had safety concerns due to a higher spinal cord dose and/or the volume of small bowel irradiated.

Another recent article by Liu et al., also compared IMRT chemoradiation 50.4 Gy with three-dimensional conformal radiotherapy (3DCRT) 45 Gy and IMRT was found to be well-tolerated with no grade 3 acute GI toxicities. As far as survival both the arms had similar results.[27]

REFERENCES

1. Takiar R, Nadayil D, Nandakumar A. Projections of number of cancer cases in India (2010-2020) by cancer groups. Asian Pac J Cancer Prev. 2010;11(4):1045-9.
2. Edge SB, Byrd DR, Compton CC, et al. American Joint Committee on Cancer, American Cancer Society. AJCC cancer staging manual, 7th edition. Springer, Berlin Heidelberg New York, 2009.
3. Ref table management overview gastric cancer: Dikken JL, Velde CJHV, Coit DG, Shah MA, Verheij M and Cats A Treatment of resectable gastric cancer. Ther Adv Gastroenterol. 2012;5:49-69.
4. Landry J, Tepper JE, Wood WC, Moulton EO, Koerner F, Sullinger J. Patterns of failure following curative resection of gastric cancer. Int J Radiat Oncol Biol Phys. 1990;19(6):1357-62.
5. Gunderson LL, Sosin H. Adenocarcinoma of the stomach: areas of failure in a re-operation series (second or symptomatic look): clinicopathologic correlation and implications for adjuvant therapy. Int J Radiat Oncol Biol Phys. 1982;8(1):1-11.
6. Earle CC, Maroun JA. Adjuvant chemotherapy after curative resection for gastric cancer in non-Asian patients: revisiting a meta-analysis of randomised trials. Eur J Cancer. 1999;35(7):1059-64.
7. Pepek JM, Willett CG, Czito BG. Technical considerations in radiation therapy for gastroesophageal junction cancer. Semin Radiat Oncol. 2013;23(1):51-9.
8. Corn BW, Coia LR, Chu JC, Hwang CC, Stafford PM, Hanks GE. Significance of prone positioning in planning treatment for esophageal cancer. Int J Radiat Oncol Biol Phys. 1991;21(5):1303-9.
9. Lowe VJ, Booya F, Fletcher JG, Nathan M, Jensen E, Mullan B, et al. Comparison of positron emission tomography, computed tomography, and endoscopic ultrasound in the initial staging of patients with esophageal cancer. Mol Imaging Biol. 2005;7(6):422-30.
10. van Vliet EP, Heijenbrok-Kal MH, Hunink MG, et al. Staging investigations for oesophageal cancer: a meta-analysis. Br J Cancer. 2008;98(3):547-57.
11. Flamen P, Lerut A, Van Cutsem E, De Wever W, Peeters M, Stroobants S, et al. Utility of positron emission tomography for the staging of patients with potentially operable esophageal carcinoma. J Clin Oncol. 2000;18(18):3202-10.
12. Dresner SM, Lamb PJ, Bennett MK, et al. The pattern of metastatic lymph node dissemination from adenocarcinoma of the esophagogastric junction. Surgery. 2001;129(1):103-9.
13. Tepper JE, Gunderson LL. Radiation treatment parameters in the adjuvant postoperative therapy of gastric cancer. Semin Radiat Oncol. 2002;12(2):187-95.
14. Milano MT, Garofalo MC, Chmura SJ, Farrey K, Rash C, Heimann R, et al. Intensity-modulated radiation therapy in the treatment of gastric cancer: early clinical outcome and dosimetric comparison with conventional techniques. Br J Radiol. 2006;79(942):497-503.
15. Wieland P, Dobler B, Mai S, Hermann B, Tiefenbacher U, Steil V, et al. IMRT for postoperative treatment of gastric cancer: covering large target volumes in the upper abdomen: a comparison of a step-and-shoot and an arc therapy approach. Int J Radiat Oncol Biol Phys. 2004;59(4):1236-44.
16. Yaremko BP, Guerrero TM, McAleer MF, Bucci MK, Noyola-Martinez J, Nguyen LT, et al. Determination of respiratory motion for distal esophagus cancer using four-dimensional computed tomography. Int J Radiat Oncol Biol Phys. 2008;70(1):145-53.
17. Zhao KL, Liao Z, Bucci MK, Komaki R, Cox JD, Yu ZH, et al. Evaluation of respiratory-induced target motion for esophageal tumors at the gastroesophageal junction. Radiother Oncol. 2007;84(3):283-9.
18. Wysocka B, Kassam Z, Lockwood G, Brierley J, Dawson LA, Buckley CA, et al. Interfraction and respiratory organ motion during conformal radiotherapy in gastric cancer. Int J Radiat Oncol Biol Phys. 2010;77(1):53-9.
19. Kelsen DP, Ginsberg R, Pajak TF, Sheahan DG, Gunderson L, Mortimer J, et al. Chemotherapy followed by surgery compared with surgery alone for localized esophageal cancer. N Engl J Med. 1998;339(27):1979-84.
20. Urba SG, Orringer MB, Turrisi A, Iannettoni M, Forastiere A, Strawderman M. Randomized trial of preoperative chemoradiation versus surgery alone in patients with locoregional esophageal carcinoma. J Clin Oncol. 2001; 19(2):305-13.
21. Hulscher JB, van Sandick JW, de Boer AG, Wijnhoven BP, Tijssen JG, Fockens P, et al. Extended transthoracic resection compared with limited transhiatal resection for adenocarcinoma of the esophagus. N Engl J Med. 2002;347(21):1662-9.
22. Gunderson LL, Sosin H. Adenocarcinoma of the stomach: areas of failure in a re-operation series (second or symptomatic look)

clinicopathologic correlation and implications for adjuvant therapy. Int J Radiat Oncol Biol Phys.1982;8(1):1-11.
23. Tepper JE, Gunderson LL. Radiation treatment parameters in the adjuvant postoperative therapy of gastric cancer. Semin Radiat Oncol. 2002;12(2):187-95.
24. Lohr F, Dobler B, Mai S, Hermann B, Tiefenbacher U, Wieland P, et al. Optimization of dose distributions for adjuvant locoregional radiotherapy of gastric cancer by IMRT. Strahlenther Onkol. 2003;179(8):557-63.
25. Wieland P, Dobler B, Mai S, Hermann B, Tiefenbacher U, Steil V, et al. IMRT for postoperative treatment of gastric cancer: covering large target volumes in the upper abdomen: a comparison of a step-and-shoot and an arc therapy approach. Int J Radiat Oncol Biol Phys. 2004;59(4):1236-44.
26. Ringash J, Perkins G, Brierley J, Lockwood G, Islam M, Catton P, et al. IMRT for adjuvant radiation in gastric cancer: a preferred plan? Int J Radiat Oncol Biol Phys. 2005;63(3):732-8.
27. Liu GF, Bair RJ, Bair E, et al. Clinical outcomes for gastric cancer following adjuvant chemoradiation utilizing intensity modulated versus three-dimensional conformal radiotherapy. PLoS ONE. 2014;9(1):e82642.

17 CHAPTER

Carcinoma of Anal Canal

Trinanjan Basu, Ruchi Singh, Tejinder Kataria

INTRODUCTION

Anal canal cancers constitute 1% of all colorectal malignancies and around 10% of all rectal cancers. These are mostly observed among those aged 60–65 years. It is one of the non-AIDS defining malignancies and has increased prevalence among HIV infected population.[1]

ETIOLOGY

Squamous cell carcinoma of the anus (SCCA) is strongly associated with human papillomavirus (HPV) infection and it is the causative agent in 80–85% of patients (usually from HPV16 or HPV18 subtypes) as its precursor lesion anal intraepithelial neoplasia (AIN) 3.[2] Anal intercourse and multiple sexual partners, men who have sex with men (MSM), HIV infection, history of HPV related cancers, long-term immunosuppressant's, auto-immune disorders all play a role in its etiology in varying proportions.

Dietary habits, chronic inflammatory diseases and hemorrhoids are not associated with increased risk of developing anal cancers.[3]

HPV and anal cancers few points:[4]

- HPV 6 and 11 are causative for benign wart. Local control achieved with a wide selection of surgical and topical techniques for them. HPV 16, 18, and 31 are found in dysplastic lesions and they have the potential for invasive anal squamous cell carcinoma.
- Following transmission, the incubation period is usually 3–4 months but can also extend up to 2 years. HPV DNA is then incorporated into the host nucleus either as free episomal form for low-risk serotypes or as incorporation into host genome for high-risk serotypes.
- HPV-associated tumors usually retain wild-type P53 and thus they respond well to concurrent chemoradiotherapy.
- Recognition and early management will be crucial to prevent morbidity and mortality associated with anal cancer.

ANATOMICAL ASPECTS

The rectum continues downward to form the anal canal, which is 3–4 cm in length and ends at the anus. The anal canal can be defined as either the surgical or the anatomical canal.

- *Anatomical anal canal:* It lies between the anal verge and the dentate line.
- *Surgical anal canal:* It is 3–4 cm section localized between the anal verge and the anorectal ring.

Anorectal ring is a muscular ring felt during a digital examination and forms the proximal end point of the internal sphincter muscle-puborectal muscle complex. It forms the border of the rectum-anal canal.

There is individual variation in the length of the anal canal (2–8 cm, mean 3.5–4 cm). These are important in cancer surgery. For instance, it is theoretically possible to conserve sphincter function when a tumor is palpated at 5 cm in a patient with a 3 cm anal canal. However, the sphincter cannot be conserved in distal rectal tumors extending into the anal canal and invading the sphincter muscles. The epithelium above the dentate line is transitional epithelium, while the epithelium below until the anal verge is a special non-keratinized squamous epithelium with no hair follicles or sweat glands, also called as anoderm (Fig. 1).[5,6]

Proximal lymphatic drainage is to perirectal nodes along the inferior mesenteric artery. Immediately above the dentate line the drainage goes into internal pudendal nodes, and to the internal iliac system. Inferior to dentate line and perianal skin the draining node are inguinal, femoral and external iliac nodes.

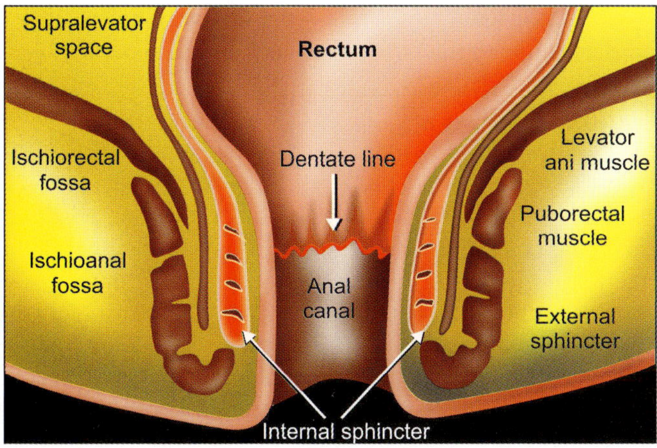

Fig. 1 Anatomy of anal canal

PATHOLOGICAL ASPECT

Most of the anal cancers are squamous cell (60%), followed by transitional cell cancers (25%) and adenocarcinomas (7%). Less frequent ones are the basaloid cell cancers (cloacogenic cancer) and malignant melanomas. Most being small cell cancers but have a high-risk of distant metastasis.[7]

Tumors of the anal margin are generally well-differentiated and mostly occur in men, in contrast to canal tumors which are poorly differentiated and more common in female.

Histological grading is variable and high-grade tumors have a comparatively worse prognosis. Some authors report that basaloid histological subtype has higher risk of metastatic potential. The biology and prognosis of keratinizing and non-keratinizing tumors of the anal canal appear to be identical. Verrucous carcinomas are a variant and also called as giant condylomas or Buschke–Lowenstein tumors and have better prognosis.[3]

CLINICAL FEATURES

Squamous cell carcinomas commonly presents with bleeding and thus other causes of per rectal bleeding needs to be excluded and this at times delay the diagnosis. Carcinomas can also present as a combination of a mass, non-healing ulcer, pain, bleeding, itching, discharge, fecal incontinence, and fistulae. Advanced lesions can also extend onto the skin at the anal margin. Inguinal lymphadenopathy is also not uncommon in anal canal cancers.[3]

STAGING INVESTIGATIONS

- *Mandatory for staging*:
  - Digital rectal examination with biopsy.
  - FNAC of enlarged inguinal lymph nodes.
  - Chest X-ray or CT scan of thorax.
  - CT/MRI of abdomen/pelvis.
- *Optional for staging*:
  - PET-CT scan.
- *Other pretreatment investigations*:
  - Patient testing positive for HIV CD4 counts.
  - Complete blood count/biochemistry.
  - Sperm banking if needed.
  - Ovarian transposition/choice of post-treatment hormone therapy.
  - Defunctioning colostomy in those with vaginal involvement.

Digital rectal examination (DRE) establishes the anal lesion and perirectal nodal involvement. In women (particularly with low anteriorly placed tumors) a vaginal examination is done to determine the site and size of the primary tumor and mucosal and/or vaginal/vaginal septal involvement. Palpation of the inguinal nodes is very important, particularly the superficial inguinal nodes, medial and close to the pubis.

Proctoscopy by a specialist surgeon or radiation oncologist and in case of painful lesions examination under anesthesia (EUA) may be appropriate. This also helps in biopsy. It is advantageous if the treating radiation oncologist has seen the lesion during EUA to document precise location, and thus can be critical for later target volume delineation in treatment planning.[3,8]

Imaging studies include MRI of the pelvis or, if not available, endo-anal ultrasound (EUS). Assessment of distant metastases with CT scan of the thorax and abdomen. MRI provides excellent contrast and spatial resolution, providing information on tumor size, local extent and spread, and invasion of adjacent organs and more accurate nodal involvement.[3,8]

Positron emission tomography (PET)/CT with [18F] fluorodeoxyglucose (FDG-PET/CT) is highly sensitive in identifying involved lymph nodes and the majority of anal carcinomas are FDG-avid. Several studies have shown that FDG-PET/CT can alter staging in approximately 20% of cases, with a trend toward upstaging and it can also influence treatment intent in approximately 3–5% of cases. The main impact of FDG-PET/CT on therapy is to distinguish between node positive and node negative anal canal cancers.[3]

TNM STAGING

The TNM clinical staging system is based on accurate assessment of size (T-stage), regional lymph node involvement (N) and metastatic spread (M). Nodal status is based on the distance from the primary site and not on the number of nodes involved (Table 1).[9]

MANAGEMENT

The primary aim of treatment would be loco-regional control and preservation of anal function keeping in mind the best possible quality of life. Though anatomically adjacent, the treatment differs significantly with that of adenocarcinomas of lower rectum. Multidisciplinary approach is warranted.

Table 1 TNM staging for carcinoma anal canal

Primary tumor (T)	
Tx	Primary tumor cannot be assessed
T0	No evidence of primary tumor
Tis	Carcinoma in situ (i.e. Bowen disease, high-grade squamous intraepithelial lesion, and anal intraepithelial neoplasia II–III)
T1	Tumor < = to 2 cm in greatest dimension
T2	Tumor > 2 cm but < 5 cm in greatest dimension
T3	Tumor > 5 cm in greatest dimension
T4	Tumor of any size invading the adjacent organ(s), e.g. vagina, urethra, and bladder
Regional lymph node (N)	
Nx	Regional lymph nodes cannot be assessed
N0	No regional lymph node metastasis
N1	Metastases in perirectal lymph node(s)
N2	Metastases in unilateral internal iliac and/or inguinal lymph node(s)
N3	Metastases in perirectal and inguinal lymph nodes and/or bilateral internal iliac and/or inguinal lymph nodes
Distant Metastasis	
M0	No distant metastasis
M1	Distant metastasis

Very small lesions (< 2 cm in diameter), involving the anal margin and not poorly differentiated may be treated by primary surgery in the form of a local excision only if adequate margins (> 5 mm) can be obtained without compromising sphincter function.[3]

The initial studies of Nigro demonstrated the curative potential of chemoradiotherapy for anal cancer.[10] Till today due to the rarity of this disease, different site of origin of the cancer (the anal margin, anal canal or dentate line) limited evidence from only six randomized trials are available.[11-16] Radical chemoradiotherapy should be considered for all patients with non-metastatic anal cancer with good performance status.

Concurrent Chemoradiation

Supporting evidence for effectiveness of concurrent chemoradiation (CRT) as a radical treatment has been provided by the results of the multiple phase II and six randomized phase III trials (EORTC 22861, UKCCCR ACT I, RTOG 87-04, RTOG 98-11, ACCORD-03, CRUK ACT II). As per chemotherapy regimen 5-FU (5-fluorouracil) with MMC (mitomycin C) combined with radiotherapy are generally recommended.

The synopses of these trials are being elaborated in Table 2. For details please refer to the individual trials separately.

Radiotherapy Techniques

Simulation

Patients can be treated both in supine and prone positions. The advantage of supine being treatment of inguinal nodes and in prone position, the displacement of small bowel from radiotherapy fields. Prone position also allows for easy visualization of anal verge which guides as starting point of target delineation once radio-opaque markers being placed.[3]

All palpable disease in the anal margin or lymph nodes is marked with radio-opaque material for identification on CT scans or simulator films. Surface boundaries of the inguinal region are marked on the skin with wire for simulation. Contrast enhanced CT scans is obtained from L2–L3 region up to mid-thigh with slice thickness varying between 3 mm and 5 mm depending upon institutional protocol.

Target Volume Definition

The CT based target delineation has its standard guidelines. The pioneer being the Myerson et. al. for ano-rectal target volume delineation and later on for anal cancer IMRT guidelines by Australasian Gastrointestinal Trials Group (AGITG). The details of them with colored atlases are available online and readers are encouraged to go through them.[17,18]

The phase 1 target volume includes all macroscopic primary tumor (GTV-T) and involved lymph nodes (GTV-N), and all microscopic disease at risk in the pelvis, inguinal and femoral nodal regions. The phase 2 target volume includes all macroscopic primary tumor (GTV-T) and involved lymph nodes if present (GTV-N) with a 10–15 mm margin for the CTV. It is always necessary to use the clinical information about the size of the tumor, its length and distance of the inferior limit from the anal verge to contour the GTV. Using radio-opaque wire on the anal verge and rectal contrast, the distance of the superior extent of the anal tumor from the anal verge can be confirmed. Diagnostic MR scans which show the extent of tumor in three dimensions can be fused with the planning CT scan.

Organs at risk (OAR) include the small bowel, bladder, femoral heads, pelvic bones and external genitals.

Phase 1 volume (all tumors):

- *Superior border*: 2 cm above inferior aspect of the sacroiliac joints is the standard border. However, it needs to be modified to include a minimum margin of 3 cm above the upper extent of GTV-T or GTV-N.
- *Lateral border* to include both inguinal nodal regions and for practical purpose this border lies lateral to the femoral head.

Table 2 Important clinical trials in carcinoma anal canal

Trial name	*Patient population and methodology*	*Main highlights*	*Toxicities*
EORTC 22861	Feasibility study to evaluate reduction of the gap between sequences to 2 weeks, to deliver mitomycin C (MMC) in each radiotherapy sequence and 5-fluorouracil (5-FU) continuously during the treatment. The first sequence was radiotherapy 36 Gy over 4 weeks. 5-FU 200 mg/m^2/days 1-26, MMC 10 mg/m(2)/day 1 gap 16 days. Then second sequence of 23.4 Gy over 17 days, 5-FU 200 mg/m^2/days 1–17 and, MMC 10 mg/m^2/day 1 was given. Total 43 patients with T2-T4, N0-N3 stages were included.	93% compliance with the planned treatment, doses and duration. The complete response rate: 90.7%.	Grade 3 toxicities were 28, 12 and 2% for skin, diarrhea and hematological toxicities, respectively.
UKCCCR ACT I	Randomization of 577 patients to receive RT alone or combined modality therapy using 5-FU and MMC. All patients received 45 Gy by external beam irradiation. Patients who responded to treatment, then further received boost RT with either Iridium implant or external beam irradiation.	With 12 years follow-up for every 100 patients treated with chemoradiation, there was an expected 25.3 fewer patients with loco-regional relapse and 12.5 fewer anal cancer deaths compared with 100 patients receiving RT alone.	Main toxicity was anorectal in both the arms at least 30%.
RTOG 87-04	To determine the importance of MMC in the treatment of anal cancer Patients received RT with concurrent fluorouracil (FU; 1,000 mg/m^2/d as a continuous infusion for 96 hours) with or without MMC (10 mg/m^2 by intravenous bolus on days 1 and 28). Radiotherapy dose was 30.6 Gy to the whole pelvis, 36 Gy to the true pelvis below the sacroiliac joints, and 45–50.4 Gy to the primary. The inguinal lymph nodes received 45 and 50.4 Gy for N0 and N+ disease respectively.	Total of 291 patients were randomly assigned and median follow-up was 3 years. Post-treatment biopsies were positive in 14% of patients in the follow-up arm versus 8% in the MMC arm. At 4 years, colostomy failure rates were lower (9% vs 22%; P 0.002), colostomy-free survival higher (71% vs 59%; P 0.014), and disease-free survival (DFS) higher (73% vs 51%; P 0.0003) in the MMC arm. There was no significant difference though in overall survival.	
RTOG 98-11	620 patients were analyzed for impact of TN category on DFS and overall (OS) survivals.	Poorest OS and DFS outcomes were for T3-4N-positive disease. Colostomy failure was lowest for T2N0 status.	
ACCORD-03	Therapeutic intensification trial. Included 119 patients for the evaluation of colostomy-free survival with induction chemotherapy and/or high dose radiotherapy. QOL was assessed both before and 2 months after treatment with the EORTC QLQ-C30 questionnaire as well as a questionnaire relating to anal sphincter conservative treatment (AS-CT).	Patients reported significant improvement in their emotional function, global health status. Constipation, appetite loss and pain. This was the first prospective study and it compared QOL of patients with advanced anal canal carcinoma, before and 2 months after conservative treatment. Induction chemotherapy and high dose radiotherapy did not provide a negative impact on QOL.	

Contd...

Contd...

Trial name	*Patient population and methodology*	*Main highlights*	*Toxicities*
CRUK ACT II	Radiotherapy dose of 50.4 Gy/28 fractions with chemotherapy of 5-FU and MMC only on day 1 while 5-FU 24 hours infusion on week 1 and week 5 for 4 days each. Digital examination for response at 11, 18 and 26 weeks and abdominopelvic CT scan at 26 weeks. If persistent disease confirmed on biopsy considered for salvage colostomy.	Positive inguinal nodes, male sex and low hemoglobin were the bad prognostic factors for loco-regional failure, anal cancer death and overall survival.	Acute grade 3 or more skin, gastro-intestinal toxicities around 75%.

- *Inferior border:* 3 cm below the anal margin (for disease confined to the anal canal only) or 3 cm below the most inferior extent of tumor (for anal margin tumors).

Phase 2 volume

The volume depends on the presence or absence of positive nodes in the inguinofemoral or pelvic regions and is defined from CT scanning. Lymph nodes that are likely to contain tumor should be treated to the full phase 2 dose.

Standard dosage

- *Phase 1:* 30.6–45 Gy in daily fractions of 1.8 Gy given in 3.5 weeks.
- *Phase 2:* 15–20 Gy in either 1.8 Gy daily fractions or hypofractionated boost (3–4 Gy per fraction) with either conformal EBRT or brachytherapy if feasible.

 or

- *Single phase:* 50.4 Gy in 28 daily fractions of 1.8 Gy given in 6 weeks.

Brachytherapy alone can be used for small T1 tumors and as a boost after chemoradiotherapy with local control rates of 80–90%. The typical planning volumes being given in Figure 2.

As per ESSO-ESMO-ESTRO consensus, it remains unclear whether increasing the radiation dose to greater than 50 Gy in

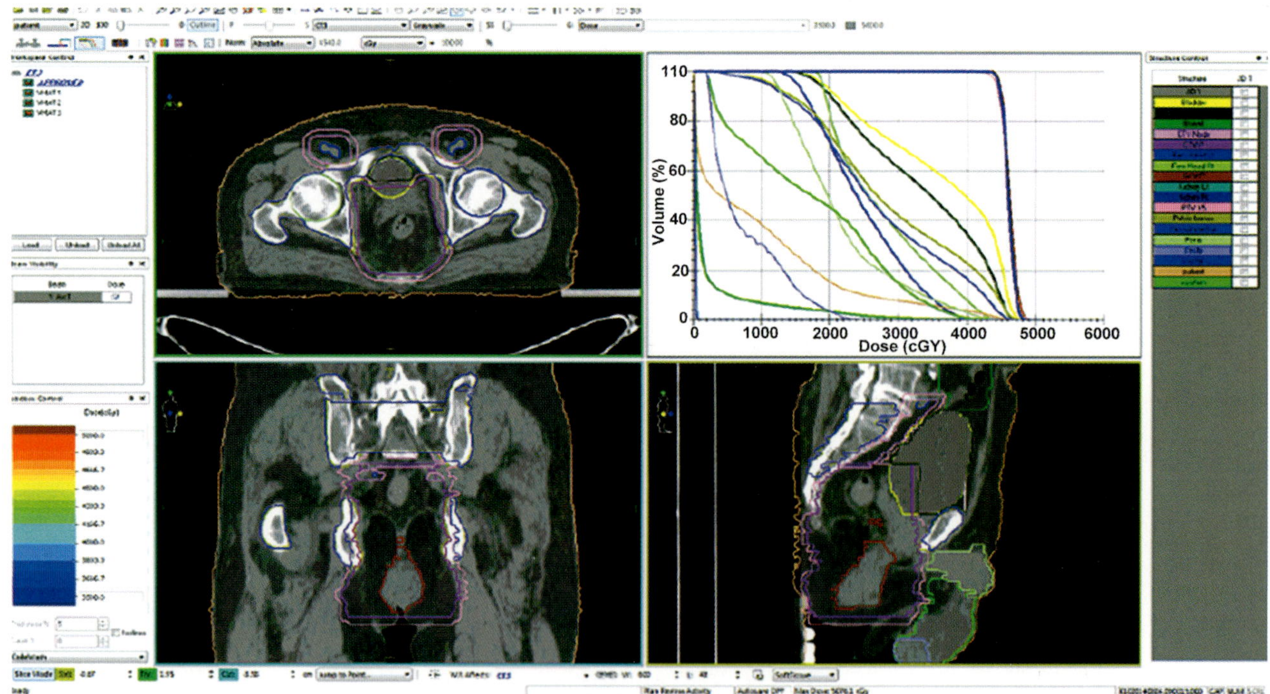

Fig. 2 Planning volumes for conformal radiotherapy in carcinoma anal canal

patients with locally advanced anal cancer receiving combined modality therapy will improve the results particularly in good responders.[3] There is Indian data which suggested that radiation dose of 56–60 Gy for T1 and T2 and 65 Gy for T3 and T4 tumors along with concurrent chemotherapy is required to achieve better local control, disease-free survival and overall survival along with acceptable toxicity.[19]

CONCLUSION

A multidisciplinary approach would be essential for the optimal management of anal cancer. Despite the results of four randomized phase III trials, radiotherapy with concurrent 5-FU and MMC developed over 30 years ago by Norman Nigro remains the standard of care.

REFERENCES

1. 4th Conference on Evidence Based Management of Cancer in India. (2006). HIV and Cancer. [online] Available from https://tmc.gov.in/clinicalguidelines/ebm/vol5/hiv_final/non-aids.htm [Accessed April, 2015].
2. Méndez-Martínez R, Rivera-Martínez NE, Crabtree-Ramírez B, Sierra-Madero JG, Caro-Vega Y, Galván SC, et.al. Multiple human papillomavirus infections are highly prevalent in the anal canal of human immunodeficiency virus-positive men who have sex with men. BMC Infect Dis. 2014;14(1):671.
3. Glynne-Jones R, Nilsson PJ, Aschele C, Goh V, Peiffert D, Cervantes A, et. al. Anal cancer: ESMO-ESSO-ESTRO clinical practice guidelines for diagnosis, treatment and follow-up. Radiother Oncol. 2014;111(3):330-9.
4. Assi R, Reddy V, Einarsdottir H, et al. Anorectal Human Papillomavirus: Current Concepts. Yale J Biol Med. 2014;87(4):537-47.
5. Agur AMR, Lee MJ, Grant JCB. Grant's Atlas of Anatomy. 10th edition. London, UK: Lippincott Williams and Wilkins; 1999.
6. Sinnatamby CS. Last's Anatomy: Regional and Applied. 10th edition. Edinburgh: Churchill Livingstone; 1999.
7. Boman BM, Moertel CG, O'Connell MJ, Scott M, Weiland LH, Beart RW, et al. Carcinoma of the anal canal. A clinical and pathologic study of 188 cases. Cancer. 1984; 54(1):114–25.
8. Goh V, Gollub FK, Liaw J, Wellsted D, Przybytniak I, Padhani AR, et al. Magnetic resonance imaging assessment of squamous cell carcinoma of the anal canal before and after chemoradiation: can MRI predict for eventual clinical outcome? Int J Radiat Oncol Biol Phys. 2010;78:715-21.
9. Edge SB, Byrd DR, Compton CC. AJCC Cancer Staging Handbook, 7th edition. New York: Springer; 2010.
10. Nigro ND, Vaitkevicius VK, Considine B Jr. Combined therapy for cancer of the anal canal: a preliminary report. 1974. Dis Colon Rectum. 1993; 36: 709-11.
11. Bartelink H, Roelofsen F, Eschwege F, Rougier P, Bosset JF, Gonzalez DG, et al. Concomitant radiotherapy and chemotherapy is superior to radiotherapy alone in the treatment of locally advanced anal cancer: results of a phase III randomized trial of the European Organization for Research and Treatment of Cancer Radiotherapy and Gastrointestinal Cooperative Groups. J Clin Oncol. 1997;15:2040-9.
12. Epidermoid anal cancer: results from the UKCCCR randomized trial of radiotherapy alone versus radiotherapy, 5-fluorouracil, and mitomycin. UKCCCR Anal Cancer Trial Working Party. UK Co-ordinating Committee on Cancer Research. Lancet. 1996;348:1049-54.
13. Flam M, John M, Pajak TF, Petrelli N, Myerson R, Doggett S, et al. Role of mitomycin in combination with fluorouracil and radiotherapy, and of salvage chemoradiation in the definitive nonsurgical treatment of epidermoid carcinoma of the anal canal: results of a phase III randomized intergroup study. J Clin Oncol. 1996;14:2527-39.
14. Ajani JA, Winter KA, Gunderson LL, Pedersen J, Benson AB 3rd, Thomas CR Jr, et al. Fluorouracil, mitomycin, and radiotherapy vs fluorouracil, cisplatin, and radiotherapy for carcinoma of the anal canal: a randomized controlled trial. JAMA. 2008;299:1914-21.
15. Peiffert D, Tournier-Rangeard L, Gérard JP, Lemanski C, François E, Giovannini M, et al. Induction chemotherapy and dose intensification of the radiation boost in locally advanced anal canal carcinoma: final analysis of the randomized UNICANCER ACCORD 03 trial. J Clin Oncol. 2012;30:1941-8.
16. James RD, Glynne-Jones R, Meadows HM, Cunningham D, Myint AS, Saunders MP, et al. Mitomycin or cisplatin chemoradiation with or without maintenance chemotherapy for treatment of squamous-cell carcinoma of the anus (ACT II): a randomised, phase 3, open label, 2x2 factorial trial. Lancet Oncol. 2013;14:516-24.
17. Myerson RJ, Garofalo MC, El Naqa I, Abrams RA, Apte A, Bosch WR, et al. Elective clinical target volumes for conformal therapy in anorectal cancer: A Radiation Therapy Oncology Group consensus panel contouring atlas. Int J Radiat Oncol Biol Phys. 2009;74:824-30.
18. Ng M, Leong T, Chander S, Chu J, Kneebone A, Carroll S, et. al. Australasian Gastrointestinal Trials Group (AGITG) Contouring Atlas and Planning Guidelines for Intensity-Modulated Radiotherapy in Anal Cancer. Int J Radiat Oncol Biol Phys. 2011;83:1455-62.
19. Engineer R, Mallik S, Mahantshetty U, et al. Impact of radiation dose on locoregional control and survival on squamous cell carcinoma of anal canal. Radiother Oncol. 2010;95(3):283-7.

18 CHAPTER

Carcinoma of Rectum

Trinanjan Basu, Nimesh Dahima, Tejinder Kataria

INTRODUCTION

Globally colorectal cancer (CRC) is one of the most common forms of gastrointestinal malignancies. In the USA, CRC ranks as third most common overall cancer for the period 1992–2001. Among Asian populations also the incidence varies widely and uniformly low in all south Asian countries and high in all developed Asian countries.[1-3]

Over the years, the management paradigm changed from primary surgery to neoadjuvant chemoradiation and a greater emphasis upon preservation of sphincter function and eventually a better quality of life (QOL).

ANATOMICAL CONSIDERATIONS

The rectum extends from the rectosigmoid junction to the puborectalis ring and ranges from 12 cm to 15 cm in length (Fig. 1).[4]

The rectum is usually divided into three portions. The lower rectum is the area approximately from 3 cm to 6 cm from the anal verge. The mid-rectum then starts and it is up to 8–10 cm and then the upper rectum extends approximately till 12–15 cm from the anal verge. The upper third of the rectum is covered with peritoneum anteriorly and on both sides. The middle one-third move deeper into the pelvis and only the anterior surface is covered with peritoneum. This forms the posterior border of the rectouterine pouch or rectovesical space. The lower one-third of the rectum has no peritoneal covering and is in close proximity to adjacent structures including the bony pelvis.

The location of a rectal tumor is most commonly indicated by the distance between the anal verge, dentate (pectinate or mucocutaneous) line, or anorectal ring and the lower edge of the tumor. These reference points differ from individual to individual and also depends on method of clinical assessment (per rectal or flexible endoscopy).

The lymphatic drainage of the upper rectum follows the course of the superior hemorrhoidal artery toward the inferior mesenteric artery. Lesions that arise in the rectum below approximately 6 cm are drained by lymphatics that follow the middle hemorrhoidal artery. Nodes involved from a cancer in this region can include the internal iliac nodes and the obturator nodes. When lesions occur below the dentate line, the lymphatic drainage is through the inguinal nodes and external iliac chain.

ETIOLOGY

Environmental and dietary factors have been established as contributing to CRC. The factors, which increase the risk of development, include increasing age, male sex, family history of CRC, increasing body mass index, processed meat intake, excessive alcohol intake and low folate consumption. Increasing age, male sex and excessive alcohol are especially contributing to rectal cancer.

Factors like high-fiber diet, consumption of fruits, nonsteroidal anti-inflammatory drugs have been recommended as preventive factors for carcinoma rectum although the data is conflicting.[5]

It has been established that CRC development is multifactorial and can arise through inactivation of the tumor suppressor genes adenomatous polyposis coli (APC) and p53 as well as mutations in the RAS proto-oncogene. Pathogenesis and heterogeneity of CRC based on the Vogelstein model of adenoma–carcinoma sequence is well understood.[6,7] The progression of adenoma to carcinoma is believed to occur over years and genetic alterations in genes such as APC, KRAS and TP53 are involved. This concept has formed the basis of screening for CRC.

However, it has become evident also that all colorectal carcinomas does not bear a “classic” molecular signature and

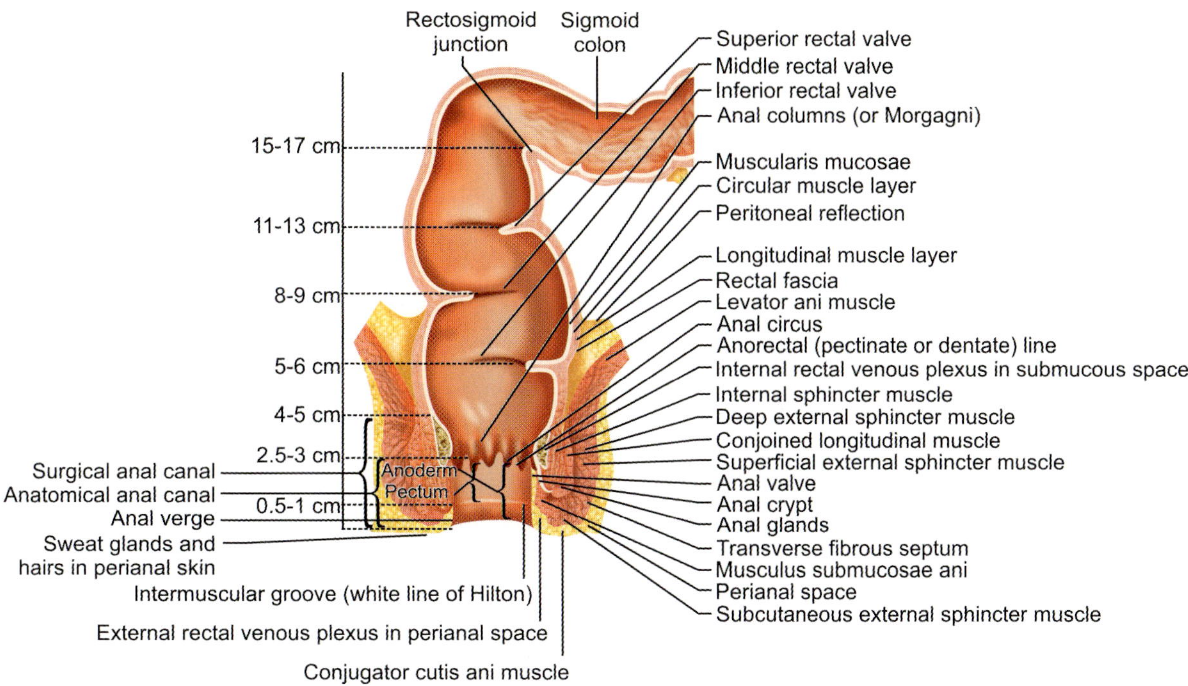

Fig. 1 Anatomical detail of rectum and anal canal

in fact only 60% of total CRCs develop along the suppressor pathway. Most of the remaining 40% of CRC occur via recently described "serrated pathway".[8]

CLINICAL PRESENTATIONS

Colorectal cancers can present in two ways in the routine OPD either as longstanding chronic symptoms or in emergency setting either with an acute obstruction or as a perforation. Various literatures reported figures of chronic symptoms are around 77–92% and for acute obstruction between 4% and 8% and for perforation 2–4%.[9-11]

The primary symptoms will also depend upon site of the lesion. Bleeding per rectum is probably the most common symptom. It is mostly frank blood in stool for rectal cancers. Beart et al. found that CRCs account for 6% of patients having rectal bleeding and diagnosed with hemorrhoids.[12]

PATHOLOGY

Most of the rectal cancers are adenocarcinomas (96%). Other types are signet-ring cell carcinoma, squamous carcinoma, undifferentiated neoplasms and medullary type adenocarcinoma (solid carcinoma with minimal glandular differentiation or slight cellular pleomorphism). These are graded into well, moderately and poorly differentiated.[13]

Conventional type adenocarcinomas are characterized by glandular formation and this forms the basis for histologic tumor grading. In well differentiated adenocarcinoma greater than 95% of the tumor is gland forming, while moderately differentiated adenocarcinoma shows 50–95% gland formation and poorly differentiated adenocarcinoma is mostly solid with less than 50% gland formation. In clinical practice mostly they are moderately differentiated (around 70%).[14]

The three main concerns regarding signet-ring cell carcinomas being younger age at presentation, locally advanced and unresectable to begin with and hence poor survival.[15] Chang et al. in Stanford University studied these early onset sporadic rectal cancers and found that signet-ring cell differentiation was the major factor leading to poor outcomes in these patients.[16]

STAGING

The TNM (tumor, node and metastasis), 7th edition staging for rectal carcinoma[17] is given in Table 1.

MANAGEMENT

Several randomized trials have demonstrated that neoadjuvant chemoradiotherapy (NACRT), when compared with postoperative CRT, downstaged tumors and improved local control, frequently permitting sphincter preservation. This was also associated with reduced toxicity.[15,18-20]

In this chapter, we have briefed about available treatment modalities with their pros and cons. A few points regarding the imaging modalities and other diagnostic tests have been highlighted before.

Table 1 The TNM staging

Primary Tumor (T)	
TX	Primary tumor cannot be assessed.
T0	No evidence of primary tumor.
Tis	Carcinoma in situ: Intraepithelial or invasion of lamina propria.
T1	Tumor invading the submucosa.
T2	Tumor invading muscularis propria.
T3	Tumor invading through the muscularis propria into the subserosa, or into non-peritonealized perirectal tissues.
T4	Tumor directly invading other organs or structures* and/or perforates visceral peritoneum (includes invasion of other segments of colon).
Regional Lymph Nodes (N)	
NX	Regional lymph nodes cannot be assessed.
N0	No regional lymph node metastasis.
N1	Metastasis in 1–3 regional lymph nodes. *N1a:* Metastasis in one regional lymph node. *N1b:* Metastasis in 2–3 regional lymph nodes. *N1c:* Tumor deposit(s) in the subserosa, mesentery, or non-peritonealized perirectal tissues without regional nodal metastasis.
N2	Metastasis in four or more regional lymph nodes (tumor nodules in the pericolonic adipose tissue without evidence of residual lymph node are classified as a regional lymph node metastases). *N2a:* Metastasis in 4–6 regional lymph nodes. *N2b:* Metastasis in 7 or more regional lymph nodes.
Distant Metastasis (M)	
MX	Distant metastasis cannot be assessed.
M0	No distant metastasis.
M1	Distant metastasis. *M1a:* Metastasis confined to one organ or site (for example, liver, lung, ovary, nonregional node). *M1b:* Metastases in more than one organ/site or the peritoneum.

*Direct invasion in T4 includes invasion of other segments of the colorectum by way of the serosa; for example, invasion of the sigmoid by a carcinoma of the cecum. Tumor that is adherent to other organs or structures, macroscopically, is classified as T4. However, if no tumor is present in the adhesion, microscopically, the classification should be pT3.

Digital Rectal Examination

A study has shown that digital rectal examination (DRE) can detect 82% of palpable rectal cancers. Lower gastrointestinal symptoms above the age of 40 years, and if anybody below this age with persistent symptoms warrant evaluation with DRE. For suspected rectal cancer in female vaginal examination should be part of the assessment. A right-sided abdominal mass is of greater diagnostic value.[21,22]

Imaging Studies

Computed tomography (CT) scan is the gold standard for preoperative evaluation and local staging of rectal tumors. There is although increasing evidence in favor of magnetic resonance imaging (MRI) from results of systematic observational studies. One of the most promising results was from the MERCURY trial (BMJ 2005) which concluded that MRI is the most reproducible method of assessing the relation of the rectal cancer to the potential circumferential resection margin (CRM).[23,24]

The role of PET-CT scan is limited in the primary staging of newly diagnosed CRC, and this is because of low sensitivity of FDG-PET for small lesions (less than 1 cm) and the chance of false positives in inflammatory bowel lesions. For suspected disease, a meta-analysis showed that FDG-PET has a sensitivity and specificity of 97% and 76%.[25]

SURGERY

In 2007, it was defined that any tumor whose distal margin is seen at 15 cm or less from the anal verge using a rigid sigmoidoscope should be classified as rectal cancer.[22]

Small early stage lesions diagnosed by colonoscopy/proctoscopy can be managed with local resection performed via colonoscopy or trans-anal excision. Resection should encompass a surrounding margin of normal mucosa and should extend into the peri-rectal fat.[26,27]

TOTAL MESORECTAL EXCISION

Total mesorectal excision (TME) has now become the standard operating procedure for radical treatment in rectal cancer. This includes dissection along the plane that separates the visceral from the parietal pelvic fascia with complete en bloc removal of the rectum so that all of the rectal mesentery remains within the envelope of the specimen. A correct TME specimen on gross pathology would have a bilobed encapsulated appearance with smooth surface and unbroken like a lipoma. TME has been shown to reduce local recurrences irrespective of associated other modalities of treatment. For stage II and stage III tumors, the survival rates with TME ranges from 80 to 85% and 65 to 70%, respectively.[28,29]

ABDOMINOPERINEAL RESECTION

Abdominoperineal resection (APR) has been considered the gold standard for surgical resection of distal rectal cancer and requires removal of the primary tumor along with a complete proctectomy, leading to a permanent colostomy. APR is associated with higher morbidity, mortality and alteration in QOL due to permanent colostomy, and there is also risk of increased margin positivity.[30]

LOW ANTERIOR RESECTION

Low anterior resection (LAR) primarily aimed at preserving the anal sphincter, but it becomes difficult for low rectal cancers. Moreover patients should have good anal sphincter continence prior to considering sphincter-preserving options. Additionally patient age, pelvic anatomy, gender and body habitus can also affect suitability for sphincter preservation. A 2 cm distal margin of preserved normal rectum is considered optimal for preservation of good bowel function. When LAR is planned following neoadjuvant radiation therapy, it is necessary to mobilize the splenic flexure to allow an unirradiated segment of the bowel to be used for an anastomosis.[5]

RADIATION THERAPY TECHNIQUE

Patients can be treated in both supine and prone position. While in prone position, small bowel can be displaced anteriorly by the use of belly board. A full bladder protocol is used for planning and treatment as this displaces small bowel superiorly. A radio-opaque marker is placed on the anal verge and a DRE performed to determine the distance from the anal verge marker to the inferior edge of the tumor.

A planning CT scan is performed with 3 mm slices from the level of L2–L3 region to mid-thigh so as to cover the beginning of common iliac vessels to coverage of inguinal nodes (low rectal or rectum with anal canal involvement).

Contrast-enhanced MRI pelvis should be used for target volume delineation, and help from radiologist should be taken for accurate gross tumor delineation. Online verification during treatment should be done using the institutional protocol.

TARGET VOLUME DEFINITION

Preoperative/Neoadjuvant Radiotherapy

Target volumes are based on the known patterns of local recurrence in rectal cancer. The details of the CT based delineation can be consulted in Myerson et al. RTOG guidelines.[31]

The gross tumor volume (GTV): It includes all gross tumors seen on the planning CT scan with reference to information from diagnostic endoscopy, MRI and DRE. Any involved lymph nodes, extrarectal extension, or extranodal deposits seen on MRI should also be included. The clinical target volume (CTV) is the primary tumor, mesorectum from the sacral promontory to insertion of levator ani into the rectal wall and the posterior presacral space. The inferior pelvic subsite, which includes the anal perineum, anal sphincter, perianal and ischiorectal space, is included if the tumor is less than 6 cm from the anal margin or if the tumor invades the anal sphincter. In all patients, mesorectal and lateral lymph nodes are included. The obturator nodes are included when the tumor is less than 10 cm from the anal margin, and the external iliac lymph nodes included if there is anterior organ involvement or skin involvement or grossly positive nodes on imaging. The inguinal lymph nodes may be included if tumor invades the lower third of the vagina, or if there is major tumor extension into the internal and external anal sphincter.[31] The CTV should reach up to 3–5 cm superiorly (limited by the L5/S1 junction), 2–3 cm inferiorly, 2 cm anteriorly and posteriorly to cover the sacrum. A boost to the primary tumor can be added. The phase 2 PTV then includes the tumor mass with a 2 cm 3D margin (Fig. 2).

Organs at risk (OAR) like small bowel, bladder, pelvic bones, bilateral femoral head and external genitalia should be contoured. The dose volume constraints are followed as per QUANTEC data.[32]

Postoperative Radiotherapy

Close collaboration with the surgical team and pathologists is essential to aid planning with a full description of the extent of residual tumor, anatomical location of clips demarcating the tumor bed and sites of close margins. The target for postoperative radiotherapy is the tumor bed, adjacent lymph nodes, presacral region and any residual tumor. The target volume should be drawn keeping in mind the standard bony landmarks as below:

- *Lateral:* 1 cm outside bony pelvis.
- *Posterior:* 1 cm behind sacrum to include sacral hollow and presacral lymph nodes.
- *Superior:* Sacral promontory, L5/S1 border.
- *Anterior:* 2 cm anterior to sacral promontory and including the anterior vaginal wall.
- *Inferior:* 3 cm below the inferior edge of the anastomosis or to the inferior obturator foramen, whichever is lower. For patients who have had an APR, the perineal scar is marked to ensure it is covered.

DOSE-FRACTIONATION

Preoperative Radiotherapy

- *Short course*: 25 Gy in 5 daily fractions of 5 Gy given in 1 week.
- *Long course*:
  - *Phase 1:* 45 Gy in 25 daily fractions of 1.8 Gy given in 5 weeks.
  - *Phase 2 (optional):* 5.4–9 Gy in 3–5 daily fractions of 1.8 Gy.

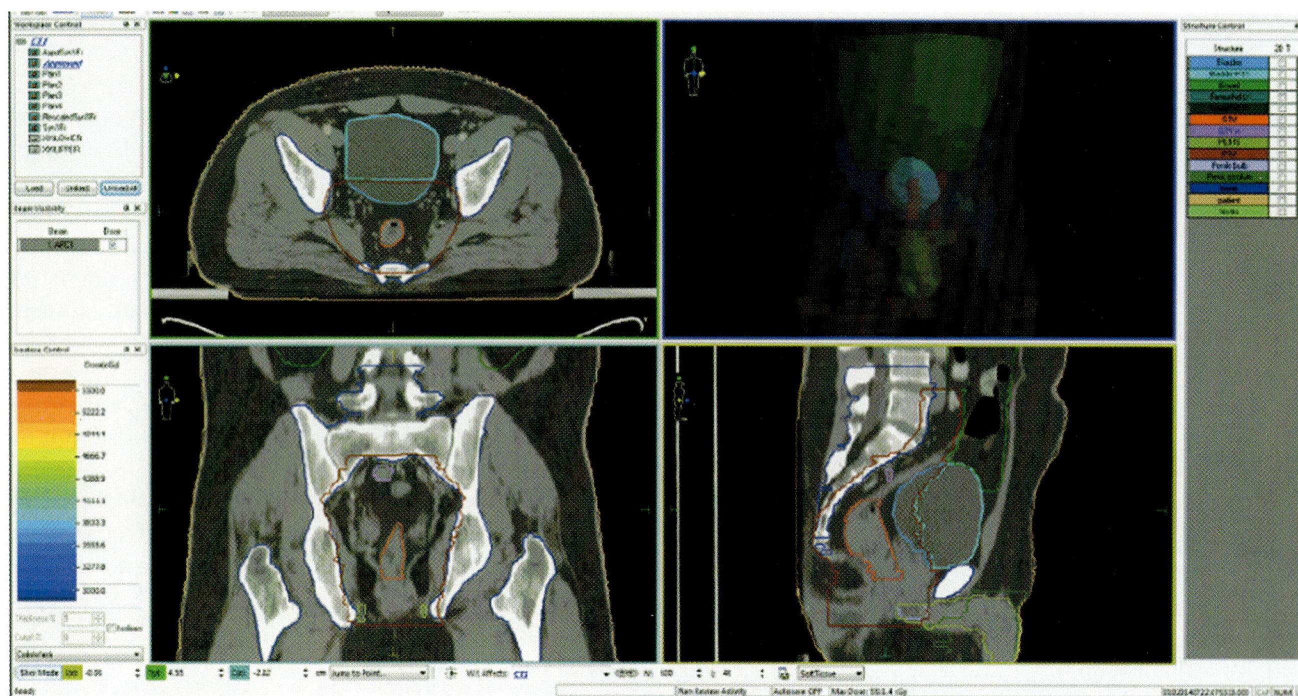

Fig. 2 Target volume in 3D for rectal carcinoma

Postoperative Radiotherapy

- *Phase 1:* 45 Gy in 25 daily fractions of 1.8 Gy given in 5 weeks.
- *Phase 2 (optional):* 5.4–9 Gy in 3–5 daily fractions of 1.8 Gy.

IMPORTANT DISCUSSIONS REGARDING RADIOTHERAPY IN RECTAL CARCINOMA

Clinical Nodal Disease Status and Risk of Recurrence

There is level 2 evidence suggesting that low-risk (T1-2N+ or T3N0) rectal cancer have a significantly favorable outcomes compared to high-risk (T3N + or T4N any). The 7-year survival (70% vs 45%) and local recurrence (9% vs 18%) and the same study showed that lymph node ratio (positive nodes divided by total number of nodes examined is a strong predictor of survival. This formed the basis for preoperative therapy for all stage II and III rectal cancers.[33,34]

Impact of Combining Chemotherapy with Preoperative Radiation Therapy in Resectable Stage II and III Rectal Cancer[35-37]

There is level 1a evidence that the addition of fluorouracil (FU) based chemotherapy (CT) to preoperative radiation (RT) significantly improved the following:

- The rate of complete pathological response (OR 2.52–5.27, $P < 0.001$).
- The incidence of local recurrence at 5 years (OR 0.39–0.72, $P < 0.001$).[35]

There is level 2 evidence to suggest that patients who achieve downstaging (ypT0-2) after preoperative CTRT: chemoradiation have improved 5-year disease-free survival and overall survival.

There is level 1b evidence that suggests preoperative CTRT: chemoradiation improves curative resection rates to up to 86–98%.

Capecitabine with Radiotherapy versus Bolus 5-FU with Radiotherapy[38-40]

There is level 1b evidence that when combined with radiation, capecitabine is non-inferior to both, bolus 5-FU and 5-FU, and leucovorin in terms of downstaging, pathological complete response rates (pCR) rates and toxicity profiles.

Is Prolonged Preoperative Chemoradiation Superior to Shorter Radiation Fractionation Schedule?

Polish randomized trial evaluated the role of short versus long course radiotherapy. Total 316 patients were randomized to receive short fractionation (5 × 5 Gy) followed by TME within 7 days or prolonged chemoradiation (50.4 Gy/28 fractions) concomitantly with two course of bolus 5-FU and leucovorin followed by TME within 4–6 weeks. It was seen that tumor downsizing was greater in prolonged chemoradiation; this did not translate into difference in sphincter preservation rates (58% vs 61% p = 0.57). There was no difference in QOL, sexual and anorectal function in either arm.[35,36]

What is the Optimal Time Between Preoperative Radiation and Surgery?

Lyon R 90-01 randomized trial evaluated the optimal time between preoperative radiotherapy and TME. The trial randomized patients into short (2 weeks) or long (6–8 weeks) interval surgery following neoadjuvant radiotherapy (39 Gy/13 fractions over 2.5 weeks). Higher pathological response rates were seen in the long interval arm (26% vs 10.3%; p = 0.005); however, this did not translate into statistically significant difference in sphincter preservation rates (75.5 vs 67.7%).[41]

Concluding Remarks from European Multidisciplinary Colorectal Cancer Congress (EMCCC) 2014[42]

The 7th EMCCC meeting in Amsterdam highlighted the following:

- Developments in screening, early detection, genetics, treatment strategies in early and advanced rectal cancer.
- The development of new biomarkers as well as biomarker-driven treatment strategies was the most prominent topics of the program.

REFERENCES

1. Boyle P, Langman JS. ABC of colorectal cancer: Epidemiology. BMJ. 2000;321:805-8.
2. Goh KL, Quek KF, Yeo GT, Hilmi IN, Lee CK, Hasnida N, et al. Colorectal cancer in Asians: a demographic and anatomic survey in Malaysian patients undergoing colonoscopy. Aliment Pharmacol Ther. 2005;22:859-64.
3. Mohandas KM. Colorectal cancer in India: controversies, enigmas and primary prevention. Indian J Gastroenterol. 2011;30(1):3-6.
4. Jorge JMN, Habr-Gama A. (2007) Anatomy and embryology of the colon, rectum and anus. In: This ASCRS Textbook of Colon and Rectal Surgery, 3rd edition (Eds Church JM, Carcia-Aguilar J, Roberts PL), pp. 1-22, Springer, New York.
5. Mohandas KM (2011). Guidelines for colorectal cancers. [Online]. Available from https://tmc.gov.in/clinicalguidelines/EBM/Vol10/Coleractal%20Final.pdf [Accessed on April, 2015].
6. Hertogh GD, Gebeoes KP. Practical and molecular evaluation of CRC. Arch path Lab Med. 2010;134:853-63.
7. Fearon ER, Vogelstein B. A genetic model for colorectal tumorigenesis. Cell. 1990;61:759-67.
8. Snover DC. Update on the serrated pathway to colorectal carcinoma. Hum Pathol. 2011;42(1):1-10.
9. Aldridge MC, Phillips RKS, Hittinger R, Fry JS, Fielding LP. Influence of tumour site on presentation, management and subsequent outcome in large bowel cancer. Br J Surg. 1986;73:663-70.
10. Mandava N, Kumar S, Pizzi WF, Aprile IJ. Perforated colorectal carcinomas. Am J Surg. 1996;172:236-8.
11. Runkel NS, Schlag P, Schwarz V, Herfarth C. Outcome after emergency surgery for cancer of the large intestine. Br J Surg. 1991;78:183-8.
12. Beart RW Jr, Melton LJ, Maruta M, Dockerty MB, Frydenberg HB, O'Fallon WM. Trends in right and left-sided colon cancers. Dis Colon Rectum. 1983;26:393-8.
13. Ponz de Leon M, Di Gregorio C. Pathology of colorectal cancer. Dig Liver Dis. 2001;33(4):372-88.
14. Fleming M, Ravula S, Tatishchev SF, Wang HL. Colorectal carcinoma: Pathologic aspects. J Gastrointest Oncol. 2012;3(3):153-73.
15. Engineer R, Basu T, Chopra S, Arya S, Patil P, Mehta S, et al. Factors influencing response to neoadjuvant chemoradiation and outcomes in rectal cancer patients: tertiary Indian cancer hospital experience. J Gastrointest Oncol. 2015;6(2):155-64.
16. Chang DT, Pai RK, Rybicki LA, Dimaio MA, Limaye M, Jayachandran P, et al. Clinicopathologic and molecular features of sporadic early-onset colorectal adenocarcinoma: an adenocarcinoma with frequent signet ring cell differentiation, rectal and sigmoid involvement, and adverse morphologic features. Mod Pathol. 2012;25:1128-39.
17. Edge S, Byrd DR, Compton CC, Fritz AG, Greene FL, Trotti A. AJCC Cancer Staging Handbook: From the AJCC Cancer Staging Manual, 7th edition. New York: Springer-Verlag; 2010.
18. Silberfein EJ, Kattepogu KM, Hu CY, Skibber JM, Rodriguez-Bigas MA, Feig B, et al. Long-term survival and recurrence outcomes following surgery for distal rectal cancer. Ann Surg Oncol. 2010;17:2863-9.
19. Dhadda AS, Zaitoun AM, Bessell EM. Regression of rectal cancer with radiotherapy with or without concurrent capecitabine--optimising the timing of surgical resection. Clin Oncol (R Coll Radiol). 2009;21:23-31.
20. Roh MS, Colangelo LH, O'Connell MJ, Yothers G, Deutsch M, Allegra CJ, et al. Preoperative multimodality therapy improves disease-free survival in patients with carcinoma of the rectum: NSABP R-03. J Clin Oncol. 2009;27:5124-30.
21. Dixon AR, Maxwell WA, Thornton Holmes J. Carcinoma of the rectum: a 10-year experience. Br J Surg. 1991;78:308-11.
22. The Association of Coloproctology of Great Britain and Ireland. Guidelines for the Management of Colorectal Cancer, 3rd edition. London: The Association of Coloproctology of Great Britain and Ireland; 2007.
23. Pomerri F, Pucciarelli S, Maretto I, Zandonà M, Del Bianco P, Amadio L, et al. Prospective assessment of imaging after preoperative chemoradiotherapy for rectal cancer. Surgery. 2011;149(1):56-64.
24. Niekel MC, Bipat S, Stoker J. Diagnostic imaging of colorectal liver metastases with CT, MR imaging, FDG PET, and/or FDG PET/CT: a meta-analysis of prospective studies including patients who have not previously undergone treatment. Radiology. 2010;257(3):674-84.
25. Lambrecht M, Deroose C, Roels S, Vandecaveye V, Penninckx F, Sagaert X, et al. The use of FDG-PET/CT and diffusion weighted magnetic resonance imaging for response prediction before, during and after preoperative chemoradiotherapy for rectal cancer. Acta Oncol. 2010;49(7):956-63.

26. Bories E, Pesenti C, Monges G, Lelong B, Moutardier V, Delpero JR, et al. Endoscopic mucosal resection for advanced sessile adenoma and early-stage colorectal carcinoma. Endoscopy. 2006;38:231-5.
27. Tytherleigh MG, Warren BF, Mortensen NJ. Management of early rectal cancer. Br J Surg. 2008;95:409-23.
28. Quirke P, Steele R, Monson J, Grieve R, Khanna S, Couture J, et al. Effect of the plane of surgery achieved on local recurrence in patients with operable rectal cancer: a prospective study using data from the MRC CR07 and NCIC-CTG CO16 randomised clinical trial. Lancet. 2009;373:821-8.
29. Peeters KC, Marijnen CA, Nagtegaal ID, Kranenbarg EK, Putter H, Wiggers T, et al. The TME trial after a median follow-up of 6 years: increased local control but no survival benefit in irradiated patients with resectable rectal carcinoma. Ann Surg. 2007;246:693-701.
30. Marr R, Birbeck KF, Garvican J, Macklin CP, Tiffin NJ, Parsons WJ, et al. The modern abdomino-perineal excision: the next challenge after total mesorectal excision. Ann Surg. 2005;242: 74-82.
31. Myerson RJ, Garofalo MC, El Naqa I, Abrams RA, Apte A, Bosch WR, et al. Elective clinical target volumes for conformal therapy in anorectal cancer: A Radiation Therapy Oncology Group consensus panel contouring atlas. Int J Radiat Oncol Biol Phys. 2009;74:824-30.
32. Marks LB, Yorke ED, Jackson A, Ten Haken RK, Constine LS, Eisbruch A, et.al. Use of normal tissue complication probability models in the clinic. Int J Radiat Oncol Biol Phys. 2010; 76(3 Suppl):S10-9.
33. Kapiteijn FMC, Nagtegaal ID. Preoperative radiotherapy combined with total mesorectal excision for resectable rectal cancer. N Eng J Med. 2001;345:638-46.
34. Gerrard JPCT, Bonnetain F. Preoperative radiotherapy with or without concurrent flourouracil and leucovorin in T3-4 rectal cancers: results of FFCD 9203. J Clin Oncol. 2006;24:4620-5.
35. Bujko KMM, Nasierowska-Guttmejer A. Long term results of a randomised trial comparing preoperative short course radiotherapy with preoperative conventionally fractionated chemoradiation for rectal cancers. Br J Surg. 2006;93:1215-23.
36. Bouslis Wasif SGA, Loygue J, Camelot D. Final Results of a randomised trial on the treatment of rectal cancer with preoperative radiotherapy alone or in combination with 5 Flououracil followed by radical surgery. Cancer. 1984;53:1811-18.
37. Wong RKTV, Desilva S. Preoperative radiotherapy and curative surgery for the management of localised rectal carcinoma. Cochrane Database Syst Rev. 2007:CD002102.
38. Dhadda AS, Zaitoun AM, Bessell EM. Regression of rectal cancer with radiotherapy with or without concurrent capecitabine--optimising the timing of surgical resection. Clin Oncol (R Coll Radiol). 2009;21:23-31.
39. Roh MS, Colangelo LH, O'Connell MJ, Yothers G, Deutsch M, Allegra CJ, et al. Preoperative multimodality therapy improves disease-free survival in patients with carcinoma of the rectum: NSABP R-03. J Clin Oncol. 2009;27:5124-30.
40. Yoon SM, Kim DY, Kim TH, Jung KH, Chang HJ, Koom WS, et al. Clinical parameters predicting pathologic tumor response after preoperative chemoradiotherapy for rectal cancer. Int J Radiat Oncol Biol Phys. 2007;69:1167-72.
41. Francois Y NC, Baulieux J, Vignal J. Influence of the interval between preoperative radiation therapy and surgery on own staging and on rate of sphincter sparing surgery for rectal cancer: The Lyon R90-01 randomised trial. J Clin Oncol. 1999;17:2396-402.
42. Punt CJA, Nagtegal ID, Van de Velde CJ, Beets-Tan R, Cats A, Hoogerbrugge N, et al. Highlights from the seventh European Multidisciplinary Colorectal Cancer Congress (EMCCC) 2014. Ecancermedicalscience. 2015;9:497.

19 CHAPTER

Surgical Principles in the Management of Pancreatic Cancer

Savio G Barreto, Adarsh Chaudhary

INTRODUCTION

Achieving a complete surgical resection remains the cornerstone in providing the patient the best chance of cure in pancreatic cancer.[1] In the past, surgical exploration was often undertaken even in patients with potentially locally advanced tumors on imaging. The aim of such an exercise was to perform a palliative surgical bypass even if a curative resection was not possible. Unnecessary surgical explorations (especially in patients with metastatic disease) must be avoided as they are fraught with the risk of morbidity and even mortality—often denying the patient the chance to receive palliative chemotherapy.

Only a small fraction of patients with pancreatic cancer present when the disease is still amenable to a curative resection.[2] Today, with the development of radiation therapy as well as a wide array of chemotherapeutic agents targeting different pathways in pancreatic carcinogenesis, there has been an increasing emphasis on a multidisciplinary approach to the management of pancreatic cancer with a common aim of improving patient survival. Better imaging modalities have enabled us to improve our preoperative selection of patients for either upfront surgery or neoadjuvant therapy prior to surgery.[3] Moreover, advancements in technical (surgical) expertise, critical care and interventional radiology have provided oncosurgeons the desired armamentarium to aggressively address this cancer that has traditionally been regarded with pessimism.

This chapter will provide the reader with a step-by-step approach to the surgical decision-making and management of pancreatic cancer based on the latest available evidence in literature.

PREOPERATIVE APPROACH TO THE PATIENT

From a surgical perspective, the most pertinent investigations in the preoperative planning include:

- *Routine blood investigations* (such as complete blood count, liver and renal function tests and coagulation profile)

  The presence of anemia (< 8 g/dL) would indicate the need for preoperative packed red cell transfusion while features of cholangitis, viz. an obstructive biliopathy profile of raised serum bilirubin and alkaline phosphatase with or without deranged transaminases along with a raised white cell count in the clinical setting of fever with or without rigors, would indicate the need for preoperative endoscopic retrograde cholangiopancreatography (ERCP) and biliary stenting along with intravenous antibiotics. Surgery would then be deferred for 4–6 weeks to permit the inflammation resulting from the procedure to settle.

  Prothrombin time and international normalized ratio (INR) should be checked prior to surgery as these are likely to be deranged in patients with obstructive jaundice—necessitating correction prior to surgery.
- *Serum tumor marker* [serum carbohydrate antigen 19-9 (CA 19-9)]

  A grossly elevated CA 19-9 that cannot be solely ascribed to the obstructive biliopathy should alert the clinician to rule out distant metastases.
- *Imaging:*[3] Preoperative radiology is the most useful aid to the surgeon in the preoperative staging of pancreatic cancer. The key features to focus on in the preoperative staging are:
  - Tumor—size, site/location, relation to surrounding vessels [superior mesenteric vein (SMV) and superior mesenteric artery (SMA), gastroduodenal artery (GDA) and hepatic artery (HA) and portal vein (PV) in pancreatic head and neck tumors; and celiac artery (CA) and splenic vein and artery (SV and SA) in body and tail tumors]

- Lymph nodes—regional or metastatic (para-aortic, interaortocaval)
- Metastases—intra- and extra-abdominal.

To date, none of the available imaging modalities is perfect. However, multidetector computed tomography (MDCT) scan of the abdomen and pelvis performed in the arterial, venous and pancreatic (triple) phase remains the most commonly performed imaging modality for the preoperative staging in patients with pancreatic cancer. Performance of an arterial phase, as part of the CT, is essential to ensure proper preoperative planning and identification of vascular anomalies.[4] Magnetic resonance imaging (MRI) and MR cholangiopancreatography (MRCP) have been suggested by some authors to be just as effective as MDCT. However, the main advantage of MDCT rests in its easier availability around the world and more importantly the widely available expertise to interpret the scans as compared to MRI.

Magnetic resonance imaging and MRCP are most useful in patients with suspected Intraductal papillary mucinous neoplasm (IPMN). Surgical resection would be warranted in the case of lesions demonstrating the presence of mural nodules, intraductal mucin, thickening of any wall and/or cytological analysis indicative of malignant cells or high-grade epithelial atypia.[5]

A chest X-ray is a useful investigation to determine the presence of lung metastases. Positron emission tomography–CT (PET-CT) may be performed in addition to MDCT or MRCP in patients in whom the tumor is large, locally advanced, or in borderline resectable tumour (BRT) in order to rule out distant metastases as this will avoid an unnecessary surgical exploration.[6]

- *Endoscopy:* Side-viewing endoscopy is useful in diagnosing periampullary lesions not clearly discernible, but suspected, on MDCT. In patients with BRTs, endoscopic ultrasonography (EUS) is useful to assess vascular involvement and/or to obtain tumor biopsies by fine needle aspiration.[7] In general, even in the presence of surgical obstructive jaundice, patients should be considered for upfront surgery so long as the disease is clearly resectable. However, in some patients with surgical obstructive jaundice an ERCP with stenting of the bile duct is advised prior to surgery. The specific indications for this include cholangitis, malnourished patients in whom it is envisaged that preoperative nutrition build-up can be achieved, coagulopathy owing to biliary obstruction, and in patients in whom delays in surgery are anticipated. While there is no clear cut-off for a serum bilirubin level at which surgery can be safely performed, patients with serum bilirubin levels more than 10 mg% are generally offered stenting prior to surgery. In all these patients surgery needs to be delayed for 4–6 weeks following stenting.[8]
- *Biopsy:*[9] Obtaining a biopsy as proof of cancer is not mandatory in a solid mass lesion of the pancreas suspected of harboring a cancer. However, a biopsy to prove cancer is essential prior to commencing neoadjuvant therapy especially in borderline resectable pancreatic cancers (BRT-*vide infra*). EUS-guided fine needle aspiration (EUS FNA) is also recommended in the evaluation of small branch-duct (BD)-IPMNs without "worrisome features" (clinical history of pancreatitis, thickened enhanced cyst walls, main pancreatic duct (MPD) size of 5–9 mm, nonenhanced mural nodules, abrupt change in the MPD caliber with distal pancreatic atrophy and lymphadenopathy).[5]

SURGICAL MANAGEMENT

Based on the above investigations, majority of the patients with pancreatic cancer can be preoperatively classified as having:

- Resectable pancreatic cancer
- BRT
- Locally advanced pancreatic cancer (LAPC)
- Metastatic disease

Resectable pancreatic cancer includes tumors regardless of the size that are nonmetastatic, are unrelated to the major vessels around the pancreas (SMV, SMA, PV, GDA and/or HA), not involving adjoining viscera (except spleen in body and tail tumors) and in whom a complete resection can be safely undertaken.

BRT as defined by the National Comprehensive Cancer Network (NCCN Version I. 2013) as follows:

- *SMV/PV*
  - Impingement and narrowing of the lumen, or
  - Encasement without encasement of nearby arteries
  - Short-segment venous occlusion due to thrombus or encasement with suitable vessel proximal and distal allowing for resection and reconstruction.
- *GDA/HA*
  - GDA encasement up to hepatic artery with either short segment encasement or direct abutment of hepatic artery, without celiac axis extension.
- *SMA*
  - not exceeding 180° of the vessel wall.

In the absence of distant metastases

LAPC—any nonmetastatic tumor involvement of the vessels more than what constitutes BRT.

Surgery offers the only chance of cure in patients with resectable cancer or BRT. However, it should only be attempted in patients in whom a complete (R0) resection is deemed feasible. Upfront surgery is reserved for patients with resectable pancreatic cancer while in patients with BRT, surgery should be undertaken after neoadjuvant therapy. The available evidence does not support the role of a palliative pancreatoduodenectomy (PD) or pancreatic resection for pancreatic cancer.[10,11] The operative treatment of choice for pancreatic head, uncinate process and/or neck cancers is a PD, a distal pancreatectomy for cancers of the body and tail and a subtotal pancreatectomy for tumors at the junction of the neck and body. The first step of any surgical exploration for pancreatic cancer involves performing a detailed laparotomy to rule out locally advanced or metastatic disease (unresectable) disease. This includes assessment of:

- The tumor—fixity to/invasion of surrounding organs, puckering at the infracolic region near the SMA or at the inferior border of the neck suggesting PV/SMV involvement, extension of the tumor to the left of the SMA
- Lymph nodes—large para-aortic or interaortocaval nodes after performing the initial Kocher's maneuver
- Metastases—liver and peritoneum, ascites.

In some centers, a diagnostic laparoscopy is performed as the first step. This may help in some patients with nonmetastatic but large tumors on imaging in whom, diagnostic laparoscopy has been shown to 'downstage' the tumor by demonstrating the potential for a curative resection.[12]

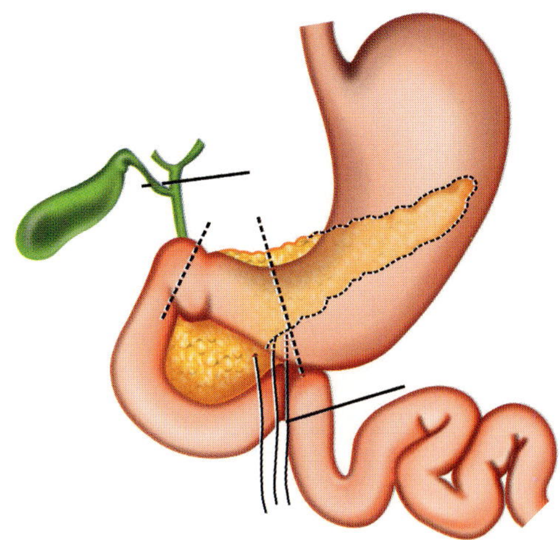

Fig. 1A Schematic representation of pancreatoduodenectomy (PD) demonstrating various organs including the stomach, duodenum and jejunum, pancreas and the extrahepatic bile duct and gallbladder with the lines of organ transection (bold lines indicating the site of transection on the bile duct and jejunum and the dashed lines indicating the level of transection of the stomach or duodenum depending on whether a classic Whipples procedure or pylorus preserving PD is being performed)

Surgery for Resectable Pancreatic Cancer

The underlying principles of surgery for pancreatic cancer are the same as for most other solid organs, viz.:

- Safe resection with negative resection margins (for cancer) on histopathological examination
- Safe reconstruction (when indicated)
- Adequate lymphadenectomy.

Head, Uncinate Process and Proximal Neck of Pancreas (Including Periampullary Cancer)

Pancreatoduodenectomy

Pancreatoduodenectomy is a technically challenging procedure associated with a high morbidity and risk of mortality[13] with a long learning curve.[14] However, standardization of the procedure within units has been shown to result in improved outcomes.[15]

Pancreatoduodenectomy entails removal of the head, uncinate process and proximal neck of the pancreas along with the duodenum (and stomach) and proximal few inches of jejunum, distal common bile duct and gallbladder.

There are principally two types of PD depending on the level of transection (Fig. 1A), viz.

1. Classical Whipple's procedure (Fig. 1B)—proximal transection at the junction of distal body and antrum of the stomach, and
2. Pylorus-preserving PD (PPPD) (Fig. 1C)—proximal transection just distal to the pyloric sphincter.

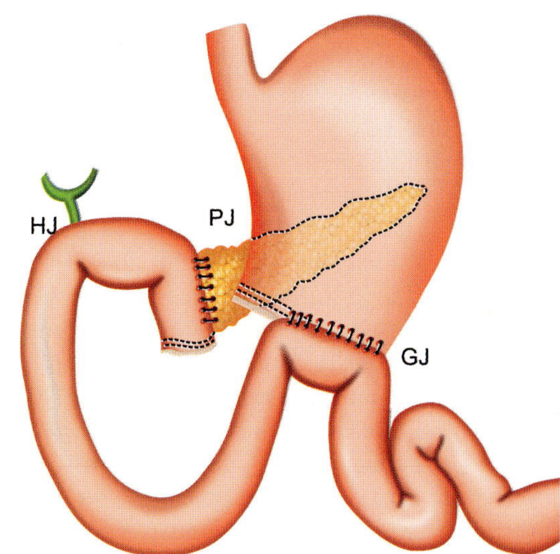

Fig. 1B Schematic representation of classic Whipples procedure clearly demonstrating the gastrojejunostomy (GJ), pancreatico-jejunostomy (PJ) and hepaticojejunostomy (HJ)

According to the available literature, there is no oncological benefit of performing a PPPD as compared to a classical Whipple's procedure.[16] However, specific indications in which only a classical Whipple procedure should be performed include duodenal cancers or large pancreatic head tumors invading the gastric antrum and/or the first part of duodenum. While PPPD takes a shorter operative time and is associated with less bleeding during surgery, it is associated

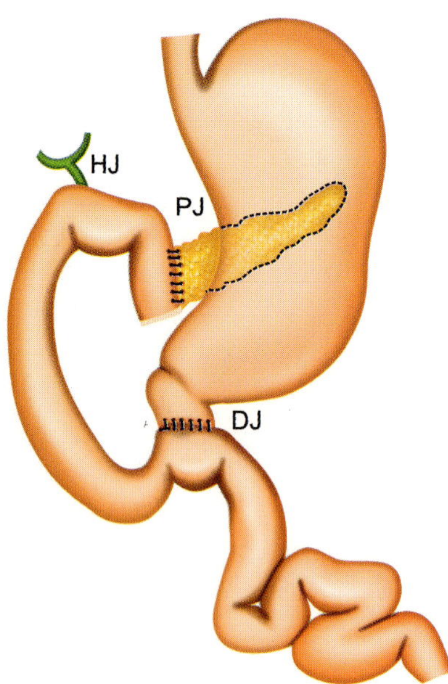

Fig. 1C Schematic representation of pylorus-preserving PD procedure clearly demonstrating the duodenojejunostomy (DJ), pancreaticojejunostomy (PJ) and hepaticojejunostomy (HJ)

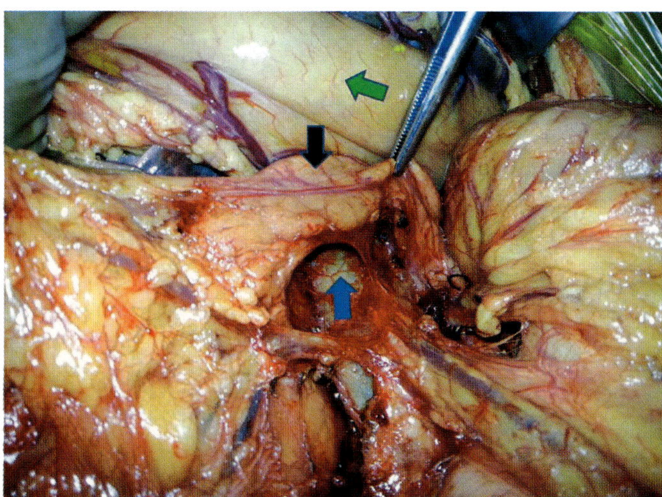

Fig. 2 Intraoperative photograph showing the step of 'tunneling' of the neck of pancreas. The stomach pointed out by the bold green arrow is reflected at the top, while the portal vein (formed by the confluence of the superior mesenteric and splenic veins) and marked by the bold blue arrow is seen traversing under the neck of the pancreas (marked by bold black arrow) which is often referred to as the tunnel

with a higher incidence of delayed gastric emptying (DGE) in the postoperative period.[17] Care must be taken to avoid injury to the important vessels in the vicinity, viz. the SMV, SV, PV and SMA (Figs 2 and 3).

A standard lymphadenectomy for pancreatic cancer involves removal of lymph nodes to the right side of the hepatoduodenal ligament (12b1, 12b1, 12c), posterior pancreaticoduodenal nodes (13a, 13b), nodes to the right side of the superior mesenteric artery from the origin of the superior mesenteric artery at the aorta to the inferior pancreaticoduodenal artery (14a, 14b) and anterior pancreaticoduodenal nodes (17a, 17b). Removal of lymph nodes beyond these is termed as an extended lymphadenectomy. Performance of extended lymphadenectomy for pancreatic cancer is not beneficial. It is not only associated with longer operating time and postoperative complications, e.g. an increased risk of intractable diarrhea as compared to a standard lymphadenectomy, but also adds no survival benefit.[18-22]

Following the complete resection (Fig. 3), the reconstruction following a PD involves three major anastomoses, viz.:

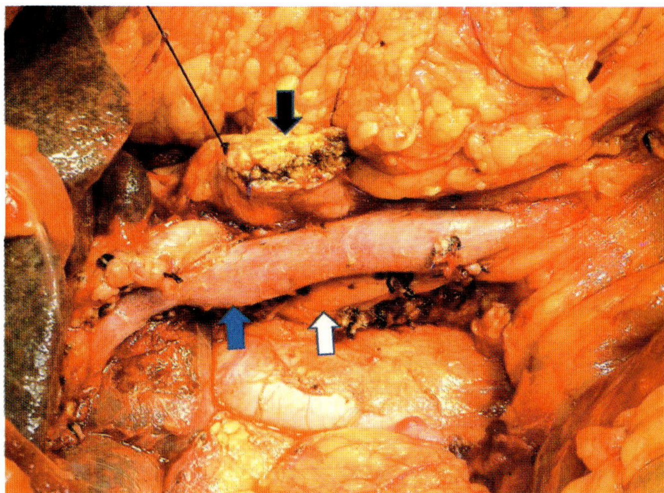

Fig. 3 Intraoperative photograph of a pancreatoduodenectomy after completion of the resection showing the relations of the pancreas stump (bold black arrow) to the underlying portal vein (formed by the confluence of the superior mesenteric and splenic veins) and marked by the bold blue arrow and the superior mesenteric artery (marked by bold white arrow)

1. Pancreatic remnant to the bowel (pancreaticoenteric)—this comprises of broadly two types:
   a. Pancreas to stomach—pancreaticogastrostomy (PG), or
   b. Pancreas to jejunum—pancreaticojejunostomy (PJ)
2. Common hepatic duct to the jejunum (hepaticojejunostomy), and
3. Stomach/duodenum to the jejunum (gastro-/duodenojejunostomy)—which can again be of two types:
   a. In front of the transverse colon—ante colic, or
   b. Behind the transverse colon, through the mesocolic window—retro colic.

The cardinal rules for a safe anastomosis remain the following: anastomosis performed with care, using fine

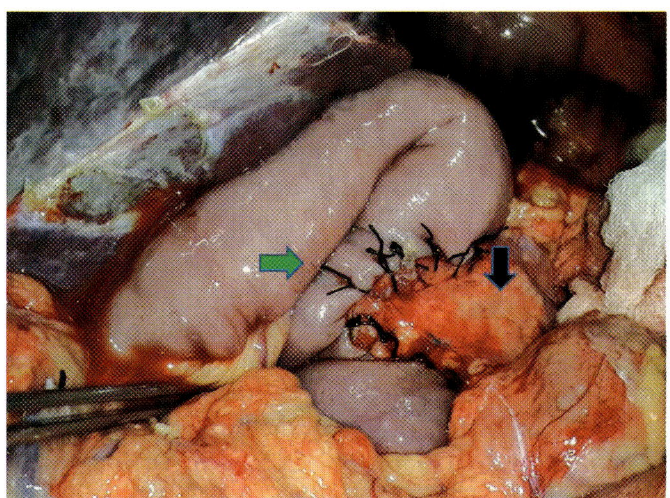

Fig. 4 Intraoperative photograph of a completed pancreatico-jejunostomy (performed in an end-to-side, duct to mucosa fashion). The liver is seen to the top end of the image while the remnant pancreas (bold black arrow) lies to the left and the jejuna roux loop lies to the right (marked by bold green arrow)

sutures (e.g. 4/0, 5/0 or 6/0 PDS), minimal handling, ensuring a good blood supply and absence of tension between the involved organs.[23]

Pancreaticoenteric Anastomosis (Pancreaticogastrostomy and Pancreaticojejunostomy)

This anastomosis remains the most challenging anastomosis in a PD, often deciding the outcome of the patient. PJ may be performed either as a duct-to-mucosa anastomosis (in end-to-side fashion—Fig. 4) or as an invagination (dunking) in either an end-to-end or an end-to-side fashion.[24,25] Similarly, PG, too, can be performed simply as an invagination of the pancreatic stump through a posterior gastrotomy using a one- or two-layer anastomosis or in the duct-to-mucosa fashion with or without additional transfixing sutures taken from the capsule of the pancreatic remnant to the gastric wall.[24,25] There have been numerous randomized controlled trials comparing PJ versus PG.[26-31] However, based on the data available from meta-analysis, there is no evidence to suggest that either technique is better than the other.[32,33] As pointed out earlier, performance of the anastomosis in a standardized manner remains the key, as does the experience of the surgeon, in achieving the best outcome.[15,34]

The most feared complication following a PD is a pancreaticoenteric anastomotic leak and pancreatic fistula (POPF).[29] Thus surgeons have resorted to numerous strategies to reduce the incidence of POPF including the perioperative use of octreotide,[35] omental wrapping of the anastomosis,[36] fibrin glue occlusion of the pancreatic duct,[37] etc. with variable outcomes. Two well-known factors influencing the development of POPF include a soft pancreatic gland and a small duct of less than 3 mm.[38] Based on a review of literature it was suggested that transanastomotic stent may be beneficial when used for patients with a soft gland and a duct size ≤ 3 mm.[38]

Gastro-/Duodenojejunostomy

An antecolic gastro-/duodenojejunostomy after PD has been shown to result in a lower incidence of DGE.[39] The postulated hypothesis for this is the avoidance of torsion or angulation that may result with a retrocolic anastomosis.

Distal Neck, Body and Tail of Pancreas

Distal/Subtotal Pancreatectomy[40]

In tumors of the neck, body, and/or tail of the pancreas, an aggressive approach has been advocated.[41] Performance of a splenectomy is considered mandatory in such procedures to achieve a complete resection.[42]

Unlike PD, in a distal pancreatectomy, the cut end of the pancreas does not need to be anastomosed to the pancreas as the proximal duct is in continuity with the duodenum. The most feared complication, however, after a distal pancreatectomy remains a pancreatic leak from the stump. Various techniques for transecting and sealing off the cut end have been advocated. The two most common techniques include cutting the pancreas with a knife of electrodiathermy and then suturing the stump or transecting the pancreas with a stapler (which achieves both functions). Both techniques are equally efficacious for closure of the pancreatic stump after a distal or subtotal pancreatectomy.[43,44] Irrespective of the technique used to transect/close the pancreatic stump, attention needs to be paid to transfixing the pancreatic duct.

Middle or central pancreatectomy should not be performed for malignant tumors.

Resectable Pancreatic Cancer Infiltrating Surrounding Organs

Unlike the head cancers, up to 30% of patients with cancers in the body and tail may have evidence of involvement of surrounding organs either as a result of direct tumor infiltration or inflammatory adhesions at the time of surgery.[45] Multivisceral resections performed in an en bloc manner should be attempted only if a complete (R0) resection can be achieved. The performance of an R0 resection following multivisceral resections has been shown to produce comparable long-term survival rates similar to patients undergoing standard resection for resectable tumors.[46-48] Moreover, the long-term survival rates in these patients are markedly improved as compared patients with unresectable locally advanced disease.[47] Since these resections have been clearly shown to be associated with an increased morbidity, they should preferably be undertaken only in high volume centers with the necessary expertise.[48,49]

Surgery for Brachytherapy

Brachytherapies are cancers that have limited involvement of the mesenteric vessels such that resection is technically possible, but which carry a high risk of margin-positive resection unless neoadjuvant therapy is employed before surgery.[50] There is currently no clear consensus on the best approach to these patients. The three options include:

1. Upfront surgery followed by adjuvant therapy (chemotherapy and/or chemoradiotherapy),
2. Neoadjuvant chemotherapy (with or without radiotherapy) followed by surgery, or
3. Neoadjuvant radiotherapy (with radiation-sensitizing chemotherapy) followed by surgery.

The benefits of upfront surgery include the lack of the need for histological proof of the cancer prior to surgery, the evidence that not all patients with BRT require vascular resections[51] and the often 'over' stated risk of disease progression in 16–21% of patients while on neoadjuvant therapy.[52,53]

However, the following points make for a strong argument for neoadjuvant chemotherapy (with or without radiotherapy) prior to surgery for patients with BRT[53-63]:

- Pancreatic cancer is a systemic disease with microscopic metastases at presentation.
- While surgery is the cornerstone for achieving cure in pancreatic cancer, chemotherapy further adds to the prospect of long-term survival. However, it is the completion of chemotherapy, which is an independent prognostic factor for survival. Patients receiving neoadjuvant chemotherapy are more likely to complete the planned cycles of chemotherapy.
- Up to 25% of patients are unable to receive adjuvant treatment following pancreatic surgery, as they do not completely recover from the effects of surgery.
- Patients receiving neoadjuvant therapy have a higher likelihood of achieving margin negative resections.
- Patients with true venous infiltration, detected on the histological examination of the specimen of vascular resections, have a significantly poorer survival. Thus using neoadjuvant therapy to achieve negative margins may help improve survival.

With regards to neoadjuvant chemoradiotherapy alone, a recent meta-analysis has confirmed that chemoradiotherapy does not achieve the amount of disease down-staging as was perceived. Moreover, it is associated with a higher toxicity rate as compared to chemotherapy alone.[64]

Thus, in patients with BRT, a useful treatment algorithm would be to offer them three cycles of neoadjuvant chemotherapy and then reassess for surgery. Patients demonstrating disease regression should be taken up for surgery while those with stable disease may be considered for extended chemotherapy[65,66] or chemoradiotherapy[67] and then reassessed for surgery.

Although technically demanding and associated with longer hospital stay, pancreatic surgery after neoadjuvant therapy is not associated with significantly increased morbidity or mortality.[68-70]

Vascular Resections

Pancreatic resections along with venous resections (SMV/PV) can be performed in expert centers without significantly increased morbidity and mortality as compared to standard resections.[71] However, these resections should be performed only if an R0 resection can be achieved, as only this will confer a survival advantage.[72,73]

Factors that determine outcomes following venous resections include the depth,[74] and length[73] of venous invasion. Involvement of tunica media and intima and length of involvement > 3 cm is associated with poor outcomes even if a complete (R0) resection is achieved.

There is currently no evidence to justify arterial resections in pancreatic cancer.[49,75,76]

Pancreatic Resection in Metastatic Disease

Although the feasibility for performance of complete pancreatic resections along with metastasectomy for stage IV cancers that have metastasized has been demonstrated,[77] to date, there exists no clear evidence to demonstrate a survival benefit of such undertakings.[49,78]

COMPLICATIONS OF PANCREATIC SURGERY

The three most frequently encountered specific complications following pancreatic surgery include POPF, DGE and postpancreatectomy hemorrhage (PPH). In an effort to standardize the reporting of these complications, a group of leading pancreatic surgeons from around the world came together under the banner, 'International Study Group of Pancreatic Surgery (ISGPS)' to provide consensus definitions which are as follows:

POPF:[29] The presence of POPF is defined by a drain output of any measurable volume of fluid on or after postoperative day 3 with an amylase content greater than three times the serum amylase activity. Three different grades of POPF (grades A, B, C) are defined according to the clinical impact on the patient's hospital course.

DGE:[79] The three grades of DGE according to the duration of nasogastric drainage requirement, include DGE grade A (up to 4–7th postoperative day), grade B (7–14th postoperative day) and grade C (beyond the 14th postoperative day).

PPH[80]: Postpancreatectomy hemorrhage is defined by three parameters—onset, location and severity. The onset is either early (< or = 24 hours after the end of the index operation) or late (> 24 hours). The location is either intraluminal or extraluminal. The severity of bleeding may be either mild or severe. Three different grades of PPH (grades A, B and C) are defined according to the time of onset, site of bleeding, severity and clinical impact.

Laparoscopy and Robotic Surgery for Pancreatic Cancer

Laparoscopic and robotic surgery have been demonstrated to be feasible for performing distal pancreatectomy with some series even demonstrating the feasibility of these procedures for PD for benign lesions of the pancreas.[81-87] However, to date there exists no evidence to suggest that laparoscopic PD or even distal pancreatectomy is equal to, or superior, to open surgery in terms of overall survival for pancreatic and periampullary cancer.[85] Also of note is the fact that pancreatic cancer surgery is complex with the morbidity associated with the procedure (POPF, DGE and PPH) generally being unrelated to the length of the abdominal incision but rather to the extensive nature of the actual intra-abdominal surgery.[88] The ability of fast-track protocols to achieve shorter duration of hospital stay after open surgery is a true reflection of this.[89] Besides, in a well-conducted trial of accelerated recovery after laparoscopic distal pancreatectomy a high readmission rate was noted.[90]

Fast-track Protocols/Enhanced Recovery after Surgery[1]

Enhanced recovery after surgery (ERAS) is an innovative approach that comprises a structured patient-care plan to reduce ambiguity, standardize patient care and prevent unnecessary delays in patient discharge. While these protocols have been tried by some centers for almost a decade, their general acceptance in pancreatic surgical units has not been low possibly related to fears of increased morbidity rates.[91] However, there is emerging evidence to support the use of ERAS protocols after pancreatic surgery. These strategies have resulted not only in improved gastric emptying and reduced postoperative stay and hospital costs[92,93] but have also contributed to significantly reduced morbidity, in general, with no increase in readmission rates.[89]

Palliative Pancreatic Resections, Gastroenterostomy and/or Biliodigestive Bypass

Patients with advanced pancreatic cancers may suffer from an obstruction to the biliary system at the lower end of the bile duct and/or the stomach or duodenum. Thus, they may clinically present with features of surgical obstructive jaundice with or without gastric outlet obstruction. In order to overcome these problems, depending on the predominant symptoms, surgical options include:

- *Double bypass:* Side-to-side hepaticojejunostomy (anastomosis of the proximal common bile duct to a Roux loop of jejunum) and a gastrojejunostomy. The Roux limb is then connected to the proximal jejunum by a side-to-side jejunojejunostomy; or
- Gastrojejunostomy—anastomosis of the stomach to a loop of jejunum in an antecolic, side-to-side, isoperistaltic manner.

Endoscopic palliation has steadily emerged as an alternative to surgical palliation, in which ERCP and stenting may help overcome biliary obstruction while a nasojejunal tube or duodenal stent may be placed to overcome gastric or duodenal outlet obstruction. These methods are preferred when the patient's general condition is poor and the anticipated survival is less than 6 months.

Over the past few decades, there has been a trend toward the performance of a double bypass, if feasible, in patients with unresectable periampullary[94] as well as pancreatic cancer[95] undergoing an exploratory laparotomy irrespective of the presence of features of gastric outlet obstruction. The rationale was based on the perceived notion while these procedures do not appear to significantly impair short-term outcomes they may contribute to avoiding long-term gastroduodenal obstruction[95] as well as be associated with reduced costs to the patients (encountered when repeated stent blocks occur necessitating frequent changes). Some data also existed to suggest that palliative resections may be associated with better survival and lesser costs as compared to palliative nonsurgical treatments. However, recent evidence from the United States has demonstrated that palliative bypass for pancreatic cancer is associated with a high rate of morbidity and mortality and this risk may be prohibitive in select patients.[11,96] These data have highlighted the importance of proper preoperative staging to avoid unnecessary surgical explorations as well as the need for proper patient selection when performing palliative bypass procedures. A recent Cochrane review has also stated that the evidence that palliative resections improve survival and reduce costs is very low compared to nonsurgical palliative treatments and that patients need to be informed of the high morbidity associated with these procedures prior to embarking on such surgeries.[10] Thus, careful patient selection is needed with surgical palliation being reserved for patients who are anticipated to have a survival more than 6 months.

SUMMARY

This chapter provided the current surgical principles in the management of pancreatic cancer. Advances in technical expertise have allowed surgeons to be more aggressive in order to achieve a complete surgical resection with microscopically negative margins. In borderline resectable pancreatic cancer, surgery should preferably be undertaken after neoadjuvant chemotherapy. Patients need to be better selected for palliative surgery avoid increasing the risk of morbidity and mortality.

ACKNOWLEDGMENT

The authors wish to acknowledge the help of Dr Ankesh Rawat, (Junior Registrar—GI Surgery, GI Oncology and Bariatric Surgery, Medanta—The Medicity) for the illustrations in this chapter.

REFERENCES

1. Shrikhande S, Barreto S. Surgery for pancreatic carcinoma: state of the art. Indian J Surg. 2012;74:79-86.
2. Krempien R, Muentier M, Harms W, et al. Neoadjuvant chemoradiation in patients with pancreatic adenocarcinoma. HPB (Oxford). 2006;8(1):22-8.
3. Shrikhande S, Barreto S, Goel M, et al. Multimodality imaging of pancreatic ductal adenocarcinoma: a review of the literature. HPB (Oxford). 2012;14(10):658-68.
4. Shukla PJ, Barreto SG, Kulkarni A, et al. Vascular anomalies encountered during pancreatoduodenectomy: do they influence outcomes? Ann Surg Oncol. 2010;17(1):186-93.
5. Tanaka M, Fernandez-Del Castillo C, Adsay V, Chari S, Falconi M, Jang JY, et al. International consensus guidelines 2012 for the management of IPMN and MCN of the pancreas. Pancreatology. 2012;12(3):183-97.
6. Farma JM, Santillan AA, Melis M, Walters J, Belinc D, Chen DT, et al. PET/CT fusion scan enhances CT staging in patients with pancreatic neoplasms. Ann Surg Oncol. 2008;15(9):2465-71.
7. Soriano A, Castells A, Ayuso C, Ayuso JR, de Caralt MT, Gines MA, et al. Preoperative staging and tumor resectability assessment of pancreatic cancer: prospective study comparing endoscopic ultrasonography, helical computed tomography, magnetic resonance imaging, and angiography. Am J Gastroenterol. 2004;99(3):492-501.
8. Jagannath P, Dhir V, Shrikhande S, Shah RC, Mullerpatan P, Mohandas KM. Effect of preoperative biliary stenting on immediate outcome after pancreaticoduodenectomy. Br J Surg. 2005;92(3):356-61.
9. Asbun HJ, Conlon K, Fernandez-Cruz L, Friess H, Shrikhande SV, Adham M, et al. When to perform a pancreatoduodenectomy in the absence of positive histology? A consensus statement by the International Study Group of Pancreatic Surgery. Surgery. 2014;155(5):887-92.
10. Gurusamy KS, Kumar S, Davidson BR, et al. Resection versus other treatments for locally advanced pancreatic cancer. Cochrane Database Syst Rev. 2014;2:CD010244.
11. Bartlett EK, Wachtel H, Fraker DL, Vollmer CM, Drebin JA, Kelz RR, et al. Surgical palliation for pancreatic malignancy: practice patterns and predictors of morbidity and mortality. J Gastrointest Surg. 2014;18(7):1292-8.
12. Hariharan D, Constantinides VA, Froeling FE, et al. The role of laparoscopy and laparoscopic ultrasound in the preoperative staging of pancreaticobiliary cancers—A meta-analysis. Eur J Surg Oncol. 2010;36(10):941-8.
13. Shrikhande SV, Barreto SG, Somashekar BA, Suradkar K, Shetty GS, Talole S, et al. Evolution of pancreatoduodenectomy in a tertiary cancer center in India: improved results from service reconfiguration. Pancreatology. 2013;13(1):63-71.
14. Tseng JF, Pisters PW, Lee JE, Wang H, Gomez HF, Sun CC, et al. The learning curve in pancreatic surgery. Surgery. 2007;141(4):456-63.
15. Shrikhande SV, Barreto G, Shukla PJ. Pancreatic fistula after pancreaticoduodenectomy: the impact of a standardized technique of pancreaticojejunostomy. Langenbecks Arch Surg. 2008;393(1):87-91.
16. Diener MK, Fitzmaurice C, Schwarzer G, Seiler CM, Antes G, Knaebel HP, et al. Pylorus-preserving pancreaticoduodenectomy (pp Whipple) versus pancreaticoduodenectomy (classic Whipple) for surgical treatment of periampullary and pancreatic carcinoma. Cochrane Database Syst Rev. 2011;5:CD006053.
17. Yang C, Wu HS, Chen XL, Wang CY, Gou SM, Xiao J, et al. Pylorus-preserving versus pylorus-resecting pancreaticoduodenectomy for periampullary and pancreatic carcinoma: a meta-analysis. PLoS One. 2014;9(3):e90316.
18. Iqbal N, Lovegrove RE, Tilney HS, Abraham AT, Bhattacharya S, Tekkis PP, et al. A comparison of pancreaticoduodenectomy with extended pancreaticoduodenectomy: a meta-analysis of 1909 patients. Eur J Surg Oncol. 2009;35(1):79-86.
19. Michalski CW, Kleeff J, Wente MN, Diener MK, Buchler MW, Friess H. Systematic review and meta-analysis of standard and extended lymphadenectomy in pancreaticoduodenectomy for pancreatic cancer. Br J Surg. 2007;94(3):265-73.
20. Sergeant G, Melloul E, Lesurtel M, et al. Extended lymphadenectomy in patients with pancreatic cancer is debatable. World J Surg. 2013;37(8):1782-8.
21. Xu X, Zhang H, Zhou P, et al. Meta-analysis of the efficacy of pancreatoduodenectomy with extended lymphadenectomy in the treatment of pancreatic cancer. World J Surg Oncol. 2013;11:311.
22. Jang JY, Kang MJ, Heo JS, Choi SH, Choi DW, Park SJ, et al. A prospective randomized controlled study comparing outcomes of standard resection and extended resection, including dissection of the nerve plexus and various lymph nodes, in patients with pancreatic head cancer. Ann Surg. 2014;259(4):656-64.
23. Shrikhande SV, Qureshi SS, Rajneesh N, et al. Pancreatic anastomoses after pancreaticoduodenectomy: do we need further studies? World J Surg. 2005;29(12):1642-9.
24. Shukla PJ, Barreto SG, Fingerhut A, Bassi C, Buchler MW, Dervenis C, et al. Toward improving uniformity and standardization in the reporting of pancreatic anastomoses: a new classification system by the International Study Group of Pancreatic Surgery (ISGPS). Surgery. 2010;147(1):144-53.
25. Shukla PJ, Barreto G, Shrikhande SV. The evolution of pancreatoduodenectomy. Hepatogastroenterology. 2011; 58(109):1409-12.
26. Wellner U, Sick O, Olschewski M, Adam U, Hopt U, Keck T. Randomized controlled single-center trial comparing pancreatogastrostomy versus pancreaticojejunostomy after partial pancreatoduodenectomy. J Gastrointest Surg. 2012;16(9):1686-95.

27. Topal B, Fieuws S, Aerts R, Weerts J, Feryn T, Roeyen G, et al. Pancreaticojejunostomy versus pancreaticogastrostomy reconstruction after pancreaticoduodenectomy for pancreatic or periampullary tumours: a multicentre randomised trial. Lancet Oncol. 2013;14(7):655-62.
28. Figueras J, Sabater L, Planellas P, Munoz-Forner E, Lopez-Ben S, Falgueras L, et al. Randomized clinical trial of pancreaticogastrostomy versus pancreaticojejunostomy on the rate and severity of pancreatic fistula after pancreaticoduodenectomy. Br J Surg. 2013;100(12):1597-605.
29. Bassi C, Dervenis C, Butturini G, Fingerhut A, Yeo C, Izbicki J, et al. Postoperative pancreatic fistula: an international study group (ISGPF) definition. Surgery. 2005;138(1):8-13.
30. Duffas JP, Suc B, Msika S, Fourtanier G, Muscari F, Hay JM, et al. A controlled randomized multicenter trial of pancreatogastrostomy or pancreatojejunostomy after pancreatoduodenectomy. Am J Surg. 2005;189(6):720-9.
31. Yeo CJ, Cameron JL, Maher MM, Sauter PK, Zahurak ML, Talamini MA, et al. A prospective randomized trial of pancreaticogastrostomy versus pancreaticojejunostomy after pancreaticoduodenectomy. Ann Surg. 1995;222(4):580-8.
32. McKay A, Mackenzie S, Sutherland FR, Bathe OF, Doig C, Dort J, et al. Meta-analysis of pancreaticojejunostomy versus pancreaticogastrostomy reconstruction after pancreaticoduodenectomy. Br J Surg. 2006;93(8):929-36.
33. Wente MN, Shrikhande SV, Muller MW, Diener MK, Seiler CM, Friess H, et al. Pancreaticojejunostomy versus pancreaticogastrostomy: systematic review and meta-analysis. Am J Surg. 2007;193(2):171-83.
34. Shukla PJ, Barreto SG, Bedi M, Bheerappa N, Chaudhary A, Gandhi M, et al. Peri-operative outcomes for pancreatoduodenectomy in India: a multi-centric study. HPB (Oxford). 2009;11(8):638-44.
35. Gurusamy KS, Koti R, Fusai G, et al. Somatostatin analogues for pancreatic surgery. Cochrane Database Syst Rev. 2010;(2):CD008370.
36. Kapoor VK, Sharma A, Behari A, et al. Omental flaps in pancreaticoduodenectomy. JOP. 2006;7(6):608-15.
37. Suc B, Msika S, Fingerhut A, Fourtanier G, Hay JM, Holmieres F, et al. Temporary fibrin glue occlusion of the main pancreatic duct in the prevention of intra-abdominal complications after pancreatic resection: prospective randomized trial. Ann Surg. 2003;237(1):57-65.
38. Shukla PJ, Barreto SG, Fingerhut A. Do transanastomotic pancreatic ductal stents after pancreatic resections improve outcomes? Pancreas. 2010;39(5):561-6.
39. Su AP, Cao SS, Zhang Y, Zhang ZD, Hu WM, Tian BL. Does antecolic reconstruction for duodenojejunostomy improve delayed gastric emptying after pylorus-preserving pancreaticoduodenectomy? A systematic review and meta-analysis. World J Gastroenterol. 2012;18(43):6315-23.
40. Barreto S, Shukla P, Shrikhande S. Tumors of the Pancreatic Body and Tail. World J Oncol. 2010;1(2):52-65.
41. Brennan MF, Moccia RD, Klimstra D. Management of adenocarcinoma of the body and tail of the pancreas. Ann Surg. 1996;223(5):506-11.
42. Shoup M, Brennan MF, McWhite K, Leung DH, Klimstra D, Conlon KC. The value of splenic preservation with distal pancreatectomy. Arch Surg. 2002;137(2):164-8.
43. Knaebel HP, Diener MK, Wente MN, et al. Systematic review and meta-analysis of technique for closure of the pancreatic remnant after distal pancreatectomy. Br J Surg. 2005;92(5):539-46.
44. Diener MK, Seiler CM, Rossion I, Kleeff J, Glanemann M, Butturini G, et al. Efficacy of stapler versus hand-sewn closure after distal pancreatectomy (DISPACT): a randomised, controlled multicentre trial. Lancet. 2011;377(9776):1514-22.
45. Christein JD, Kendrick ML, Iqbal CW, et al. Distal pancreatectomy for resectable adenocarcinoma of the body and tail of the pancreas. J Gastrointest Surg. 2005;9(7):922-7.
46. Sasson AR, Hoffman JP, Ross EA, Kagan SA, Pingpank JF, Eisenberg BL. En bloc resection for locally advanced cancer of the pancreas: is it worthwhile? J Gastrointest Surg. 2002;6(2):147-57.
47. Shoup M, Conlon KC, Klimstra D, et al. Is extended resection for adenocarcinoma of the body or tail of the pancreas justified? J Gastrointest Surg. 2003;7(8):946-52.
48. Hartwig W, Hackert T, Hinz U, Hassenpflug M, Strobel O, Buchler MW, et al. Multivisceral resection for pancreatic malignancies: risk-analysis and long-term outcome. Ann Surg. 2009;250(1):81-7.
49. Shrikhande SV, Barreto SG. Extended pancreatic resections and lymphadenectomy: An appraisal of the current evidence. World J Gastrointest Surg. 2010;2(2):39-46.
50. Katz MH, Pisters PW, Evans DB, et al. Fleming JB, et al. Borderline resectable pancreatic cancer: the importance of this emerging stage of disease. J Am Coll Surg. 2008;206(5):833-46.
51. Shrikhande SV, Arya S, Barreto SG, Ingle S, D'Souza MA, Hawaldar R, et al. Borderline resectable pancreatic tumors: is there a need for further refinement of this stage? Hepatobiliary Pancreat Dis Int. 2011;10(3):319-24.
52. Andriulli A, Festa V, Botteri E, Valvano MR, Koch M, Bassi C, et al. Neoadjuvant/preoperative gemcitabine for patients with localized pancreatic cancer: a meta-analysis of prospective studies. Ann Surg Oncol. 2012;19(5):1644-62.
53. Gillen S, Schuster T, Buschenfelde CMZ, et al. Preoperative/neoadjuvant therapy in pancreatic cancer: systematic review and meta-analysis of response and resectino percentages. PLoS Med. 2010;7(4):e1000267.
54. Tzeng CW, Tran Cao HS, Lee JE, Pisters PW, Varadhachary GR, Wolff RA, et al. Treatment sequencing for resectable pancreatic cancer: influence of early metastases and surgical complications on multimodality therapy completion and survival. J Gastrointest Surg. 2014;18(1):16-24.
55. Valle JW, Palmer D, Jackson R, Cox T, Neoptolemos JP, Ghaneh P, et al. Optimal duration and timing of adjuvant chemotherapy after definitive surgery for ductal adenocarcinoma of the pancreas: ongoing lessons from the ESPAC-3 study. J Clin Oncol. 2014;32(6):504-12.
56. Liao WC, Chien KL, Lin YL, Wu MS, Lin JT, Wang HP, et al. Adjuvant treatments for resected pancreatic adenocarcinoma: a systematic review and network meta-analysis. Lancet Oncol. 2013;14(11):1095-103.
57. Papavasiliou P, Chun YS, Hoffman JP. How to define and manage borderline resectable pancreatic cancer. Surg Clin North Am. 2013;93(3):663-74.
58. Haeno H, Gonen M, Davis MB, Herman JM, Iacobuzio-Donahue CA, Michor F. Computational modeling of pancreatic

cancer reveals kinetics of metastasis suggesting optimum treatment strategies. Cell. 2012;148(1-2):362-75.
59. Rhim AD, Mirek ET, Aiello NM, Maitra A, Bailey JM, McAllister F, et al. EMT and dissemination precede pancreatic tumor formation. Cell. 2012;148(1-2):349-61.
60. Sohn TA, Yeo CJ, Cameron JL, Koniaris L, Kaushal S, Abrams RA, et al. Resected adenocarcinoma of the pancreas-616 patients: results, outcomes, and prognostic indicators. J Gastrointest Surg. 2000;4(6):567-79.
61. Pingpank JF, Hoffman JP, Ross EA, Cooper HS, Meropol NJ, Freedman G, et al. Effect of preoperative chemoradiotherapy on surgical margin status of resected adenocarcinoma of the head of the pancreas. J Gastrointest Surg. 2001;5(2):121-30.
62. Krempien R, Muenter MW, Harms W, et al. Neoadjuvant chemoradiation in patients with pancreatic adenocarcinoma. HPB (Oxford). 2006;8(1):22-8.
63. Raut CP, Tseng JF, Sun CC, Wang H, Wolff RA, Crane CH, et al. Impact of resection status on pattern of failure and survival after pancreaticoduodenectomy for pancreatic adenocarcinoma. Ann Surg. 2007;246(1):52-60.
64. Festa V, Andriulli A, Valvano MR, Uomo G, Perri F, Andriulli N, et al. Neoadjuvant chemo-radiotherapy for patients with borderline resectable pancreatic cancer: a meta-analytical evaluation of prospective studies. JOP. 2013;14(6):618-25.
65. Rose JB, Rocha FG, Alseidi A, Biehl T, Moonka R, Ryan JA, et al. Erratum to: Extended neoadjuvant chemotherapy for borderline resectable pancreatic cancer demonstrates promising postoperative outcomes and survival. Ann Surg Oncol. 2014;21(5):1538.
66. Rose JB, Rocha FG, Alseidi A, Biehl T, Moonka R, Ryan JA, et al. Extended neoadjuvant chemotherapy for borderline resectable pancreatic cancer demonstrates promising postoperative outcomes and survival. Ann Surg Oncol. 2014;21(5):1530-7.
67. Heinemann V, Haas M, Boeck S. Neoadjuvant treatment of borderline resectable and non-resectable pancreatic cancer. Ann Oncol. 2013;24(10):2484-92.
68. Araujo RL, Gaujoux S, Huguet F, Gonen M, D'Angelica MI, DeMatteo RP, et al. Does pre-operative chemoradiation for initially unresectable or borderline resectable pancreatic adenocarcinoma increase post-operative morbidity? A case-matched analysis. HPB (Oxford). 2013;15(8):574-80.
69. Barugola G, Partelli S, Crippa S, Capelli P, D'Onofrio M, Pederzoli P, et al. Outcomes after resection of locally advanced or borderline resectable pancreatic cancer after neoadjuvant therapy. Am J Surg. 2012;203(2):132-9.
70. Massucco P, Capussotti L, Magnino A, Sperti E, Gatti M, Muratore A, et al. Pancreatic resections after chemoradiotherapy for locally advanced ductal adenocarcinoma: analysis of perioperative outcome and survival. Ann Surg Oncol. 2006;13(9):1201-8.
71. Yu XZ, Li J, Fu DL, Di Y, Yang F, Hao SJ, et al. Benefit from synchronous portal-superior mesenteric vein resection during pancreaticoduodenectomy for cancer: a meta-analysis. Eur J Surg Oncol. 2014;40(4):371-8.
72. Tang D, Zhang JQ, Wang DR. Long term results of pancreatectomy with portal-superior mesenteric vein resection for pancreatic carcinoma: a systematic review. Hepatogastroenterology. 2011;58(106):623-31.
73. Kaneoka Y, Yamaguchi A, Isogai M. Portal or superior mesenteric vein resection for pancreatic head adenocarcinoma: prognostic value of the length of venous resection. Surgery. 2009;145(4):417-25.
74. Fukuda S, Oussoultzoglou E, Bachellier P, Rosso E, Nakano H, Audet M, et al. Significance of the depth of portal vein wall invasion after curative resection for pancreatic adenocarcinoma. Arch Surg. 2007;142(2):172-9.
75. Kato H, Usui M, Isaji S, Nagakawa T, Wada K, Unno M, et al. Clinical features and treatment outcome of borderline resectable pancreatic head/body cancer: a multi-institutional survey by the Japanese Society of Pancreatic Surgery. J Hepatobiliary Pancreat Sci. 2013;20(6):601-10.
76. Ravikumar R, Holroyd D, Fusai G. Is there a role for arterial reconstruction in surgery for pancreatic cancer? World J Gastrointest Surg. 2013;5(3):27-9.
77. Niess H, Conrad C, Kleespies A, Haas F, Bao Q, Jauch KW, et al. Surgery for metastasis to the pancreas: is it safe and effective? J Surg Oncol. 2013;107(8):859-64.
78. Michalski CW, Erkan M, Huser N, Muller MW, Hartel M, Friess H, et al. Resection of primary pancreatic cancer and liver metastasis: a systematic review. Dig Surg. 2008;25(6):473-80.
79. Wente MN, Bassi C, Dervenis C, Fingerhut A, Gouma DJ, Izbicki JR, et al. Delayed gastric emptying (DGE) after pancreatic surgery: a suggested definition by the International Study Group of Pancreatic Surgery (ISGPS). Surgery. 2007;142(5):761-8.
80. Wente MN, Veit JA, Bassi C, Dervenis C, Fingerhut A, Gouma DJ, et al. Postpancreatectomy hemorrhage (PPH): an International Study Group of Pancreatic Surgery (ISGPS) definition. Surgery. 2007;142(1):20-5.
81. Kendrick ML, Cusati D. Total laparoscopic pancreaticoduodenectomy: feasibility and outcome in an early experience. Arch Surg. 2010;145(1):19-23.
82. Palanivelu C, Rajan PS, Rangarajan M, Vaithiswaran V, Senthilnathan P, Parthasarathi R, et al. Evolution in techniques of laparoscopic pancreaticoduodenectomy: a decade long experience from a tertiary center. J Hepatobiliary Pancreat Surg. 2009;16(6):731-40.
83. Ammori BJ. Laparoscopic hand-assisted pancreaticoduodenectomy: initial UK experience. Surg Endosc. 2004; 18(4):717-8.
84. Staudacher C, Orsenigo E, Baccari P, et al. Laparoscopic assisted duodenopancreatectomy. Surg Endosc. 2005;19(3):352-6.
85. Kendrick ML. Laparoscopic and robotic resection for pancreatic cancer. Cancer J. 2012;18(6):571-6.
86. Boggi U, Signori S, De Lio N, Perrone VG, Vistoli F, Belluomini M, et al. Feasibility of robotic pancreaticoduodenectomy. Br J Surg. 2013;100(7):917-25.
87. Strijker M, van Santvoort HC, Besselink MG, van Hillegersberg R, Borel Rinkes IH, Vriens MR, et al. Robot-assisted pancreatic surgery: a systematic review of the literature. HPB (Oxford). 2013;15(1):1-10.
88. Shrikhande SV, Barreto SG, Shukla PJ. Laparoscopy in pancreatic tumors. J Minim Access Surg. 2007;3(2):47-51.
89. Coolsen MM, van Dam RM, van der Wilt AA, Slim K, Lassen K, Dejong CH. Systematic review and meta-analysis of enhanced recovery after pancreatic surgery with particular emphasis on pancreaticoduodenectomies. World J Surg. 2013;37(8):1909-18.

90. Baker MS, Bentrem DJ, Ujiki MB, et al. Adding days spent in readmission to the initial postoperative length of stay limits the perceived benefit of laparoscopic distal pancreatectomy when compared with open distal pancreatectomy. Am J Surg. 2011;201(3):295-9.
91. Ypsilantis E, Praseedom RK. Current status of fast-track recovery pathways in pancreatic surgery. JOP. 2009;10(6):646-50.
92. Balzano G, Zerbi A, Braga M, Rocchetti S, Beneduce AA, Di Carlo V. Fast-track recovery programme after pancreaticoduodenectomy reduces delayed gastric emptying. Br J Surg. 2008;95(11):1387-93.
93. Kennedy EP, Rosato EL, Sauter PK, Rosenberg LM, Doria C, Marino IR, et al. Initiation of a critical pathway for pancreaticoduodenectomy at an academic institution—the first step in multidisciplinary team building. J Am Coll Surg. 2007;204(5):917-23.
94. Gurusamy K, Kumar S, Davidson B. Prophylactic gastrojejunostomy for unresectable periampullary carcinoma. Cochrane Database Syst Rev. 2010;10:CD008533.
95. Huser N, Michalski C, Schuster T, et al. Systematic review and meta-analysis of prophylactic gastroenterstomy for unresectable advanced pancreatic cancer. Br J Surg. 2009;96(7):711-9.
96. Spanheimer PM, Cyr AR, Liao J, Johlin FC, Hoshi H, Howe JR, et al. Complications and survival associated with operative procedures in patients with unresectable pancreatic head adenocarcinoma. J Surg Oncol. 2014;109(7):697-701.

20 CHAPTER

Pancreatic Cancer

Shikha Goyal, Tejinder Kataria, Vikraman Subramani

EPIDEMIOLOGY

Pancreatic cancer is the 10th most common cancer in both men and women and the 4th most common cause of cancer death. Most patients present with advanced disease. Incidence increases with age, and nearly 70% cases occur in patients older than 60 years. Incidence is higher in Western hemisphere, and correlates with cigarette smoking, high dietary fat intake, diabetes mellitus and chronic pancreatitis. Nearly 10% cases may be familial. Risk of cancer is 18-fold greater in first-degree relatives of familial cases (at least two first-degree relatives with pancreatic cancer). Associations have been seen with other syndromes such as the familial breast, ovarian, pancreas cancer syndrome associated with *BRCA2*, the familial pancreas cancer syndrome associated with *CDKN2A* abnormalities, the Peutz-Jeghers polyposis gastrointestinal malignancy syndrome associated with mismatched repair genes, *LKB1/STK11*, and the hereditary nonpolyposis colon cancer (HNPCC) syndrome.[1,2]

PREVENTION AND EARLY DETECTION

Till date, no simple, cost-effective test is available for early detection even in high-risk groups. Endoscopic ultrasound (EUS) detects smaller lesions than those detected with thin-section, dual-phase spiral CT and may be the imaging modality of choice for early detection. In combination with fine-needle aspiration (FNA), EUS can provide a cytologic diagnosis of lesions as small as 2–5 mm not visualized by CT, ultrasonography (USG), or magnetic resonance imaging (MRI). Endoscopic retrograde cholangiopancreatography (ERCP) is less likely to detect small tumors, is relatively more invasive owing to the risk of developing pancreatitis, but may help in detailed characterization of ductal anomalies.

No routinely available blood test qualifies as a screening tool. CA19-9 (carbohydrate antigen 19-9) is a tumor-associated antigen that is frequently elevated in patients with pancreatic adenocarcinoma, but is not specific, and thus used mainly in following treatment response in proven pancreatic cancers.

Biomarkers for early detection targeting, including DNA, RNA and protein-based approaches are being developed.[3-5]

BIOLOGY AND MOLECULAR MECHANISMS

Prognosis is determined by resectability (possible in 15–20% cases). Pathologic features related to prognosis include tumor size and differentiation, DNA content and margin and nodal status. The CDKN2A tumor suppressor gene (chromosome 9p) is inactivated in 95% of pancreatic cancers.[6] The most frequently activated oncogene is KRAS (90%). Molecular abnormalities may be used to define the precursors of pancreatic adenocarcinoma, to help characterize histologically ambiguous lesions, as the basis for new screening tests, and as important epidemiologic tools.[7]

PATHOLOGY AND PATHOGENESIS

Pathology

Infiltrating ductal adenocarcinoma is the most common histologic type (75%) for malignant tumors of exocrine pancreas. These malignant epithelial neoplasms show glandular or ductal differentiation, most arising in the periampullary region. Other rare histologies include adenosquamous carcinoma, acinic cell carcinoma, giant cell carcinomas and serous or mucinous cystadenocarcinomas. Metastases may occur in the pancreas from primary tumors of the breast, lung, colon/rectum, stomach and melanoma. Lymphomas constitute 1–2% of all primary pancreatic neoplasms, the most common type being diffuse large B-cell tumors.

Pathways of Spread

The pancreas is a retroperitoneal organ and lies in close proximity to stomach, duodenum, jejunum, kidneys, spleen, celiac trunk, superior mesenteric artery (SMA) and vein, common bile duct (CBD), and portal vein (PV). At diagnosis, over 85% of pancreas tumors have extended into adjacent organs, lymph nodes, fat, or soft tissue, allowing early metastases to regional and distant lymph nodes.

Frequently involved nodal sites include the posterior pancreaticoduodenal, superior or inferior pancreatic head, superior pancreatic body and porta hepatis. There is also a relationship between para-aortic lymph node involvement and involvement of posterior pancreaticoduodenal nodes by direct interlymphatic communication. Venous drainage of the pancreas is to the liver via PV.

Following resection, nearly 50% develop local recurrence, 42% show peritoneal dissemination and 62% liver metastases. The lung is the most commonly involved extra-abdominal organ. Retroperitoneal margin, poor differentiation, and lymph node involvement determine risk of relapse, especially local. Local recurrence may be responsible for death in up to 30% of patients with overt metastatic disease.[8-10]

CLINICAL EVALUATION

Pancreatic cancers usually present with locally advanced or metastatic disease. Tumors arising in the periampullary region of the pancreas (head, neck, uncinate process) cause obstructive jaundice (pruritus, dark urine, clay-colored stools and steatorrhea), pain or gastric outlet obstruction through duodenal compression or invasion. Nearly 20% patients present with recently diagnosed diabetes.

In contrast, tumors in the body or tail of pancreas usually present much later, achieve larger sizes before detection, with symptoms of jaundice, severe back pain (usually denoting posterior extension or unresectability). Tumors in the tail of pancreas may give rise to "left-sided" portal hypertension with upper gastrointestinal bleeding and/or splenomegaly from splenic vein obstruction/thrombosis. Laboratory results may show elevated serum bilirubin, alkaline phosphatase, gamma-glutamyl transpeptidase and aminotransferases. CA19-9 may be used to assess prognosis and follow patients postoperatively to guide response to treatment. Some early data suggest that monitoring levels of KRAS after treatment may indicate tumor response in patients treated with gefitinib and chemoradiation.[3,11]

Patient Evaluation

Staging and baseline data include history and physical examination, complete blood cell counts, liver and renal function tests, CA19-9, chest X-ray or chest contrast-enhanced CT (CECT), and CECT of abdomen and pelvis.

For patients with apparently resectable lesions, preoperative biopsy is not required. Biopsy to confirm diagnosis is required if neoadjuvant therapy is being planned or in patients with locoregionally unresectable or metastatic disease. Biopsy may be performed under USG, CT or ERCP guidance. CECT helps identify pancreatic masses, pancreatic duct dilatation, local invasion, liver metastases and vascular invasion of the great vessels. EUS is more effective in detecting vascular invasion of pancreatic cancer when CT is inconclusive.[12] In addition to enabling biopsy, ERCP may help decompress the biliary tree, and localize the source of obstruction. Percutaneous and transhepatic cholangiography may also help relieve biliary obstruction. Visceral angiography is selectively used to address concerns regarding vascular invasion, which may deem a tumor unresectable.

CA19-9 has limited use for diagnosis or screening because it may be elevated in pancreatitis, poorly-controlled diabetes, or obstruction of the pancreaticobiliary tree and may be falsely negative in patients lacking Lewis antigens. However, when elevated in known pancreatic cancer, it assists in following the treatment response and progression.

Positron emission tomography (PET) may be helpful in detecting distant metastases that would be missed with CT, but its role in pancreatic cancer is still evolving.[13]

STAGING

Tumors staged as T1, T2 or T3 are usually considered resectable. Unresectable pancreatic tumors are those in which the tumor cannot be separated from the adjacent large arterial structures (celiac axis or SMA). The extent of resection (R0 vs R1 or R2) carries prognostic significance. Recent data suggest that margins more than 1.5 mm optimize locoregional control, and the extent of clear margins in R0 resections may potentially be used to estimate risk of locoregional failure.[14]

PRIMARY THERAPY

Surgery is the primary therapy; however, 2-year survival rates with surgery alone are only 20–40% in resectable cases. Up to 80–90% develop local recurrence and/or distant metastases, commonest sites being liver, regional tissues and nodes, peritoneum and lung. At presentation, the outcome appears to be determined primarily by the extent of evident disease, resectability and performance status. Most (75–80%) pancreatic adenocarcinomas present in the head, neck, and/or uncinate process (periampullary region), and most clinical data on management is available for this subset. Body and tail presentation is less common, more advanced at diagnosis, with less robust data limited to this subset.

Surgery

The standard procedure for carcinoma head of pancreas is Whipple's pancreaticoduodenectomy, wherein the gallbladder, CBD, duodenum (second to fourth part), and head of pancreas are resected along with the postpyloric duodenum (pylorus-preserving pancreaticoduodenectomy) or resection is continued proximally to include the distal stomach (classic pancreaticoduodenectomy), along with regional lymph node dissection. Surgical mortality is only 1-3% in large volume centers.[15,16] Morbidity of pancreaticoduodenectomy may include pancreatic leak and infection, delayed gastric emptying and pancreatic fistula. Understanding the postoperative anatomy is imperative to planning adjuvant local therapy.

Cancers of body or tail of pancreas present late, with larger and more locally advanced masses or evidence of overt metastatic disease, hence most cases are unresectable. When resectable, a distal pancreatectomy with en bloc splenectomy is performed.

Prognostic Factors Associated with Surgery

Resectability itself is the most important prognostic factor. 5-year overall survival (OS) for patients undergoing resection is 24% versus 0% for those not undergoing resection.[17]

For patient undergoing curative resection and surviving perioperative period, tumor size, tumor differentiation, presence of lymphovascular invasion, capillary invasion, perineural microinvasion, lymph node status, or type of procedure (pancreaticoduodenectomy vs total pancreatectomy) do not affect survival.[18] Perioperative survival, however, is better with intraoperative blood loss less than 700 mL, tumor location (duodenum or ampulla vs bile duct or pancreas), tumor diameter less than 3 cm, negative margins, negative nodes and well-differentiated tumors. Resurgery for complications is significantly associated with decreased survival. For long-term survival, negative nodal involvement, extent of lymph node involvement, tumor differentiation, and resected margin status are all important prognostic factors for periampullary tumors.[19-22]

Brennan et al. developed a nomogram to predict outcome at 1, 2 or 3 years.[23]

Patterns of Failure after Surgery

For patients undergoing surgery alone, nearly 50–75% develop local relapses while another 15–20% develop distant failures. Most failures, even distant, are intra-abdominal (peritoneum, liver) while less than 25% of failures are extra-abdominal and never the only site of failure. In those treated with adjuvant chemoradiation, liver and peritoneum constitute major relapse sites while reported local failures are fewer than 10%. Prognostic factors for local control include T stage (T1/T2 vs T3/T4), N stage (N+ vs N-), tumor differentiation (moderate vs. poor) and resection margins.[24-26]

The observed patterns of failure indicate the need for adjuvant interventions to address locoregional, peritoneal, and hepatic failure patterns.

ADJUVANT THERAPY

After surgical resection, adjuvant chemotherapy with gemcitabine has shown survival advantage versus observation; however, role of adjuvant chemoradiation is controversial. Some nonrandomized studies have shown a benefit of radiation therapy (RT) in addition to chemotherapy after surgery. Neoadjuvant therapy is being evaluated in both resectable and borderline resectable disease.

Adjuvant Chemotherapy and Irradiation after Resection, Randomized Data

Gastrointestinal Tumor Study Group (GITSG) established the role of adjuvant 5FU-based chemoradiation in a prospective randomized trial, with a superior OS. External beam RT (EBRT) was given as two courses of 20 Gy in ten fractions, 2 weeks apart with concurrent 5FU bolus given on first 3 days of each RT course. Performance status and extent of tumor were the only independently significant prognostic variables. The study was terminated prematurely because of poor accrual.[27]

To address concerns related to poor accrual, GITSG registered additional 30 patients in a nonrandomized fashion to receive the same adjuvant therapy. Results in these patients recapitulated the results of the treatment arm in the randomized study. Local recurrence rate was 30–50% in all patients regardless of whether they received adjuvant treatment and the incidence of hepatic metastases was 40–50%. These results, although strongly suggesting a treatment effect, imply that the dose of RT was too low to deal with the regional burden of disease and the efficacy of 5FU alone was inadequate to sterilize disease outside the treatment fields for most patients.[28]

The European Organization for Research and Treatment of Cancer (EORTC), in a multi-institutional, randomized trial in periampullary cancers, including pancreatic adenocarcinoma, randomized to receive surgery alone or surgery plus postoperative 5FU-based chemoradiation, showed no benefit for the overall group but survival trends favored adjuvant postoperative chemoradiation for pancreatic cancer. There were several flaws in the trial design and the study was underpowered.[29]

The European Study for Pancreatic Cancer (ESPAC)-1 study attempted to evaluate the independent effects of adjuvant chemotherapy and chemoradiation, with a complex design (three separate but concurrent phase III trials) with a 2 × 2 factorial design: (1) observation; (2) concomitant chemoradiation alone (20 Gy in 10 fractions over 2 weeks with 500 mg/m^2 5FU IV bolus during first 3 days of RT and then repeated after a planned 2-week break); (3) chemotherapy alone (leucovorin 20 mg/m^2 bolus followed by 5FU 425 mg/m^2 day 1–5 every 28 days for six cycles); and (4) chemoradiation followed by six cycles of adjuvant 5FU/leucovorin. Patients randomized to receive adjuvant chemotherapy had a survival benefit (5-year OS, 21% vs 8%; p = 0.009). Local recurrence was a component of failure in 34% patients at risk and 63% patients with relapse. Major concerns regarding the design and execution of this trial include more than one randomization scheme, patients allowed to receive "background" therapy in addition to protocol therapy in two of the three trials, no restaging of disease after resection and before adjuvant therapy, and no Quality Assurance (QA) guidelines for the delivery of RT (i.e. no section in the protocol on appropriate field design, no central audit of radiation fields).[30]

Radiation therapy oncology group (RTOG) 97-04, a randomized phase III trial, evaluated the role of adjuvant gemcitabine versus 5FU in addition to 5FU-based chemoradiation (50.4 Gy in 28 fractions over 5.5 weeks plus concurrent 5FU infusion). Gemcitabine arm showed a trend toward better OS, with a higher grade 4 neutropenia rate but no difference in febrile neutropenia or in the ability to complete chemotherapy or RT.[31]

Retrospective and Prospective Adjuvant Chemoradiation Studies, Nonrandomized

Most nonrandomized studies suggest a benefit for adjuvant chemoradiation in pancreatic cancers. Data from University of Pennsylvania showed a decrease in local recurrence from 85% in patients treated with surgery alone to 25% in patients treated with RT and 5FU infusion. Inferior survival was noted in presence of positive surgical margins. Among patients with negative margins, 3-year survival was 22% for surgery alone, 11% for surgery plus RT with or without bolus 5FU and 47% for patients receiving postoperative RT with 5FU infusion.[32] Additionally, this study emphasized the role of nutritional support and CT-based RT planning.

The Johns Hopkins Hospital data demonstrated that patients receiving GITSG-style chemoradiation with maintenance 5FU truncated at 6 months (rather than 2 years) or a more intensive regimen (involving higher doses of RT as well as hepatic irradiation administered without interruption and with continuous infusion 5FU/leucovorin chemotherapy) did better than patients receiving no postsurgical therapy. The median survival rates for the standard, intensive and control arms were 21 months, 17.5 months and 13.5 months, respectively, with respective 2-year survivals of 44%, 22% and 30%. Intensive therapy had no survival advantage over standard therapy, but there was a statistically significant difference between the standard versus control arms (p < 0.0002). Multivariate analysis confirmed that prognostic factors for disease relapse included margin and lymph node status, tumor size and degree of differentiation.[33]

Investigators at Johns Hopkins have updated their prospective cohort of patients who underwent resection of proximal pancreatic cancer between 1993 and 2005. Patients who received chemoradiation had better median, and 5-year OS compared with patients with no chemoradiation (median 21.2 vs 14.4 months, 5-year OS 32% vs 15%; p < 0.001). This survival advantage persisted even after controlling for age, medical comorbidities and surgical complications.[34]

A Johns Hopkins Hospital—Mayo Clinic collaborative analysis in patients who had pancreaticoduodenectomy for pancreatic adenocarcinoma consisted of over 1,000 patients treated with curative intent with half receiving adjuvant 5FU-based chemoradiation (median RT dose, 50.4 Gy). OS was significantly longer among patients who received adjuvant chemoradiation versus pancreaticoduodenectomy alone (median 21.1 vs 15.5 months; 5-year OS 22.3% vs 16.1%, p < 0.001).[35]

Adjuvant Chemotherapy

Adjuvant therapy for pancreatic cancer has focused on both chemoradiation and chemotherapy in the United States, while in Europe, most studies have focused on adjuvant chemotherapy alone, based on the results of ESPAC-1. Historically, the most commonly used regimes include 5FU, and more recently, gemcitabine.

Gemcitabine has shown superior symptom palliation as well as longer median survival compared with 5FU in symptomatic advanced pancreatic cancer.[36] In the adjuvant setting (CONKO-001 trial), gemcitabine showed significantly better disease-free survival (DFS) and OS in patients with postoperative CA19-9 values less than or equal to 2.5 times normal and with R0 or R1 resections.[37] Applicability of these results to patients with higher postoperative CA19-9 levels is uncertain.

In metastatic and locally advanced disease, doublets have not proved superior to gemcitabine alone. A statistically significant, small improvement in median survival and 1-year OS has been seen with gemcitabine and erlotinib combination compared to gemcitabine alone.[38] The largest trial comparing adjuvant 5FU/leucovorin to adjuvant gemcitabine in resected pancreatic cancer, ESPAC-3, shows no survival benefit with gemcitabine.[39]

Newer Chemoradiation Regimens

Although the historic trials previously discussed used 5FU-based chemoradiation in the adjuvant setting, new systemic agents have been coupled with RT over the past decade. Many feasibility studies have shown that these regimens can be given safely, and now randomized trials are needed to see if they lead to improved results.

Interferon-based Chemoradiation

External beam RT (45–54 Gy with standard fractionation) and concurrent chemotherapy (5FU infusion, weekly cisplatin, and interferon-alpha 3 million units on alternate days) followed by two 6-week courses of chemotherapy (5FU infusion) during weeks 9 to 14 and 17 to 22, showed higher grade 3/4 gastrointestinal toxicities, requiring hospitalization in 35%. Majority of patients were still able to receive more than 80% of planned therapy, with a superior median OS and 2-year OS versus GITSG-based chemoradiation.[40] The American College of Surgeons Oncology Group (ACOSOG) initiated a multi-institutional phase II study of a similar adjuvant chemoradiation regimen. Patients received postoperative RT to 50.4 Gy with 1.8 Gy fractions given concurrently with 5FU infusion (days 1 to 38), cisplatin (30 mg/m^2 IV weekly), and interferon-alpha (3 million units on alternate days), followed by continuous infusion 5FU for two cycles. RT fields included just the regions at highest risk for local recurrence, namely, the surgical margins, celiac axis and SMA/uncinate regions. Results showed promising 2-year OS (84% vs. 54%).[41] The study was closed early owing to high severe acute toxicity rates. These results were also replicated in subsequent studies at other centers.[42]

Gemcitabine-based Chemoradiation

Gemcitabine-based chemoradiation utilizes the radiosensitizing properties of gemcitabine in pancreatic carcinoma cells. Various regimes have explored full-dose gemcitabine, twice-weekly low-dose gemcitabine and reduced-dose weekly gemcitabine. EORTC 40013, a phase II trial, compared gemcitabine alone or gemcitabine followed by gemcitabine-based chemoradiation. Patients were randomized to receive either four cycles of gemcitabine alone or two cycles of gemcitabine, followed by weekly gemcitabine with concurrent irradiation (50.4 Gy in 28 fractions). Both arms had similar rates of distant progression, but the rate of first local recurrence was lower in the chemoradiation arm (11% vs 24%, $p = 0.16$).[43]

Present Status of Adjuvant Therapy for Pancreatic Cancer

It is established that surgery alone does not accomplish cure in pancreatic cancers. CONKO-001 trial established a role for gemcitabine in adjuvant setting, but did not explore the role of adjuvant RT. Subsequent trials exploring role of RT have invited criticism due to design flaws (GITSG, EORTC, ESPAC-1, RTOG 97-04), hence the issue remains unresolved. National Comprehensive Cancer Network guidelines for pancreatic cancer include chemotherapy (gemcitabine, capecitabine, or 5FU based) or chemotherapy followed by chemoradiation.

In late 2009, the RTOG in cooperation with Southwest Oncology Group (SWOG) and EORTC opened RTOG 08-48, a randomized phase III trial designed to address two questions—whether gemcitabine plus erlotinib produces superior survival results compared to gemcitabine alone, and whether addition of RT in combination with 5FU or capecitabine enhances survival for patients remaining disease-free after chemotherapy. The trial stratifies for known prognostic variables, QA for both surgical and radiotherapy components and requires enrollment of more than 900 patients over 4 years.[44]

Neoadjuvant Strategies

Neoadjuvant chemotherapy or RT in resectable or borderline resectable disease carries the theoretical advantages of superior radiobiologic effect with improved blood flow, avoiding omission of chemoradiation secondary to postoperative recovery, and allowing patients destined for early systemic failures to declare themselves to avert futile surgery. EBRT did not improve resectability, though it produced better 1-year OS and reduced early regional failures.[45]

Neoadjuvant chemoradiation for periampullary tumors (EBRT 50.4 Gy concurrent with 5FU/ mitomycin C infusions) has been attempted, and on historical comparison with similar postoperative regimens, has shown no difference in intraoperative management or length of postoperative stay, but with fewer involved nodes and higher proportion with negative resection margins. No benefit in relapse-free survival or OS was observed. However, the patients treated preoperatively tended to have more advanced tumors than those treated postoperatively and to be more debatable surgical candidates to begin with, so the similar OS and DFS may still favor the use of preoperative treatment in certain subsets of patients.[46,47] Use of RT concurrent with gemcitabine neoadjuvantly for resectable pancreatic cancer has shown promising early data on survival.[48-50]

In summary, for established resectable disease, it is extremely difficult to directly compare the results of neoadjuvant and adjuvant approaches. In the neoadjuvant approach, the effects of prior therapy alter pathologic staging. It assures the use of chemotherapy with or without radiotherapy before surgery, provides a window of opportunity for rapidly progressive disease to declare itself, and probably enhances the chances for an R0 resection. The adjuvant approach allows for the more definitive approach of surgery to be performed upfront, with the goal of cure or best anatomic palliation, provides unambiguous pathologic staging with respect to disease site (pancreas, distal CBD, ampulla of Vater and periampullary duodenum), tumor grade and nodal involvement. Many operations performed with curative intent may fail their intent in both contexts and the choice between the two approaches remains with the treating surgeon or oncologist.

Neoadjuvant Therapy for Borderline Resectable Disease

Most recent data on neoadjuvant therapy has focused on borderline resectable tumors, that is, tumors at high risk postoperatively for having microscopic residual disease, especially at the uncinate or SMA margins. Positive margins after surgery have been associated with significantly worse survival.[51] To achieve a higher probability of R0 resection in this subset, neoadjuvant therapy has been integrated into some treatment regimes.

Researchers at M.D. Anderson Cancer Center have proposed objective CT-based anatomic criteria to classify borderline resectable disease. Tumors with severe unilateral superior mesenteric vein/portal impingement, large area of contact with superior mesenteric artery, encasement of gastroduodenal artery up to hepatic artery origin, short superior mesenteric vein occlusion, or adrenal, colon, or kidney invasion are termed borderline resectable while those with distant metastases, encasement of superior mesenteric, celiac or hepatic arteries, occlusion of superior mesenteric or portal veins, invasion or encasement of aorta or inferior vena cava, invasion of superior mesenteric vein below transverse mesocolon or invasion to rib or vertebra are deemed unresectable.[52] Surgery with gross negative margins was possible in 41% of patients treated with neoadjuvant therapy, and 94% of these had negative margins on pathology. Median survival was 40 months for the patients undergoing resection, compared with 13 months to those not receiving surgery ($p < 0.001$). Similar results from the Fox Chase Cancer Center showed that patients who underwent neoadjuvant therapy followed by surgery had an 85% rate of margin-negative resections.[53] These data suggest that neoadjuvant therapy for borderline-resectable pancreatic cancer may improve the likelihood of an R0 resection, but randomized trials are needed to formally test this approach.

LOCALLY ADVANCED DISEASE

For unresectable disease, RT with concurrent 5FU has shown a survival benefit, and is effective in pain palliation. Gemcitabine and RT combinations are promising. Chemoradiation, chemotherapy alone, intraoperative RT (IORT), radioactive implants, and stereotactic radiosurgery have been evaluated in this context. Therapeutic selection among these options depends on patient presentation, performance status and physician and institution preference.

Palliative Surgery

Palliative surgery for periampullary tumors could include hepaticojejunostomy, gastrojejunostomy, or both, to relieve biliary obstruction and gastric outlet obstruction. Patients undergoing palliative pancreaticoduodenectomy fare significantly better than patients undergoing palliative bypass (2-year OS 30% vs 10%; $p < 0.02$). Addition of adjuvant chemoradiation further extends survival. Even in patients who undergo bypass therapy, postoperative RT extends survival.[54,55]

Chemoradiation for Locoregional Unresectable Disease

For locoregionally unresectable disease, GITSG has shown that split-course RT (40–60 Gy) with concurrent 5FU bolus is superior to RT alone (60 Gy).[56] Another study showed that chemoradiation followed by SMF chemotherapy (streptozotocin, mitomycin C, 5FU) is superior to chemotherapy alone.[57]

Only 10% tumors become operable after chemoradiation, but most patients experience pain relief. Treatment toxicity is related to EBRT volume, total dose, fraction size, use or absence of a planned split, as well as the intensity of the chemotherapy regime. In adequately nourished patients with absent or bypassed hepatic or gastric obstruction, toxicities such as nausea and mucositis, are readily manageable.

Gemcitabine concurrent with EBRT (50.4 Gy in 28 fractions) in various schedules (20 mg/m^2 twice a week, 40 mg/m^2 twice a week) with or without additional gemcitabine cycles has shown encouraging response rates, albeit at the cost of significant hematologic (60–70%) and gastrointestinal (40%) toxicities.[58-60]

An Eastern Cooperative Oncology Group (ECOG) phase III trial attempted to assess the benefit of RT combined with gemcitabine in unresectable pancreatic cancer but was closed early because of poor accrual. Published as an abstract, 50.4 Gy of RT with weekly gemcitabine significantly improved median survival compared with weekly gemcitabine alone, but with higher grade 4 toxicity.[61]

Gemcitabine has also been combined with cisplatin and RT. A phase I study at Mayo Clinic gave twice-weekly gemcitabine and cisplatin for 3 weeks during EBRT (50.4 Gy in 28 fractions). Dose-limiting toxicities were grade 4 nausea and vomiting. The recommended phase II dose was gemcitabine 30 mg/m^2 and cisplatin 10 mg/m^2.[62] Another trial used strictly time-scheduled gemcitabine (dosing on days 2, 5, 26 and 33) and cisplatin (days 1 to 5 and 29 to 33) combined with RT, with a recommended phase II dose of 20 mg/m^2 for cisplatin and 300 mg/m^2 for gemcitabine. Chemoradiation enabled 10 of 30 patients with initially unresectable disease to undergo surgery, with an R0 resection in nine cases.[63]

Because the ESPAC-3 study showed no survival difference in patients treated adjuvantly with 5FU versus gemcitabine, the question of which agent to use in the locally advanced setting is debatable. A retrospective review of MD Anderson data in locally advanced disease treated with RT (30 Gy in 10 fractions) with either concurrent 5FU or gemcitabine, showed higher acute toxicity with gemcitabine, higher resectability rates with gemcitabine-based chemoradiation but a similar median survival in both groups.[64]

Bevacizumab is being tested as a radiosensitizer in unresectable pancreatic cancer. Early reports showed a higher rate of duodenal bleed; hence further studies have excluded cases with duodenal involvement. RTOG 04-11 tested RT concurrent with bevacizumab and capecitabine followed by gemcitabine and bevacizumab in unresectable pancreatic cancer while excluding tumors with duodenal invasion. This regime was tolerated well with no duodenal bleeds.[65]

Use of single-fraction stereotactic body RT (SBRT) sequentially with gemcitabine-based chemotherapy for locally unresectable pancreatic cancer has shown promise, but the short follow up period precludes definite recommendations. Dose used was 25 Gy to gross tumor plus a margin of 2–3 mm.[66]

Chemotherapy

Since the benefit of chemoradiation is relatively modest, some oncologists recommend chemotherapy alone for locally advanced disease. Gemcitabine is the most commonly used agent, extrapolating from the metastatic disease setting, with good symptom control and modest survival improvement. ECOG phase III trial (E4201) comparing gemcitabine/irradiation versus gemcitabine alone, though closed prematurely for inadequate accrual, showed that patients in the chemoradiation arm had superior median survival (11.0 months vs 9.2 months, p = .044).[61]

Only one doublet (gemcitabine and erlotinib) has shown modest survival benefit compared with gemcitabine alone (median survival 6.24 vs 5.91 months; p = .038). Progression-free survival and 1-year OS were also significantly improved with the addition of erlotinib. Erlotinib arm had more adverse reactions, but most were grade 1 and 2.[38]

Intraoperative Irradiation or Brachytherapy ± External Beam Radiation Therapy (EBRT)

The combination of EBRT plus brachytherapy or intraoperative electron irradiation (IOERT) has resulted in better local control in series from Thomas Jefferson University Hospital, Massachusetts General Hospital, and Mayo Clinic, but this does not reflect in better median OS or 2-year OS owing to high rates of abdominal relapse (liver, peritoneal).[67-70] The delivery of EBRT plus concurrent chemotherapy before restaging and laparotomy plus IOERT or brachytherapy or resection plus IOERT translates into improved patient selection and some improvement in median and 2-year OS.[71,72]

Stereotactic Body Radiotherapy

Linear accelerator or CyberKnife-based stereotactic body radiotherapy (SBRT) has recently gained popularity in management of locally advanced, nonmetastatic pancreatic cancer. Requisite criteria include a life expectancy of 12 weeks or higher, tumor size less than 7.5 cm, absence of extensive vascular involvement, portal vein occlusion and aorta or inferior vena cava invasion. The treatment is challenging since the tumor lies in close proximity to duodenum, stomach, liver and kidneys. The earliest experience from Stanford studied single fraction doses ranging from 15 Gy to 25 Gy, and later the 25 Gy single fraction regime was integrated with sequential gemcitabine-based chemotherapy, with encouraging local control.[73,74] However, due to reports of grade 3-4 duodenal toxicity with this schedule, later studies used three fractions of 8–15 Gy each, depending on proximity of tumor to duodenum, stomach and small bowel.[75]

PALLIATION AND SUPPORT

Median survival with metastatic disease (liver, lung and peritoneum) is 3–5 months. Important issues during all phases of management include pain, nausea, dehydration, depression, malabsorption, weight loss, hyperglycemia, electrolyte balance and jaundice. Endoscopic stenting may help bypass obstructive disease, but sometimes surgery may be required to achieve gastric and/or biliary bypass.

Best Supportive Care

The supportive care needs of patients with locoregionally advanced, periampullary pancreatic cancer can be substantial, and attention to these forms the foundation of excellent palliation and care, regardless of whether intervention with antineoplastic therapy (chemotherapy with or without RT) is selected. Presence of unrelieved jaundice, gastric outlet obstruction or weight loss will compromise tolerance to any antineoplastic therapy. RT in patients with gastric outlet obstruction is associated with severe nausea, vomiting and anorexia.

IRRADIATION TECHNIQUES

Adjuvant therapy: High-energy photons (6–10 MV) are preferred. Clinical target volume (CTV) includes the tumor bed, peripancreatic lymph nodes and para-aortic lymph nodes between the T11 and L3 vertebrae.

CT-based treatment planning is preferred. Hepaticojejunostomy, the pancreaticojejunostomy, the pancreatic remnant, the celiac axis, the superior mesenteric artery, and critical normal structures, such as liver, spinal cord, and kidneys are contoured on RT planning CT. Coregistration with preoperative CT images help assess the preoperative tumor location.

For critical structure tolerance, the RTOG 97-04 protocol offers some guidelines.[76] Efforts should be made to exclude the small bowel and liver as much as possible. Not more than 60% of liver should receive greater than 30 Gy. The spinal cord dose is limited to less than 45 Gy. The equivalent of one kidney should receive below 20 Gy, or at least the equivalent of two thirds of one kidney must be spared from the RT fields. If only a single functioning kidney is present, at least two thirds of the functioning kidney must be excluded from any radiation port. For either head or tail lesions, at least 2/3 of the contralateral kidney should be shielded. Sites of surgical anastomoses are difficult to identify or localize; however, these sites represent potential areas of residual microscopic tumor either by direct or lymphatic extension. Care must be taken to allow for adequate margins that account for beam edge penumbra, daily setup variation and respiratory or physiologic movements.

In RTOG 08-48, the principles utilized in two-dimensional RT planning have been extended to three-dimensional conformal radiotherapy (3D-CRT) and intensity-modulated radiotherapy (IMRT) planning. A detailed atlas of these principles is available. This protocol targets the areas of greatest subclinical tumor concentration based on anatomic landmarks not readily apparent in two-dimensional imaging (celiac and superior mesenteric arteries, portal vein, pancreaticojejunostomy, gross tumor volume location of the resected tumor) and also specifies more precisely suggested tolerance parameters for critical normal organs. The CTV and PTV resulting are significantly smaller than those utilized in the past with 2D planning.

With use of potent systemic agents, the use of limited fields has gained momentum. Many full-dose gemcitabine studies exclude elective nodal irradiation. Use of 4D planning with assessment of pancreatic motion may help reduce treatment volumes further.

Treatment planning considerations for locoregional unresectable tumors are similar but can be complicated by the size of the mass and by extension of gross tumor superiorly into the retrogastric region. Size can be a problem for avoiding excessive renal parenchyma exposure, and extension into the retrogastric area increases the amount of stomach, especially the posterior antrum, that is treated. The importance of covering para-aortic lymph nodes has not been well studied.

The advent of IMRT has sparked interest in the treatment of both resected and unresectable pancreatic adenocarcinomas. Two studies analyzed the use of IMRT to treat patients with malignancies of the pancreas. The majority of patients received concurrent chemotherapy. Compared with conventional RT, IMRT reduced the mean dose to the liver, kidneys, stomach and small bowel. These dosimetric improvements may allow safer delivery of larger, systemic doses of concurrent chemotherapy.[77]

Figure 1A shows the target volume and normal structures for a case of unresectable adenocarcinoma pancreas with SMA encasement. Figure 1B shows a single arc volumetric-modulated arc therapy (VMAT) plan.

Figure 2A shows the target volumes and organs at risks (OARs) for a case of adenocarcinoma pancreas, post-Whipple's procedure, pT2N0. Figure 2B shows the respective conformal plan.

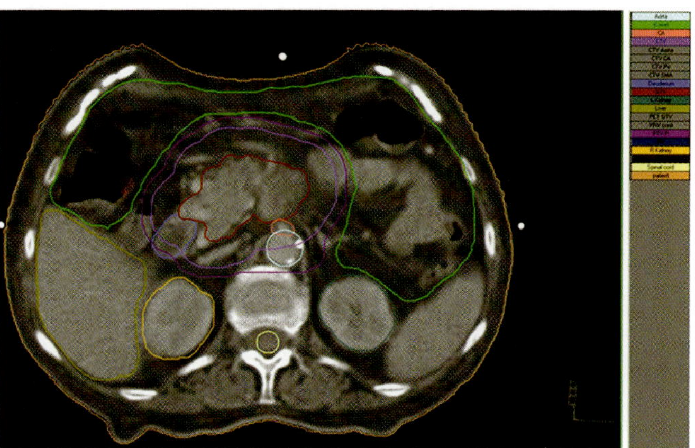

Fig. 1A The target volume and normal structures for a case of unresectable adenocarcinoma pancreas with SMA encasement

For SBRT, the gross disease is identified as GTV. CTV is the same as GTV, and PTV is defined as a 3–5 mm margin around GTV and dose is prescribed typically at 65–85% isodose. The total dose and fractional dose is defined by proximity to critical structures. Linear accelerator (LINAC)-based SBRT employs either IMRT or forward noncoplanar 3D-CRT planning. Availability of the various image guidance technologies available is mandatory for verification and execution of SBRT treatment. CyberKnife is one of the most advanced SBRT delivery systems. Tumor tracking is enabled either by spine tracking for paravertebral tumors whose movements mimic spinal movements or by fiducial tracking wherein three to six cylindrical solid gold markers 3–5 mm in length are placed within and around the tumor at a minimum interfiducial distance of 2 cm and their motion is monitored and corrected automatically throughout treatment delivery in real time in conjunction with creating a respiratory model linking tumor movement with chest wall movement detected by infrared trackers placed on the body surface.

Figure 3 shows the beam profile, isodose distribution and dose-volume histograms for a patient with carcinoma pancreas who received radical chemoradiation of 45 Gy in 25 fractions with EBRT, and was subsequently taken up for CyberKnife boost to residual tumor. GTV was marked in both end-exhale and end-inhale CT datasets, and an ITV was generated. A dose of 18 Gy in three fractions was prescribed to 87% isodose. Spine tracking was used for localization during treatment delivery.

TREATMENT ALGORITHM, CONTROVERSIES AND FUTURE POSSIBILITIES

For resectable disease, surgical therapy is clearly required for any chance at cure. However, controversies abound regarding the most appropriate adjuvant therapy. The rate of local and distant relapse in both retrospective and prospective studies support the role of chemoradiation; however, the available

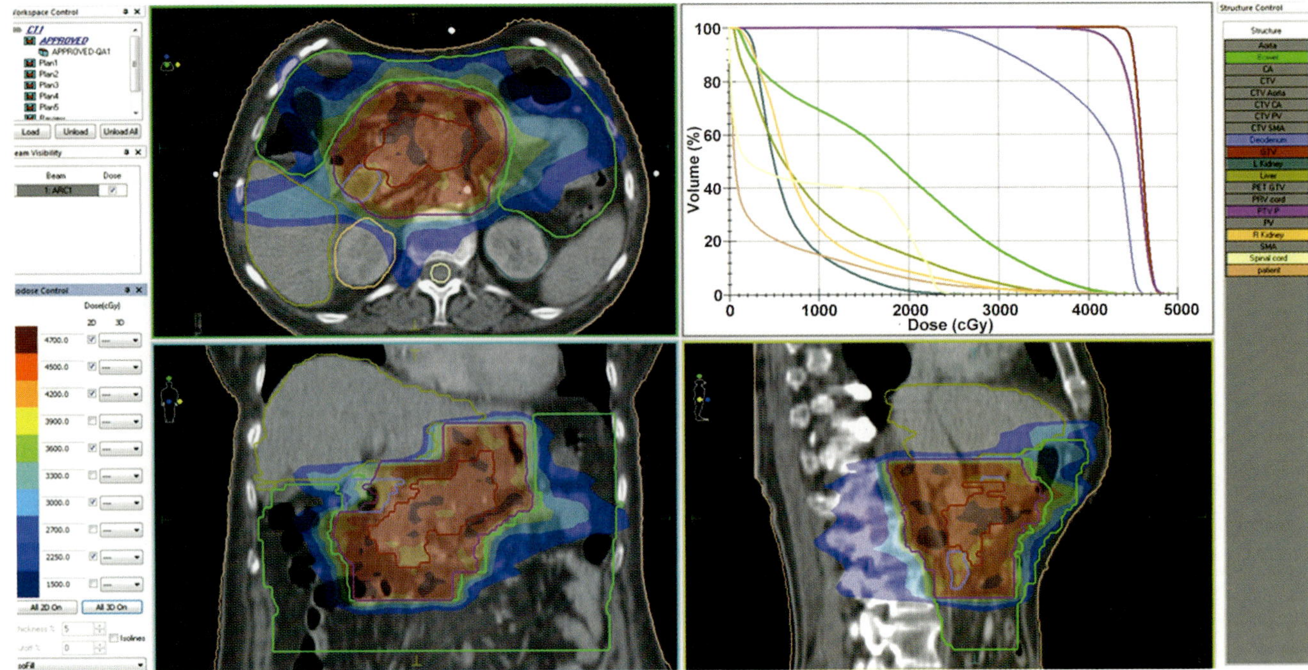

Fig. 1B A single arc volumetric-modulated arc therapy (VMAT) plan

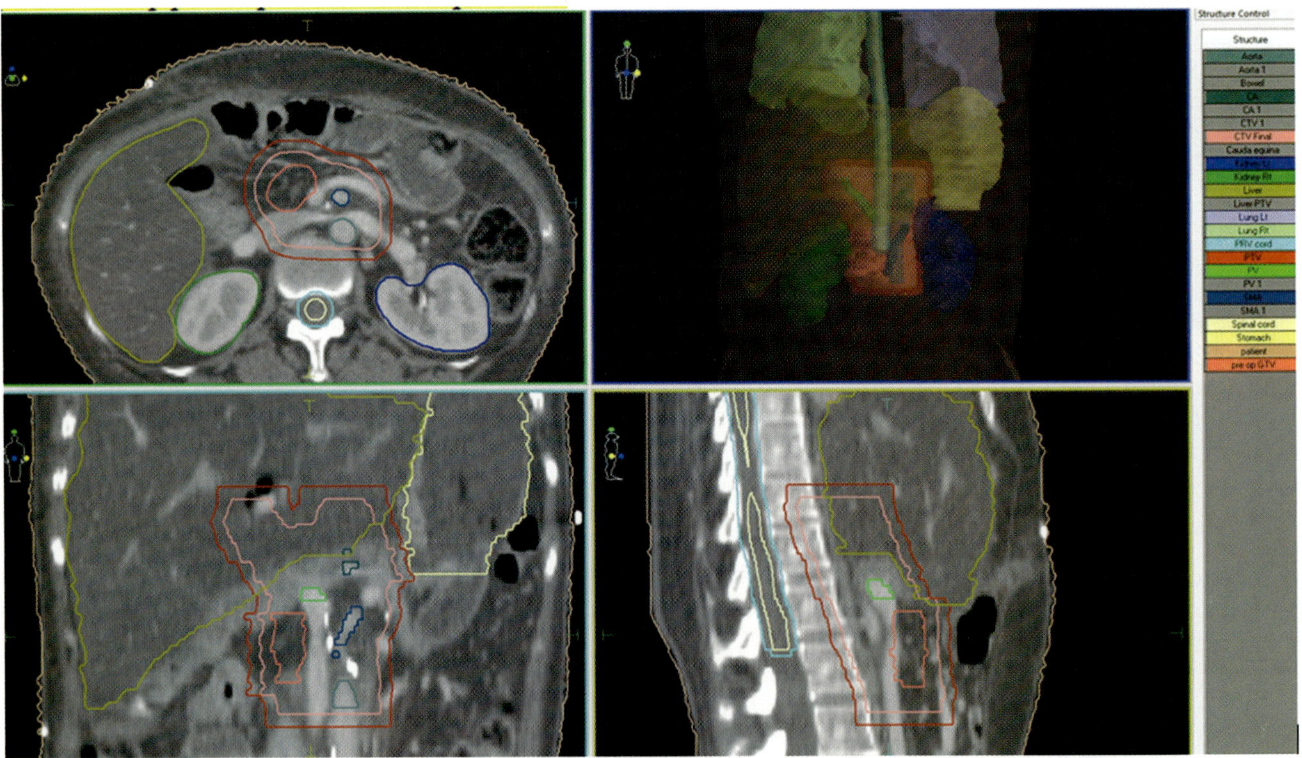

Fig 2A The target volumes and organs at risks (OARs) for a case of adenocarcinoma pancreas, post-Whipple's procedure, pT2N0

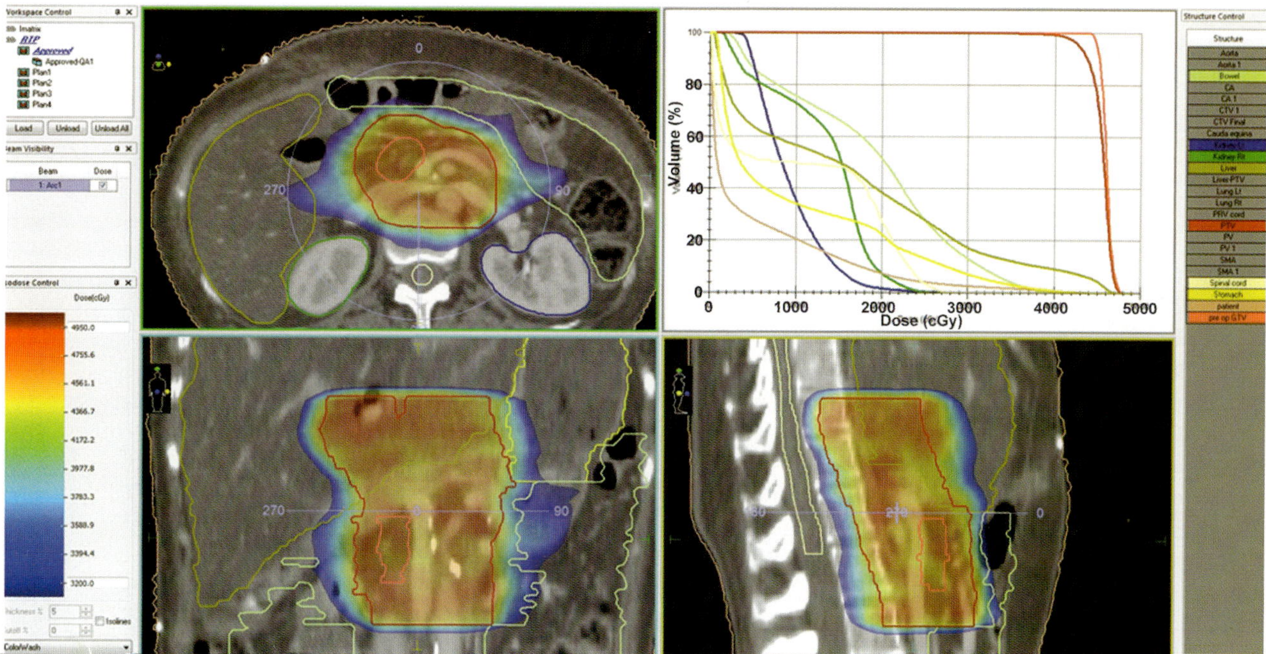

Fig. 2B The respective conformal plan

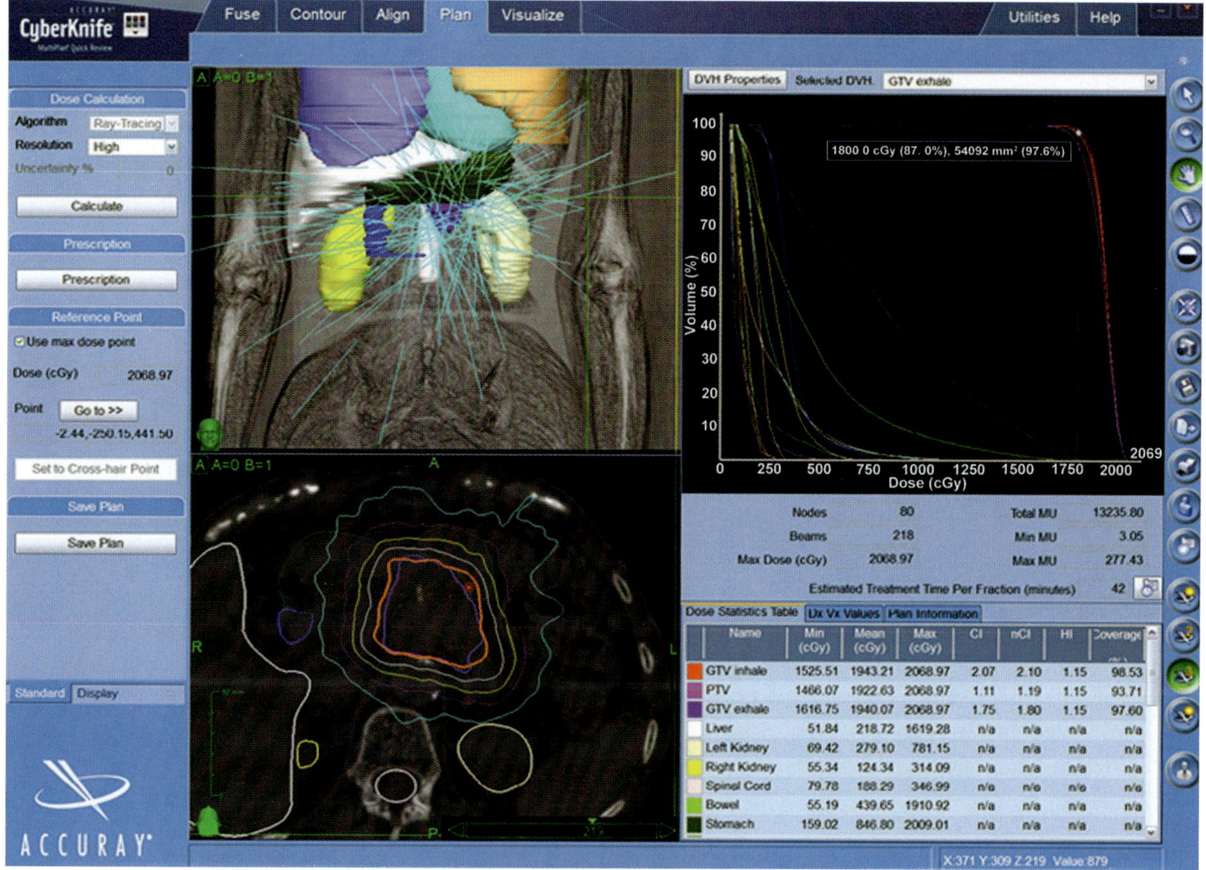

Fig. 3 The beam profile, isodose distribution and dose-volume histograms for a patient with carcinoma pancreas who received radical chemoradiation of 45 Gy in 25 fractions with EBRT, and was subsequently taken up for CyberKnife boost to residual tumor

phase III data (both in support and challenging this assertion) are flawed by study limitations. Neither RTOG 97-04 nor CONKO-001 tested the question of chemoradiation versus chemotherapy. EORTC trial was statistically underpowered and the ESPAC-1 trial was criticized for negating the role of chemoradiation in adjuvant therapy of resected pancreatic cancer due to design issues relating to lack of QA, inadequate toxicity reporting and nonadherence to the protocol.[78,79]

Future possibilities for improvement in survival for patients with locally advanced pancreatic cancer need to involve more effective systemic therapy and RT. The evaluation of high-dose preoperative EBRT plus concurrent and maintenance chemotherapy is reasonable in both borderline and unresectable pancreas cancers in good performance status patients, if metastatic disease has been excluded. In patients who have surgical exploration, dose escalation with IOERT should be evaluated; and for nonsurgical patients, EBRT boosts with SBRT or IMRT should be evaluated. The results of RTOG 97-04 support the use of gemcitabine as the chemotherapeutic agent of choice before and after 5FU-based EBRT, confirms the importance of differentiating between results of pancreatic head versus body or tail tumors, as well as extent of lymph node involvement. It also demonstrated that postoperative CA 19-9 levels and adherence to RT guidelines might significantly affect survival outcomes.[31]

The most optimal results for patients with potentially curable pancreatic cancer (gross total resection with negative margins) will likely be achieved with trimodality treatment (surgery, chemotherapy and RT). The safest, most effective combination of all three components is still being explored. Future trials would address sequencing of systemic therapy with concurrent chemoradiation.[80,81] Future treatment possibilities include molecular-based regimens utilizing gene targeting exploring antibody-based approaches designed to target and kill pancreatic cancer cells.[82]

REFERENCES

1. Greenhalf W, Malats N, Nilsson M, et al. International registries of families at high risk of pancreatic cancer. Pancreatology. 2008;8(6):558-65.
2. Shi C, Hruban RH, Klein AP. Familial pancreatic cancer. Arch Pathol Lab Med. 2009 Mar;133(3):365-74.
3. Berger AC, Garcia M Jr, Hoffman JP, Regine WF, Abrams RA, Safran H, et al. Postresection CA 19-9 predicts overall survival in patients with pancreatic cancer treated with adjuvant chemoradiation: a prospective validation by RTOG 9704. J Clin Oncol. 2008;26(36):5918-22.
4. Tang S, Bonaroti J, Unlu S, Liang X, Tang D, Zeh HJ, et al. Sweating the small stuff: microRNAs and genetic changes define pancreatic cancer. Pancreas. 2013;42(5):740-59.
5. Hinton J, Callan R, Bodine C, Glasgow W, Brower S, Jiang SW, et al. Potential epigenetic biomarkers for the diagnosis and prognosis of pancreatic ductal adenocarcinomas. Expert Rev Mol Diagn. 2013;13(5):431-43.
6. Schutte M, Hruban RH, Geradts J, Maynard R, Hilgers W, Rabindran SK, et al. Abrogation of the Rb/p16 tumor-suppressive pathway in virtually all pancreatic carcinomas. Cancer Res. 1997;57(15):3126-30.
7. Hruban RH, Offerhaus GJ, Kern SE, Goggins M, Wilentz RE, Yeo CJ. Tumor-suppressor genes in pancreatic cancer. J Hepatobiliary Pancreat Surg. 1998;5(4):383-91.
8. Asiyanbola B, Gleisner A, Herman JM, Choti MA, Wolfgang CL, Swartz M, et al. Determining pattern of recurrence following pancreaticoduodenectomy and adjuvant 5-flurouracil-based chemoradiation therapy: effect of number of metastatic lymph nodes and lymph node ratio. J Gastrointest Surg. 2009;13(4):752-9.
9. Van den Broeck A, Sergeant G, Ectors N, Van Steenbergen W, Aerts R, Topal B. Patterns of recurrence after curative resection of pancreatic ductal adenocarcinoma. Eur J Surg Oncol. 2009;35(6):600-4.
10. Winter JM, Tang LH, Klimstra DS, Liu W, Linkov I, Brennan MF, et al. Failure patterns in resected pancreas adenocarcinoma: lack of predicted benefit to SMAD4 expression. Ann Surg. 2013;258(2):331-5.
11. Olsen CC, Schefter TE, Chen H, Kane M, Leong S, McCarter MD, et al. Results of a phase I trial of 12 patients with locally advanced pancreatic carcinoma combining gefitinib, paclitaxel, and 3-dimensional conformal radiation: report of toxicity and evaluation of circulating K-ras as a potential biomarker of response to therapy. Am J Clin Oncol. 2009;32(2):115-21.
12. Nawaz H, Fan CY, Kloke J, Khalid A, McGrath K, Landsittel D, et al. Performance characteristics of endoscopic ultrasound in the staging of pancreatic cancer: a meta-analysis. JOP. 2013;14(5):484-97.
13. Wang Z, Chen JQ, Liu JL, et al. FDG-PET in diagnosis, staging and prognosis of pancreatic carcinoma: a meta-analysis. World J Gastroenterol. 2013;19(29):4808-17.
14. Chang DK, Johns AL, Merrett ND, Gill AJ, Colvin EK, Scarlett CJ, et al. Margin clearance and outcome in resected pancreatic cancer. J Clin Oncol. 2009;27(17):2855-62.
15. Grace PA, Pitt HA, Tompkins RK, DenBesten L, Longmire WP Jr. Decreased morbidity and mortality after pancreatoduodenectomy. Am J Surg. 1986;151(1):141-9.
16. Vollmer CM Jr, Sanchez N, Gondek S, et al. Pancreatic Surgery Mortality Study Group, et al. A root-cause analysis of mortality following major pancreatectomy. J Gastrointest Surg. 2012;16(1):89-102.
17. Geer RJ, Brennan MF. Prognostic indicators for survival after resection of pancreatic adenocarcinoma. Am J Surg. 1993;165(1):68-72.
18. Michelassi F, Erroi F, Dawson PJ, Pietrabissa A, Noda S, Handcock M, et al. Experience with 647 consecutive tumors of the duodenum, ampulla, head of the pancreas, and distal common bile duct. Ann Surg. 1989;210(4):544-54.
19. Yeo CJ, Cameron JL, Sohn TA, Lillemoe KD, Pitt HA, Talamini MA, et al. Six hundred fifty consecutive pancreaticoduodenectomies in the 1990s: pathology, complications, and outcomes. Ann Surg. 1997;226(3):248-57.
20. Yeo CJ, Sohn TA, Cameron JL, Hruban RH, Lillemoe KD, Pitt HA. Periampullary adenocarcinoma: analysis of 5-year survivors. Ann Surg. 1998;227(6):821-31.

21. Hurtuk MG, Hughes C, Shoup M, et al. Does lymph node ratio impact survival in resected periampullary malignancies? Am J Surg. 2009;197(3):348-52.
22. Riediger H, Keck T, Wellner U, zur Hausen A, Adam U, Hopt UT, et al. The lymph node ratio is the strongest prognostic factor after resection of pancreatic cancer. J Gastrointest Surg. 2009;13(7):1337-44.
23. Brennan MF, Kattan MW, Klimstra D, et al. Prognostic nomogram for patients undergoing resection for adenocarcinoma of the pancreas. Ann Surg. 2004;240(2):293-8.
24. Griffin JF, Smalley SR, Jewell W, Paradelo JC, Reymond RD, Hassanein RE, et al. Patterns of failure after curative resection of pancreatic carcinoma. Cancer. 1990;66(1):56-61.
25. Foo ML, Gunderson LL, Nagorney DM, McLlrath DC, van Heerden JA, Robinow JS, et al. Patterns of failure in grossly resected pancreatic ductal adenocarcinoma treated with adjuvant irradiation ±5 fluorouracil. Int J Radiat Oncol Biol Phys. 1993;26(3):483-9.
26. Willett CG, Warshaw AL, Convery K, et al. Patterns of failure after pancreaticoduodenectomy for ampullary carcinoma. Surg Gynecol Obstet. 1993;176(1):33-8.
27. Kalser MH, Ellenberg SS. Pancreatic cancer. Adjuvant combined radiation and chemotherapy following curative resection. Arch Surg. 1985;120(8):899-903.
28. Gastrointestinal Tumor Study Group. Further evidence of effective adjuvant combined radiation and chemotherapy following curative resection of pancreatic cancer. Cancer. 1987;59(12):2006-10.
29. Klinkenbijl JH, Jeekel J, Sahmoud T, van Pel R, Couvreur ML, Veenhof CH, et al. Adjuvant radiotherapy and 5-fluorouracil after curative resection of cancer of the pancreas and periampullary region: phase III trial of the EORTC gastrointestinal tract cancer cooperative group. Ann Surg. 1999;230(6):776-82.
30. Neoptolemos JP, Dunn JA, Stocken DD, Almond J, Link K, Beger H, et al. Adjuvant chemoradiotherapy and chemotherapy in resectable pancreatic cancer: a randomised controlled trial. Lancet. 2001;358(9293):1576-85.
31. Regine WF, Winter KA, Abrams RA, Safran H, Hoffman JP, Konski A, et al. Fluorouracil vs gemcitabine chemotherapy before and after fluorouracil-based chemoradiation following resection of pancreatic adenocarcinoma: a randomized controlled trial. JAMA. 2008;299(9):1019-26.
32. Whittington R, Bryer MP, Haller DG, et al. Adjuvant therapy of resected adenocarcinoma of the pancreas. Int J Radiat Oncol Biol Phys. 1991;21(5):1137-43.
33. Yeo CJ, Abrams RA, Grochow LB, Sohn TA, Ord SE, Hruban RH, et al. Pancreaticoduodenectomy for pancreatic adenocarcinoma: postoperative adjuvant chemoradiation improves survival. A prospective, single-institution experience. Ann Surg. 1997;225(5):621-33.
34. Herman JM, Swartz MJ, Hsu CC, Winter J, Pawlik TM, Sugar E, et al. Analysis of fluorouracil-based adjuvant chemotherapy and radiation after pancreaticoduodenectomy for ductal adenocarcinoma of the pancreas: results of a large, prospectively collected database at the Johns Hopkins Hospital. J Clin Oncol. 2008;26(21):3503-10.
35. Hsu CC, Herman JM, Corsini MM, Winter JM, Callister MD, Haddock MG, et al. Adjuvant chemoradiation for pancreatic adenocarcinoma: the Johns Hopkins Hospital-Mayo Clinic collaborative study. Ann Surg Oncol. 2010;17(4):981-90.
36. Burris HA 3rd, Moore MJ, Andersen J, Green MR, Rothenberg ML, Modiano MR, et al. Improvements in survival and clinical benefit with gemcitabine as first-line therapy for patients with advanced pancreas cancer: a randomized trial. J Clin Oncol. 1997;15(6):2403-13.
37. Oettle H, Neuhaus P, Hochhaus A, Hartmann JT, Gellert K, Ridwelski K, et al. Adjuvant chemotherapy with gemcitabine and long-term outcomes among patients with resected pancreatic cancer: the CONKO-001 randomized trial. JAMA. 2013;310(14):1473-81.
38. Moore MJ, Goldstein D, Hamm J, Figer A, Hecht JR, Gallinger S, et al. Erlotinib plus gemcitabine compared with gemcitabine alone in patients with advanced pancreatic cancer: a phase III trial of the National Cancer Institute of Canada Clinical Trials Group. J Clin Oncol. 2007;25(15):1960-6.
39. Neoptolemos JP, Stocken DD, Bassi C, Ghaneh P, Cunningham D, Goldstein D, et al. Adjuvant chemotherapy with fluorouracil plus folinic acid vs gemcitabine following pancreatic cancer resection: a randomized controlled trial. JAMA. 2010;304(10):1073-81.
40. Nukui Y, Picozzi VJ, Traverso LW. Interferon-based adjuvant chemoradiation therapy improves survival after pancreaticoduodenectomy for pancreatic adenocarcinoma. Am J Surg. 2000;179(5):367-71.
41. Picozzi VJ, Abrams RA, Decker PA, Traverso W, O'Reilly EM, Greeno E, et al. Multicenter phase II trial of adjuvant therapy for resected pancreatic cancer using cisplatin, 5-fluorouracil, and interferon-alfa-2b-based chemoradiation: ACOSOG Trial Z05031. Ann Oncol. 2011;22(2):348-54.
42. Linehan DC, Tan MC, Strasberg SM, Drebin JA, Hawkins WG, Picus J, et al. Adjuvant interferon-based chemoradiation followed by gemcitabine for resected pancreatic adenocarcinoma: a single-institution phase II study. Ann Surg. 2008; 248(2):145-51.
43. Van Laethem JL, Hammel P, Mornex F, Azria D, Van Tienhoven G, Vergauwe P, et al. Adjuvant gemcitabine alone versus gemcitabine-based chemoradiotherapy after curative resection for pancreatic cancer: a randomized EORTC-40013-22012/FFCD-9203/GERCOR phase II study. J Clin Oncol. 2010;28(29):4450-6.
44. Abrams RA. A phase IIR and a phase III trial evaluating both erlotinib (Ph IIR) and chemoradiation (Ph III) as adjuvant treatment for patients with resected head of pancreas adenocarcinoma (2014). [online] Available from http://www.rtog.org/ClinicalTrials/ProtocolTable/StudyDetails.aspx?study=0848 [Accessed February 2014].
45. Ishikawa O, Ohigashi H, Imaoka S, Sasaki Y, Iwanaga T, Matayoshi Y, et al. Is the long-term survival rate improved by preoperative irradiation prior to Whipple's procedure for adenocarcinoma of the pancreatic head? Arch Surg. 1994;129(10):1075-80.
46. Hoffman JP, Weese JL, Solin LJ, Agarwal P, Engstrom P, Scher R, et al. A single institutional experience with preoperative chemoradiotherapy for stage I-III pancreatic adenocarcinoma. Am Surg. 1993;59(11):772-80.

47. Meszoely IM, Wang H, Hoffman JP. Preoperative chemoradiation therapy for adenocarcinoma of the pancreas: The Fox Chase Cancer Center experience, 1986-2003. Surg Oncol Clin N Am. 2004;13(4):685-96.
48. Talamonti MS, Small W Jr, Mulcahy MF, Wayne JD, Attaluri V, Colletti LM, et al. A multi-institutional phase II trial of preoperative full-dose gemcitabine and concurrent radiation for patients with potentially resectable pancreatic carcinoma. Ann Surg Oncol. 2006;13(2):150-8.
49. Evans DB, Varadhachary GR, Crane CH, Sun CC, Lee JE, Pisters PW, et al. Preoperative gemcitabine-based chemoradiation for patients with resectable adenocarcinoma of the pancreatic head. J Clin Oncol. 2008;26(21):3496-502.
50. Small W Jr, Berlin J, Freedman GM, Lawrence T, Talamonti MS, Mulcahy MF, et al. Full-dose gemcitabine with concurrent radiation therapy in patients with nonmetastatic pancreatic cancer: a multicenter phase II trial. J Clin Oncol. 2008;26(6):942-7.
51. Springett GM, Hoffe SE. Borderline resectable pancreatic cancer: on the edge of survival. Cancer Control. 2008;15(4): 295-307.
52. Katz MH, Pisters PW, Evans DB, Sun CC, Lee JE, Fleming JB, et al. Borderline resectable pancreatic cancer: the importance of this emerging stage of disease. J Am Coll Surg. 2008; 206(5):833-46.
53. Brown KM, Siripurapu V, Davidson M, Cohen SJ, Konski A, Watson JC, et al. Chemoradiation followed by chemotherapy before resection for borderline pancreatic adenocarcinoma. Am J Surg. 2008;195(3):318-21.
54. Lillemoe KD, Pitt HA. Palliation. surgical and otherwise. Cancer. 1996;78(3 Suppl):605-14.
55. Ouchi K, Sugawara T, Ono H, Fujiya T, Kamiyama Y, Kakugawa Y, et al. Palliative operation for cancer of the head of the pancreas: significance of pancreaticoduodenectomy and intraoperative radiation therapy for survival and quality of life. World J Surg. 1998;22(4):413-6.
56. Moertel CG, Frytak S, Hahn RG, O'Connell MJ, Reitemeier RJ, Rubin J, et al. Therapy of locally unresectable pancreatic carcinoma: a randomized comparison of high dose (6000 rads) radiation alone, moderate dose radiation (4000 rads + 5-fluorouracil), and high dose radiation + 5-fluorouracil: The Gastrointestinal Tumor Study Group. Cancer. 1981; 48(8): 1705-10.
57. Gastrointestinal Tumor Study Group. Treatment of locally unresectable carcinoma of the pancreas: comparison of combined-modality therapy (chemotherapy plus radiotherapy) to chemotherapy alone. J Natl Cancer Inst. 1988;80(10):751-5.
58. Blackstock AW, Bernard SA, Richards F, Eagle KS, Case LD, Poole ME, et al. Phase I trial of twice-weekly gemcitabine and concurrent radiation in patients with advanced pancreatic cancer. J Clin Oncol. 1999;17(7):2208-12.
59. Blackstock AW, Tepper JE, Niedwiecki D, Hollis DR, Mayer RJ, Tempero MA. Cancer and leukemia group B (CALGB) 89805: phase II chemoradiation trial using gemcitabine in patients with locoregional adenocarcinoma of the pancreas. Int J Gastrointest Cancer. 2003;34(2-3):107-16.
60. Blackstock AW, Mornex F, Partensky C, Descos L, Case LD, Melin SA, et al. Adjuvant gemcitabine and concurrent radiation for patients with resected pancreatic cancer: a phase II study. Br J Cancer. 2006;95(3):260-5.
61. Loehrer PJ, Powell ME, Cardenes HR, Wagner L, Brell JM, Ramanathan RK, et al. A randomized phase III study of gemcitabine in combination with radiation therapy versus gemcitabine alone in patients with localized, unresectable pancreatic cancer: E4201. J Clin Oncol, 2008 ASCO Annual Meeting Proceedings (Post-Meeting Edition). Vol 26, No 15S (May 20 Supplement), 2008: 4506.
62. Martenson JA, Vigliotti AP, Pitot HC, Geeraerts LH, Sargent DJ, Haddock MG, et al. A phase I study of radiation therapy and twice-weekly gemcitabine and cisplatin in patients with locally advanced pancreatic cancer. Int J Radiat Oncol Biol Phys. 2003;55(5):1305-10.
63. Brunner TB, Grabenbauer GG, Klein P, Baum U, Papadopoulos T, Bautz W, et al. Phase I trial of strictly time-scheduled gemcitabine and cisplatin with concurrent radiotherapy in patients with locally advanced pancreatic cancer. Int J Radiat Oncol Biol Phys. 2003;55(1):144-53.
64. Crane CH, Abbruzzese JL, Evans DB, Wolff RA, Ballo MT, Delclos M, et al. Is the therapeutic index better with gemcitabine-based chemoradiation than with 5-fluorouracil-based chemoradiation in locally advanced pancreatic cancer? Int J Radiat Oncol Biol Phys. 2002;52(5):1293-302.
65. Crane CH, Winter K, Regine WF, Safran H, Rich TA, Curran W, et al. Phase II study of bevacizumab with concurrent capecitabine and radiation followed by maintenance gemcitabine and bevacizumab for locally advanced pancreatic cancer: Radiation Therapy Oncology Group RTOG 0411. J Clin Oncol. 2009;27(25):4096-102.
66. Chang DT, Schellenberg D, Shen J, Kim J, Goodman KA, Fisher GA, et al. Stereotactic radiotherapy for unresectable adenocarcinoma of the pancreas. Cancer. 2009;115(3):665-72.
67. Willett CG, Del Castillo CF, Shih HA, Goldberg S, Biggs P, Clark JW, et al. Long-term results of intraoperative electron beam irradiation (IOERT) for patients with unresectable pancreatic cancer. Ann Surg. 2005;241(2):295-9.
68. Shipley WU, Wood WC, Tepper JE, Warshaw AL, Orlow EL, Kaufman SD, et al. Intraoperative electron beam irradiation for patients with unresectable pancreatic carcinoma. Ann Surg. 1984;200(3):289-96.
69. Roldan GE, Gunderson LL, Nagorney DM, Martin JK, Ilstrup DM, Holbrook MA, et al. External beam versus intraoperative and external beam irradiation for locally advanced pancreatic cancer. Cancer. 1988;61(6):1110-6.
70. Mohiuddin M, Regine WF, Stevens J, Rosato F, Barbot D, Biermann W, et al. Combined intraoperative radiation and perioperative chemotherapy for unresectable cancers of the pancreas. J Clin Oncol. 1995;13(11):2764-8.
71. Garton GR, Gunderson LL, Nagorney DM, Donohue JH, Martin JK, McIlrath DC, et al. High-dose preoperative external beam and intraoperative irradiation for locally advanced pancreatic cancer. Int J Radiat Oncol Biol Phys. 1993;27(5):1153-7.
72. Ashman JB, Moss AA, Rule WG, Callister MG, Reddy KS, Mulligan DC, et al. Preoperative chemoradiation and IOERT for unresectable or borderline resectable pancreas cancer. J Gastrointest Oncol. 2013;4(4):352-60.

73. Koong AC, Le QT, Ho A, Fong B, Fisher G, Cho C, et al. Phase I study of stereotactic radiosurgery in patients with locally advanced pancreatic cancer. Int J Radiat Oncol Biol Phys. 2004;58(4):1017-21.
74. Schellenberg D, Kim J, Christman-Skieller C, Chun CL, Columbo LA, Ford JM, et al. Single-fraction stereotactic body radiation therapy and sequential gemcitabine for the treatment of locally advanced pancreatic cancer. Int J Radiat Oncol Biol Phys. 2011;81(1):181-8.
75. Mahadevan A, Jain S, Goldstein M, Miksad R, Pleskow D, Sawhney M, et al. Stereotactic body radiotherapy and gemcitabine for locally advanced pancreatic cancer. Int J Radiat Oncol Biol Phys. 2010;78(3):735-42.
76. RTOG Protocol 97-04. Available online at http://www.rtog.org/ClinicalTrials/ProtocolTable/StudyDetails.aspx?action=openFile&FileID=7546.
77. Ben-Josef E, Shields AF, Vaishampayan U, Vaitkevicius V, El-Rayes BF, McDermott P, et al. Intensity-modulated radiotherapy (IMRT) and concurrent capecitabine for pancreatic cancer. Int J Radiat Oncol Biol Phys. 2004;59(2):454-9.
78. Milano MT, Chmura SJ, Garofalo MC, Rash C, Roeske JC, Connell PP, et al. Intensity-modulated radiotherapy in treatment of pancreatic and bile duct malignancies: toxicity and clinical outcome. Int J Radiat Oncol Biol Phys. 2004;59(2):445-53.
79. Koshy MC, Landry JC, Cavanaugh SX, Fuller CD, Willett CG, Abrams RA, et al. A challenge to the therapeutic nihilism of ESPAC-1. Int J Radiat Oncol Biol Phys. 2005;61(4):965-6.
80. Ko AH, Quivey JM, Venook AP, Bergsland EK, Dito E, Schillinger B, et al. A phase II study of fixed-dose rate gemcitabine plus low-dose cisplatin followed by consolidative chemoradiation for locally advanced pancreatic cancer. Int J Radiat Oncol Biol Phys. 2007;68(3):809-16.
81. Krishnan S, Rana V, Janjan NA, Varadhachary GR, Abbruzzese JL, Das P, et al. Induction chemotherapy selects patients with locally advanced, unresectable pancreatic cancer for optimal benefit from consolidative chemoradiation therapy. Cancer. 2007;110(1):47-55.
82. Choti MA. Adjuvent therapy for pancreatic cancer—the debate continues. M Engl J Med. 2004;350(12):1249-51.

21

CHAPTER

Hepatobiliary Malignancies

Shikha Goyal, Tejinder Kataria

INTRODUCTION

Malignant disease of the hepatobiliary system includes hepatocellular carcinoma (HCC), gallbladder cancer, extrahepatic cholangiocarcinoma (EHCC), and intrahepatic cholangiocarcinoma (IHCC). HCC is the fifth most common malignancy with increasing incidence in the United States, partly related to the parallel increase in hepatitis C. Although surgery is the mainstay of management, very few people present with resectable disease. Various systemic agents (chemotherapy, targeted therapy), chemoembolization, immunotherapy, and ablation techniques have been tried for managing unresectable or borderline resectable disease, but no standards exist till date. Role of radiation therapy, earlier limited by the treatment volumes and attendant toxicity especially in liver tumors, has been evolving in the last 2 decades owing to sophistication in imaging, treatment planning and delivery techniques, as well as improved understanding on the dose-volume equation in the context of radiation-induced liver disease (RILD).

EPIDEMIOLOGY

Hepatobiliary cancers occur primarily in the elderly and the incidence increases with age. The most common hepatobiliary cancer is HCC, followed by gallbladder cancer, EHCC, and IHCC. Approximately one-fourth of cholangiocarcinomas occur at the bifurcation of the common hepatic duct (hilar or Klatskin tumors). Other rare hepatic neoplasms include carcinoid tumors, hepatoblastoma, angiosarcoma, and leiomyosarcoma. HCC and IHCC are more common in men than women, whereas gallbladder cancer is more common in women and EHCC occurs with equal frequency.[1]

In Asia, Southeast Asia, and sub-Saharan Africa, HCC is 15–100 times more common than in North America, although the incidence is increasing in the United States and Europe. Carcinoma of the gallbladder also has shown a substantial geographic variation, and the incidence in some areas, such as Northeastern Europe, is more than 20 times higher than in the United States. EHCC has a fairly uniform incidence, while IHCC is more common in Southeast Asia, parallel to the higher incidence of liver fluke infestation in this region.[2-4]

ETIOLOGY

Hepatocellular Carcinoma

Infection with hepatitis B and C viruses has been established as the most important causative factor for HCC, especially in Asian countries. Conversely, in the United States, cirrhosis without hepatitis infection is a more common causative factor.[2] Aflatoxin B has been implicated as another agent in certain Asian and African countries.[5]

Gallbladder Cancer

Gallbladder cancer is more common in regions with high incidence of cholelithiasis, although the direct causal association for malignancy has not been established. The incidence is higher in the setting of calcified gallbladder.[4,6]

Cholangiocarcinoma

Various environmental associations have been described, such as liver fluke infestation, hepatolithiasis, pyogenic cholangitis, congenital bile duct cysts, past exposure to thorium dioxide, a typhoid carrier state, and ulcerative colitis. Patients with primary sclerosing cholangitis (PSC) have an increased risk. EHCCs possibly share a common pathway of carcinogenesis with gallbladder cancer because the risk reduces 10 years after cholecystectomy.[7,8]

PREVENTION AND EARLY DETECTION

Awareness of risk factors and poor treatment results have made preventive and early detection strategies more important. Hepatitis B vaccination programs have been successful in controlling the incidence rates in Taiwan.[9]

Early detection tools in endemic areas include serum alpha-fetoprotein (AFP) for screening but with low detection rates. Liver ultrasonography has also been used for screening with better detection rates but it is expensive. National Comprehensive Cancer Network (NCCN) practice guidelines recommend screening with AFP and ultrasound every 6–12 months in high-risk populations.[10]

Carbohydrate antigen 19-9 (CA 19-9) has been investigated for screening cholangiocarcinomas, however, with moderate sensitivity and specificity.[11]

There are no known preventive measures for the biliary tract cancers. Even though cholelithiasis may be a risk factor for gallbladder cancer and EHCCs, role of preventive cholecystectomy is unknown.[4]

BIOLOGIC CHARACTERISTICS

It has been postulated that hepatitis B viral integration activates oncogenes or interferes with tumor suppressor genes. However, sites of viral DNA integration are not consistent and do not occur near any known oncogenes or tumor suppressor genes, nor does the viral DNA contain any known oncogenes. If the integration of viral DNA is necessary for carcinogenesis, the mechanism may be caused by genomic instability from deletions and chromosomal rearrangement rather than specific oncogene activation or disruption of a tumor suppressor gene pathway.[12]

Carcinogenesis may be related to the ability of the liver to respond to damage by regeneration. The continuous liver damage seen with chronic hepatitis or cirrhosis leads to increased turnover of hepatocytes. During normal hepatocyte regeneration, both proto-oncogene activation and inactivation of suppressor genes occur. Chronic liver damage leads to a nearly continuous cellular reproduction, which may allow carcinogenic molecular changes to accumulate without repair.[12]

PATHOLOGY AND PATHOGENESIS

Hepatocellular Carcinoma

On gross examination, HCC can appear as expanding or spreading, with discrete or poorly defined margins, or may be multifocal, with multiple tumors scattered throughout the liver. Microscopically, it appears similar to normal liver tissue, both in cytologic findings and in its characteristic plate-like growth. A four-grade system is used for nuclear grading—cells are either low grade (grade 1 or 2) or high grade (grade 3 or 4). It is difficult to differentiate grade 1 tumors from adenomas or atypical hyperplastic nodules. Similarly, grade 4 tumors may resemble other anaplastic cancers.[13,14]

Hepatocellular carcinoma may locally invade the portal vein, hepatic vein, or diaphragm. Nearly a third of patients have regional disease at presentation, with metastases to the porta hepatis and celiac axis lymph node chains. Intra-abdominal metastases to peritoneum or liver or extra-abdominal spread to the lungs and bone are found in another third.[15] Metastases to other sites, such as the brain or muscle, are uncommon.

Fibrolamellar carcinoma is a subtype of HCC, constituting 5% of cases. It is found in younger women and is associated with favorable survival. Grossly, fibrolamellar carcinoma is classified as an expanding, sclerosing tumor, characterized by septa of retracted collagenous structures radiating from a central region. On cytologic examination, the tumor cells are large and polygonal, with a granular cytoplasm resulting from numerous mitochondria. The abundant fibrous stroma is characteristic and is arranged in parallel lamellae around nests, cords, and sheets of tumor cells.[13]

Gallbladder Cancer

Most gallbladder cancers are adenocarcinomas. The gross appearance can vary from localized nodular growths to entire organ involvement. Histologically, both grade and vascular invasion have prognostic value.[16] Papillary adenocarcinoma is a variant histologic type, found in 6% with a much better outcome. Mucinous carcinoma is another variant, occurring in about 5% of cases and associated with gallbladder perforation.

Direct liver invasion is common due to the thin wall and single muscular layer of the gallbladder, the presence of Rokitansky-Aschoff sinuses, and contiguous location of perimuscular connective tissue of the gallbladder with the interlobular connective tissue of the liver. Nearly, 40–50% patients have distant metastases at presentation, usually to the liver or peritoneum. Lymphatic spread to the cystic, pericholedochal, hilar, and celiac lymph nodes is seen in 45% patients, but in tumors confined to gallbladder, only 5% of patients have positive regional lymph nodes.[6,16]

Cholangiocarcinoma

Biliary cancer is typically divided according to the site of origin into intrahepatic tumors, extrahepatic tumors, or hilar (Klatskin) tumors. Nearly all biliary tree carcinomas are mucin-producing adenocarcinomas. As with gallbladder cancer, papillary adenocarcinoma has a better prognosis.

Cholangiocarcinoma typically spreads by direct extension along the biliary tree, although separate tumor nodules may represent either multifocal tumor development or metastatic deposits. Direct invasion of adjacent organs is more common for intrahepatic and hilar tumors than for extrahepatic tumors. Involvement of the cystic, hilar, or celiac lymph nodes is found in 30–50%. The incidence of distant metastases is about 30%, with a lower incidence of peritoneal disease than for gallbladder cancer.[15,17,18]

CLINICAL EVALUATION

Symptoms and Signs

Clinical presentation depends on the site of origin. Patients with primary liver tumors, whether HCC or IHCC, frequently present with right upper abdominal or epigastric pain. Rarely, patients with HCC complain of a sudden, sharp, severe pain related to acute bleeding into the tumor or rupture of the tumor with intra-abdominal bleeding. The patient may also be aware of an abdominal mass or increased girth related to ascites.

Nearly 70% patients with HCC have cirrhosis.[19] Jaundice is unusual with primary liver tumors and may be obstructive because of tumor compression of the biliary system or hepatocellular because of end-stage hepatic replacement with tumor.

In contrast to the primary liver tumors, patients with hilar or distal cholangiocarcinomas almost always present with jaundice. Abdominal pain and the nonspecific complaints of weight loss, anorexia, fatigue, fever, and night sweats are common in patients with either biliary or hepatic tumors. Patients with gallbladder cancer commonly complain of both abdominal pain and jaundice and may also have weight loss, anorexia, and fatigue but are usually undiagnosed before an attempted cholecystectomy.

The most common physical finding in patients with primary hepatic tumors is tender hepatomegaly. The liver may be nodular due to tumor or cirrhosis. Occasionally, patients with HCC may have a hepatic bruit because of high vascularity. Ascites is a particularly ominous finding because it represents either hepatic dysfunction resulting from cirrhosis or tumor replacement, Budd-Chiari syndrome from malignant invasion of the hepatic veins, or peritoneal spread of cancer.

Patients with EHCC or gallbladder cancer usually have icterus but may also have hepatomegaly or tenderness in the right upper quadrant.

Laboratory Studies

Workup for hepatobiliary tumors helps define the extent of disease as well as assess liver function. Laboratory tests include a complete blood count, routine biochemistry panel, and coagulation studies. Serum CA 19-9 is a tumor marker for cholangiocarcinoma. Serum AFP is a tumor marker for HCC; levels more than 400 μg/L (4,000 μg/L in presence of hepatitis) are diagnostic of HCC, though lower levels do not rule out smaller and perhaps curable HCC. AFP levels are prognostic for patients with tumors 5 cm or smaller as well as those with more than 50% involvement of the liver.[20] It is recommended that patients with known cirrhosis and/or hepatitis and a rise in AFP levels undergo retesting in 1–3 months, after resolution of hepatitis. AFP has a false-negative rate of 10–15%, in anaplastic or well-differentiated tumors.

Patients negative for hepatitis B or C respond better to systemic therapy with fewer side effects. Paraneoplastic syndromes such as hypoglycemia, erythrocytosis, hypercalcemia, or hypercholesterolemia may be seen in 5% HCC patients.

Radiographic Studies

The primary imaging modalities for liver tumors include ultrasonography (USG), computed tomography (CT), and magnetic resonance imaging (MRI). Patients suspected of hepatic disease, whether IHCC or HCC, are typically first evaluated with USG. Doppler imaging may help define vascular flow patterns. USG is operator dependent in addition to being affected by obesity, bowel distension, or scars. For potentially resectable cases, CT and MRI discern segmental anatomy of liver in addition to defining hepatic and extrahepatic spread. A dynamic CT study with acquisition of three contrast phases (arterial hepatic, portal venous, and equilibrium) is very important for assessing lesion vascularity. HCC is hypervascular and typically displays intense enhancement during the arterial-hepatic phase with postcontrast washout, while cholangiocarcinoma demonstrates delayed enhancement. Even more sophisticated methodologies are CT arterial portography and CT hepatic arteriography, which are considered the most sensitive methods of detecting small liver cancers, detecting lesions as small as 0.2 cm in diameter, albeit with a high false-positive rate.[21]

MRI is a modality of choice for evaluating lesions in cirrhotic patients owing to its better contrast resolution and capability of multiplanar imaging. Modern MRI protocols usually include parenchymal imaging with one or more types of contrast agents, magnetic resonance (MR) angiography, and magnetic resonance cholangiopancreatography (MRCP). MRCP is a noninvasive technique that has obviated the need for ERCP only to situations where cytopathology or biopsy evidence is needed or procedures to decompress the biliary obstruction. Unlike ERCP, it provides additional information regarding portal vein and regional lymph nodes.[22,23]

EHCC typically appears as a stricture at the site of involvement with upstream dilatation of the biliary tract. The tumor itself may extend for some distance along the biliary tract. PSC, occasionally indistinguishable from EHCC usually shows diffuse rather than focal biliary narrowing. Imaging frequently shows no discernible mass, but intrahepatic biliary dilatation may provide clues to location of disease.[24]

Diagnosis

National Comprehensive Cancer Network guidelines recommend a biopsy or fine-needle aspiration cytology (FNAC) to confirm HCC if AFP level is 400 μg/L or less (≤ 4,000 μg/L in patients with hepatitis). In patients with high AFP or larger lesions, characteristic imaging alone may be sufficient for diagnosis.[25]

Establishing the diagnosis of cholangiocarcinoma is more difficult, due to extensive sclerosis. Cytology may help confirm cancer in 50–90% cases.[26]

Staging

The American Joint Committee on Cancer Staging Manual, 7th edition, has defined separate tumor, node and metastasis (TNM) staging systems for hepatic tumors, IHCCs, gallbladder tumors, and EHCCs, divided into perihilar and distal bile duct lesions. The staging for both gallbladder cancers and EHCC tumors is primarily surgical, reflecting the role of resection.

Follow-up

After transplant or locoregional therapy such as resection or radiofrequency ablation, imaging is recommended every 3–6 months for 2 years, and then annually. If pretreatment AFP is high, it should be repeated every 3 months for 2 years, and then every 6 months afterward.

PRIMARY THERAPY

Hepatocellular Carcinoma

Potentially curative treatments include partial hepatectomy, total hepatectomy with a liver transplant, and nonsurgical ablative therapies. No randomized controlled trials comparing these treatments are available. Best results are obtained with resection and transplantation in well-selected candidates (5-year survival rate of 60–70%). Percutaneous treatments may be chosen for cases unsuitable for resection with 5-year survival rate of 40–50%. Patients with carcinoma in situ or single small tumors may be suitable for either treatment with similar outcome.[27-29]

Resection

Hepatic resection is the treatment of choice for HCC in noncirrhotic patients. However, patients with cirrhosis are more prone to liver failure, hence strict selection criteria are necessary. Relapse rates are as high as 70%, predictive factors being positive surgical margins, microvascular invasion, poorly differentiated histology, and presence of satellite lesions.[30,31]

Efficacy of adjuvant therapies is still unclear. A 2002 review of randomized controlled trials identified 13 trials with relapse or survival endpoints reported at 3 years or longer. Three studies involved adjuvant chemotherapy; four involved arterial chemotherapy or embolization; and six used other therapeutic modalities, including immunotherapy, differentiation agents, and hepatic artery infusion of lipiodol labeled with iodine-131. Better disease-free survival (DFS) or overall survival (OS) rates were noted in six trials, five of which involved modalities other than systemic or hepatic artery chemotherapy or embolization. The authors concluded that adjuvant systemic and hepatic artery chemotherapy or chemoembolization has resulted in better OS or DFS.[32] A 2009 Cochrane systematic review of 12 randomized studies concluded that there is limited evidence that adjuvant lipiodol therapy or immunotherapy may improve DFS.[33] Another meta-analysis of adjuvant interferon found a lower mortality and recurrence risk compared with curative local therapy alone in patients with viral hepatitis.[34]

Liver Transplantation

Total hepatectomy with orthotopic liver transplantation for cirrhotic patients removes the entire organ, and with it, all gross, microscopic and premalignant disease in addition to managing cirrhosis. Limitations include the shortage of donor organs, high procedure costs and high perioperative mortality rates (10–25%). Outcomes have improved with use of strict selection criteria (one lesion < 5 cm in diameter or up to three lesions < 3 cm in diameter) with 5-year OS of 70% and relapse rates under 15%.[2,27] Most centers advocate the use of chemotherapy, chemoembolization, percutaneous ablation, stereotactic radiation therapy or a combination during the waiting periods, but with doubtful usefulness.

Percutaneous Ablation

Resectable disease is seen in only a third of HCC patients. Percutaneous ablation is the most common management option for small unresectable lesions. Ablation could be chemical (alcohol, acetic acid), thermal [radiofrequency ablation (RFA), microwave, laser coagulation or cryoablation]. Best results with RFA are seen with tumors less than 4 cm.[35] Needle-track seeding is a complication with subcapsular and poorly differentiated tumors. Cryoablation has high complication rate and inferior outcomes. Microwave and laser coagulation are still experimental.

Intrahepatic Cholangiocarcinoma

Complete resection is the only potentially curative treatment. Most tumors are often large at presentation, and negative margins are difficult to achieve, even with major hepatic resections. Median survival is 12–28 months with 5-year survival of 22–36%.[36,37] Poor prognostic factors include large tumor size, multiple tumors, vascular involvement, and positive margins. Prognostic value of lymph node involvement and role of lymphadenectomy in improving outcomes is unclear.

Gallbladder Carcinoma

Resection is the only curative therapy, but possible in only 10–30%. Surgical options (depending on stage) include simple cholecystectomy; radical or extended cholecystectomy, involving removal of the gallbladder with at least 2 cm of the gallbladder bed and dissection of lymph nodes from the hepatoduodenal ligament behind the second part of duodenum, the head of the pancreas, and the celiac axis; radical cholecystectomy with liver (segmental or lobar) resection; radical cholecystectomy with extensive lymph node (para-aortic) dissection; and radical cholecystectomy with resection of the bile duct or pancreaticoduodenectomy. Patients initially treated by laparoscopic cholecystectomy require additional port site resection.

In 1–2% cases, carcinoma may be detected after cholecystectomy for benign disease. Management in such scenarios depends on depth of tumor invasion. If the tumor has invaded the muscularis propria (T1b and beyond), radical cholecystectomy is recommended.[38,39]

Surgical management of gallbladder carcinoma diagnosed preoperatively depends on the extent of the disease. Patients with organ-confined disease should have a radical cholecystectomy. Management of T3 and T4 disease is more controversial, but cures are still possible with radical surgery. The role of more extensive surgery, including pancreaticoduodenectomy, right colectomy, and nephrectomy is unclear. Patients with locally advanced disease may have para-aortic lymph node involvement in 20% cases, but para-aortic lymphadenectomy is not routinely recommended.[38,40,41]

Adjuvant Therapy

Surgery alone is associated with high local failure rates. Limited data exist on the role of adjuvant radiotherapy (RT) or chemoradiation.

Mayo Clinic data on adjuvant concurrent external beam radiation therapy (EBRT) (54 Gy to tumor bed and regional lymphatics) with bolus 5-fluorouracil (5-FU) showed 5-year OS and local control of 33% and 73%, respectively. This data was updated later with no significant difference between surgery along and adjuvant chemoradiation arms, possibly owing to inclusion of higher stage patients in adjuvant group. Increasing T and N classification as well as histologic type other than adenocarcinoma were significant predictors for worse OS. Adjuvant chemoradiation became statistically significant for improved OS after adjusting for these multivariate prognostic factors.[42,43]

Extrahepatic Cholangiocarcinoma

Hilar or common bile duct tumors are treated with resection and reconstruction using a Roux-en-Y hepaticojejunostomy; surgery is possible in 14–40% cases, with reported 5-year OS of 10–40%, higher OS for R0 resections. En bloc partial hepatectomy ensures higher negative margins. Tumors of the distal biliary tract have better operability rates (nearly 90%) with pancreaticoduodenectomy, 5-year OS of 30–40%.[18,43-45]

Adjuvant Therapy

Positive surgical margins are common for hilar tumors and denote poor prognosis. Positive margins are less common in distal biliary tumors. Nearly half of operable patients have lymph node involvement. Local failure rates after complete resection are 25–40%.[18,46,47]

Cholangiocarcinomas have a much greater tendency for local relapse, the proportion of patients with a locoregional failure as the first site of failure being 59% for cholangiocarcinoma and 15% for gallbladder cancer. Multivariate analysis confirmed the independent predictive value of positive regional lymph node involvement, moderate to poor tumor differentiation, and a positive resection margin for relapse at any site; diagnosis of cholangiocarcinoma was the only independent predictor of isolated locoregional recurrence.[48]

Limited data is available on role of adjuvant RT or chemoradiation in cholangiocarcinoma. A retrospective report of European Organization for Research and Treatment of Cancer (EORTC) in nearly 95% patients with positive margins, showed a statistically significant survival benefit with adjuvant RT (3-year OS 31% vs 10%, and median survival 19 months vs 8 months, favoring RT).[47,49] In a retrospective review of patients with hilar cholangiocarcinoma resected at the University of Amsterdam, the median survival time was significantly longer in patients who received postoperative RT than in patients who had surgery alone (24 months vs 8 months; $p < 0.01$). Brachytherapy did not improve survival and had significantly higher complication rate.[50] Possibly, the benefit suggested is limited to patients with noncurative resection, and, indeed, the survival of patients who received postoperative RT in this series matches that of patients from other series with R0 resection and no adjuvant therapy. Additionally, selection bias is a concern because patients with a poor performance status would not likely receive adjuvant therapy.

In general, approximately a third of resected patients have gross residual disease, and addition of RT in this setting gives median survival of about 13 months.[51]

Liver Transplant Alone or with Neoadjuvant Chemoradiation or Brachytherapy

A large majority of patients have extensive disease or advanced PSC with severe fibrosis and cirrhosis, making them poor candidates for surgical resection. Patients with PSC often have multifocal cholangiocarcinoma and have a high risk for developing additional tumors following standard surgery. For such cases, orthotopic liver transplantation has been proposed as an alternative, but with 5-year OS of only 2–23%.[52]

Mayo Clinic have published their experience with transplantation for small (<3 cm) perihilar cholangiocarcinomas. Patients received preoperative EBRT (45 Gy in 1.5-Gy fractions twice daily) with concurrent 5-FU followed by an intraluminal brachytherapy boost (20–30 Gy). Protracted venous infusion (PVI) of 5-FU was initiated with brachytherapy and continued until the time of transplantation. PVI 5-FU was later replaced by capecitabine. Subsequently, patients underwent exploratory laparotomy with biopsy of perihilar lymph nodes. Only patients with disease confined to the liver and uninvolved lymph nodes were eligible for transplantation. 5-year OS was 58% for all patients intended for transplant and 82% for those who underwent transplant. 5-year OS was 21% for patients who underwent standard resection ($p = 0.02$ favoring neoadjuvant therapy and orthotopic liver transplantation).[53,54]

LOCALLY ADVANCED DISEASE AND PALLIATION

Hepatocellular Carcinoma

The prognosis for unresectable disease is poor. Liver dysfunction, gastrointestinal hemorrhage, and spontaneous bacterial peritonitis are terminal events. The high incidence of liver dysfunction, whether resulting either from the tumor or cirrhosis, has limited the potential role of palliative liver RT. A number of prognostic factors have been identified for patients with unresectable HCC, including albumin levels, AFP levels, portal vein obstruction, Child's class, the presence of serologic markers for hepatitis B or C virus, and the size of the tumor or presence of multiple tumors.

Systemic Treatment

Sorafenib, an oral multikinase inhibitor, has improved OS and time to radiologic progression in patients with advanced HCC in the Sorafenib Hepatocellular Carcinoma Assessment Randomized Protocol (SHARP trial).[55] Side effects are mild, including diarrhea, hand-foot skin reaction, and weight loss. Systemic chemotherapy or tamoxifen have shown no benefit.[56,57]

Since hepatic neoplasms derive 80% of their blood supply from the hepatic artery, higher concentrations of anticancer drugs can be delivered to the tumor by hepatic artery infusion than by the systemic intravenous route. Regional chemotherapy series have indeed shown higher response rates and longer median survival in small series but the result has not been replicated in terms of survival benefit in a randomized trial.[58,59]

Since blood supply to HCCs is derived from the hepatic artery and normal parenchyma from the portal vein, transarterial chemoembolization (TACE) can target disease with some specificity, without causing liver necrosis. Delivery of the embolization material (typically, gelatin sponge, polyvinyl alcohol, or starch microspheres) with or without chemotherapy is accomplished by injection into the right or left hepatic artery or a first-, second-, or third-order branch, depending on disease extent. Two randomized trials have demonstrated improved survival rates using TACE, compared with symptomatic therapy alone and blind embolization.[60,61] Multiple sessions are applied until imaging shows no contrast enhancement. Common complications include abdominal pain, nausea, fever, fatigue, and transient elevation of liver enzymes. Rare complications include exacerbation of liver failure, liver abscess, gastrointestinal bleeding, and bile duct injury.

Intrahepatic Cholangiocarcinoma

Limited data are available on treatment of unresectable IHCC. Survival rates with or without treatment are poor; the median survival time is approximately 7 months, with no 5-year survivors.[18] Studies including radiolabeled anti-carcinoembryonic antigen (CEA) antibodies combined with whole-liver RT and chemotherapy or yttrium-90 (90Y) radioembolization have been reported, but there is no standard approach to treatment.[62] In an Australian study of 25 patients treated with 90Y radioembolization, median survival was 9.3 months. About 24% of patients had a partial response, 48% had stable disease, and 20% had progressive disease. Side effects were fatigue and transient abdominal pain, with rare grade 3 bilirubin, albumin, or alkaline phosphatase abnormalities.[63] In another series of 24 patients from Northwestern University, 27% of patients had a partial response, 68% had stable disease, and 5% had progressive disease. Median survival was 15 months.[64]

Conformal Irradiation for Intrahepatic Tumors

Development in three dimensional conformal radiotherapy (3D CRT) planning techniques has expanded the role of EBRT for patients with unresectable primary hepatobiliary cancers. In a series of prospective studies at the University of Michigan, doses well above the whole-liver tolerance dose were delivered safely to focal lesions.[65] This was enabled by the development of a normal tissue complication probability (NTCP) model that quantitatively described the relationship between dose and volumes irradiated and the probability of developing RILD and by the use of conformal techniques.[66] The radiation dose was individualized based on the volume of normal liver that could be spared without exceeding a 10–15% risk of RILD. The prescribed dose was 40–90 Gy. The total irradiation dose was the most important predictor of survival in multivariate analysis, and patients who received doses of 75 Gy or more had a significantly higher OS.

The use of lower doses of radiation with TACE in unresectable HCC has been reported, mostly by Asian investigators. A recent systematic review of 17 trials involving almost 1,500 patients found that patients treated with TACE and RT had improved survival rates compared with patients treated with TACE alone. Because only five of these trials were randomized, selection bias could have affected these results, but they are promising.[67] Recently, chemotherapy, including capecitabine, has been added to RT in this setting, with encouraging results.[68]

Stereotactic body radiotherapy (SBRT) is also being investigated, both with and without TACE, at fractional dose of 6–15 Gy and total dose of 30–50 Gy.[69-71] In contrast to patients with metastatic disease to the liver, who typically have normal liver function and tolerate SBRT well, patients with HCC often have liver dysfunction, and radiation tolerance is not established. Considerable variability in patient selection and treatment details, as well as the nonprospective nature of these analyses, makes the interpretation of these results difficult. Nevertheless, similar to the University of Michigan experience, a common finding was that the RT dose was a major determinant of survival rates.

Gallbladder Cancer

Patients with unresectable gallbladder cancer have a median survival of approximately 5 months and a 2-year OS of less than 5%.[72] A large number of agents, including fluorouracil, mitomycin, methotrexate, etoposide, doxorubicin, and cisplatin, have been tested as single or combination therapies with little effect.[63-72] Short-lived partial responses lasting from weeks to months have been observed in approximately 10–20% of cases. Combination chemotherapy regimes such as CEF (cisplatin, epirubicin, and 5-FU) and gemcitabine-cisplatin are associated with relatively high response rates of 30–60%, but their impact on survival is not known.[73,74] Similarly, the efficacy of palliative RT for unresectable gallbladder cancer is unknown.

Extrahepatic Cholangiocarcinoma

Unresectable EHCC is typically located in the hilum; distal tumors are usually resectable. Most patients die from hepatic dysfunction resulting from biliary obstruction or cholangitis, or both. The median survival time of patients treated with palliative intent is approximately 6 months, with 3-year survival rates of less than 10%.[17,43] Palliation can be performed either with a biliary enteric bypass or nonsurgically, using transhepatic percutaneous drainage catheters or endoscopically placed indwelling biliary stents.[43,75] Cholangitis is frequent after both of these procedures. Complications related to catheters include frequent exchanges, septic deaths in presence of indwelling catheters or stents or recurrent obstruction due to progressive tumor growth or biliary sludge.[75]

Chemotherapy for unresectable cholangiocarcinoma is largely ineffective. A review of 65 clinical trials of nonsurgical therapies did not show any survival benefit either in the setting of unresectable disease or adjuvant therapy.[76]

External Beam Irradiation with or without Chemotherapy or Brachytherapy

The median survival of patients treated with EBRT to a total dose of 45–50 Gy, alone or with chemotherapy, has been reported to be 9–12 months. Both intraoperative radiation therapy (IORT) with electrons or high-dose-rate brachytherapy, and transcatheter brachytherapy have been used alone or in combination with EBRT to focally irradiate the bile duct to higher total doses of RT. Brachytherapy as a component of overall treatment produces median survival rates of 10–24 months and 3-year OS of 10–30%. Local failure is still common despite the high total dose of RT.[47] This finding may be related to the difficulty in fully covering unresectable biliary tumors, which are often larger than 2 cm. The combination of EBRT, brachytherapy, and 5-FU shows promise. In a Mayo Clinic analysis of 24 patients with proximal extrahepatic bile duct carcinoma treated with EBRT and brachytherapy, 9 patients received concurrent 5-FU. Three patients survived for over 5 years, and two of them had received 5-FU.[77] Mayo Clinic results with neoadjuvant chemoradiation/brachytherapy followed by liver transplantation have been discussed earlier.[54] Patients who undergo percutaneous transhepatic biliary drainage (PTBD) for malignant obstructive jaundice to EHCC or IHCC may benefit from brachytherapy for prolonging stent patency and preventing reocclusion, either as a single modality or as boost along with sequential EBRT for larger tumors. The initial experience at our institute with intraluminal brachytherapy doses of 10–14 Gy enabled a stent patency of 84% with a median patency duration of 9.8 months (range 5–22 months).[78]

IRRADIATION TECHNIQUES

Dose-Limiting Organs

Liver is the major dose-limiting organ. RILD occurs 4–8 weeks after RT completion and clinically resembles veno-occlusive disease. Patients complain of fatigue and vague right upper quadrant discomfort. Signs and symptoms of ascites, with rapid weight gain and increased girth may be evident. Laboratory studies show 3–10 fold increase in alkaline phosphatase levels and moderate elevations of transaminase levels but minimal increase in bilirubin or lactate dehydrogenase (LDH) levels. It may be difficult to differentiate recurrent disease from radiation change within the liver on CT scan. Although the use of axial beam arrangements shows typical straight-line borders between the liver and areas of radiation change, nonaxial beam arrangements can lead to poorly defined borders and can be confused with infiltrative recurrent disease. RILD can be treated conservatively using diuretics and steroids, and in some cases, anticoagulation.[79,80]

Radiation-induced liver disease risk depends on the volume of liver irradiated. Whole liver irradiation to 30 Gy in 15 fractions or less carries little risk, while at 42 Gy, there is an approximately 50% risk for symptoms.[66,81] Partial liver volume irradiation to high doses is possible without clinically relevant toxicity. Trials from the University of Michigan using 3D treatment planning have shown that approximately one-third of normal liver can tolerate up to 72.6 Gy. Although the use of concurrent hepatic arterial fluorodeoxyuridine was not found to increase the risk of RILD, case reports suggest that previous alkylator therapy increases the chances of such disease.[79]

The other major dose-limiting organs are the kidneys, stomach, and small bowel. Kidney irradiation can especially be of concern when palliative whole-liver treatment is given, because opposed anterior-posterior fields, which irradiate all or a major portion of the right kidney, are frequently used. If the patient has hepatomegaly, tangential fields may be required to avoid treating the entire left kidney. Even with tangential fields, the entire right kidney is frequently irradiated. 3D treatment planning helps to ensure that the left kidney is appropriately spared.

The stomach and duodenum are of concern when the left lobe of the liver or the extrahepatic biliary tract is treated to high doses. Although some authors suggest that a dose of 60 Gy to one third of the stomach carries a 5% risk of ulceration or perforation, the Mayo Clinic data for biliary tract cancer suggest that a dose of 55 Gy or less to the stomach or duodenum carries a 5–10% risk of severe gastrointestinal complications; with doses exceeding 55 Gy, the risk of severe gastrointestinal complications in the stomach or duodenum increases to 30–40%.[82]

Irradiation Technique

Liver

Palliative liver RT may be indicated for both locally advanced hepatic tumors and metastatic disease. The appropriate dose and schedule for palliation were examined in a prospective, nonrandomized trial of more than 100 patients with symptomatic liver metastases. Six different doses and fractionation options ranging from 21 Gy in 7 fractions to 25.6 Gy in 16 fractions were tested. Palliation of pain was achieved in 55% of patients, with no difference among the treatment regimens. Although RILD was not observed, the short median survival time of these patients and the problem of distinguishing this complication from progressive disease make interpretation of this finding difficult.[83] Field arrangement may include opposed anterior-posterior or tangential approaches.

Irradiation of locally unresectable hepatic tumors to doses above the whole-liver tolerance requires 3D treatment planning. The gross tumor volume (GTV) is typically defined as radiographically abnormal areas seen on CT or MRI. The clinical target volume (CTV) is defined as GTV plus 1 cm based on surgical reports that at least a 1 cm resection margin is necessary for a successful partial hepatectomy. The planning target volume (PTV) includes CTV plus 0.5 cm for daily patient setup variation and between 0.5 cm and 2.5 cm (determined under fluoroscopy or four-dimensional CT scanning) in the cranial-caudal dimension to account for liver motion from respiration. The normal liver is defined as the GTV subtracted from the total liver volume. Using 3D treatment planning, it has been possible to safely irradiate two-thirds of the normal liver to 48–52.8 Gy and one-third of the liver to 66–72.6 Gy (Figs 1A and B).[66,84]

Gallbladder and Extrahepatic Cholangiocarcinoma

In the case of gallbladder cancer, the treatment fields should be designed to include the gallbladder fossa and the hilar and celiac lymph node-bearing areas. Accurate definition of the gallbladder fossa can be difficult in the absence of preoperative CT scans or surgical clips placed at the time of resection. Doses of 45–50 Gy (1.8–2 Gy per fraction) for subclinical disease and 60–65 Gy for microscopically positive margins are appropriate, although caution must be exercised because irradiation of the gallbladder fossa can include large volumes of liver (Figs 2A and B).

The target volume for EHCC can require inclusion of large portions of normal liver if the tumor is located in the hilum, extending to 3–5 cm within the liver to include subclinical spread along the biliary tree. Distal EHCC requires considerably less irradiation of the hepatic parenchyma, but higher duodenal or distal gastric doses may be necessary. On the basis of Mayo Clinic tolerance data, if doses greater than 55 Gy are indicated for tumor control (i.e. unresectable or residual disease), 3D treatment planning should be used to decrease normal tissue high-dose volumes.

Brachytherapy has frequently been used for EHCC. Usually, brachytherapy is given as a supplement to 45–50 Gy (1.8- to 2-Gy fractions) of EBRT. The external biliary drainage

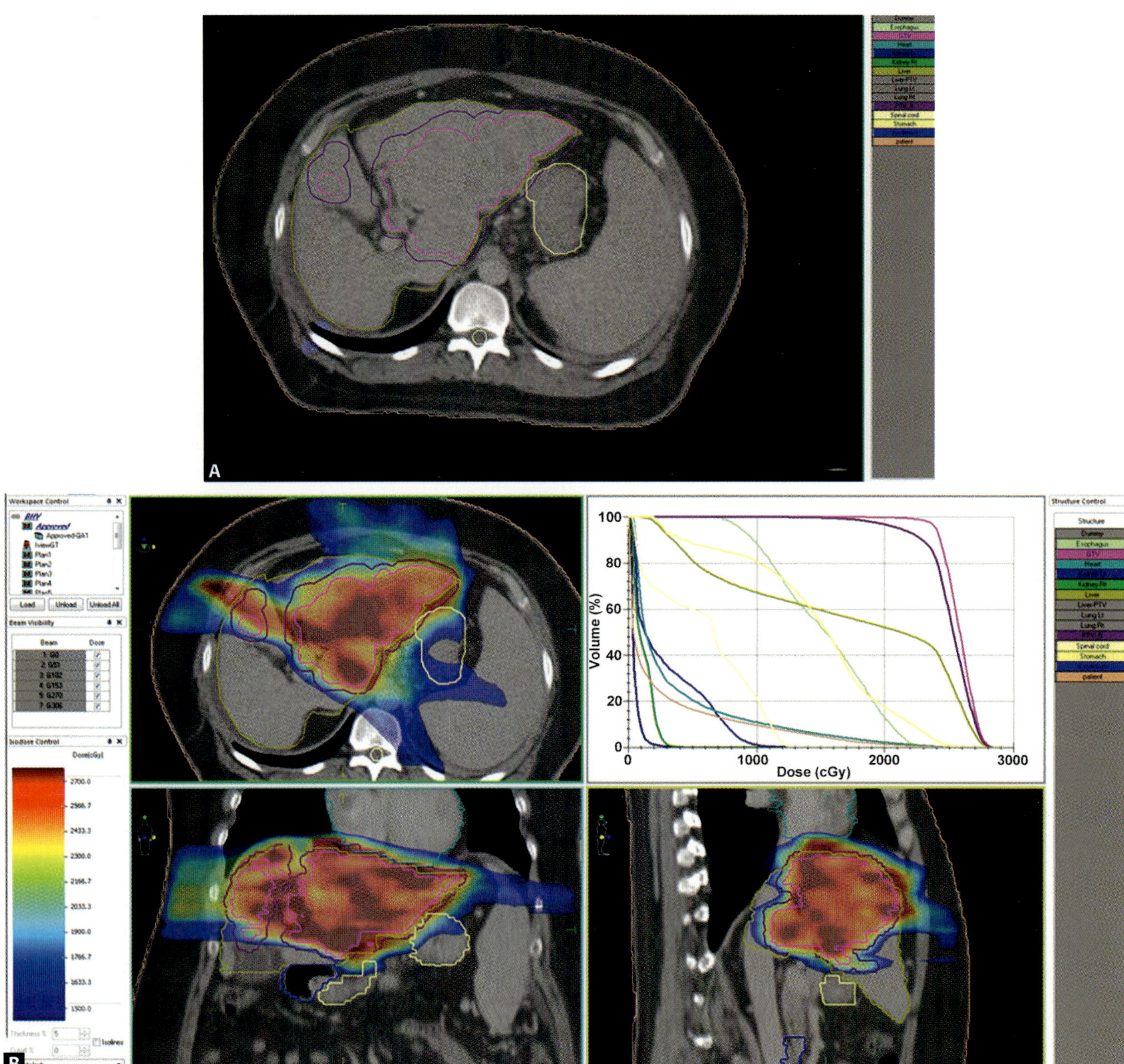

Figs 1A and B (A) The target volume and normal structures for a case of hepatocellular carcinoma involving almost the entire left lobe and part of right lobe of liver; (B) The 7-beam intensity-modulated radiotherapy (IMRT) plan for palliative RT showing optimum sparing of surrounding normal liver, lung and duodenum

Courtesy: Dr Tejinder Kataria, Division of Radiation Oncology, Medanta—The Medicity, Haryana, India

catheter is then used to gain access, and fluoroscopy helps to place a guidewire in the treatment area. In general, a boost dose of 15–20 Gy is prescribed to a radius of 0.5–1 cm from the brachytherapy catheter, although some have suggested an evaluation of boost doses of 30 Gy to a 1-cm radius, depending on the disease location relative to the stomach and duodenum (Figs 3 A to F).[77,85]

TREATMENT ALGORITHM AND FUTURE DIRECTIONS

Improvements in RT for intrahepatic malignancies have been made possible with advent of 3D conformal planning, which have enabled the delivery of high radiation doses. Brachytherapy has added to the advantage of EBRT in EHCC. Improved accuracy of treatment delivery using modern

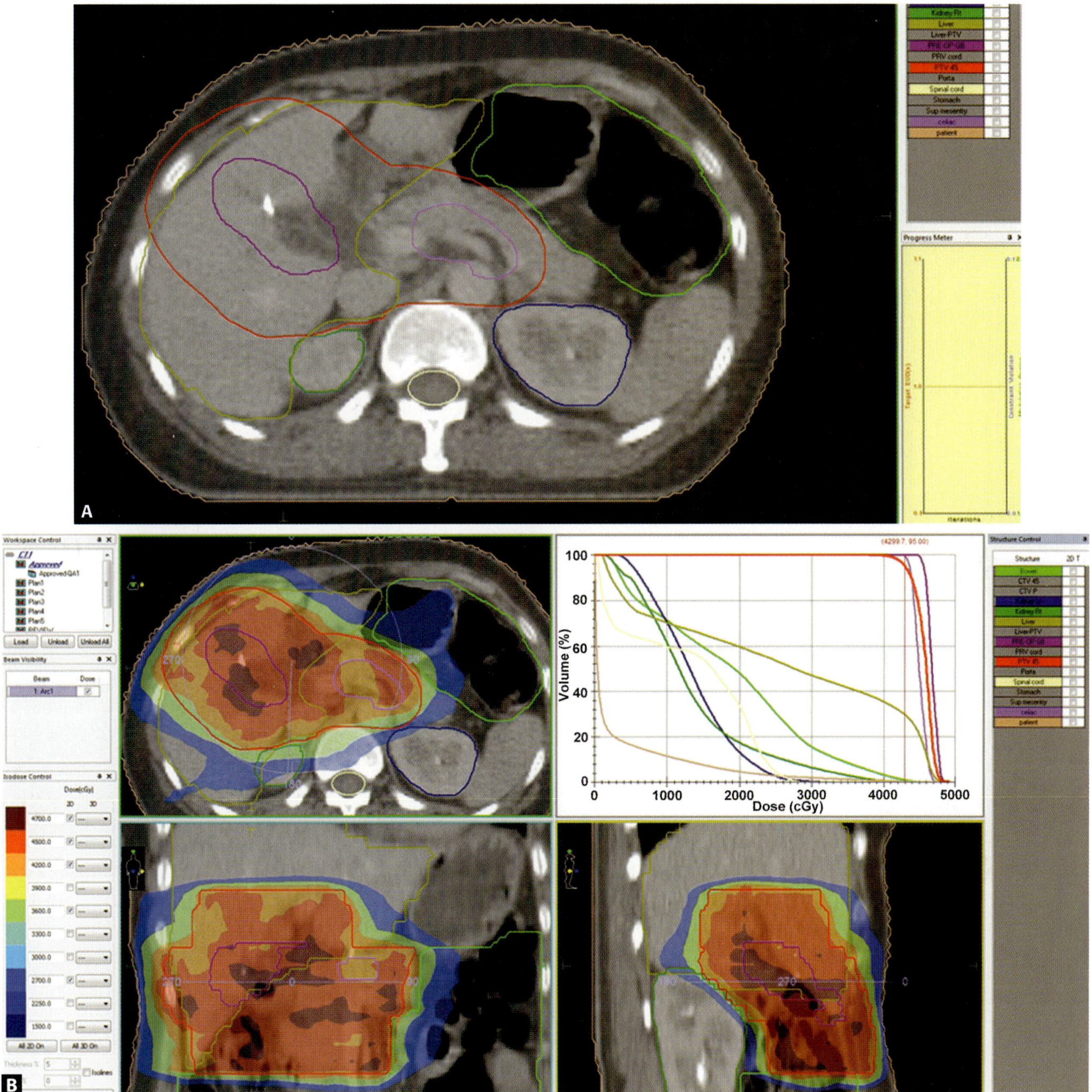

Figs 2A and B (A) The normal structure and target volume contours for a case of adenocarcinoma gallbladder, post-radical cholecystectomy, pT3N0; (B) A single arc volumetric modulated arc therapy (VMAT) plan for the same volumes

Courtesy: Dr Tejinder Kataria, Division of Radiation Oncology, Medanta—The Medicity, Haryana, India

techniques, image guidance to reduce PTV margins and better imaging allowing for accurate target delineation have added to the safety and efficacy of treatment. Use of radiation sensitizers or radioprotectors during hepatic irradiation could help improve the therapeutic index.

Improved understanding of RILD should eventually help in preventing and treating it. Better understanding of pathways whereby cytokines such as transforming growth factor-beta may participate in the process leading to veno-occlusive disease, will help develop appropriate remedial measures.

To summarize, improved outcomes for patients with hepatobiliary tumors would be achievable with combination of better dose delivery using 3D treatment planning and

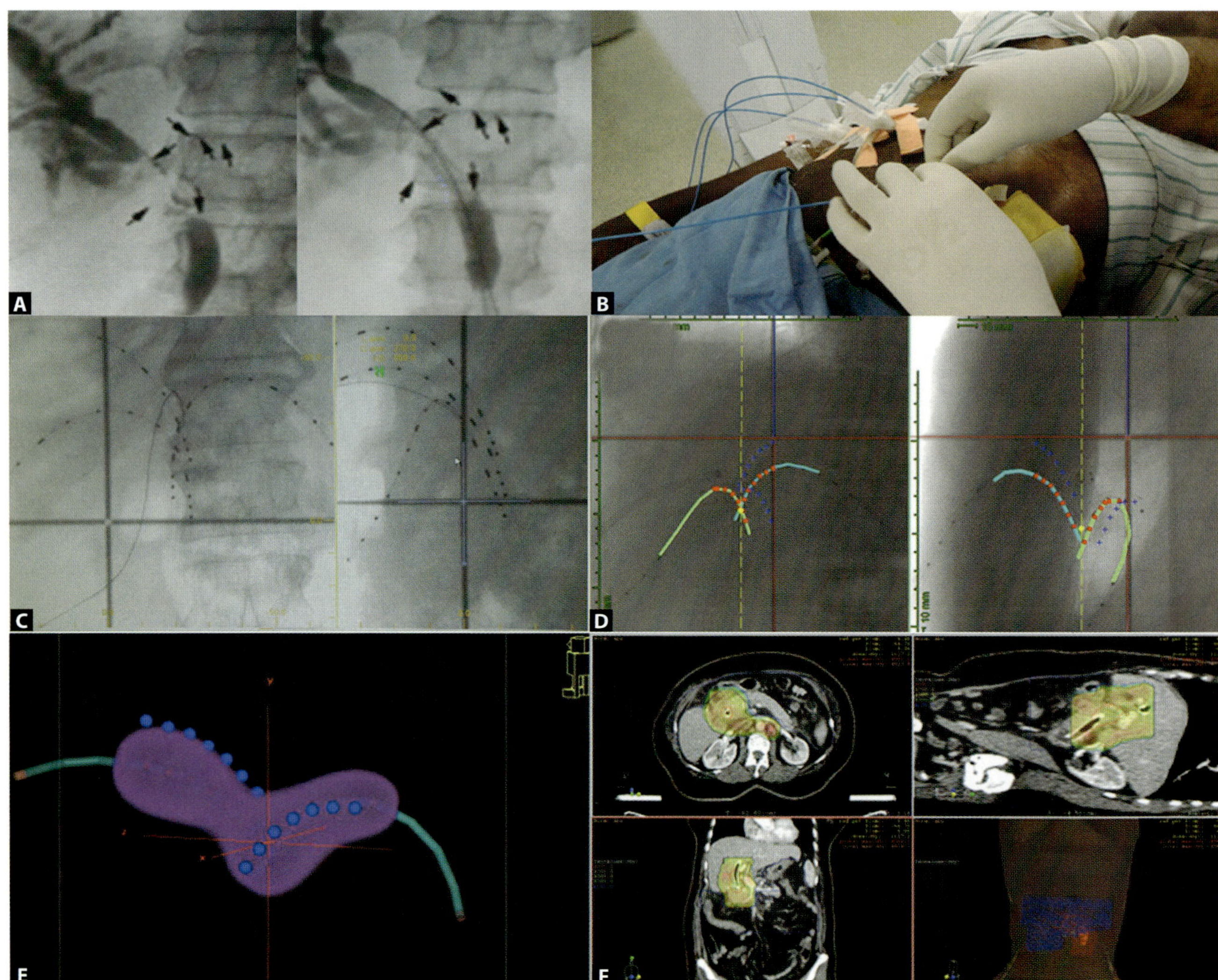

Figs 3A to F Steps of percutaneous transhepatic cholangiography (PTC)-assisted brachytherapy: (A) PTC with fluoroscopy helps visualize the stricture or bile duct narrowing and stent is deployed across. Brushing cytology may be taken at same sitting; (B) After 7–10 days, after bilirubin reduces and cytology conforms malignancy, 10 F external-internal drainage catheter is placed with its distal tip across the stricture under fluoroscopy guidance. The applicator 6F luminacath with dummy sources is placed through the sheath; (C) Orthogonal images are taken with dummy sources in situ and the catheters are reconstructed digitally; (D) Dose (10–14 Gy) is prescribed at 1 cm from surface of applicator; (E) Irradiated volume is customized to cover 1 cm proximal, distal and radial to the maximum length of the stricture as determined by PTC; (F) In situations where the disease is inoperable and there is a significant volume of the tumor beyond bile ducts, CT-based planning for external beam radiation therapy (EBRT) may be used to deliver additional dose, in which case brachytherapy serves as local boost

Courtesy: Dr Tejinder Kataria, Division of Radiation Oncology, Medanta—The Medicity, Haryana, India

brachytherapy, improved imaging, more effective use of radiosensitizers, and evaluation of both chemical and biologic protectors of normal liver.

REFERENCES

1. Wharton JT, Delclos L, Gallager S, et al. Radiation hepatitis induced by abdominal irradiation with the cobalt 60 moving strip technique. Am J Roentgenol Radium Ther Nucl Med. 1973;117(1):73-80.
2. Nagorney DM, Gigot JF. Primary epithelial hepatic malignancies: etiology, epidemiology, and outcome after subtotal and total hepatic resection. Surg Oncol Clin N Am. 1996;5(2):283-300.
3. El-Serag HB. Hepatocellular carcinoma: recent trends in the United States. Gastroenterology. 2004;127(5):S27-34.
4. Diehl AK. Epidemiology of gallbladder cancer: a synthesis of recent data. J Natl Cancer Inst. 1980;65(6):1209-14.
5. Khakoo SI, Grellier LF, Soni PN, et al. Etiology, screening, and treatment of hepatocellular carcinoma. Med Clin North Am. 1996;80(5):1121-45.

6. Abi-Rached B, Neugut AI. Diagnostic and management issues in gallbladder carcinoma. Oncology (Williston Park). 1995;9(1):19-24; discussion 24, 27, 30.
7. Rosen CB, Nagorney DM. Cholangiocarcinoma complicating primary sclerosing cholangitis. Semin Liver Dis. 1991;11(1):26-30.
8. Ekbom A, Hsieh CC, Yuen J, Trichopoulos D, McLaughlin JK, Lan SJ, et al. Risk of extrahepatic bile duct cancer after cholecystectomy. Lancet. 1993;342(8882):1262-5.
9. Chang MH, You SL, Chen CJ, Liu CJ, Lee CM, Lin SM, et al. Decreased incidence of hepatocellular carcinoma in hepatitis B vaccinees: a 20-year follow-up study. J Natl Cancer Inst. 2009;101(19):1348-55.
10. National Comprehensive Cancer Network®. NCCN Clinical Practice Guidelines in Oncology 2014. Hepatobiliary cancers. [online] Available from www.nccn.org/professionals/physician_gls/f_guidelines.asp#hepatobiliary. [Accessed April, 2015].
11. Nichols JC, Gores GJ, LaRusso NF, Wiesner RH, Nagorney DM, Ritts RE. Diagnostic role of serum CA 19-9 for cholangiocarcinoma in patients with primary sclerosing cholangitis. Mayo Clin Proc. 1993;68(9):874-9.
12. Okuda K. Hepatocellular carcinoma: recent progress. Hepatology. 1992;15(5):948-63.
13. Okuda K, Peters RL, Simson IW. Gross anatomic features of hepatocellular carcinoma from three disparate geographic areas. Proposal of new classification. Cancer. 1984;54(10):2165-73.
14. Nzeako UC, Goodman ZD, Ishak KG. Comparison of tumor pathology with duration of survival of North American patients with hepatocellular carcinoma. Cancer. 1995;76(4):579-88.
15. Carriaga MT, Henson DE. Liver, gallbladder, extrahepatic bile ducts, and pancreas. Cancer. 1995;75(1):171-90.
16. Henson DE, Albores-Saavedra J, Corle D. Carcinoma of the gallbladder. Histologic types, stage of disease, grade, and survival rates. Cancer. 1992;70(6):1493-7.
17. Henson DE, Albores-Saavedra J, Corle D. Carcinoma of the extrahepatic bile ducts. Histologic types, stage of disease, grade, and survival rates. Cancer. 1992;70(6):1498-501.
18. Nakeeb A, Pitt HA, Sohn TA, Coleman J, Abrams RA, Piantadosi S, et al. Cholangiocarcinoma. A spectrum of intrahepatic, perihilar, and distal tumors. Ann Surg. 1996;224(4):463-73; discussion 473-5.
19. American Cancer Society: Cancer facts and Figures 2004. American Cancer Society, 2004.
20. Nomura F, Ohnishi K, Tanabe Y. Nomura F, Ohnishi K, Tanabe Y. Cancer. 1989;64(8):1700-7.
21. Hori M, Murakami T, Kim T, Takahashi S, Oi H, Tomoda K, et al. Sensitivity of double-phase helical CT during arterial portography for detection of hypervascular hepatocellular carcinoma. J Comput Assist Tomogr. 1998;22(6):861-7.
22. Braga L, Guller U, Semelka RC. Modern hepatic imaging. Surg Clin North Am. 2004;84(2):375-400.
23. Hann LE, Winston CB, Brown KT, et al. Diagnostic imaging approaches and relationship to hepatobiliary cancer staging and therapy. Semin Surg Oncol. 2000;19(2):94-115.
24. Van Leeuwen DJ, Huibregtse K, Tytgat GN. Carcinoma of the hepatic confluence 25 years after Klatskin's description: diagnosis and endoscopic management. Semin Liver Dis. 1990;10(2):102-13.
25. Anthony B. Tumours and tumour-like lesions of the liver and biliary tract. In: Macsween RN, Anthony PP, Scheur PJ, et al. Pathology of the Liver, 3rd edition. Edinburgh: Churcill Livingstone; 1994.
26. González González D, Gerard JP, Maners AW, De la Lande-Guyaux B, Van Dijk-Milatz A, Meerwaldt JH, et al. Results of radiation therapy in carcinoma of the proximal bile duct (Klatskin tumor). Semin Liver Dis. 1990;10(2):131-41.
27. Llovet JM, Fuster J, Bruix J. Intention-to-treat analysis of surgical treatment for early hepatocellular carcinoma: resection versus transplantation. Hepatology. 1999;30(6):1434-40.
28. Mazzaferro V, Regalia E, Doci R, Andreola S, Pulvirenti A, Bozzetti F, et al. Liver transplantation for the treatment of small hepatocellular carcinomas in patients with cirrhosis. N Engl J Med. 1996;334(11):693-9.
29. Arii S, Yamaoka Y, Futagawa S, Inoue K, Kobayashi K, Kojiro M, et al. Results of surgical and nonsurgical treatment for small-sized hepatocellular carcinomas: a retrospective and nationwide survey in Japan. The Liver Cancer Study Group of Japan. Hepatology. 2000;32(6):1224-9.
30. Bismuth H, Majno PE. Hepatobiliary surgery. J Hepatol. 2000;32(1):208-24.
31. Nagasue N, Uchida M, Makino Y, Takemoto Y, Yamanoi A, Hayashi T, et al. Incidence and factors associated with intrahepatic recurrence following resection of hepatocellular carcinoma. Gastroenterology. 1993;105(2):488-94.
32. Schwartz JD, Schwartz M, Mandeli J, et al. Neoadjuvant and adjuvant therapy for resectable hepatocellular carcinoma: review of the randomised clinical trials. Lancet Oncol. 2002;3(10):593-603.
33. Samuel M, Chow PK, Chan Shih-Yen E, et al. Neoadjuvant and adjuvant therapy for surgical resection of hepatocellular carcinoma. Cochrane Database Syst Rev. 2009;(1):CD001199.
34. Breitenstein S, Dimitroulis D, Petrowsky H, Puhan MA, Müllhaupt B, Clavien PA. Systematic review and meta-analysis of interferon after curative treatment of hepatocellular carcinoma in patients with viral hepatitis. Br J Surg. 2009;96(9):975-81.
35. Tanabe KK, Curley SA, Dodd GD, et al. Radiofrequency ablation: the experts weigh in. Cancer. 2004;100(3):641-50.
36. Inoue K, Makuuchi M, Takayama T, Torzilli G, Yamamoto J, Shimada K, et al. Long-term survival and prognostic factors in the surgical treatment of mass-forming type cholangiocarcinoma. Surgery. 2000;127(5):498-505.
37. Weber SM, Jarnagin WR, Klimstra D, DeMatteo RP, Fong Y, Blumgart LH. Intrahepatic cholangiocarcinoma: resectability, recurrence pattern, and outcomes. J Am Coll Surg. 2001;193(4):384-91.
38. Shirai Y, Yoshida K, Tsukada K, et al. Inapparent carcinoma of the gallbladder. An appraisal of a radical second operation after simple cholecystectomy. Ann Surg. 1992;215(4):326-31.
39. Bartlett DL, Fong Y, Fortner JG, et al. Long-term results after resection for gallbladder cancer. Implications for staging and management. Ann Surg. 1996;224(5):639-46.
40. Fahim RB, McDonald JR, Richards JC, et al. Carcinoma of the gallbladder: a study of its modes of spread. Ann Surg. 1962;156:114-24.

41. Kondo S, Nimura Y, Hayakawa N, Kamiya J, Nagino M, Uesaka K. Regional and para-aortic lymphadenectomy in radical surgery for advanced gallbladder carcinoma. Br J Surg. 2000;87(4):418-22.
42. Kresl JJ, Schild SE, Henning GT, Gunderson LL, Donohue J, Pitot H, et al. Adjuvant external beam radiation therapy with concurrent chemotherapy in the management of gallbladder carcinoma. Int J Radiat Oncol Biol Phys. 2002;52(1):167-75.
43. Gold DG, Miller RC, Haddock MG, Gunderson LL, Quevedo F, Donohue JH, et al. Adjuvant therapy for gallbladder carcinoma: the Mayo Clinic Experience. Int J Radiat Oncol Biol Phys. 2009;75(1):150-5.
44. Wade TP, Prasad CN, Virgo KS, et al. Experience with distal bile duct cancers in U.S. Veterans Affairs hospitals: 1987-1991. J Surg Oncol. 1997;64(3):242-5.
45. Nagorney DM, Donohue JH, Farnell MB, et al. Outcomes after curative resections of cholangiocarcinoma. Arch Surg. 1993;128(8):871-7; discussion 877-9.
46. Cameron JL, Pitt HA, Zinner MJ, et al. Management of proximal cholangiocarcinomas by surgical resection and radiotherapy. Am J Surg. 1990;159(1):91-7; discussion 97-8.
47. Fritz P, Brambs HJ, Schraube P, Freund U, Berns C, Wannenmacher M. Combined external beam radiotherapy and intraluminal high dose rate brachytherapy on bile duct carcinomas. Int J Radiat Oncol Biol Phys. 1994;29(4):855-61.
48. Jarnagin WR, Ruo L, Little SA, Klimstra D, D'Angelica M, DeMatteo RP, et al. Patterns of initial disease recurrence after resection of gallbladder carcinoma and hilar cholangiocarcinoma: implications for adjuvant therapeutic strategies. Cancer. 2003;98(8):1689-700.
49. González González D, Gerard JP, Maners AW, De la Lande-Guyaux B, Van Dijk-Milatz A, Meerwaldt JH, et al. Results of radiation therapy in carcinoma of the proximal bile duct (Klatskin tumor). Semin Liver Dis. 1990;10(2):131-41.
50. Gerhards MF, van Gulik TM, González González D, et al. Results of postoperative radiotherapy for resectable hilar cholangiocarcinoma. World J Surg. 2003;27(2):173-9.
51. Mahe M, Romestaing P, Talon B, Ardiet JM, Salerno N, Sentenac I, et al. Radiation therapy in extrahepatic bile duct carcinoma. Radiother Oncol. 1991;21(2):121-7.
52. Shimoda M, Farmer DG, Colquhoun SD, Rosove M, Ghobrial RM, Yersiz H, et al. Liver transplantation for cholangiocellular carcinoma: analysis of a single-center experience and review of the literature. Liver Transpl. 2001;7(12):1023-33.
53. Heimbach JK, Haddock MG, Alberts SR, Nyberg SL, Ishitani MB, Rosen CB, et al. Transplantation for hilar cholangiocarcinoma. Liver Transpl. 2004;10(10):S65-8.
54. Rea DJ, Heimbach JK, Rosen CB, Haddock MG, Alberts SR, Kremers WK, et al. Liver transplantation with neoadjuvant chemoradiation is more effective than resection for hilar cholangiocarcinoma. Ann Surg. 2005;242(3):451-8; discussion 458-61.
55. Llovet JM, Ricci S, Mazzaferro V, Hilgard P, Gane E, Blanc JF, et al. Sorafenib in advanced hepatocellular carcinoma. N Engl J Med. 2008;359(4):378-90.
56. Simonetti RG, Liberati A, Angiolini C, et al. Treatment of hepatocellular carcinoma: a systematic review of randomized controlled trials. Ann Oncol. 1997;8(2):117-36.
57. Chow PK, Tai BC, Tan CK, Machin D, Win KM, Johnson PJ, et al. High-dose tamoxifen in the treatment of inoperable hepatocellular carcinoma: A multicenter randomized controlled trial. Hepatology. 2002;36(5):1221-6.
58. Yamashita T. Chemotherapy for advanced hepatocellular carcinoma: systemic chemotherapy or hepatic arterial infusion chemotherapy? J Gastroenterol. 2004;39(4):404-6.
59. Tzoracoleftherakis EE, Spiliotis JD, Kyriakopoulou T, et al. Intra-arterial versus systemic chemotherapy for non-operable hepatocellular carcinoma. Hepatogastroenterology. 1999; 46(26):1122-5.
60. Lo CM, Ngan H, Tso WK, Liu CL, Lam CM, Poon RT, et al. Randomized controlled trial of transarterial lipiodol chemoembolization for unresectable hepatocellular carcinoma. Hepatology. 2002;35(5):1164-71.
61. Llovet JM, Real MI, Montaña X, Planas R, Coll S, Aponte J, et al. Arterial embolisation or chemoembolisation versus symptomatic treatment in patients with unresectable hepatocellular carcinoma: a randomised controlled trial. Lancet. 2002;359(9319):1734-9.
62. Stillwagon GB, Order SE, Haulk T, Herpst J, Ettinger DS, Fishman EK, et al. Variable low dose rate irradiation (131I-anti-CEA) and integrated low dose chemotherapy in the treatment of nonresectable primary intrahepatic cholangiocarcinoma. Int J Radiat Oncol Biol Phys. 1991;21(6):1601-5.
63. Saxena A, Bester L, Chua TC, et al. Yttrium-90 radiotherapy for unresectable intrahepatic cholangiocarcinoma: a preliminary assessment of this novel treatment option. Ann Surg Oncol. 2010;17(2):484-91.
64. Ibrahim SM, Mulcahy MF, Lewandowski RJ, Sato KT, Ryu RK, Masterson EJ, et al. Treatment of unresectable cholangiocarcinoma using yttrium-90 microspheres: results from a pilot study. Cancer. 2008;113(8):2119-28.
65. Robertson JM, McGinn CJ, Walker S, Marx MV, Kessler ML, Ensminger WD, et al. A phase I trial of hepatic arterial bromodeoxyuridine and conformal radiation therapy for patients with primary hepatobiliary cancers or colorectal liver metastases. Int J Radiat Oncol Biol Phys. 1997;39(5):1087-92.
66. Dawson LA, Normolle D, Balter JM, McGinn CJ, Lawrence TS, Ten Haken RK. Analysis of radiation-induced liver disease using the Lyman NTCP model. Int J Radiat Oncol Biol Phys. 2002;53(4):810-21. Erratum in: Int J Radiat Oncol Biol Phys. 2002;53(5):1422.
67. Meng MB, Cui YL, Lu Y, She B, Chen Y, Guan YS, et al. Transcatheter arterial chemoembolization in combination with radiotherapy for unresectable hepatocellular carcinoma: a systematic review and meta-analysis. Radiother Oncol. 2009;92(2):184-94.
68. McIntosh A, Hagspiel KD, Al-Osaimi AM, Northup P, Caldwell S, Berg C, et al. Accelerated treatment using intensity-modulated radiation therapy plus concurrent capecitabine for unresectable hepatocellular carcinoma. Cancer. 2009;115(21):5117-25.
69. Choi BO, Choi IB, Jang HS, Kang YN, Jang JS, Bae SH, et al. Stereotactic body radiation therapy with or without transarterial chemoembolization for patients with primary hepatocellular carcinoma: preliminary analysis. BMC Cancer. 2008;8:351.

70. Takeda A, Takahashi M, Kunieda E, Takeda T, Sanuki N, Koike Y, et al. Hypofractionated stereotactic radiotherapy with and without transarterial chemoembolization for small hepatocellular carcinoma not eligible for other ablation therapies: Preliminary results for efficacy and toxicity. Hepatol Res. 2008;38(1):60-9.
71. Tse RV, Hawkins M, Lockwood G, Kim JJ, Cummings B, Knox J, et al. Phase I study of individualized stereotactic body radiotherapy for hepatocellular carcinoma and intrahepatic cholangiocarcinoma. J Clin Oncol. 2008;26(4):657-64.
72. Chao TC, Greager JA. Primary carcinoma of the gallbladder. J Surg Oncol. 1991;46(4):215-21.
73. Ellis PA, Norman A, Hill A, O'Brien ME, Nicolson M, Hickish T, et al. Epirubicin, cisplatin and infusional 5-fluorouracil (5-FU) (ECF) in hepatobiliary tumours. Eur J Cancer. 1995;31A(10):1594-8.
74. Doval DC, Sekhon JS, Gupta SK, Fuloria J, Shukla VK, Gupta S, et al. A phase II study of gemcitabine and cisplatin in chemotherapy-naive, unresectable gall bladder cancer. Br J Cancer. 2004;90(8):1516-20.
75. Lokich JJ, Kane RA, Harrison DA, et al. Biliary tract obstruction secondary to cancer: management guidelines and selected literature review. J Clin Oncol. 1987;5(6):969-81.
76. Hejna M, Pruckmayer M, Raderer M. The role of chemotherapy and radiation in the management of biliary cancer: a review of the literature. Eur J Cancer. 1998;34(7):977-86.
77. Foo ML, Gunderson LL, Bender CE, et al. External radiation therapy and transcatheter iridium in the treatment of extrahepatic bile duct carcinoma. Int J Radiat Oncol Biol Phys. 1997;39(4):929-35.
78. Jain S, Kataria T, Bisht SS, Gupta D, Vikraman S, Baijal S, et al. Malignant obstructive jaundice -brachytherapy as a tool for palliation. J Contemp Brachytherapy. 2013;5(2):83-8.
79. Lawrence TS, Robertson JM, Anscher MS, Jirtle RL, Ensminger WD, Fajardo LF. Hepatic toxicity resulting from cancer treatment. Int J Radiat Oncol Biol Phys. 1995;31(5):1237-48.
80. Yamasaki SA, Marn CS, Francis IR, et al. High-dose localized radiation therapy for treatment of hepatic malignant tumors: CT findings and their relation to radiation hepatitis. AJR Am J Roentgenol. 1995;165(1):79-84.
81. Jackson A, Ten Haken RK, Robertson JM, Kessler ML, Kutcher GJ, Lawrence TS. Analysis of clinical complication data for radiation hepatitis using a parallel architecture model. Int J Radiat Oncol Biol Phys. 1995;31(4):883-91.
82. Buskirk SJ, Gunderson LL, Schild SE, Bender CE, Williams HJ, McIlrath DC, et al. Analysis of failure after curative irradiation of extrahepatic bile duct carcinoma. Ann Surg. 1992;215(2):125-31.
83. Borgelt BB, Gelber R, Brady LW, et al. The palliation of hepatic metastases: results of the Radiation Therapy Oncology Group pilot study. Int J Radiat Oncol Biol Phys. 1981;7(5):587-91.
84. Dawson LA, McGinn CJ, Normolle D, Ten Haken RK, Walker S, Ensminger W, et al. Escalated focal liver radiation and concurrent hepatic artery fluorodeoxyuridine for unresectable intrahepatic malignancies. J Clin Oncol. 2000;18(11):2210-8.
85. Hayes JK, Sapozink MD, Miller FJ. Definitive radiation therapy in bile duct carcinoma. Int J Radiat Oncol Biol Phys. 1988;15(3):735-44.

22

CHAPTER

Radiation Therapy in Hematologic Malignancies

Manoj Tayal, Tejinder Kataria, Kushal Narang

INTRODUCTION

Hematologic malignancies are broadly divided into myeloid neoplasms, lymphoid neoplasms (leukemias and lymphomas), lymphoproliferative disorders, and histiocytic/ dendritic cell neoplasms. They are widely recognized as arising out of specific stages of myeloid or lymphoid development or specific subsets of these types of cells.

By definition, "leukemia" is any myeloid or lymphoid malignancy that largely involves the peripheral blood and bone marrow (BM).[1] They may be classified as acute or chronic, depending on maturity of the cell of origin (acute = blasts and chronic = more mature cells), which also tends to correlate with the clinical acuity (acute = weeks and chronic = years).

A lymphoma is a lymphoid malignancy that involves lymph nodes and/or other extramedullary sites. They are broadly classified as being Hodgkin or non-Hodgkin and are treated with very different therapies.

Histiocytic and dendritic cell neoplasms generally are rare except for Langerhans cell histiocytosis (an entity whose neoplastic nature is controversial), which is seen relatively more commonly, especially in children.

Although morphology and clinical history are very helpful in the initial differential diagnosis, detailed immunophenotyping by either flow cytometry or immunohistochemistry is usually needed to classify a leukemia or lymphoma according the cell lineage [myeloid, B, T, natural killer (NK)] and stage of maturation.[1]

ACUTE LEUKEMIAS

The immature, clonally proliferating cells that form blasts may be derived from myeloid or lymphoid cell lines. Transformation of granulocyte, red blood cell (RBC), or platelet (myeloid) precursors results in acute myelogenous leukemia (AML). Acute lymphoblastic leukemia (ALL) originates from B or T lymphocytes. Acute leukemias have traditionally been classified using the French-American-British (FAB) morphologic and cytologic criteria of classification.[2] AML and its subtypes can most often be identified microscopically by the presence of Auer rods, staining for myeloperoxidase or monocyte-associated esterases, and other cytologic features of differentiation.

Acute myelogenous leukemia with minimal or no myeloid differentiation (M1 and M0 subtypes) can be confused with ALL but for flow cytometric identification of early myeloid antigens. The more differentiated AML subtypes M2-M6 are usually recognizable by morphology and cytochemistry.

The World Health Organization (WHO) proposed a new classification scheme for myeloid neoplasms.[3] The WHO classification creates three new subgroups based on the presence of recurring genetic abnormalities, dysplastic features, or history of alkylator or topoisomerase therapy. Leukemias bearing none of these features are grouped according to maturation features, similar to the traditional FAB classification, in a fourth subgroup termed AML, not otherwise categorized.

The FAB classification for ALL has three subtypes based on morphology. L1 is the predominant type in 85% of childhood ALL. It is characterized by small cells with scanty cytoplasm and inconspicuous nucleoli. L2 is common in ALL of adults and is identified morphologically by blasts that show prominent nucleoli, abundant cytoplasm and more variability in size.

L3 lymphoblasts are large cells with cytoplasmic basophilia and vacuolization, similar to Burkitt's lymphoma cells.

Clinical prognostic features of B-cell leukemias have been commonly used to place patients into risk groups. Standard risk has been generally understood to include patients whose age at diagnosis is between 1 year and 10 years as well as a presenting leukocyte count of less than 50,000/μL, in the absence of central nervous system (CNS) involvement. Current clinical practice is for T-cell leukemias to be treated on different protocols than B-cell lineage ALL.[4] Assessment of CNS involvement at diagnosis in acute leukemia is critical as to risk stratification, which is, of course, of particular importance to the radiation oncologist.

Central nervous system involvement has been unequivocally defined[5] by a cerebrospinal fluid (CSF) leukocyte count of 5 or more white blood cells (WBCs) per microliter along with either blast cells on cytospin or the presence of cranial nerve palsy. By convention, this is now classified as CNS-3. CNS-1 is defined as no blast cells on CSF cytology and CNS-2 is less than 5 WBCs per microliter with blast cells present.

Epidemiology

In 2012, leukemia developed in 3,52,000 people globally and caused 265,000 deaths.[6] It is the most common type of cancer in children, with three quarters of leukemia cases in children being ALL.[7] However, about 90% of all leukemias are diagnosed in adults, with AML and chronic lymphocytic leukemia (CLL) being most common in adults.[7] It occurs more commonly in the developed world.[6]

Risk Factors

Men are more likely to develop chronic myelogenous leukemia (CML), CLL and AML than women. The risk of most leukemias, with the exception of ALL, typically increases with age. Among adults, the known causes are natural and artificial ionizing radiation, a few viruses such as human T-lymphotropic virus (HTLV), and some chemicals, notably benzene and alkylating chemotherapy agents for previous malignancies.[8-10] Viruses have also been linked to some forms of leukemia. The first human retrovirus identified was HTLV-1, which is known to cause adult T-cell leukemia.[11] Chromosomal abnormalities or certain other genetic conditions have a greater risk of leukemia.[9] For example, people with Down's syndrome have a significantly increased risk of developing forms of acute leukemia (especially acute myeloid leukemia), and Fanconi anemia is a risk factor for developing acute myeloid leukemia.[8] Exposure to high levels of radiation: exposure to high-energy radiation[8] and intense exposure to low-energy radiation from electromagnetic fields (e.g. power lines).[12]

Clinical Presentation

- Frequent infections, ranging from infected tonsils, sores in the mouth, or diarrhea to life-threatening pneumonia or opportunistic infections.
- Flu-like symptoms, nausea or a feeling of fullness due to hepatomegaly and splenomegaly.
- Anemia, which may cause dyspnea and pallor.
- The patient may have easy bruisability, abnormal excessive bleeding, or petechiae.
- Neurological symptoms (notably headaches) can occur if CNS is involved.

Some leukemias particularly common in hairy cell leukemia,[13] do not have high WBC counts. This condition is called as aleukemia. The leukemic cells in BM disrupt the normal production of blood cells. For an aleukemic patient, the WBC counts in the bloodstream can be normal or low.

Diagnostic Evaluation

Morphology and clinical history are very helpful in the initial differential diagnosis, a detailed immunophenotyping by either flow cytometry or immunohistochemistry is usually needed to classify a leukemia to the cell lineage and stage of maturation[1] and specific monoclonal antibodies can be used to assay for a panel of antigens, known as cluster of differentiation (CD) molecules. For instance, positivity for CD13, CD33, and cytoplasmic myeloperoxidase are correlated with myeloid cells and other markers defining different degrees of differentiation and maturation, ALL is divided into T-cell and B-cell lineage.[1] Cytogenetic or chromosomal abnormalities have distinct prognostic and therapeutic implications. Adult and childhood forms of ALL have distinctly different patterns of genetic abnormalities as well as immunophenotyping.[14]

Treatment of Leukemias

Treatment involves combination of chemotherapy, radiation therapy, targeted therapy, and BM transplant, in addition to supportive care and palliative care as needed. Certain types of leukemia may be managed with watchful waiting.[7] The success of treatment depends on the type of leukemia and the age of the person. The average 5-year survival rate is 60% in the United States.[7] In children under 15 years, the 5-year survival is up to 85%, depending on the type of leukemia.[15]

Treatment of Acute Myelocytic Leukemias

Prognostic factors: Those patients who are older (older than 60 years) and those with an elevated blast count at diagnosis (> 20,000) have a worse prognosis. Chemotherapy-related AML and prior history of myelodysplasia (MDS) imparts a lower chance of obtaining complete remission (CR) and long-term survival. A history of trisomy 21 may impart a good prognosis. The advent of molecular diagnostics has heralded an explosion in new prognostic factors, including gene mutations in KIT, feline McDonough sarcoma (FMS)-like tyrosine kinase 3 (FLT3), nucleophosmin 1 (NPM1) and CCAAT enhancer-binding protein D (CEBPA).[16]

Treatment of AML consists of induction and post-remission therapy.[17] The goal of induction is to produce a CR and that of post-remission therapy to maintain it by eliminating residual disease. Once in a morphologic CR, there are still as many as 10^9 leukemia cells present below the threshold of detection by light microscopy (minimal residual disease).[18] Further therapy is, therefore, necessary to reduce this number and minimize the chances of relapse.[19] All FAB subtypes except M3 are usually given induction chemotherapy with cytarabine (ara-C) and an anthracycline (most often daunorubicin). The M3 subtype of AML, also known as acute promyelocytic leukemia (APL), is almost universally treated with the drug all-trans-retinoic acid (ATRA) in addition to induction chemotherapy, usually an anthracycline.

Post-remission therapy consists of repeated cycles of chemotherapy or hematopoietic stem cell transplantation (HSCT) in its various forms (autologous, allogeneic, haploidentical, cord blood, reduced intensity). At this moment, there is no accepted role for maintenance therapy in AML. The role of CNS prophylaxis is not well-defined for AML, as CNS relapse rates are relatively infrequent (at about 5–10%).[20]

Treatment of Acute Lymphoblastic Leukemia

Prognostic factors: Females have better prognosis than males. Children between 1 year and 10 years of age are most likely to be cured of it. Older patients are more likely to have chromosomal abnormalities (e.g. the Philadelphia chromosome) and have a poorer prognosis. A high WBC count at presentation and CNS involvement have a worse outcome. Presence of genetic disorders such as Down's syndrome, marrow blast percentage and remission status at the end of induction therapy are significant predictors of outcome. Among karyotype abnormalities with an independent influence on prognosis, high hyperdiploidy (>50 chromosomes) was shown to be favorable, whereas near haploidy (23–29 chromosomes), presence of the Philadelphia chromosome, t (4;11) and abnormalities affecting the short arm of chromosome 9 [abn (9p)] were adverse risk factors.[14]

The four components of specific ALL therapy are:

1. Induction of remission
2. Intensification and/or consolidation
3. Maintenance therapy
4. CNS prophylaxis.[17]

The remission induction and consolidation phases typically involve blocks of monthly treatment for 6–8 months followed by long-term maintenance, which is given for up to 3 years.[17]

Induction regimens include combination of prednisolone or dexamethasone, vincristine, asparaginase (better tolerance in pediatric patients), and daunorubicin (used in adult ALL) is used. Current multiagent induction regimens result in complete response rates that range from 60% to 90%.[21,22]

Intensification protocols use vincristine, cyclophosphamide, cytarabine, daunorubicin, etoposide, thioguanine or mercaptopurine given as blocks.

Central nervous system prophylaxis is typically administered by multiple rounds of intrathecal chemotherapy that are staggered over the entire treatment duration. Cranial radiotherapy (RT) may be used to prevent CNS relapse of leukemia. From a historical perspective, its use has been well documented for ALL. With concerns about late sequel and improvements in systemic therapy including agents that can better penetrate the blood-brain barrier, prophylactic cranial RT is used less frequently.[23] Several cooperative group trials have demonstrated that low-risk ALL could be effectively managed without cranial radiation, substituting intrathecal methotrexate (IT MTX) throughout induction, consolidation, and maintenance therapy in place of cranial radiation. High-risk ALL patients have generally continued to receive cranial radiation. In order to reduce the toxicity of prophylactic cranial radiation, several investigations have explored a reduction in radiation dose.[24] The use of 18 Gy in 9 or 10 fractions along with IT MTX yields comparable disease control rates as 24 Gy. Nevertheless, a dose of 18 Gy for prophylactic cranial irradiation has become more or less standard for pediatric ALL. For adults with ALL, various protocols have used 24 Gy and others employ 18 Gy.[25-27]

Bone Marrow Transplant (or Hematopoietic Stem Cell Transplant)

Autologous transplant: Autologous transplant is a further consolidation for patients with poor-risk disease who have no donors for allogeneic transplant. It is an option after intensive consolidation chemotherapy. It can also be performed in older patients (up to 70 years).[28]

Allogeneic transplant: Allogeneic transplant has the added benefit of graft versus leukemia effect. It is considered for all patients with relapsed or refractory disease, as it is the option that may yield long-term survival. It is performed in the first CR or early in the course for those patients with poor risk cytogenetics, t (9; 21), or MDS, especially with a matched-related donor. It may be associated with increased failure-free survival. When transplanted in first CR, overall survival (OS) is 60%; it decreases to less than 35% when performed for patients with relapsed disease, and is lower than 10% for patients with refractory disease.

Nonmyeloablative transplantation is being explored for those patients unable to proceed with ablative treatment secondary to age or illness.[28]

The results of a series of retrospective and prospective studies published between 1987 and 1994 suggest that allo-bone marrow transplantation (BMT) or auto-BMT as post-remission therapy offers no survival advantage over intensive chemotherapy, except perhaps for patients with high-risk or Ph1-positive ALL.[29]

Total Body Irradiation

Total body irradiation (TBI) is one of the essential treatment modalities used in certain hematologic, oncologic, and immunologic diseases and has been used in conjunction with chemotherapy as a conditioning regimen, principally for BMT or peripheral blood stem cell transplantation.[30,31] Allogeneic stem cell transplantation cures hematologic malignancies through two major mechanisms. The pre-transplantation conditioning regimen kills leukemic cells directly, either eradicating the malignancy or reducing it to a minimal residual disease state. The second mechanism is a graft-versus-tumor effect. The relative importance of these two mechanisms differs from disease to disease: graft-versus-tumor effects are most important in CML and less important, although demonstrable, in AML and ALL.[32]

Goals of TBI are:

- Eradicating diseased marrow,
- Reducing tumor burden,
- Immunosuppression,
- Deplete the BM to allow physical space for engraftment of healthy donor marrow. TBI may be particularly important in the setting of matched-unrelated donor transplants, when adequate immunosuppression is essential. The total dose of fractionated TBI needs to be increased to have a similar immunosuppressive effect as single-dose TBI. There are some suggestions that AML is not (or only slightly) sensitive to fractionation. In such a case, one should favor the fractionated schemes. For CML, in contrast, available data suggest a significant fractionation sensitivity, which should lead to favor an increase in total dose for fractionated schemes (or again to resort to single dose TBI). For ALL and lymphomas, data remain too few and controversial to allow firm conclusions.[33] TBI in daily or twice-daily fractions appears to improve the therapeutic ratio, allowing higher radiation doses. Myeloablative regimens delivering 12 Gy at 2 Gy/fraction, twice daily, over 3 days, in combination with chemotherapy are most commonly employed. Dose of 15–16 Gy showed no improvement in OS (may be due to increased mortality unrelated to relapse).[34]

CHRONIC LEUKEMIAS

Chronic Myelogenous Leukemia

Chronic myelogenous leukemia is the clonal expansion of the primitive hematopoietic stem cells. It involves myeloid, erythroid, megakaryocytic, and, sometimes, lymphoid elements. Clinically, the disease may manifest in one of its several phases: an initial chronic indolent phase of 3–4 years with progression to an accelerated phase and finally an acute transformation to blast phase, which occurs in 75–85% of patients, with a survival of 3–6 months. Imatinib is a relatively nontoxic oral medication that has been shown to be effective in inducing remissions of CML in chronic and accelerated phases. Allogeneic transplantation can cure a substantial proportion of patients with CML. Palliative RT may be of benefit in those patients with massive splenomegaly; chloromas (which may also occur with AML) are responsive to modest doses of RT.[35] Symptomatic problems from chloromas or leukemic infiltration of the spleen may be readily relieved with RT to doses of 10–20 Gy.[36]

Chronic Lymphocytic Leukemia

Ninety-five percent of cases of CLL are B cell in origin.[37] The usual course is characterized by gradual progression from no significant physical findings to lymphadenopathy, gradual increase in peripheral blood count with increasing splenomegaly, sometimes, massive in size. Nonlymphoid organ involvement may occur with advanced stage of disease. As disease progression occurs, anemia and thrombocytopenia occur. Asymptomatic early-stage patients may be followed without therapy. About 20% of such patients will have an indolent course indefinitely.

Because this disease is generally not curable, occurs in an elderly population and often progresses slowly, it is most often treated in a conservative fashion.[38] In asymptomatic patients, treatment may be deferred until the patient becomes symptomatic as the disease progresses. Treatment ranges from periodic observation with treatment of infectious, hemorrhagic, or immunologic complications to a variety of therapeutic options, including steroids, alkylating agents, purine analogs, combination chemotherapy, monoclonal antibodies, and transplant options.[38] Radiotherapy is used in the management of painful splenomegaly or occasionally for cytopenias associated with splenomegaly when splenectomy is not an option. It is also indicated in instances of unresponsive disease to alleviate symptomatic adenopathy or nonlymphoid organ involvement.[37]

LYMPHOMAS

A lymphoma is a lymphoid malignancy that involves lymph nodes and/or other extramedullary sites. They are broadly classified as being Hodgkin or non-Hodgkin and are treated with very different therapies (Table 1).[1]

Epidemiology

Non-Hodgkin's lymphoma (NHL) is the most common in the developed world, with the highest incidence in USA, Australia and New Zealand, Europe and the lowest in eastern and south-central Asia.[39] The median age of NHL in Asian

Table 1: Important features of Non-Hodgkin's Lymphomas and Hodgkin's Lymphomas[1]

Non-Hodgkin lymphomas	*Hodgkin lymphomas*
• **Precursor lymphoid neoplasms** – May arise as leukemias or lymphomas (B or T lymphoblastic leukemia/lymphoma) – Composed of immature B or T cells • **Mature B-cell lymphomas** – Small B-cell lymphomas (most are low grade except mantle cell) ◆ Chronic lymphocytic leukemia/small lymphocytic lymphoma - Usually presents as a leukemia - In lymph nodes, vaguely nodular pattern with proliferation centers - Some risk of transformation to diffuse large B-cell lymphoma (DLBCL) ◆ Follicular lymphoma (FL) - Usually presents in lymph nodes with widespread disease at presentation - Nodular proliferation of monotonous crowded abnormal germinal centers - Some risk of transformation to DLBCL ◆ Mantle cell lymphoma (MCL) - Usually present in lymph nodes with widespread disease at presentation - Diffuse sheets of monotonous small lymphocytes - Unlike other small B cell lymphomas, it behaves aggressively clinically ◆ Marginal zone lymphoma (MZL) - Three settings—nodal, splenic, or mucosa-associated lymphoid tissue (MALT) – More aggressive B-cell lymphomas ◆ Diffuse large B-cell lymphoma - Usually involves lymph nodes, but commonly involves extranodal sites - Subdivided into various subtypes based on clinical setting, immunophenotype, associations with viruses, morphology - May be de novo or arise out of a lower grade lymphoma ◆ Burkitt's lymphoma - Extranodal involvement very common (especially GI in the Western world) - Sheets of medium size lymphoid cells with a "starry sky" - Some cases are Epstein-Barr virus (EBV) related - Very aggressive and very rapid doubling time - Three clinical and genetic subtypes: endemic, sporadic, and immunodeficiency-related. • **Mature T/natural killer (NK) cell lymphomas** – Peripheral T-cell lymphoma, not otherwise specified (PTCL-NOS) ◆ Most commonly nodal, but may be extranodal ◆ Aggressive clinical course ◆ Diffuse sheets of small, medium, and large atypical lymphoid cells admixed with histiocytes and eosinophils – Anaplastic large cell lymphoma ◆ Most cases are anaplastic lymphoma kinase (ALK) positive ◆ Sinusoidal infiltrate of large atypical cells with reniform or horseshoe-shaped nuclei	• Characterized by contiguous spread • Neoplastic cells are the Reed-Sternberg (RS) cells and Hodgkin cells • Majority of cells seen are reactive lymphocytes, histiocytes, granulocytes, and eosinophils with only relatively few neoplastic cells • Classified as classical or nodular lymphocyte predominant based on immunophenotype of the neoplastic cells **REAL** (Revised European American Lymphoma) **Classification (1994):** • Classical Hodgkin lymphoma (HL): – Nodular sclerosis HL. – Mixed-cellularity HL. – Lymphocyte depletion HL. – Lymphocyte-rich classical HL. • Nodular lymphocyte—predominant HL. *Nodular sclerosis HL*: It is the most common subtype and is composed of large tumor nodules showing scattered lacunar classical RS cells set in a background of reactive lymphocytes, eosinophils and plasma cells with varying degrees of collagen fibrosis/sclerosis. *Mixed-cellularity HL*: This subtype is composed of numerous classic RS cells admixed with numerous inflammatory cells including lymphocytes, histiocytes, eosinophils, and plasma cells without sclerosis. This type is most often associated with EBV infection. *Lymphocyte depletion HL*: This is a rare subtype, composed of large numbers of often pleomorphic RS cells with only few reactive lymphocytes which may easily be confused with diffuse large cell lymphoma. Many cases previously classified within this category would now be reclassified under anaplastic large cell lymphoma. *Lymphocyte-rich classical HL*: This is a rare subtype. It has many features which may cause diagnostic confusion with nodular lymphocyte predominant B-cell non-Hodgkin's lymphoma (B-NHL). This form also has the most favorable prognosis.

countries is significantly lower, compared to the population-based registration in western countries. The Hematological Malignancy Research Network reported that the median age of their patients was 68 years.[40] However, the median age in Asian countries is younger, about 52–66 years.[41,42] In most of the countries, there has been an increase in the incidence of NHL, there is also statistically significant increase in the incidence of NHL in all the Indian registries.[43]

Hodgkin's lymphoma (HL) is among the most common malignancies of young adults. HL is rare in children younger than 10 years of age; the median age of patients at the time of diagnosis is 26 years. The incidence of HL has a bimodal peak as a function of age.[44] The early peak, from ages 25–30 years, shows an incidence of approximately 5.5 per 100,000 per year. A second peak, from ages 75 to 80 years, shows a similar incidence.

Diagnostic Confirmation and Staging Work-Up (Table 2)

- Excision biopsy of an enlarged lymph node: Evaluation of the specimen by a hematopathologist including immunophenotyping. Generally, needle biopsies are insufficient for a proper diagnosis.
- History with attention to B symptoms.
- Complete physical examination and documentation of measurable disease.
- Laboratory tests include:
  - Complete blood count (CBC), erythrocyte sedimentation rate (ESR)
  - Biochemical tests of liver function, renal function, and serum uric acid, lactate dehydrogenase (LDH), serum albumin.
- Computed tomography (CT) scan of the chest, abdomen, and pelvis are used for evaluation. CT scan of the neck is useful, particularly, if the neck or upper chest is involved.
- Baseline gallium scans or positron emission tomography (PET) scans can be useful. PET scan is increasingly favored for staging because of evidence of higher sensitivity and accuracy, particularly, in the spleen.
- Bone marrow biopsy of at least one posterior iliac crest for those with abnormal CBC or clinical stage IIB, III, or IV.
- Lumbar puncture with cytology in patients at risk for CNS disease; diffuse large B-cell lymphoma (DLBCL) with elevated LDH level and more than one extranodal site and/or aggressive lymphoma in the BM. All Burkitt's lymphoma and AIDS-related lymphoma (ARL) cases should be assessed.

PET-CT: PET-CT is accurate for baseline staging and yields important prognostic information for determining the most appropriate initial treatment (Table 3). Used for evaluation of treatment response, PET-CT can depict residual viable malignant lesions with greater accuracy than can other imaging techniques.[45]

Table 2 Staging [Ann Arbor/American Joint Committee for Cancer (AJCC) and Cotswold]

Stage I	Involvement of single lymph node region or lymphoid structure (spleen, thymus, Waldeyer's ring), or involvement of a single extralymphatic site (IE)
Stage II	Involvement of two or more lymph node regions on the same side of the diaphragm (II), which may be accompanied by localized contiguous involvement of an extralymphatic organ or site (IIE). The number of anatomic sites may be indicated by numeric subscript
Stage III	Involvement of lymph node regions on both sides of the diaphragm (III), which may also be accompanied by localized involvement of an associated extralymphatic organ or site (IIIE), by involvement of the spleen (IIIS), or both (IIIE + S)
Stage IV	Disseminated involvement of one or more extralymphatic organs, with or without associated lymph node involvement, or isolated extralymphatic organ involvement with distant (nonregional) nodal involvement Each stage is divided into A and B categories: B for those with defined systemic symptoms and A for those without
X	A mass > 10 cm or a mediastinal mass larger than one third of the thoracic diameter
E	Involvement of a single extranodal site contiguous to a known nodal site
B symptoms	B symptoms: Unexplained weight loss of more than 10% of body weight over the previous 6 months, explained fever of > 35°C, and drenching night sweats

Management of Newly Diagnosed Hodgkin's Lymphoma

Hodgkin's lymphoma is considered to be a curable malignancy, but therapies for this disease can have significant long-term toxicity. Therefore, advances in treatment protocols have sought to minimize the treatment given to patients with early-stage, low-risk disease and safely maximize the treatment given to patients with disease that is likely to be refractory to standard therapies.[46]

Standard HL treatment protocols for both adult and pediatric HL patients have employed risk-adapted therapy, in which patients with more adverse prognostic factors receive more intensive therapy (Table 4). Differences in treatment between adult and pediatric protocols are largely related to age-specific concerns regarding the late effects of alkylating agents, anthracycline, and radiation.

Clinical Features

More than 80% of patients present with cervical lymph node enlargement, and more than 50% have mediastinal

Table 3 International Harmonization Project Criteria for Assessment of Response to Therapy for Lymphoma[47]

Response	*FDG-avid at baseline*	*Not FDG-avid at baseline*
Complete remission	Complete resolution of FDG-avid lesions and negative result of bone marrow biopsy	Return to normal size of lymphadenopathy with complete resolution of extranodal disease
Partial remission	> 50% decrease in sum or product of diameters of lesions with persistent residual FDG uptake in at least one site	> 50% decrease in sum or product of diameters of lesions
Progressive disease	Any new FDG-avid lesion; ≥ 50% increase in sum or product of diameters of previously involved sites with respect to nadir sum or product of diameters associated with abnormal FDG uptake; or new or recurrent bone marrow involvement	Any new lesion > 1.5 cm in any axis; ≥ 50% increase in sum or product of diameters of previously involved sites with respect to nadir sum or product of diameters; or new or recurrent bone marrow involvement
Stable disease	No complete remission, partial remission, or progressive disease	No complete remission, partial remission, or progressive disease

Abbreviation: FDG, fludeoxyglucose

Table 4 Risk groups employed in selected trials of pediatric and adult HL

Study group	*Risk features (RF)*	*Low risk*	*Intermediate/Early unfavorable risk*	*High risk*
Pediatric				
Children's Oncology Group		IA/IIA no bulk or extranodal extension	IA bulk or "E" extension IB IIA bulk or "E" extension IIB, IIIA, IVA	IIIB, IVB
German Multicenter Studies		IA/B IIA	IIB IIIEA IIIB	IIEB IIIEA/B IIIB, IVA/B
St. Jude/Stanford/ Dana Farber	Categorized as favorable or unfavorable risk by IPS	IA/IIA no bulk		IA bulk IB IIA bulk IIB, III, IV
Children's Cancer Group	Hilar lymphadenopathy > 4 sites nodal disease Bulky disease	IA/B without RFs IIA without RFs	IA/B with RFs IIA with RFs IIB IIIA/B	IV
Adult				
EORTC	Large mediastinal mass Age > 50 years Elevated ESR > 4 involved regions	I/II supradiaphragmatic without RFs	I/II supradiaphragmatic with RFs	III/IV
GHSG	Large mediastinal mass Elevated ESR Extranodal disease > 3 involved regions	I/IIA without RFs	I/IIA with > 1 risk factor IIB with elevated ESR or > 3 involved regions	IB/IIIA with large mediastinal mass or with extranodal lesions III/IV
ECOG-NCIC	Histology (LD or MC) Age > 40 years Elevated ESR or B symptoms Four or more involved regions	I/II without risk factors	I/II with > 1 risk factors	I/II with massive mediastinal disease III/IV

Abbreviations: IPS, International Prognostic Score; EORTC, European Organization for Research and Treatment of Cancer; GHSG, German Hodgkin Study Group; ESR, erythrocyte sedimentation rate; ECOG-NCIC, Eastern Cooperative Oncology Group-National Cancer Institute of Canada

adenopathy. Lymph nodes are usually nontender, firm, and rubbery.

Constitutional Symptoms (B Symptoms)

- Unexplained fever (temperature, > 38°C)
- Drenching night sweats
- Unexplained weight loss (> 10% of body weight, more than 6 months before the diagnosis)

Other symptoms important to note are fatigue, weakness, anorexia, alcohol-induced nodal pain, and pruritus.

Unfavorable Prognostic Features

The most important unfavorable prognostic features for Hodgkin's disease (HD) are advanced stage, B symptoms, and presence of bulky disease.

- Advanced stage (IIIB and IV)
- Presence of B symptoms
- Bulky disease defined as greater than 10-cm diameter, particularly in the mediastinum (more than one third of chest diameter)
- Extranodal involvement (liver, spleen, and BM)
- Patients older than 40 years
- Increased ESR (B symptoms + ESR > 30, or no B symptoms and ESR > 70)
- Histology
  - *Unfavorable:* Mixed cellularity and lymphocyte depletion
  - *Favorable:* Lymphocyte-predominant and nodular sclerosis
- Low serum albumin.

Initial treatment success in HL was observed with extended field RT alone at doses of 35–45 Gy in early stage disease.[48-50] This was followed by the introduction of a non-cross-resistant chemotherapy regimen MOPP (nitrogen mustard, vincristine, procarbazine, prednisone) for advanced stage disease in adults[51,52] and then children.[49,53-55] The MOPP regimen was replaced with ABVD (adriamycin, bleomycin, vinblastine, dacarbazine), a regimen initially developed for use as a salvage therapy in adults relapsing after MOPP or RT.[56] ABVD is more effective at curing HL than MOPP; it is significantly less likely to induce second leukemias or permanent gonadal toxicity.[57-59]

Treatment of Favorable Risk Disease

Adult Patients

- The standard treatment of stage IA/IIA nonbulky adult HL: combined modality therapy (CMT) with two to four cycles of ABVD followed by 30 Gy involved-field radiotherapy (IFRT) (Table 5).[46,60]
- Excellent disease-free survival (DFS) and OS have been reported in the combined modality setting using IFRT fields limited to lymph node regions with radiologically enlarged nodes, and the dose can be decreased from 40 Gy to 30 Gy (and possibly lower) without compromising outcome.[61-63]

Efforts to eliminate RT from the treatment of all adults with favorable risk disease have not been uniformly followed as there is superior recurrence-free survival (RFS) with CMT.[64,65]

Pediatric Patients

- Several multi-institutional trials demonstrate that children and adolescents with stage IA/IIA nonbulky HL can be effectively treated with two to four cycles of chemotherapy followed by 15–25 Gy IFRT.[66]
- The German-Austrian Multicenter Trial DAL-HD-95 treated favorable risk patients with two cycles of chemotherapy,[67] RT was omitted among patients achieving a complete response with the remaining patients receiving 20–35 Gy IFRT demonstrated relapse rates less than 10%.
- The chemotherapy protocols in children differ from adult protocols by modifying chemotherapy exposure according to sex to minimize the gonadotoxic effects of alkylating agents on males. Several regimens have successfully eliminated the use of alkylating agents altogether for favorable risk disease.[68,69]
- Efforts to eliminate RT in children with favorable risk disease have been studied in The Children's Oncology Group low-risk HL protocol (AHOD 0431) and EORTC/GELA H9F trial;[70] the results have shown that CT-evaluated complete response to a full course of chemotherapy is not a sufficiently accurate indicator of long-term disease control to omit IFRT without increasing the risk of relapse. The use of advanced imaging techniques including interim PET may help define those patients in whom RT can be omitted.

Treatment of Intermediate or High Risk Disease

Adult Patients

- *Low stage unfavorable HL:* The standard of care is CMT. Multi-institutional studies have examined type of chemotherapy [MOPP-ABV or ABVD or BEACOPP (Bleomycin, Etoposide, Adriamycin, Cyclophosphamide, Oncovin, Procarbazine, Prednisolone)], number of cycles, and radiation dose and fields. Practice guidelines recommend therapy with ABVD for four to six cycles followed by IFRT, for low-stage unfavorable/intermediate risk HL.[71]
- *Advanced stage (IIIB/IV):* The standard treatment for advanced-stage disease is combination chemotherapy. ABVD for six to eight cycles has been shown to be superior and improved toxicity profile over MOPP.[58,59,71] The role of RT in adults with advanced stage HL

Table 5 Trials of therapy for favorable Hodgkin lymphoma

Trial	*Treatment regimens*	*#Pts*	*Outcome*		*Follow-up (y)*
Adult					
SWOG[60]			FFTF	OS	3
	3 AV STNI (36–40 Gy)	165	94%	98%	
	STNI (36–40 Gy)	161	81%	96%	
EORTC/GELA			P < 0.0001	P NS	
H8F[46]			EFS (5 y)	OS (10 y)	7.5
	3 MOPP/ABV IFRT (36 Gy)	271	98%	97%	
	STNI	272	74%	92%	
HD10[72]	2 ABVD IFRT (20 Gy)	210	OS (all)	99%	
	4 ABVD IFRT (30 Gy)	218			
	4 ABVD IFRT (20 Gy)	215			
Pediatric					
SFOP MDH90[73]	4 VBVP IFRT (20 Gy) (good responders)	202	EFS 91%	97.5% (all)	5
	4 VBVP 1-2 OPPA IFRT (20-40 Gy) (poor responders)		OS	78%	
Stanford/St. Jude Dana Farber[74]	4 VAMP IFRT (15–25.5 Gy)	110	EFS	96.1%	10
			OS	89.4%	
Children's Cancer			EFS	OS	3
Group[75]	4 COPP/ABV	46	91%	100%	
	4 COPP/ABV IFRT (21 Gy)	54	97%	100%	
GPOH HD90[76]	2 OPPA/OEPA IFRT (20–35 Gy)	267	EFS	OS	5
			94%	99.6%	
GPOH HD90[77]		281	DFS	OS	3
	2 OPPA/OEPA (no RT if CR)	(28%)	97%	97% (all)	
	2 OPPA/OEPA IFRT (20–35Gy)		94%		

Abbreviations: SWOG, Southwest Oncology Group; AV, adriamycin and vinblastine; STNI, subtotal nodal irradiation; FFTF, freedom from treatment failure; OS, overall survival; EORTC/GELA, European Organisation for Research and Treatment of Cancer/Group d'Etude des Lymphome d'Adulte; MOPP/ABV, mechlorethamine, vincristine, prednisone, procarbazine/adriamycin, bleomycin, vinblastine; IFRT, involved field radiotherapy; EBVP, epirubicin, bleomycin, vinblastine, prednisone; ABVD, adriamycin, bleomycin, vinblastine, dacarbazine; VBVP, vinblastine, bleomycin, etoposide, prednisone; VPPA, vincristine, procarbazine, prednisone, adriamycin; VAMP, vinblastine, adriamycin, methotrexate, prednisone; CVPP/ABV, cyclophosphamide, vincristine, procarbazine, prednisone/adriamycin, bleomycin, vinblastine; VEPA, vincristine, etoposide, prednisone, adriamycin; DFS, disease-free survival

seems limited. Several randomized trials of adults in CR following chemotherapy for advanced stage HL found no benefit to the addition of RT in this context. Current guidelines recommend considering the use of IFRT after chemotherapy only to sites of initial bulky disease or remaining PET avid disease at the completion of chemotherapy.[71,78] Randomized trials have established that consolidation of first CR with high-dose therapy and autologous stem-cell transplantation has no benefit in progression-free or overall survival.[79]

Pediatric Patients

The outcome of pediatric patients with unfavorable risk factors is also substantially improved with intensification of chemotherapy, although the use of IFRT in advanced stage disease in children differs from that in adults in that several pediatric protocols use IFRT to all initially involved sites after chemotherapy.[80]

Response adapted therapy: Interim ^{18}F-FDG PET in advanced-stage disease has high sensitivity and specificity[81] and is better than the international prognostic score in prediction of outcome.[82] Treatment can be tailored according to the results of interim PET scans in advanced disease. However, the optimal time to evaluate treatment response with FDG-PET is unclear, and the outcome of patients with discordant CT and FDG-PET results is unknown.

GENERAL RADIATION THERAPY GUIDELINES

Radiotherapy in the treatment of lymphoma remains the most effective single modality. Success of RT as single modality requires treatment of all clinically involved lymph nodes and regions at risk (nodal and extranodal). In order to minimize late sequelae, one should consider to reduce both treatment volume and overall treatment dose but without compromising the excellent disease control.

In the current era of combined modality treatment, modern imaging should be integrated with three-dimensional planning and advanced techniques of RT treatment delivery, so that the role of reduced volume and reduced doses is addressed. The classic wide-fields and involved-field techniques should be complemented by the use of CT and PET imaging and volumes are defined based on the International Commission on Radiation Units and Measurements (ICRU) concepts of gross tumor volume (GTV), clinical target volume (CTV) and planning target volume (PTV). Contrast enhanced 3-mm CT should be done to delineate the target volumes.[83]

CLASSIC RADIATION FIELDS

Mantle Field

The radiation field that covers most lymph node areas above the diaphragm is called the "mantle".[84] Extending from the base of the mandible to the diaphragm, the mantle field covers the submandibular, cervical, supraclavicular, infraclavicular, axillary, mediastinal, and hilar nodal areas. Individually contoured blocks shield the lungs and the cardiac apex. In addition, depending on anatomy and disease location, supplementary blocks are placed over the humeral heads, occiput, and mouth, posteriorly and anteriorly. Blocks are inserted to shield the larynx anteriorly and the cervical cord posteriorly throughout the treatment course. If high cervical lymph nodes (above the thyroid notch) are involved, the preauricular nodes are treated prophylactically to a dose of 30–36 Gy.

Subdiaphragmatic Fields

The classic subdiaphragmatic radiation field for HD is the inverted Y (Fig. 1), which includes the major lymph node regions from the diaphragm to the femoral area. Sequential treatment to the mantle and inverted Y fields is termed "total lymphoid irradiation" (TLI). The upper field, called the "para-aortic field," includes all the para-aortic lymph nodes between the aortic bifurcation and the bottom of the mantle field. This field also includes the spleen and the splenic hilar nodes. If the spleen has been removed, only the splenic pedicle is included. Attention should be paid to the location of the kidneys, and proper shielding can decrease the irradiated renal volume. The inferior border of the para-aortic field is placed at the bottom of the L4 vertebral body.

The pelvic field encompasses the iliac, inguinal, and femoral nodes. The superior border is at the level of L5, matched with an appropriate gap to the bottom of the para-aortic field. A customized block shields the midline structures that are not at risk. The large central block covers the bladder, rectum, and the centrally transposed ovaries in female patients and the testes in male patients. A scrotal shield can be used to decrease the dose to the testes or the centrally placed ovaries to 3–8% of the fractionated total dose. Iliac wing blocks are placed to spare BM.

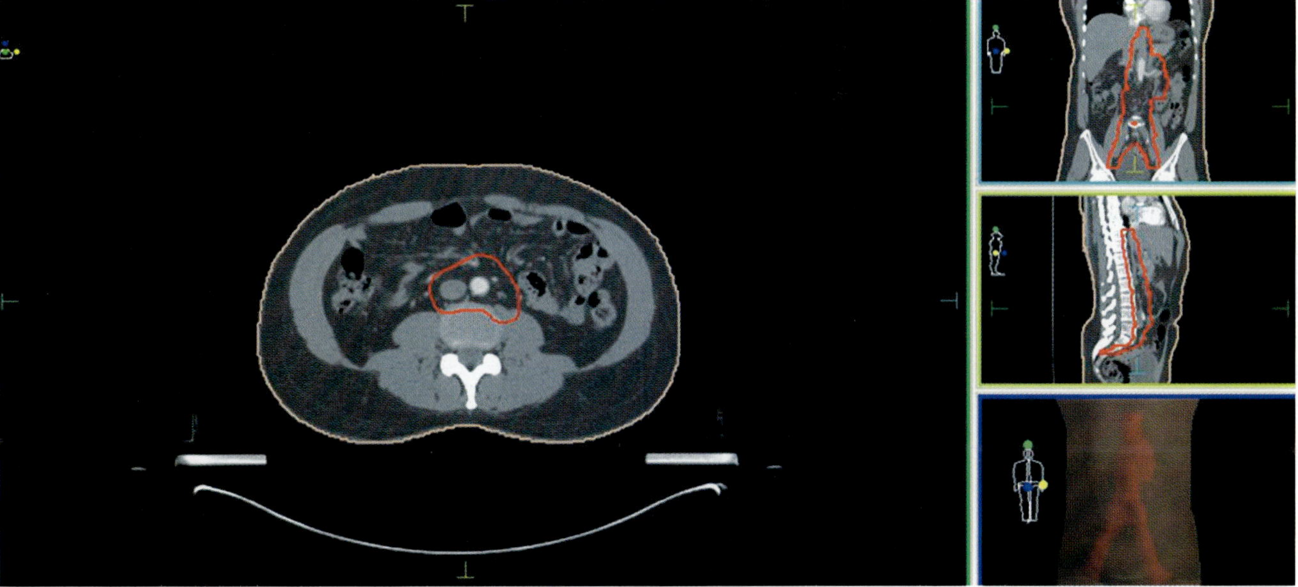

Fig. 1 Subdiaphragmatic radiation field for Hodgkin's disease (HD) is the inverted Y, which includes the major lymph node regions from the diaphragm to the femoral area

Often, it is not necessary to treat the pelvic lymph nodes, and only the mantle and the para-aortic fields are irradiated in sequence subtotal lymphoid irradiation (STLI).

The large field techniques although appear elegant (as used with the given technology of the 1970s), such techniques are no longer relevant to modern RT. These wide-field RT have limited role in the salvage treatment in patients who fail chemotherapy and are unsuitable for more intensive treatment schedules. For first-line treatment, randomized controlled trials in HL have shown that IFRT along with multiagent chemotherapeutic agents is equivalent to extended-field RT for survival.[46,61]

Short-course chemotherapy with IFRT for early-stage low-risk NHL, is also equivalent to more extended combination chemotherapy schedules and there is no role for extended-field treatment.[85]

The two main variables in radiation treatment are treatment volume and treatment dose. Radiotherapy guidelines for lymphoma based on involved fields defined by anatomical landmarks are no longer applicable in the modern era. There is increasing concern about the late effects of treatment and there is a strong impetus to minimize radiation exposure.

Involved-Field Radiotherapy

Radiation delivery is limited to the lymph node region involved with macroscopic lymphoma (Fig. 2). IFRT is based on pre-chemotherapy anatomical node region involved, thus the involved field includes the entire neck including the supraclavicular fossa when a neck node was involved; the entire mediastinum and supraclavicular nodes for mediastinal involvement; the entire para-aortic chain for para-aortic node disease and typically inguinal and ipsilateral iliac nodes for groin node disease.[86]

In the last decade, IFRT has changed from a two-dimensional field to a three-dimensional volume as CT planning has been introduced, although the principles are the same, the nodal volume are defined more accurately on an individual basis.[87]

Involved-Site Radiotherapy

This is based on a modified involved field, defining the site of gross disease before chemotherapy, the GTV and using a CT-based volume with an expansion to form a CTV in the cranio-caudal direction (Fig. 3). The post-chemotherapy involved nodal chain and residual disease form the CTV in all other directions as used in recent pediatric HL protocols.[77]

Involved-Node Radiotherapy

This is similar to involved-site RT basing the definition of the CTV on pre-chemotherapy imaging, including PET.[88] The principal distinction between involved-node RT and involved-site RT is that no additional margin around the node volume is added in involved-node RT. The CTV is defined by the pre-chemotherapy node volume and image fusion is recommended to reproduce this at the time of RT planning. Normal tissue structures, such as muscle previously displaced by an enlarged node, are excluded from the CTV, as are other normal structures, such as large vessels, whenever possible. The PTV is then defined by adding the necessary margin for set-up error and organ motion.

Immobilization and Imaging Techniques

Modern lymphoma planning should incorporate the current conventions defined in International Commission on Radiation Units and Measurements Report (ICRU-50) based on defining a GTV, a CTV, and a PTV.[83] The PTV is

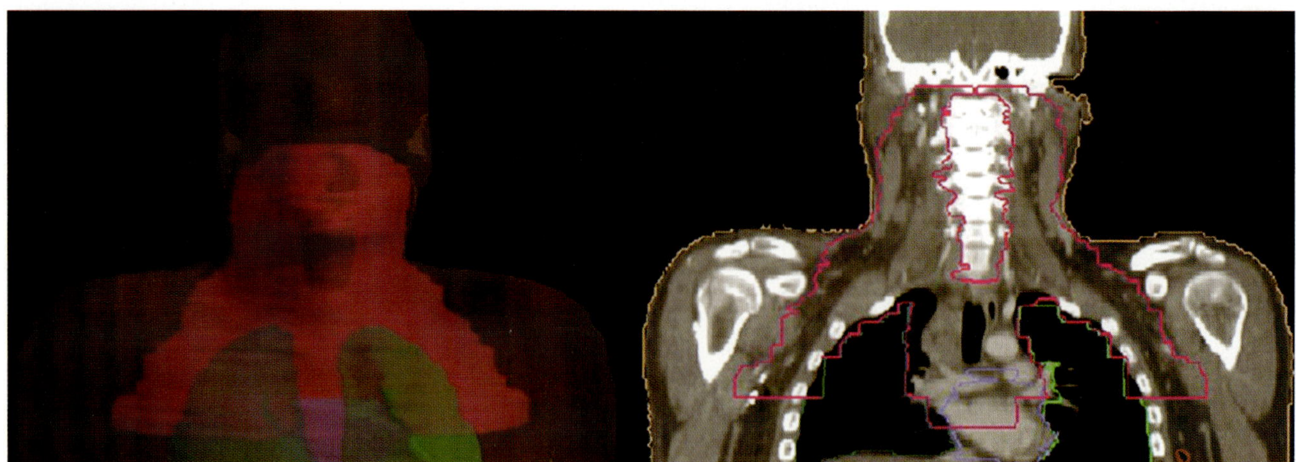

Fig. 2 Involved-field radiotherapy has been changing from a two-dimensional field defined by anatomical structures to a three-dimensional volume as CT-planning has been introduced

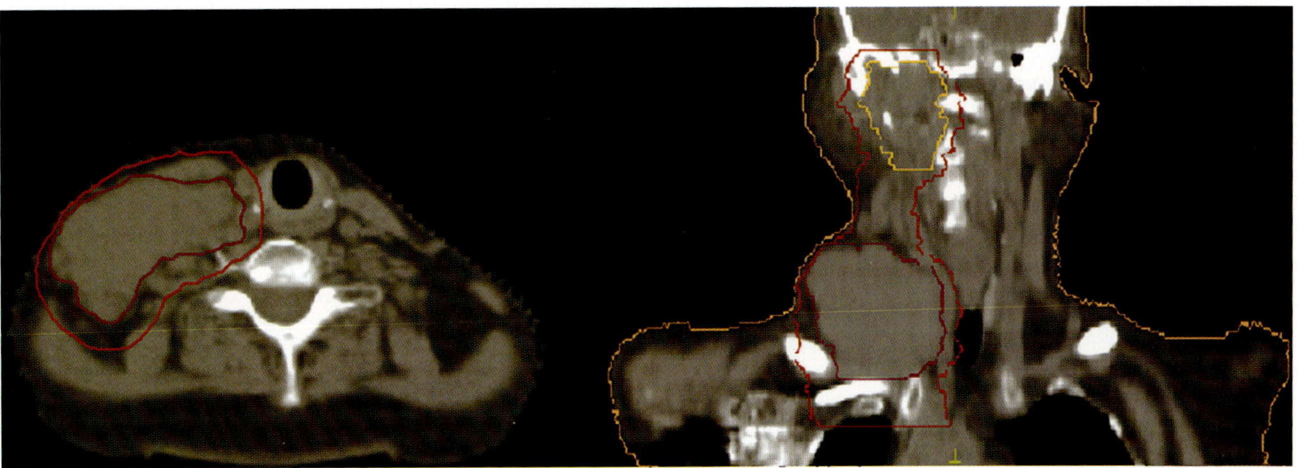

Fig. 3 Involved-site radiotherapy, based on a modified involved field. The post-chemotherapy involved nodal chain and residual disease form the CTV

then used to define beam coverage. Well-defined atlases[89-91] should be referred to when outlining lymph node anatomy on CT. Planning CT should be taken with the patient having appropriate immobilization. Contiguous slices with a slice thickness of no more than 3 mm should be taken through the region of interest. It is recommended that intravenous contrast be given to improve identification of the node chains.

Gross Tumor and Clinical Target Volumes

Imaging done prior to starting chemotherapy is used to define the superior and inferior extent of original disease, and it expanded craniocaudally by a margin of 1.5 cm in the direction of potential lymphatic spread. These margins are added because prechemotherapy imaging is not carried out in the RT treatment position and does not use the same immobilization techniques. The margins allow for both positional and anatomical changes as well as the uncertainties in image co-registration. It is not always necessary to encompass entire nodal regions or adjacent areas. In the transverse plane, the GTV will include the involved lymph nodes (or organ) only with any residual disease, not the whole pre-chemotherapy disease volume. The GTV should not extend into muscle planes or bone or air, unless there is invasion of the muscle or bone. The CTV should be expanded by hand as a direct three-dimensional volumetric expansion.

When pre-chemotherapy imaging is unavailable, the patient should be treated using anatomical landmarks for the involved-site RT.

Examples of involved-site radiotherapy CTVs can be seen below:

- Supradiaphragmatic sites: These include cervical nodal chains, supraclavicular fossae, axillae, mediastinum and hilum. If disease is confined to the superior mediastinum, only the superior mediastinum is treated. The entire pericardial and pleural cavities are *not* irradiated if the pericardial or pleural effusions present initially resolve after chemotherapy. Similarly, when there is parenchymal involvement of the lung then it is recommended that only residual disease, i.e. the post-chemotherapy GTV, be treated using an appropriate margin.
- *Infradiaphragmatic sites:* These include para-aortic nodes, mesenteric nodes, spleen and splenic hilum and iliac and inguinal lymph nodes. When para-aortic lymph nodes are to be treated with the spleen/splenic hilum, a single volume encompassing all sites may be used.
- Radiotherapy field may be enlarged if adjacent nodal regions are involved. Alternatively, sequential supra- and infra-diaphragmatic fields may be treated consecutively, with a calculated gap between the two and leaving a 2–3 weeks interval between treatments. Care is needed when matching the adjacent fields to avoid overlap.

Planning Target Volume

To account for organ motion and set-up errors, the CTV is expanded further to create the PTV. The margins are defined individually for each disease site and treatment center depending upon their technique, setup accuracy and consideration of internal organ motion.

Dose

It has been well-known that durable control is achieved with much lower doses of RT than those required for epithelial tumors.[92] All RT treatment schedules assume daily fractionation, 1.8–2 Gy per day, 5 days per week.

- *Hodgkin lymphoma*: The basis for modern dose prescriptions in HL results from the trials of the German Hodgkin Study Group HD1,[93] HD5,[94] HD10,[95] and HD11.[96]

The conclusion from these studies was that after four cycles of ABVD, 30 Gy is recommended for early-stage unfavorable HL, whereas 20 Gy is adequate for early-stage favorable HL after two cycles of ABVD. If early-stage unfavorable disease is treated using BEACOPP rather than ABVD, the dose may be reduced to 20 Gy.

- *Non-Hodgkin lymphoma*: Historically, doses for NHL have varied between 30 Gy and 40 Gy, with lower doses tending to be chosen for low-grade indolent lymphomas. Cohort studies have suggested that doses as low as 24 Gy in 12 fractions for "low-grade" and 30 Gy in 15 fractions for "high-grade" lymphomas are effective.[97] One exception to the results reported by Lowry et al.[98] is NK cell lymphoma, which has been shown to require higher doses of at least 50 Gy.[74] Current evidence-based recommendations for radiation dose for NHL is 24 Gy in 12 fractions for indolent lymphomas (follicular, marginal zone, small lymphocytic or chronic lymphocytic lymphoma). In the palliative setting, follicular lymphoma (FL) patients will respond to 4 Gy in two fractions.[99]

Radiation Toxicity

Late complications of mantle irradiation include lung, heart, and thyroid dysfunction; second malignancies; growth abnormalities.

Age-adjusted risk of death from myocardial infarction increases modestly in mediastinal irradiation.[100] Mediastinal doses of more than 30 Gy increases the relative risk of cardiac death to 3.5 at an average follow-up time of 9.5 years. The risk can be reduced by subcarinal blocking after 30–35 Gy.[101]

The incidence of breast cancer is increased among women who were younger than 30 years at the time of mantle irradiation; the younger the patient and the greater the radiation dose, the higher the relative risk.[102-104] The cumulative risk of developing a solid tumor such as osteosarcoma or carcinoma of the breast, thyroid, lung, stomach or colon is approximately 0.3–0.5% per year[11,12] and increases with time, particularly 10 years or more after the irradiation. Irradiated patients also have an increased risk of developing NHL[103] but not acute non-lymphocytic leukemia.

NON-HODGKIN'S LYMPHOMA

The WHO classification divides NHL into B-cell neoplasms and T-cell neoplasms, with 31 different and distinct lymphomas delineated. These specific entities are distinguished on the basis of morphologic, immunologic, and genetic characteristics. The most common ones in order of decreasing frequency, namely DLBCL, FL, marginal zone lymphoma (MZL), mantle cell lymphoma (MCL), peripheral T-cell lymphoma (PTCL), and small lymphocytic lymphoma B-cell/chronic lymphocytic leukemia (SLLB-CLL).

Clinical Features

Non-Hodgkin's lymphoma may involve lymph nodes in almost any area of the body but may also present in extranodal sites. Approximately two-thirds of NHL is nodal at presentation[97] and one-third is extranodal, in contrast to HD, where extranodal presentation is rare. NHL is primarily a disease of older adults (in contrast to HD), with a median age at presentation from 55 years to 65 years.[97,105]

Staging Evaluation

The pretreatment evaluation for NHL is similar to that for HL and should include physical examination, with attention to node-bearing areas, including Waldeyer's ring, and the size of liver and spleen; assessment of B symptoms (i.e. fever, night sweats, weight loss) and performance status.

To identify subgroups of patients most likely to relapse, an international prognostic index was compiled for 2,031 patients with aggressive NHL.[106] One point is assigned for presence of each of the following risk factors:

- Age (< 60 years vs > 60 years).
- Serum LDH (normal vs elevated).
- Performance status [Eastern Cooperative Oncology Group (ECOG) or Zubrod's 0 or 1 vs 2–4].
- Stage (stage I or stage II vs stage III or stage IV).
- Extranodal site involvement (0 or 1 vs 2–4).

The sum of the points allotted correlates with the following risk groups (Table 6).

Diffuse Large B-Cell Lymphoma

Immunophenotypically, DLBCL expresses various pan-B markers such as CD19, CD20, CD22, and CD79a. Proliferation rates, measured by immunohistochemical staining with the antibody Ki-67, are usually high, and tumors in which 90% or more of the cells are positive for Ki-67 have been linked with particularly poor outcome.[107] The molecular heterogeneity of these tumors, reflected in differences in their gene expression patterns, may account for some of the variation in tumor proliferation rate, host response to therapy, and differentiation state of the tumor. Patients who have an elevated serum LDH level and more than one extranodal site of disease are at high risk for recurrent disease in the CNS, which carries a poor prognosis.[108] Patients with testicular involvement are also at increased risk for CNS involvement.[109]

Table 6 International Prognostic Index risk score[106]

Risk	*Points*	*5-year survival*
Low risk	0–1	73%
Low-intermediate risk	2	51%
High-intermediate risk	3	43%
High risk	4–5	26%

Table 7 Drug combinations are used in aggressive NHL

ACVBP	doxorubicin + cyclophosphamide + vindesine + bleomycin + prednisone
CHOP	cyclophosphamide + doxorubicin + vincristine + prednisone
CNOP	cyclophosphamide + mitoxantrone + vincristine + prednisone
m-BACOD	methotrexate + bleomycin + doxorubicin + cyclophosphamide + vincristine + dexamethasone + leucovorin
MACOP-B	methotrexate + doxorubicin + cyclophosphamide + vincristine + prednisone fixed dose + bleomycin + leucovorin
ProMACE CytaBOM	prednisone + doxorubicin + cyclophosphamide + etoposide + cytarabine + bleomycin + vincristine + methotrexate + leucovorin
R-CHOP	rituximab, an anti-CD20 monoclonal antibody, + cyclophosphamide + doxorubicin + vincristine + prednisone

The most common treatment strategy for stage I or II disease has been anthracycline-based chemotherapy followed by radiation (Table 7). In 1993, the National High Priority Intergroup Phase III trial compared CHOP (consisting of cyclophosphamide, hydroxydaunomycin, vincristine, and prednisone), MACOP-B (methotrexate + doxorubicin + cyclophosphamide + vincristine + prednisone fixed dose + bleomycin + leucovorin), ProMACE-CytaBOM (prednisone + doxorubicin + cyclophosphamide + etoposide + cytarabine + bleomycin + vincristine + methotrexate + leucovorin), and m-BACOD (methotrexate + bleomycin + doxorubicin + cyclophosphamide + vincristine + dexamethasone + leucovorin), demonstrating that the outcomes of the four regimens were equivalent and that CHOP was associated with the most modest toxicity. Thus, following this trial, CHOP chemotherapy emerged as the standard regimen.[109] The addition of the anti-CD20 antibody rituximab to chemotherapy (CHOP regimen) became the standard of care after showing benefit in terms of time to progression and OS time compared with CHOP alone.[110,111] The following drug combinations are used in aggressive NHL as shown in Table 7.

Whether radiation therapy has a role in the treatment of bulky stage III or IV large B-cell lymphoma remains a matter of debate. Some groups see no benefit[112,113] and others suggest that delivery of involved-field radiation to lymphomas measuring 4 cm or more before induction chemotherapy may improve disease-free and overall survival rates[114,115] but all these are retrospective studies. A prospective randomized study[116] demonstrated that addition of radiation therapy produced significant improvements in 5-year DFS rates (72% and 35%, $P < 0.01$) and OS rates (5-year rates of 81% and 55%, $P < 0.01$) in patients who experienced a complete response to anthracycline-based chemotherapy were randomly assigned to receive or not receive involved-field radiation therapy (40–50 Gy) to initially bulky sites of disease.

Follicular Lymphoma

Morphologically, these lymphomas are composed of follicles containing a mixture of centrocytes (i.e. cleaved follicle center cells or small cells) and centroblasts (i.e. noncleaved follicle center cells or large cells) that proliferate within a network of nonmalignant follicular dendritic cells and T cells. Two factors influence the course of treatment in FL. The first is the considerable variability in the course of the disease (i.e. indolent, characterized by waxing and waning versus rapid growth and massive tumors that produce symptoms that require treatment), and the second is the tendency for histologic transformation to DLBCL, which occurs at rates of 5–10% per year depending on the initial percentage of large cells in the specimen.[117]

Unlike aggressive lymphoma, FL is usually considered incurable with conventional treatment. Some investigators have concluded that deferring therapy might be appropriate in selected cases.[85] At many institutions, patients with stage I or II FLs are treated with involved-field radiation therapy. This approach has led to freedom from treatment failure rates of 41–49% and OS rates of 43–79%.[118,119] Central lymphatic irradiation is administered for clinical stage I to III FLs at some institutions,[120] central lymphatic irradiation differs from TLI in that all of the mesenteric lymph nodes are included in the CTV, consequently, wider abdominal and pelvic portals are irradiated than in TLI. Treatment with central lymphatic irradiation produced 5-year, 10-year, and 15-year RFS rates of 75%, 58%, and 58% for patients with stage I to III FLs.[121]

Chemotherapy alone is commonly recommended for patients with stage III FLs that are bulky or are causing symptoms or organ dysfunction. The use of combined-modality therapy remains controversial for patients with stage I to III FLs.[122,123] In stage III or IV FLs smaller than 10 cm, that are not causing symptoms or organ dysfunction, most oncologists advocate a watch-and-wait philosophy for previously untreated patients.[124]

Marginal Zone or Mucosa-Associated Lymphoid Tissue Lymphoma

Mucosa-associated lymphoid tissue (MALT) lymphoma can manifest as extranodal, nodal, or splenic disease. The most common presentation, extranodal, represents an infiltration of extranodal zone B cells into epithelial tissues in the gastrointestinal tract, salivary glands, breast, thyroid, prostate, skin, orbit, conjunctiva, lung, kidney, brain, or soft tissues. Microbial agents that have been linked with the development of MALT lymphoma include *Helicobacter pylori, Borrelia burgdorferi, Campylobacter jejuni*, and *Chlamydia psittaci*. Autoimmune disorders, such as Hashimoto's thyroiditis in thyroid MALT lymphoma and Sjögren's syndrome in thymic or salivary-gland MALT lymphoma, have also been implicated. The National Comprehensive Cancer Network Practice Guidelines recommend that stages IE and IIE, nongastric and *H. pylori*-negative or antibiotic-resistant gastric MALT lymphomas be treated with involved-field radiation therapy to 30–33 Gy. Rituximab, alone or in combination with chemotherapy, is used for advanced disease.[125]

Extranodal NK Cell/T-Cell Lymphoma, Nasal and Nasal Type

Pathologically, nasal NK/T-cell lymphomas show a broad morphologic spectrum, frequent angioinvasion and angiocentricity with zone necrosis, and nearly ubiquitous association with Epstein-Barr virus infection. Clinically, this entity is characterized by its predominance in young males, its tendency to manifest as localized stage I or stage II disease, its resistance to conventional chemotherapy, and its sensitivity to radiation therapy.[126] The current recommendation is that the target volume plus a generous margin should be treated to 54 Gy.[127]

Burkitt's Lymphoma

Burkitt's lymphoma is an uncommon, highly aggressive tumor of B-cell origin that often arises in extranodal sites. Treatment for Burkitt's lymphoma consists largely of dose-intensive multiagent chemotherapy, with high-dose systemic methotrexate and cytosine arabinoside used to control CNS and systemic disease. The use of radiation for CNS prophylaxis has been abandoned by most groups. For patients with stage IV disease, the recommended dose of craniospinal radiation is 24 Gy in 12 fractions over 2.5 weeks. This protocol can also be used to palliate symptoms in patients with a chemorefractory CNS recurrence.[128]

Mycosis Fungoides

Mycosis fungoides, also known as Sézary syndrome or cutaneous T-cell lymphoma, is a clinicopathologic diagnosis. Treatments used for early-stage disease have included topical steroids, topical mechlorethamine, topical retinoids, phototherapy, and total-skin electron-beam radiation therapy. Localized radiation therapy (e.g. 30 Gy in 15 fractions over 3 weeks using a 2-cm margin for visible and palpable disease)[129] and psoralen activated with ultraviolet-A light (PUVA) are effective treatment options for patients with early-stage mycosis fungoides. Total-skin electron-beam radiation therapy is typically recommended for patients who present with thick plaques or have a recent history of rapid progression of cutaneous disease and are no longer responding to topical mechlorethamine or PUVA.[130,131] At Medanta Cancer Institute, total-skin electron-beam radiation therapy is administered by using a Stanford dual fixed-angle six-field technique[129] with a Lucite scatter plate to improve dose homogeneity.

REFERENCES

1. Swerdlow SH, Campo E, Harris NL, Jaffe ES, Pileri SA, Stein H, Thiele J, Vardiman JW (Eds). WHO Classification of Tumours of the Haematopoietic and Lymphoid Tissues. IARC: Lyon; 2008.
2. Bennett JM, Catovsky D, Daniel MT, Flandrin G, Galton DA, Gralnick HR, et al. Proposals for the classification of the acute leukaemias. French-American-British (FAB) co-operative group. Br J Haematol. 1976;33(4):451-8.
3. Vardiman JW, Thiele J, Arber DA, Brunning RD, Borowitz MJ, Porwit A, et al. The 2008 revision of the World Health Organization (WHO) classification of myeloid neoplasms and acute leukemia: rationale and important changes. Blood. 2009;114(5):937-51.
4. Smith M, Arthur D, Camitta B, Carroll AJ, Crist W, Gaynon P, et al. Uniform approach to risk classification and treatment assignment for children with acute lymphoblastic leukemia. J Clin Oncol. 1996;14(1):18-24.
5. Bürger B, Zimmermann M, Mann G, Kühl J, Löning L, Riehm H, et al. Diagnostic cerebrospinal fluid examination in children with acute lymphoblastic leukemia: significance of low leukocyte counts with blasts or traumatic lumbar puncture. J Clin Oncol. 2003;21(2):184-8.
6. World Health Organization. World Cancer Report 2014. Chapter 5.13.
7. National Cancer Institute. (2014) SEER Cancer Statistics Review (CSR) 1975-2011. [online] Available from seer.cancer.gov/csr/1975_2011/. [Accessed April, 2015].
8. Wiernik PH. Adult Leukemias. New York: BC Decker; 2001. pp. 3-15.
9. Robinette MS, Cotter S, Van de Water. Quick Look Series in Veterinary Medicine: Hematology. Teton NewMedia; 2001. p. 105.
10. Stass SA, Schumacher HR, Rock WR. Handbook of Hematologic Pathology. New York, NY: Marcel Dekker; 2000. pp. 193-4.
11. Leonard B. Leukemia: A Research Report. Diane Publishing; 1998. p. 7.
12. Non-Ionizing Radiation, Part 1: Static and Extremely Low-Frequency (ELF) Electric and Magnetic Fields (IARC Monographs on the Evaluation of the Carcinogenic Risks). Geneva: World Health Organization; 2002. pp. 332-3, 338.
13. Naik RR, Saven A. My treatment approach to hairy cell leukemia. Mayo Clin Proc. 2012;87(1):67-76.

14. Hann I, Vora A, Harrison G, Harrison C, Eden O, Hill F, et al. Determinants of outcome after intensified therapy of childhood lymphoblastic leukaemia: results from Medical Research Council United Kingdom acute lymphoblastic leukaemia XI protocol. Br J Haematol. 2001;113(1):103-14.
15. American Cancer Society. (2014). Survival rates for childhood leukemia. [online] Available from www.cancer.org/acs/groups/cid/documents/webcontent/003044-pdf.pdf. [Accessed April, 2015].
16. ASH Education Book. 2010:1 47-55.
17. Kebriaei P, Champlin R, deLima M, et al. Management of acute leukemias. In: DeVita VT Jr, Lawrence TS, Rosenberg SA (Eds). Cancer: Principles and Practice of Oncology, 9th edn. Philadelphia, PA: Lippincott Williams & Wilkins; 2011. pp. 1928-54.
18. de Greef GE, van Putten WL, Boogaerts M, Huijgens PC, Verdonck LF, Vellenga E, et al. Criteria for defining a complete remission in acute myeloid leukaemia revisited. An analysis of patients treated in HOVON-SAKK co-operative group studies. Br J Haematol. 2005;128(2):184-91.
19. Cassileth PA, Lynch E, Hines JD, Oken MM, Mazza JJ, Bennett JM, et al. Varying intensity of postremission therapy in acute myeloid leukemia. Blood. 1992;79(8):1924-30.
20. Morrison FS, Kopecky KJ, Head DR, Athens JW, Balcerzak SP, Gumbart C, et al. Late intensification with POMP chemotherapy prolongs survival in acute myelogenous leukemia--results of a South west Oncology Group study of rubidazone versus adriamycin for remission induction, prophylactic intrathecal therapy, late intensification, and levamisole maintenance. Leukemia. 1992;6(7):708-14.
21. Goldstone AH, Richards SM, Lazarus HM, Tallman MS, Buck G, Fielding AK, et al. In adults with standard-risk acute lymphoblastic leukemia, the greatest benefit is achieved from a matched sibling allogeneic transplantation in first complete remission, and an autologous transplantation is less effective than conventional consolidation/maintenance chemotherapy in all patients: final results of the International ALL Trial (MRC UKALL XII/ECOG E2993). Blood. 2008;111(4):1827-33.
22. Kantarjian H, Thomas D, O'Brien S, Cortes J, Giles F, Jeha S, et al. Long-term follow-up results of hyperfractionated cyclophosphamide, vincristine, doxorubicin, and dexamethasone (Hyper-CVAD), a dose-intensive regimen, in adult acute lymphocytic leukemia. Cancer. 2004;101(12):2788-801.
23. Clarke M, Gaynon P, Hann I, Harrison G, Masera G, Peto R, et al. CNS-directed therapy for childhood acute lymphoblastic leukemia: Childhood ALL Collaborative Group overview of 43 randomized trials. J Clin Oncol. 2003;21(9):1798-809.
24. Nesbit ME, Sather HN, Robison LL, Ortega J, Littman PS, D'Angio GJ, et al. Presymptomatic central nervous system therapy in previously untreated childhood acute lymphoblastic leukaemia: comparison of 1800 rad and 2400 rad. A report for Children's Cancer Study Group. Lancet. 1981;1(8218):461-6.
25. Cortes J. Central nervous system involvement in adult acute lymphocytic leukemia. Hematol Oncol Clin North Am. 2001;15(1):145-62.
26. Larson RA, Dodge RK, Burns CP, Lee EJ, Stone RM, Schulman P, et al. A five-drug remission induction regimen with intensive consolidation for adults with acute lymphoblastic leukemia: cancer and leukemia group B study 8811. Blood. 1995;85(8):2025-37.
27. Möricke A, Reiter A, Zimmermann M, Gadner H, Stanulla M, Dördelmann M, et al. Risk-adjusted therapy of acute lymphoblastic leukemia can decrease treatment burden and improve survival: treatment results of 2169 unselected pediatric and adolescent patients enrolled in the trial ALL-BFM 95. Blood. 2008;111(9):4477-89.
28. Fière D, Lepage E, Sebban C, Boucheix C, Gisselbrecht C, Vernant JP, et al. Adult acute lymphoblastic leukemia: a multicentric randomized trial testing bone marrow transplantation as postremission therapy. The French Group on Therapy for Adult Acute Lymphoblastic Leukemia. J Clin Oncol. 1993;11(10):1990-2001.
29. Goldstone AH, Richards SM, Lazarus HM, Tallman MS, Buck G, Fielding AK, et al. In adults with standard-risk acute lymphoblastic leukemia, the greatest benefit is achieved from a matched sibling allogeneic transplantation in first complete remission, and an autologous transplantation is less effective than conventional consolidation/maintenance chemotherapy in all patients: final results of the International ALL Trial (MRC UKALL XII/ECOG E2993). Blood. 2008;111(4):1827-33.
30. Appelbaum FR. The influence of total dose, fractionation, dose rate, and distribution of total body irradiation on bone marrow transplantation. Semin Oncol. 1993;20(4):3-10; quiz 11.
31. Gilson D, Taylor RE. Total body irradiation. Report on a meeting organized by the BIR Oncology Committee, held at The Royal Institute of British Architects, London, 28 November 1996. Br J Radiol. 1997;70(840):1201-3.
32. Passweg JR, Tiberghien P, Cahn JY, Vowels MR, Camitta BM, Gale RP, et al. Graft versus leukemia effects in T-lineage and B-lineage acute lymphoblastic leukemia. Bone Marrow Transplant. 1998;21(2):153-8.
33. Cosset JM, Socié G, Girinsky T, Dubray B, Fourquet A, Gluckman E. Radiobiological and Clinical Bases for Total Body Irradiation in the Leukemias and Lymphomas. Semin Radiat Oncol. 1995;5(4):301-15.
34. Homans AC, Barker BE, Forman EN, Cornell CJ Jr, Dickerman JD, Truman JT. Immunophenotypic characteristics of cerebrospinal fluid cells in children with acute lymphoblastic leukemia at diagnosis. Blood. 1990;76(9):1807-11.
35. Bakst R, Wolden S, Yahalom J. Radiation therapy for chloroma (granulocytic sarcoma). Int J Radiat Oncol Biol Phys. 2012;82(5):1816-22.
36. Shrimali RK, Correa PD, O'Rourke N. Low-dose palliative splenic irradiation in haematolymphoid malignancy. J Med Imaging Radiat Oncol. 2008;52(3):297-302.
37. Halperin EC, Perez CA, Brady LW (Eds). Perez and Brady's Principles and Practice of Radiation Oncology, 5th edn. 2008, pp 1784-5.
38. Gribben JG, O'Brien S. Update on therapy of chronic lymphocytic leukemia. J Clin Oncol. 2011;29(5):544-50.
39. Ekström-Smedby K. Epidemiology and etiology of non-Hodgkin lymphoma – a review. Acta Oncol. 2006;45(3):258-71.
40. Smith A, Roman E, Howell D, Jones R, Patmore R, Jack A. The Haematological Malignancy Research Network (HMRN): a new information strategy for population based epidemiology and health service research. Br J Haematol. 2010;148(5):739-53.

41. Ko YH, Kim CW, Park CS, Jang HK, Lee SS, Kim SH, et al. REAL classification of malignant lymphomas in the Republic of Korea. Cancer. 1998;83(4):806-12.
42. Aoki R, Karube K, Sugita Y, Nomura Y, Shimizu K, Kimura Y, et al. Distribution of malignant lymphoma in Japan: analysis of 2260 cases, 2001–2006. Pathol Int. 2008;58(3):174-82.
43. Yeole BB. Trends in the incidence of Non-Hodgkin's lymphoma in India. Asian Pac J Cancer Prev. 2008;9(3):433-6.
44. Mauch P, Armitage J, Diehl V, Hoppe R, Weiss L. Hodgkin's Disease. Lippincott Williams & Wilkins; 1999. pp. 62-4.
45. Cronin CG, Swords R, Truong MT, Viswanathan C, Rohren E, Giles FJ, et al. Clinical Utility of PET/CT in lymphoma. AJR Am J Roentgenol. 2010;194(1):W91-W103.
46. Ferme C, Eghbali H, Meerwaldt JH. Chemotherapy plus involved- field radiation in early-stage Hodgkin's disease. N Engl J Med. 2007;357(19):1916-27.
47. Cheson BD1, Pfistner B, Juweid ME, Gascoyne RD, Specht L, Horning SJ, et al. The International Harmonization Project on Lymphoma: revised response criteria for malignant lymphoma. J Clin Oncol. 2007;25(5):579-86
48. Bayle-Weisgerber C, Lemercier N, Teillet F, Asselain B, Gout M, Schweisguth O. Hodgkin's disease in children. Results of therapy in a mixed group of 178 clinical and pathologically staged patients over 13 years. Cancer. 1984;54(2):215-22.
49. Gehan EA, Sullivan MP, Fuller LM, Johnston J, Kennedy P, Fryer C, et al. The intergroup Hodgkin's disease in children. A study of stages I and II. Cancer. 1990;65(6):1429-37.
50. Donaldson SS, Glatstein E, Rosenberg SA, et al. Pediatric Hodgkin's disease. II. Results of therapy. Cancer. 1976;37(5):2436-47.
51. Devita VT Jr, Serpick AA, Carbone PP. Combination chemotherapy in the treatment of advanced Hodgkin's disease. Ann Intern Med. 1970;73(6):881-95.
52. Longo DL, Young RC, Wesley M, Hubbard SM, Duffey PL, Jaffe ES, et al. Twenty years of MOPP therapy for Hodgkin's disease. J Clin Oncol. 1986;4(9):1295-306.
53. Donaldson SS, Link MP. Combined modality treatment with low-dose radiation and MOPP chemotherapy for children with Hodgkin's disease. J Clin Oncol. 1987;5(5):742-9.
54. Jenkin D, Doyle J, Berry M, Blanchette V, Chan H, Doherty M, et al. Hodgkin's disease in children: treatment with MOPP and low-dose, extended field irradiation without laparotomy. Late results and toxicity. Med Pediatr Oncol. 1990;18(4):265-72.
55. Oberlin O, Leverger G, Pacquement H, Raquin MA, Chompret A, Habrand JL, et al. Low-dose radiation therapy and reduced chemotherapy in childhood Hodgkin's disease: The experience of the French Society of Pediatric Oncology. J Clin Oncol. 1992;10(10):1602-8.
56. Bonadonna G, Zucali R, Monfardini S, et al. Combination chemotherapy of Hodgkin's disease with adriamycin, bleomycin, vinblastine, and imidazole carboxamide versus MOPP. Cancer. 1975;36(1):252-9.
57. Canellos GP, Anderson JR, Propert KJ, Nissen N, Cooper MR, Henderson ES, et al. Chemotherapy of advanced Hodgkin's disease with MOPP, ABVD, or MOPP alternating with ABVD. N Engl J Med. 1992;327(21):1478-84.
58. Duggan DB, Petroni GR, Johnson JL, Glick JH, Fisher RI, Connors JM, et al. Randomized comparison of ABVD and MOPP/ABV hybrid for the treatment of advanced Hodgkin's disease: report of an intergroup trial. J Clin Oncol. 2003;21(4):607-14.
59. Santoro A, Bonadonna G, Valagussa P, Zucali R, Viviani S, Villani F, et al. Long-term results of combined chemotherapy-radiotherapy approach in Hodgkin's disease: superiority of ABVD plus radiotherapy versus MOPP plus radiotherapy. J Clin Oncol. 1987;5(1):27-37.
60. Press OW, LeBlanc M, Lichter AS, Grogan TM, Unger JM, Wasserman TH, et al. Phase III randomized intergroup trial of subtotal lymphoid irradiation versus doxorubicin, vinblastine, and subtotal lymphoid irradiation for stage IA to IIA Hodgkin's disease. J Clin Oncol. 2001;19(22):4238-44.
61. Engert A, Schiller P, Josting A, Herrmann R, Koch P, Sieber M, et al. Involved-field radiotherapy is equally effective and less toxic compared with extended-field radiotherapy after four cycles of chemotherapy in patients with early-stage unfavorable Hodgkin's lymphoma: Results of the HD8 trial of the German Hodgkin's Lymphoma Study Group. J Clin Oncol. 2003;21(19):3601-8.
62. Bonadonna G, Bonfante V, Viviani S, Di Russo A, Villani F, Valagussa P. ABVD plus subtotal nodal versus involved-field radiotherapy in early-stage Hodgkin's disease: long-term results. J Clin Oncol. 2004;22(14):2835-41.
63. Eich H, Mueller R, Engert A. Comparison of 30 Gy versus 20 Gy involved field radiotherapy after two versus four cycles of ABVD in early stage Hodgkin's lymphoma: Interim analysis of the German Hodgkin Study Group Trial HD10. Int J Radiat Oncol Biol Phys. 2005;63(suppl 1):S1.
64. Meyer RM. Is there convincing evidence for the use of chemotherapy alone in patients with limited stage Hodgkin's lymphoma? Eur J Haematol. 2005;(66):115-20.
65. Yahalom J. Don't throw out the baby with the bathwater: On optimizing cure and reducing toxicity in Hodgkin's lymphoma. J Clin Oncol. 2006;24(4):544-8.
66. Hodgson DC, Hudson MM, Constine LS. Pediatric Hodgkin lymphoma: Maximizing efficacy and minimizing toxicity. Semin Radiat Oncol. 2007;17(3):230-42.
67. Ruehl U. The German GPOH-HD 95 Trial on Pediatric Hodgkin's Disease: 10 Year Results and Analysis of Treatment Failures. Int J Rad Onc Bio Phys. 2008;72(1):S77.
68. Hodgson DC, Hudson MM, Constine LS. Pediatric Hodgkin lymphoma: Maximizing efficacy and minimizing toxicity. Semin Radiat Oncol. 2007;17(3):230-42.
69. Tebbi CK, Mendenhall N, London WB, Williams JL, de Alarcon PA, Chauvenet AR, et al. Treatment of stage I, IIA, IIIA(1) pediatric Hodgkin's disease with doxorubicin, bleomycin, vincristine and etoposide (DBVE) and radiation: A Pediatric Oncology Group (POG) study. Pediatr Blood Cancer. 2006;46(2):198-202.
70. Thomas J, Ferme C, Noordijk EM. Results of the EORTC-GELA H9 randomized trials: The H9-F trial (comparing 3 radiation dose levels) and H9-U trial (comparing 3 chemotherapy schemes) in patients with favorable or unfavorable early stage Hodgkin's lymphoma. Haematologica. 2007;92:27.

71. National Comprehensive Cancer Network. The NCCN Clinical Practice Guidelines in Oncology. Hodgkin's Disease/ Lymphoma. [online] Available from www.nccn.org. [Accessed April, 2015].
72. Diehl V, Fuchs M. Early, intermediate and advanced Hodgkin's lymphoma: Modern treatment strategies. Ann Oncol. 2007; 18(suppl 9):ix71-9.
73. Landman-Parker J1, Pacquement H, Leblanc T, Habrand JL, Terrier-Lacombe MJ, Bertrand Y, et al. Localized childhood Hodgkin's disease: Response-adapted chemotherapy with etoposide, bleomycin, vinblastine, and prednisone before low-dose radiation therapy-results of the French Society of Pediatric Oncology Study MDH90. J Clin Oncol. 2000;18(7):1500-7.
74. Donaldson SS1, Link MP, Weinstein HJ, Rai SN, Brain S, Billett AL, et al. Final results of a prospective clinical trial with VAMP and low-dose inolved-field radiation for children with low-risk Hodgkin's disease. J Clin Oncol. 2007;25(3):332-7.
75. Nachman JB1, Sposto R, Herzog P, Gilchrist GS, Wolden SL, Thomson J, et al. Randomized comparison of low-dose involved-field radiotherapy and no radiotherapy for children with Hodgkin's disease who achieve a complete response to chemotherapy. J Clin Oncol. 2002;20(18):3765-71.
76. Schellong G, Pötter R, Brämswig J, Wagner W, Prott FJ, Dörffel W, et al. High cure rates and reduced longterm toxicity in pediatric Hodgkin's disease: The German-Austrian multicenter trial DAL-HD-90. The German-Austrian Pediatric Hodgkin's Disease Study Group. J Clin Oncol. 1999;17(12):3736-44.
77. Dörffel W, Lüders H, Rühl U, Albrecht M, Marciniak H, Parwaresch R, et al. Preliminary results of the multicenter trial GPOH-HD 95 for the treatment of Hodgkin's disease in children and adolescents: Analysis and outlook. Klin Padiatr. 2003;215(3):139-45.
78. Eichenauer DA, Engert A, Dreyling M. ESMO Guidelines Working Group. Hodgkin's lymphoma: ESMO clinical recommendations for diagnosis, treatment and follow-up. Ann Oncol. 2011;22 Suppl 6:vi55-8.
79. Proctor SJ, Mackie M, Dawson A, et al. A population-based study of intensive multi-agent chemotherapy with or without autotransplant for the highest risk Hodgkin's disease patients identified by the Scotland and Newcastle Lymphoma Group (SNLG) prognostic index. A Scotland and Newcastle Lymphoma Group study (SNLG HD III). Eur J Cancer. 2002;38:795-806.
80. Shankar A, Visaduraki M, Hayward J, Morland B, McCarthy K, Hewitt M. Clinical outcome in children and adolescents with Hodgkin lymphoma after treatment with chemotherapy alone—The results of the United Kingdom HD3 national cohort trial. Eur J Cancer. 2012;48(1):108-13.
81. Terasawa T, Lau J, Bardet S, Couturier O, Hotta T, Hutchings M, et al. Fluorine-18-18F-FDG positron emission tomography for interim response assessment of advanced-stage Hodgkin's lymphoma and diffuse large B-cell lymphoma: a systematic review. J Clin Oncol. 2009;27(11):1906-14.
82. Cerci JJ, Pracchia LF, Linardi CC, Pitella FA, Delbeke D, Izaki M, et al. 18F-FDG PET after 2 cycles of ABVD predicts event-free survival in early and advanced Hodgkin lymphoma. J Nucl Med. 2010;51(9):1337-43.
83. Hoskin PJ, Díez P, Williams M, et al. Participants of the Lymphoma Radiotherapy Group. Recommendations for the use of radiotherapy in nodal lymphoma. Clin Oncol (R Coll Radiol). 2013;25(1):49-58.
84. Kaplan HS. Hodgkin's Disease, 2nd edn. Cambridge, MA: Harvard University Press; 1980. p. 375e407.
85. Miller TP, Dahlberg S, Cassady JR, Adelstein DJ, Spier CM, Grogan TM, et al. Chemotherapy alone compared with chemotherapy plus radiotherapy for localized intermediate and high grade non-Hodgkin's lymphoma. N Engl J Med. 1998;339(1):21-6.
86. Yahalom J, Mauch P. The involved field is back: issues in delineating the radiation field in Hodgkin's disease. Ann Oncol. 2002;13(Suppl 1):79-83.
87. Díez P, Hoskin PJ, Aird EG. Treatment planning and delivery of involved field radiotherapy in advanced Hodgkin's disease: results from a questionnaire-based audit for the UK Stanford V regimen vs ABVD clinical trial quality assurance programme. Br J Radiol. 2007;80(958):816-21.
88. Girinsky T, van der Maazen R, Specht L, Aleman B, Poortmans P, Lievens Y, et al. Involved-node radiotherapy (INRT) in patients with early Hodgkin lymphoma: concepts and guidelines. Radiother Oncol. 2006;79(3):270-7.
89. Taylor A, Rockall AG, Powell ME. An atlas of the pelvic lymph node regions to aid radiotherapy target volume definition. Clin Oncol (R Coll Radiol). 2007;19(7):542-50.
90. Lengelé B, Hamoir M, Scalliet P, et al. Anatomical bases for the radiological delineation of lymph node areas. Major collecting trunks, head and neck. Radiother Oncol. 2007;85(1):146-55.
91. Lengele B, Nyssen-Behets C, Scalliet P. Anatomical bases for the radiological delineation of lymph node areas. Upper limbs, chest and abdomen. Radiother Oncol. 2007;84(3):335-47.
92. Kaplan HS. Evidence for a tumouricidal dose level in the radiotherapy of Hodgkin's disease. Cancer Res 1966; 26(6):1221-4.
93. Loeffler M, Diehl V, Pfreundschuh M, Rühl U, Hasenclever D, Nisters-Backes H, et al. Dose-response of complementary radiotherapy following four cycles of combination chemotherapy in intermediate stage Hodgkin's disease. J Clin Oncol 1997;15(6):2275-87.
94. Sieber M, Tesch H, Pfistner B, Rueffer U, Lathan B, Brosteanu O, et al. Rapidly alternating COPP/ ABV/IMEP is not superior to conventional alternating COPP/ ABVD in combination with extended-field radiotherapy in intermediate-stage Hodgkin's lymphoma: final results of the German Hodgkin's Lymphoma Study Group Trial HD5. J Clin Oncol. 2002;20(2):476-84.
95. Engert A, Plütschow A, Eich HT, Lohri A, Dörken B, Borchmann P, et al. Reduced treatment intensity in patients with early stage Hodgkin's lymphoma. New Engl J Med. 2010;363(7): 640-52.
96. Eich HT, Diehl V, Görgen H, Pabst T, Markova J, Debus J, et al. Intensified chemotherapy and dose reduced involved field

radiotherapy in patients with early unfavourable Hodgkin's lymphoma: final analysis of the German Hodgkin Study Group HD11 trial. J Clin Oncol. 2010;28(27):4199-206.

97. Sutcliffe SB, Gospodarowicz MK, Bush RS, Brown TC, Chua T, Bean HA, et al. Role of radiation therapy in localised non-Hodgkins lymphoma. Radiother Oncol. 1985;4(3):211-23.
98. Lowry L, Smith P, Qian W, Falk S, Benstead K, Illidge T, et al. Reduced dose radiotherapy for local control in non-Hodgkin lymphoma: a randomised phase III trial. Radiother Oncol. 2011;100(1):86-92.
99. Hoskin PJ, Kirkwood AA, Popova B, Smith P, Robinson M, Gallop-Evans E, et al. 4 Gy versus 24 Gy radiotherapy for patients with indolent lymphoma (FORT): a randomised phase 3 non-inferiority trial. Lancet Oncol. 2014;15(4):457-63.
100. Boivin JF, Hutchison GB, Lubin JH, Mauch P. Coronary artery disease mortality in patients treated for Hodgkin's disease. Cancer. 1992;69(5):1241-7.
101. Hancock SL, Tucker MA, Hoppe RT. Factors affecting late mortality from heart disease after treatment of Hodgkin's disease. JAMA. 1993;270(16):1949-55.
102. Hancock S, Tucker M, Hoppe R. Breast cancer after treatment of Hodgkin's disease. J Natl Cancer Inst. 1993;85(1):25-31.
103. Aisenberg AC, Finkelstein DM, Doppke KP, Koerner FC, Boivin JF, Willett CG. High risk of breast carcinoma after irradiation of young women with Hodgkin's disease. Cancer. 1997;79(6):1203-10.
104. Bhatia S, Robison LL, Oberlin O, Greenberg M, Bunin G, Fossati-Bellani F, et al. Breast cancer and other second neoplasms after childhood Hodgkin's disease. N Engl J Med. 1996;334(12):745-51.
105. Straus DJ, Filippa DA, Lieberman PH, Koziner B, Thaler HT, Clarkson BD. The non-Hodgkin's lymphomas. I. A retrospective clinical and pathologic analysis of 499 cases diagnosed between 1958 and 1969. Cancer. 1983;51(1):101-9.
106. A predictive model for aggressive non-Hodgkin's lymphoma. The International Non-Hodgkin's Lymphoma Prognostic Factors Project. N Engl J Med. 1993;329(14):987-94.
107. Miller TP, Grogan TM, Dahlberg S, Spier CM, Braziel RM, Banks PM, et al. Prognostic significance of the Ki-67-associated proliferative antigen in aggressive non-Hodgkin's lymphomas: a prospective Southwest Oncology Group trial. Blood. 1994;83(6):1460-6.
108. van Besien K, Ha CS, Murphy S, McLaughlin P, Rodriguez A, Amin K, et al. Risk factors, treatment, and outcome of central nervous system recurrence in adults with intermediate-grade and immunoblastic lymphoma. Blood. 1998;91(4):1178-84.
109. Touroutoglou N, Dimopoulos MA, Younes A, Hess M, Pugh W, Cox J, et al. Testicular lymphoma: late relapses and poor outcome despite doxorubicin-based therapy. J Clin Oncol. 1995;13(6):1361-7.
110. Fisher RI, Gaynor ER, Dahlberg S, Oken MM, Grogan TM, Mize EM, et al. A Phase III comparison of CHOP vs. m-BACOD vs.ProMACE-CytaBOM vs. MACOP-B in patients with intermediate or high grade non-Hodgkin's lymphoma: results of SWOG- 8516 (Intergroup 0067), the national high priority lymphoma study. Ann Oncol. 1994;5:591-5
111. Coiffier B, Lepage E, Briere J, Herbrecht R, Tilly H, Bouabdallah R, et al. CHOP chemotherapy plus rituximab compared with CHOP alone in elderly patients with diffuse large-B-cell lymphoma. N Engl J Med. 2002;346(4):235-42.
112. Coiffier B, Thieblemont C, Van Den Neste E, Lepeu G, Plantier I, Castaigne S, et al. Long-term outcome of patients in the LNH-98.5 trial, the first randomized study comparing rituximab-CHOP to standard CHOP chemotherapy in DLBCL patients: a study by the Groupe d'Etudes des Lymphomes de l'Adulte. Blood. 2010;116(12):2040-5.
113. Coiffier B. Treatment of aggressive non-Hodgkin's lymphoma. Semin Oncol. 1999;26(5):12-20.
114. Schlembach PJ, Wilder RB, Tucker SL, Ha CS, Rodriguez MA, Hess MA, et al. Impact of involved field radiotherapy after CHOP-based chemotherapy on stage III-IV, intermediate grade and large-cell immunoblastic lymphomas. Int J Radiat Oncol Biol Phys. 2000;48(4):1107-10.
115. Ferreri AJ, Dell'Oro S, Reni M, Ceresoli GL, Cozzarini C, Ponzoni M, et al. Consolidation radiotherapy to bulky or semibulky lesions in the management of stage III-IV diffuse large B cell lymphomas. Oncology. 2000;58(3):219-26.
116. Avilés A, Delgado S, Nambo MJ, Alatriste S, Díaz-Maqueo JC. Adjuvant radiotherapy to sites of previous bulky disease in patients stage IV diffuse large cell lymphoma. Int J Radiat Oncol Biol Phys. 1994;30(4):799-803.
117. Longo DL. What's the deal with follicular lymphomas? J Clin Oncol. 1993;11(2):202-8.
118. Lawrence TS, Urba WJ, Steinberg SM, Sundeen JT, Cossman J, Young RC, et al. Retrospective analysis of stage I and II indolent lymphomas at the National Cancer Institute. Int J Radiat Oncol Biol Phys. 1988;14(3):417-24.
119. Wilder RB, Jones D, Tucker SL, Fuller LM, Ha CS, McLaughlin P, et al. Long-term results with radiotherapy for stage I-II follicular lymphomas. Int J Radiat Oncol Biol Phys. 2001;51(5):1219-27.
120. Ha CS, Kong JS, Tucker SL, McLaughlin P, Wilder RB, Hess MA, et al. Central lymphatic irradiation for stage I-III follicular lymphoma: report from a single-institutional prospective study. Int J Radiat Oncol Biol Phys. 2003;57(2):316-20.
121. De Los Santos JF, Mendenhall NP, Lynch JW. Is comprehensive lymphatic irradiation for low-grade non-Hodgkin's lymphoma curative therapy? Long-term experience at a single institution. Int J Radiat Oncol Biol Phys. 1997;38(1):3-8.
122. Peterson BA. Current treatment of follicular low-grade lymphomas. Semin Oncol 1999;26(5):2-11.
123. Ha CS, Kong JS, McLaughlin P, Tucker SL, Fayad LE, Hess MA, et al. Stage III follicular lymphoma: long-term follow-up and patterns of failure. Int J Radiat Oncol Biol Phys. 2003;57(3):748-54.
124. Horning SJ, Rosenberg SA. The natural history of initially untreated low-grade non-Hodgkin's lymphomas. N Engl J Med. 1984;311(23):1471-5.
125. National Comprehensive Cancer Network. The NCCN Clinical Practice Guidelines in Oncology for Non-Hodgkin's

Lymphoma V2.2014. [online] Available from www.nccn.org. [Accessed April, 2015].
126. Cheung MM, Chan JK, Lau WH, et al. Early stage nasal T/NK-cell lymphoma: clinical outcome, prognostic factors, and the effect of treatment modality. Int J Radiat Oncol Biol Phys. 2002;54(1):182-90.
127. Li YX, Yao B, Jin J, Wang WH, Liu YP, Song YW, et al. Radiotherapy as primary treatment for stage IE and IIE nasal natural killer/T-cell lymphoma. J Clin Oncol. 2006;24(1):181-9.
128. Ostronoff M, Soussain C, Zambon E, Ibrahim A, Bosq J, Bayle C, et al. Burkitt's lymphoma in adults: a retrospective study of 46 cases. Nouv Rev Fr Hematol. 1992;34(5):389-97.
129. Micaily B, Miyamoto C, Kantor G, Lessin S, Rook A, Brady L, et al. Radiotherapy for unilesional mycosis fungoides. Int J Radiat Oncol Biol Phys. 1998;42(2):361-4.
130. Kim YH, Hoppe RT. Mycosis fungoides and the Sezary syndrome. Semin Oncol 1999;26(3):276-89.
131. Hoppe RT, Fuks Z, Bagshaw MA. Radiation therapy in the management of cutaneous T-cell lymphomas. Cancer Treat Rep. 1979;63(4):625-32.

23 CHAPTER

Principles of Care of Pediatric Malignancies

Ruchira Misra

INCIDENCE

Children's cancers are relatively much less common than those seen in the adults. The incidence of childhood cancer in the United States is approximately 1–2 children in every 10,000 children aged 14 years and younger.[1] In India, this incidence is approximately 38–124 per million children aged less than 18 years of age.[2] However, this data is biased as most of the information comes from urban centers. Despite having lesser numbers to work with, children's cancers are more curable than adult cancers. Most pediatric cancers have an overall survival that is more than 70%, and in some cancers like Wilms' tumor and Hodgkin's lymphomas (HLs) the survival rates are over 95%.

Amongst the cancers, acute lymphoblastic leukemia (ALL) is the commonest cancer seen in the pediatric age-group. It accounts for approximately 36% of the pediatric cancers. It is followed by brain tumors which account for 17% of the cases and followed by neuroblastoma (14%).[1]

GENETIC BASIS FOR CANCER

Usually, no cause has been found with most pediatric malignancies, though a few tumors are reported to have an increased incidence with some genetic conditions. For example, children with Down's syndrome have an increased risk of leukemia—an estimated cumulative incidence of 2.1% by 5 years.[3,4] Beckwith-Wiedemann syndrome and other overgrowth disorders are linked with Wilms' tumors and hepatoblastomas.[5] Other tumors that have a genetic basis are adrenocortical carcinoma (50–80% are inherited or have a hereditary component), optic gliomas (45%), retinoblastomas (40%), pheochromocytomas (40%) and atypical teratoid/rhabdoid tumors (ATRT) (25%).[6-11] Li and Fraumeni reported an inherited cancer predisposition syndrome, later named after them, in which p53 mutations are inherited and this leads to an increased incidence/risk of cancers—namely, lymphomas, sarcomas, premenopausal breast cancers, colorectal cancers and brain tumors.

Cancer occurs because of changes in the genome of the cell. These changes may occur at the germ line level (constitutional) or at the somatic level (acquired). Figure 1 summarizes the common genomic and genetic alterations found in cancer.

These translocations and inversions lead to activation of proto-oncogenes which may carry a prognostic impact or may even affect the management. Hence, doing molecular testing especially in the cases of leukemia becomes important in today's practice. TEL-AML fusion gene [t(12;21)] in pro-B ALL has a good prognosis in ALL.[12,13] Similarly, a 9;21 translocation carries a poor prognosis. In acute myeloid leukemia (AML), those with inversion (16)/t(16;16), t(8;21) carry a good prognosis while those with monosomy 5 or 7 and FLT3/ITD mutations carry a poor prognosis. Acute promyelocytic leukemia (APML) is characterized by the presence of PML-RARA mutation and carries a good prognosis, and a treatment plan that is different from the AML protocol of management.

PRINCIPLES OF ASSESSMENT AND INVESTIGATIONS IN A CHILD WITH SUSPECTED CANCER

It is always difficult and challenging to assess an unwell/sick child. Despite these challenges, a timely diagnosis is extremely important as early stage disease is more curable than advanced or metastatic disease. This requires an astute pediatrician who is aware of the clinical signs and symptoms of childhood malignancies. Most of the early symptoms of cancer are common to a number of illnesses; hence, persistence of symptoms or no improvement within a

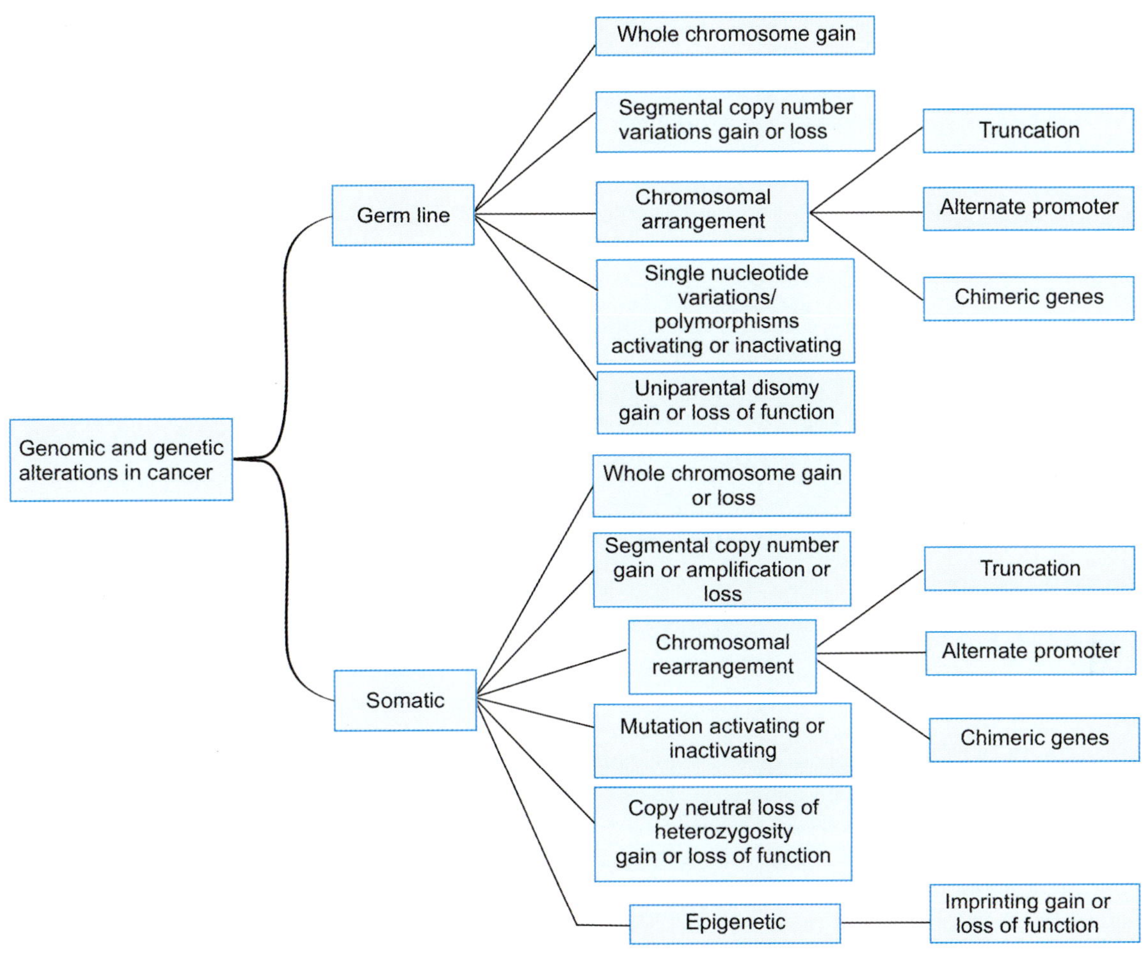

Fig. 1 Summary of the common genetic alterations found in cancer

Source: Principles and Practice of Pediatric Oncology by Pizzo and Poplack, 6th edition.

few days must preclude a workup for malignancies. Certain children as mentioned above are predisposed to cancer. Premature children born preterm may have an increased risk of hepatoblastoma.[14] Infections like Epstein-Barr virus (EBV) infection may predispose to lymphomas, especially post-transplant lymphoproliferative disorders. Those children who have survived cancer are at risk of developing secondary cancers, especially those that have received radiation and certain chemotherapeutic agents. There is an increased risk of breast cancer, bone tumors and thyroid cancer in HL patients.

The common symptoms at presentation may be fever for a few days, not responding to antipyretics and antibiotics; lymphadenopathy; or bleeding from any point. These would indicate a leukemia or a lymphoma. Some children with massive lymphadenopathy may present with snoring or with features of superior vena cava syndrome.

Solid tumors generally present as "lumps and bumps". Wilms' tumor commonly presents as an abdominal mass noticed in an apparently well child, whereas a neuroblastoma presents as an abdominal mass in an irritable and unwell child who may also have bleeding manifestations. Children with brain tumors present with recurring or persistent headaches, visual difficulties as blurring or loss of vision, vomiting and neurological deficits like ataxia or paresis.

Bone marrow aspiration and biopsy are indicated if there is:

- Depression of two or more cell lines
- Presence of blasts on the peripheral smear
- Unexplained hepatosplenomegaly or lymphadenopathy
- Anterior mediastinal mass.

To stage solid tumors like neuroblastoma and Ewing's tumors, it is recommended to take bone marrow biopsy from two sites, generally bilateral iliac crests in patients with solid tumors or lymphomas.

Positron emission tomography (PET) scans are forming an important part in the staging investigations for children with malignancies, and have been proven to be of use in Ewing's sarcomas, germ cell tumors, lymphomas and neuroblastomas. In a country like India where metaiodobenzylguanidine

(MIBG) scans may not be readily available, a PET scan and a bone scan may help to stage the disease. PET scans are also proving to be a good investigational tool for graft-versus-host disease (GVHD) of the gut where they have helped to delineate the involved areas which can then be biopsied by endoscopy.

Specific Tests for Some Pediatric Cancers

Acute Lymphoblastic Leukemia

- Bone marrow aspiration and biopsy. To send the sample for cytogenetics and for molecular genetics, especially breakpoint cluster region-abelson mutation (BCR-ABL), mixed lineage leukemia (MLL) gene re-arrangements [t(4;11)], t(8;21) and t(1;19). These molecular tests are especially useful in pre or pro-B ALL.
- Cerebrospinal fluid (CSF) examination to look for blast cells
- Testicular examination
- Fundus examination.

Acute Myeloid Leukemia

- Bone marrow aspiration and biopsy. To send the sample for cytogenetics and for molecular genetics, especially FLT3/ITD mutations and PML-RARA mutations
- Cerebrospinal fluid examination for blast cells
- Magnetic resonance imaging (MRI) brain with contrast if there is any neurological dysfunction
- Coagulation studies in those suspected to have APML.

Brain Tumors

- Magnetic resonance imaging of the brain and the spine with contrast
- Cerebrospinal fluid to be done within 3 days of surgery
- Tumor tissue to be sent for integrase interactor 1 (INI1) mutation studies in children less than 5 years with brain tumors, especially if they are posterior fossa tumors to rule out ATRT brain.
- Alpha-fetoprotein (AFP) and beta-human chorionic gonadotropin (beta-hCG) of both serum and CSF in cases of germinomas.

Lymphomas

- Tissue biopsy of the mass
- Bone marrow aspiration and biopsy
- Positron emission tomography-Contrast-enhanced computed tomography PET-CECT/MRI whole body
- Cerebrospinal fluid examination.

Germ Cell Tumors

- Alpha-fetoprotein and beta-hCG
- Positron emission tomography-CECT/MRI whole body.

PRINCIPLES IN THE MANAGEMENT OF CHILDHOOD CANCERS

Most cancers in the pediatric age-group are treatable. The importance is to have a high index of suspicion and to treat them early. Here, we describe the treatments of a few common types of pediatric cancers.

Acute Lymphoblastic Leukemia

Acute lymphoblastic leukemia, as is commonly known, is the commonest pediatric malignancy. The incidence of ALL is approximately 3–4 cases in every 100,000 children in the United States.[15,16] Acute leukemia was initially classified on the basis of morphology of the cells (Fig. 2), but now immunophenotyping plays an important role both in the diagnosis as well as in the follow-up (Table 1). More than 200 different monoclonal antibodies are now available which can detect antigens with different hematopoietic lineages. Using these antigens, the leukemia cells can be segregated according to their degree of maturation.

Once the bone marrow examination and the CSF have been done and investigations have been sent, treatment is initiated with aggressive fluid management to prevent tumor lysis and steroids. Allopurinol or rasburicase may be considered depending on the risk of tumor lysis. Daily weight monitoring and blood sugar testing are recommended.

There are various protocols in circulation for the treatment of ALL; all divide patients into different risk categories and intensify the treatment based on the risk. Some of these risk factors are:

- A white cell count of more than 50,000 at diagnosis
- Male sex

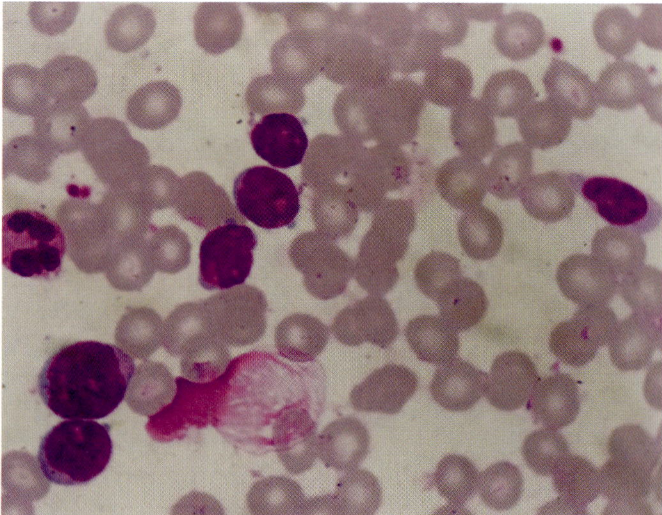

Fig. 2 Morphology of lymphoblasts

Source: Department of Haematology and Blood Transfusion Medicine, Medanta—The Medicity, Haryana, India

Table 1 General guide to the classification of acute lymphoblastic leukemia including common stains, immunophenotype and cytogenetics

B cell	*T cell*	*Myeloid*
Tdt+, PAS+/– FAB L1, L2	PAS (block positivity)	Granules, Auer rods, Sudan Black+, esterase+/-
Pro-B/early Pre-B CD34+/CD19+ t(4;11)+, t(9;22) hyperdiploid	Pro-T CD3+/CD7+ Multiple TF/TCR translocations	Further classification based on CD+ cells classify the subtype
Common ALL (cALL) CD34+/–, CD19+/CD10+ FAB L1(occasionally L2) Hyperdiploid, t (12;21), t (9;22), 6q–	Pre-T CD2+/CD5+/CD8+ Multiple TF/TCR	
Pre-B ALL CD34–/CD19+/CD20+/CD22+ FAB L1/L2 Cytogenetics similar to cALL but have t(1;19) or (9;22)	Common T CD2+/CD5+/CD8+ Multiple TF /TCR	
B cell ALL CD10+/–, CD19+,Tdt–, FAB L3 t(8;14) and t (2;8), t(8;20) between Ig receptors and c-myc		

Source: Principles and Practice of Pediatric Oncology by Pizzo and Poplack, 6th edition

- High risk cytogenetics like MLL rearrangement of Ph+ ALL
- More than 1,000 blast cells/mm^3 in peripheral blood on day 8
- Prednisolone response
- Number of blasts in the marrow at the end of induction.

Induction therapy generally consists of combination therapy using steroids, vincristine, L-asparaginase and daunorubicin. The aim is to have less than 5% blasts in a recovering marrow at the end of induction. Minimal residual disease (MRD) testing is also being used as a marker to monitor response to therapy. MRD measures the presence of the leukemic cells via flow cytometry and it has been found that those who become MRD-negative at an early stage have a better prognosis. Some protocols test for MRD on day 14/15, while others test at the end of induction between day 29 and day 33.

Steroids are the mainstay for treatment of ALL. The use of steroids and vincristine induce remission in about 80% of the cases; however, this effect is short-lived without the addition of L-asparaginase and/or daunorubicin. Prednisolone has been the most common glucocorticoid used in ALL induction but there is data available to say that dexamethasone has a better central nervous system (CNS) penetration and can prolong remission status.[17-20] However, dexamethasone may increase life-threatening infections; cause avascular necrosis, sleep disturbances, fatigue; and have detrimental neurocognitive sequelae.[21]

The addition of L-asparaginase has not only improved induction response rates but also significantly prolonged remission duration.[22] Asparaginase preparations are derived from bacteria, and therefore, have the potential to be highly immunogenic. Hypersensitivity reactions to L-asparaginase occur in up to 30% of patients and are frequently associated with the development of neutralizing antibodies. Other asparaginase-associated toxicities include pancreatitis (in 5–10% of patients) and thrombosis (in 2–5% of patients). Patients who receive a truncated course of asparaginase because of intolerable side effects may have an inferior outcome compared with those who receive all intended doses.[23] Patients treated with PEG-asparaginase had more rapid clearance of lymphoblasts from day 7 and day 14 bone marrow aspirates and more prolonged asparaginase activity than those treated with native asparaginase. Half-lives of asparaginase were 5.5 days and 0.65 days for PEG-asparaginase and native asparaginase, respectively. Patients treated with PEG-asparaginase had lower rates of antibody formation and hence lesser side effects.[23] Current practices are moving away from radiation therapy in the treatment of ALL. Instead of craniospinal radiation, high dose methotrexate is used as CNS preventive therapy.[24]

About 20% of the children will relapse. Depending on the time of relapse, they are again classified as standard risk, intermediate risk or high risk. An allogenic bone marrow transplant offers a chance of cure for those who have relapsed

Table 2 Risk stratification of acute lymphoblastic leukemia relapse

	Non-T			*T-cell*		
	Isolated EM	*Combined*	*Isolated marrow*	*Isolated EM*	*Combined*	*Isolated marrow*
Very early	H	H	H	H	H	H
Early	I	I	H	I	H	H
Late	S	I	I	S	H	H

Very early: Within 18 months of diagnosis; *Early:* After 18 months of diagnosis but within 6 months of stopping treatment; *Late:* More than 6 months after stopping treatment. EM = Extramedullary. Combined = Marrow and extramedullary involvement

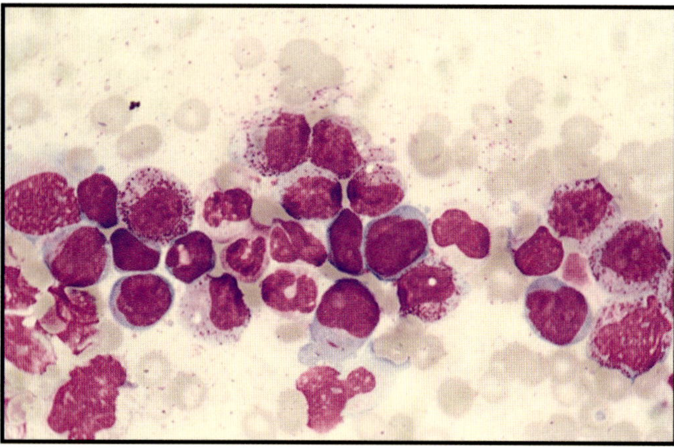

Fig. 3 Acute myeloid leukemia with Auer rods

Source: Department of Hematology and Blood Transfusion Medicine, Medanta—The Medicity, Haryana, India

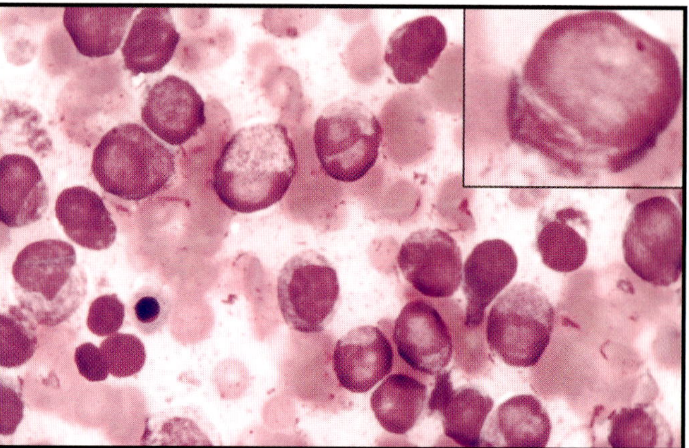

Fig. 4 Acute promyelocytic leukemia

Source: Department of Hematology and Blood Transfusion Medicine, Medanta—The Medicity, Haryana, India

early or very early. Relapse may be isolated marrow, CNS, testicular or combined (Table 2).

Those who relapse late may benefit from rechallenge with chemotherapy. Cladribine and nelarabine are being evaluated for those cases that have relapsed and show some promise.

Acute Myeloid Leukemia

Acute myeloid leukemia is a more aggressive form of blood malignancy and is seen in 5–7 cases per million population per year. It is about five times less common than ALL.[25] The survival rates are also inferior to that seen in ALL. The French-American-British (FAB) classification divides AML into eight subtypes (M0 to M7). Immunophenotyping is also used to confirm the diagnosis (Figs 3 and 4). There are certain molecular markers that are characteristics of certain subtypes, e.g. PML-RARA translocations t(15;17) are seen in 95% of AML M3 subtype.

Treatment for AML, except for AML M3, includes 4–5 cycles of chemotherapy using adriamycin, cytarabine, etoposide and mitoxantrone. The CNS preventive therapy is through intrathecal chemotherapy alone. Radiation is not used in the treatment of AML unless there is extramedullary disease. The importance of good supportive care cannot be stressed as the maximum mortality is seen in the induction period and usually as a result of uncontrolled infection. The use of posaconazole in induction has decreased the incidence of fungal infections in AML and hence the mortality. Survival rates are about 60–65% as reported from various centers.[26]

Acute promyelocytic leukemia often presents with uncontrolled bleeding and disseminated intravascular coagulation (DIC). Once controlled, this form of AML has the best prognosis. Use of all-trans-retinoic acid (ATRA) and arsenic has improved survival in APML.[27,28]

Though the adults continue to consider autologous stem cell transplant in AML, there is no role of autologous stem cell transplant in the pediatric population. A matched sibling bone marrow transplant is offered to those that have intermediate risk cytogenetics in first remission. Those with high-risk features are offered an allogeneic transplant from a matched related or unrelated donor as soon as they achieve complete remission (CR).

Gemtuzumab ozogamicin (GO), an anti-CD33 monoclonal antibody, was tried in the treatment of new cases of AML. It, however, produced inferior outcome as there were higher incidences of veno-occlusive disease.[29]

Relapsed cases, unfortunately, do not do well. Clofarabine is presently being evaluated for the management of such cases of AML.

Hodgkin's Lymphoma

Hodgkin's lymphoma is one of the success stories in pediatric malignancies. Cure rates have risen from 70% to more than 95% over the years. It is also one of the diseases where infections like EBV are considered as a causative factor.[30] Two large Indian studies from Mumbai and Vellore reported EBV association in 78% and 82% of all age HL, while two smaller studies from Chennai and Bangalore (now Bengaluru) reported 31% and 55% association, respectively. Ninety-six to 98% of pediatric cases from Mumbai, Vellore and Delhi have EBV genome detectable in tumor cells.[31]

The current World Health Organization (WHO) classification of HL is based on the Rye modification of the Luke's and Butler classification schema (Boxes 1 and 2).

Positron emission tomography scans have become the favored modality of investigation for staging of HL. It is also a great tool for monitoring disease response and the combination of PET-CT helps to characterize residual disease as fibrosis or active disease (Fig. 5). Bone marrow involvement at the time of presentation is rare in HL but may be seen in stage III or IV disease or those with B symptoms or disease recurrence.

Treatment of pediatric HL has changed from radiotherapy for all patients to risk-adapted therapy. Those with favorable characteristics are treated with chemotherapy alone (Table 3).

Those with unfavorable disease would benefit from intensive chemotherapy and radiation.

Most relapses would occur within 3 years of treatment though late relapses are also known. These patients are still salvageable and can be treated with chemotherapy, followed by autologous bone marrow transplant or chemotherapy and radiation therapy. Transplant associated mortality occurs in

Box 1 World Health Organization classification of Hodgkin's lymphoma

Nodular lymphocytic predominant Hodgkin's lymphoma

Classic Hodgkin's lymphoma

- Nodular sclerosis
- Mixed cellularity
- Lymphocyte rich
- Lymphocyte depleted.

Source: Principles and Practice of Pediatric Oncology by Pizza and Poplack, 6th edition

Box 2 Ann Arbor staging/classification of Hodgkin's lymphoma

Stage I: Involvement of a single lymph node region (I) or of a single extralymphatic organ or site (IE)*

Stage II: Involvement of two or more lymph node regions or lymphatic structures on the same side of the diaphragm alone (II) or with involvement of limited, contiguous extralymphatic organ or tissue (IIE)

Stage III: Involvement of lymph node regions on both sides of the diaphragm (III) which may include the spleen (IIIS) or limited, contiguous extralymphatic organ or site (IIIE) or both (IIIES)

Stage IV: Diffuse or disseminated foci of involvement of one or more extralymphatic organs or tissues, with or without associated lymphatic involvement.

*In addition, each stage is further classified as A or B depending on the presence or absence of fever higher than 38°C for three consecutive days drenching night sweats or weight loss more than 10% in the last 6 months. The suffix S is also used to indicate the involvement of the spleen. The designation "E" generally refers to *extranodal contiguous extension* (i.e. proximal or contiguous extranodal disease) that can be encompassed within an irradiation field appropriate for nodal disease of the same anatomic extent.

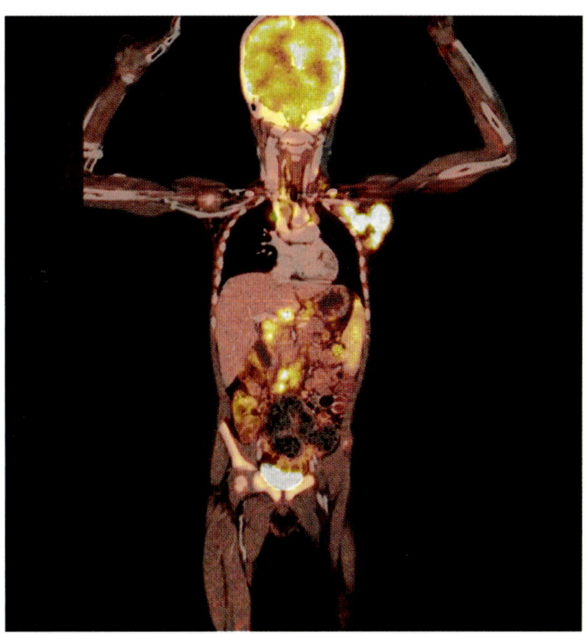

Fig. 5 PET-CECT showing areas of involvement of organs and nodes with Hodgkin's lymphoma rods

Source: Department of Nuclear Medicine, Medanta—The Medicity, Hayana, Inda

Table 3 Favorable and unfavorable classification of Hodgkin's lymphoma

Favorable characteristics	*Unfavorable disease*
Localized nodal disease in the absence of B symptoms and bulky disease	Presence of B symptoms Bulky mediastinal disease or peripheral lymphadenopathy Extranodal extension of disease Stage IIIB or IV disease

Source: Adopted from Principles and practice of pediatric oncology by Pizza and Poplack, 6th edition.

approximately 10% of the patients and is usually a result of infections or cardiopulmonary complications.[32]

Since the cure rates of HL are very good, a lot of work has been done in studying the late effects of chemotherapy or radiation on children. Prepubertal children who received high dose radiation to the axial skeleton showed an alteration in their sitting heights as compared with standing heights.[33] Other musculoskeletal abnormalities observed included narrowing of the thoracic apex, atrophy of the soft tissues of the neck, retroperitoneal fibrosis and brachial plexopathy. There is also an increased risk of breast cancer and thyroid cancer as well as secondary AML in the survivors of HL.

Non-Hodgkin's Lymphoma

Non-Hodgkin's lymphoma (NHL) is more common than HL in children less than 10 years, though the incidence of HL increases in children above 10 years of age. Burkitt's lymphoma characteristically occurs in children between the age of 5 and 15 years while lymphoblastic lymphoma is seen across all age-groups. Anaplastic lymphomas, diffuse large B cell lymphomas are seen more commonly in adolescents and young adults (Box 3).

Lymphoblastic lymphomas are very similar to leukemia in their cell structure as well as in immunophenotyping. Hence, these are treated on the same lines of ALL and have good survival outcomes.

Box 3 St Jude's staging for childhood non-Hodgkin's lymphoma

Stage I

- A single tumor (extranodal) or single anatomical area (nodal) with the exclusion of the mediastinum or abdomen

Stage II

- A single tumor (extranodal) with regional node involvement
- Two or more nodal areas on the same side of the diaphragm
- Two single (extranodal) tumors with or without regional node involvement on the same side of the diaphragm
- A primary gastrointestinal tract tumor, usually in the ileocecal area, with or without involvement of associated mesenteric nodes only, grossly completely resected

Stage III

- Two single tumors (extranodal) on opposite sides of the diaphragm
- Two or more nodal areas above and below the diaphragm
- All the primary intrathoracic tumors (mediastinal, pleural, thymic)
- All extensive primary intra-abdominal disease, unresectable
- All paraspinal or epidural tumors, regardless of other tumor site (s).

Stage IV

- Any of the above with initial CNS and/or bone marrow involvement.

Burkitt's lymphoma is characterized by CD20+ cells which also show CD19, CD22 and CD10 positivity and an absence of Bcl-2 protein. These cells also show a t (8;14) (q24;q32) rearrangement.

Positron emission tomography scan is used as a common modality for staging of NHL in addition to a bone marrow aspiration and biopsy. Those with more than 25% blasts are classified as leukemia.

Rituximab is an anti-CD20 antibody that has shown a remarkable improvement in the survival of adults with Burkitt's lymphomas. There is an ongoing Children's Oncology Group (COG) trial to see its effectiveness in the pediatric population. At present, the event free survival (EFS) is 70–90% for most lymphomas.[1]

Relapses are treated with rituximab and intensive chemotherapy like ICE (ifosfamide, carboplatin and etoposide), followed by autologous stem cell therapy.

Brain Tumors

Brain tumors are the second commonest malignancies seen in the pediatric age-group. Of these, medulloblastomas are the most common. These are primitive neuroectodermal tumors that are found in the posterior fossa region. Survival outcomes are best with radiation therapy, followed by high dose chemotherapy and stem cell rescue. The St Jude's protocols have survival rates of 80–85% with this combination therapy.[34]

Recent literature also suggests that radiation may play an important role in anaplastic ependymomas even in children less than 3 years of age.

Atypical teratoid/rhabdoid tumor brain, till very recently, classified as medulloblastomas. However, with the current research, it has been detected that these tumors are characterized by a loss of the SMARCB1/INI1 protein expression. In children less than 3 years of age, this tumor may account for up to 20% of the cases. Overall survivals are poor with a median survival of 17 months in one study. Intensive chemotherapy and radiation therapy may have a beneficial role in these patients.[35]

SUPPORTIVE CARE IN PEDIATRIC MALIGNANCIES

Supportive care plays a major role in improving survival in the pediatric population. The children are at an increased risk of infections, both bacterial and viral, as they are constantly exposed to the same.

Patients with solid tumors are known to have subclinical abnormalities at the time of diagnosis itself. Chemotherapy decreases the neutrophil count which does recover rapidly but places the patient at risk of bacterial infections.

Corticosteroids are commonly used in the treatment of leukemia and lymphomas, and as antiemetic therapy with emetogenic chemotherapy or brain tumors and radiation, but predispose to fungal infections. Children are also susceptible to *Pneumocystis carinii* pneumonia.

Most children would be placed on medications to prevent these infections, hence cotrimoxazole-trimethoprim combinations and antifungals are part of the medications that these children receive. Addition of posaconazole in the induction phase of AML has decreased the mortality related to breakthrough fungal infections.

Chemotherapy induces vomiting. Control of emesis using effective medication can decrease the emotional trauma that the children have to face. Drugs like aprepitant have helped in this area though it is important to know its interactions.

Good nutrition is also important especially in children who have to use the energy not only to fight disease but also to grow. Consider early intervention in the form of Ryle's tube feeding or parenteral nutrition in children.

Children will also need blood and blood product support during chemotherapy. It is important to maintain adequate hemoglobin levels to avoid fatigue and also to give platelet transfusions whenever there is a risk of bleeding. It is also important to give controlled weight-based volumes of these products so as to avoid fluid overload.

Supportive care would also include decreasing the pain especially during procedures, either with the use of local anesthetic creams or injections, or with mild sedation.

Psychosocial support of children is an often neglected area in the treatment of children. Children often lose out on their studies, feel isolated from their peers and appear to be more mature than their peers or siblings. Play therapy needs to be a part of their overall management even during their hospital stay as well as schooling.

CONCLUSION

Pediatric malignancies are not the same as their adult counterparts. They have a different biology and respond differently to treatment. Most cancers originate from the embryonal cells. These tumors are more chemoresponsive and hence offer the opportunity for better survival. With improved survival, the focus also needs to shift to decrease side effects, especially the long-term sequelae of therapy. Focus is now shifting to preventing infertility and decreasing the risk of secondary cancers in the survivors. Some treatment protocols are now considering reduction in the chemotherapy or elimination/reduction of radiation. However, a lot of work still needs to done so that we can guarantee cure for all children with cancer.

REFERENCES

1. Ries LAG, Smith MA, Gurney JG, Linet M, Tamra T, Young JL, Bunin GR (Eds). Cancer incidence and survival among children and adolescents: United States SEER program 1975-1995. Bethesda, MD: National Cancer Institute, SEER Program. NIH Pub. No. 99-4649; 1999.
2. Arora RS, Eden TO, Kapoor G. Epidemiology of childhood cancer in India. Indian J Cancer. 2009;46(4):264-73.
3. Rabin KR, Whitlock JA. Malignancy in children with trisomy 21. Oncologist. 2009;14(2):164-73.
4. Hasle H, Clemmensen IH, Mikkelsen M. Risks of leukaemia and solid tumours in individuals with Down's syndrome. Lancet. 2000;355(9199):165-9.
5. Elliott M, Bayly R, Cole T, Temple IK, Maher ER. Clinical features and natural history of Beckwith-Wiedemann syndrome: presentation of 74 new cases. Clin Genet. 1994;46(2):168-74.
6. Wagner J, Portwine C, Rabin K, Leclerc JM, Narod SA, Malkin D. High frequency of germline p53 mutations in childhood adrenocortical cancer. J Natl Cancer Inst. 1994;86(22):1707-10.
7. Varley JM, McGown G, Thorncroft M, James LA, Margison GP, Forster G, et al. Are there low-penetrance TP53 Alleles? Evidence from childhood adrenocortical tumors. Am J Hum Genet. 1999;65(4):995-1006.
8. Rush JA, Younge BR, Campbell RJ, MacCarty CS. Optic glioma. Long-term follow-up of 85 histopathologically verified cases. Ophthalmology. 1982;89(11):1213-9.
9. Lohmann DR, Gallie BL. Retinoblastoma: revisiting the model prototype of inherited cancer. Am J Med Genet C Semin Med Genet. 2004;129C(1):23-8.
10. Neumann HP, Bausch B, McWhinney SR, Bender BU, Gimm O, Franke G, et al. Germ-line mutations in nonsyndromic pheochromocytoma. N Engl J Med. 2002;346(19):1459-66.
11. Biegel JA, Zhou JY, Rorke LB, Stenstrom C, Wainwright LM, Fogelgren B. Germ-line and acquired mutations of INI1 in atypical teratoid and rhabdoid tumors. Cancer Res. 1999;59(1):74-9.
12. Rubnitz JE, Downing JR, Pui CH, Shurtleff SA, Raimondi SC, Evans WE, et al. TEL gene rearrangement in acute lymphoblastic leukemia: a new genetic marker with prognostic significance. J Clin Oncol. 1997;15(3):1150-7.
13. Rubnitz JE, Shuster JJ, Land VJ, Link MP, Pullen DJ, Camitta BM, et al. Case-control study suggests a favorable impact of TEL rearrangement in patients with B-lineage acute lymphoblastic leukemia treated with antimetabolite-based therapy: a Pediatric Oncology Group study. Blood. 1997;89(4):1143-6.
14. Tanimura M, Matsui I, Abe J, Ikeda H, Kobayashi N, Ohira M, et al. Increased risk of hepatoblastoma among immature children with a lower birth weight. Cancer Res. 1998;58(14):3032-5.
15. Jemal A, Tiwari RC, Murray T, Ghafoor A, Samuels A, Ward E, et al. Cancer statistics, 2004. CA Cancer J Clin. 2004;54(1):8-29.
16. Jemal A, Siegel R, Ward E, Hao Y, Xu J, Thun MJ. Cancer statistics, 2009. CA Cancer J Clin. 2009;59(4):225-49.

17. Schrappe M, Zimmermann M, Moricke A, et al. Dexamethasone in induction can eliminate one third of all relapses in childhood acute lymphoblastic leukemia (ALL): results of an International randomized trial in 3655 patients (Trial AIEOP-BFM ALL 2000). Blood. 2008;112(11):Abstract 7.
18. Teuffel O, Kuster SP, Hunger SP, Conter V, Hitzler J, Ethier MC, et al. Dexamethasone versus prednisone for induction therapy in childhood acute lymphoblastic leukemia: a systematic review and meta-analysis. Leukemia. 2011;25(8):1232-8.
19. Ito C, Evans WE, McNinch L, Coustan-Smith E, Mahmoud H, Pui CH, et al. Comparative cytotoxicity of dexamethasone and prednisolone in childhood acute lymphoblastic leukemia. J Clin Oncol. 1996;14(8):2370-6.
20. Hurwitz CA, Silverman LB, Schorin MA, Clavell LA, Dalton VK, Glick KM, et al. Substituting dexamethasone for prednisone complicates remission induction in children with acute lymphoblastic leukemia. Cancer. 2000;88(8):1964-9.
21. Mitchell CD, Richards SM, Kinsey SE, Lilleyman J, Vora A, Eden TO, et al. Benefit of dexamethasone compared with prednisolone for childhood acute lymphoblastic leukaemia: results of the UK Medical Research Council ALL97 randomized trial. Br J Haematol. 2005;129(6):734-45.
22. Silverman LB, Gelber RD, Dalton VK, Asselin BL, Barr RD, Clavell LA, et al. Improved outcome for children with acute lymphoblastic leukemia: results of Dana-Farber Consortium Protocol 91-01. Blood. 2001;97(5):1211-8.
23. Avramis VI, Sencer S, Periclou AP, Sather H, Bostrom BC, Cohen LJ, et al. A randomized comparison of native *Escherichia coli* asparaginase and polyethylene glycol conjugated asparaginase for treatment of children with newly diagnosed standard-risk acute lymphoblastic leukemia: a Children's Cancer Group study. Blood. 2002;99(6):1986-94.
24. Pui CH, Campana D, Pei D, Bowman WP, Sandlund JT, Kaste SC, et al. Treating childhood acute lymphoblastic leukemia without cranial irradiation. N Engl J Med. 2009;360(26):2730-41.
25. Goubin A, Auclerc MF, Auvrignon A, Patte C, Bergeron C, Hémon D, et al. Survival in France after childhood acute leukaemia and non-Hodgkin's lymphoma (1990-2000). Eur J Cancer. 2006;42(4):534-41.
26. Kaspers GJ, Creutzig U. Pediatric acute myeloid leukemia: international progress and future directions. Leukemia. 2005;19(12):2025-9.
27. Ghavamzadeh A, Alimoghaddam K, Ghaffari SH, Rostami S, Jahani M, Hosseini R, et al. Treatment of acute promyelocytic leukemia with arsenic trioxide without ATRA and/or chemotherapy. Ann Oncol. 2006;17(1):131-4.
28. Shen ZX, Shi ZZ, Fang J, Gu BW, Li JM, Zhu YM, et al. All-trans retinoic acid/As_2O_3 combination yields a high quality remission and survival in newly diagnosed acute promyelocytic leukemia. Proc Natl Acad Sci U S A. 2004;101(15):5328-35.
29. Wadleigh M, Richardson PG, Zahrieh D, Lee SJ, Cutler C, Ho V, et al. Prior gemtuzumab ozogamicin exposure significantly increases the risk of veno-occlusive disease in patients who undergo myeloablative allogeneic stem cell transplantation. Blood. 2003;102(5):1578-82.
30. Mueller N, Evans A, Harris NL, Comstock GW, Jellum E, Magnus K, et al. Hodgkin's disease and Epstein-Barr virus. Altered antibody pattern before diagnosis. N Engl J Med. 1989;320(11):689-95.
31. Dinand V, Dawar R, Arya LS, Unni R, Mohanty B, Singh R. Hodgkin's lymphoma in Indian children: prevalence and significance of Epstein-Barr virus detection in Hodgkin's and Reed-Sternberg cells. Eur J Cancer. 2007;43(1):161-8.
32. Baker KS, Gordon BG, Gross TG, Abromowitch MA, Lyden ER, Lynch JC, et al. Autologous hematopoietic stem-cell transplantation for relapsed or refractory Hodgkin's disease in children and adolescents. J Clin Oncol. 1999;17(3):825-31.
33. Papadakis V, Tan C, Heller G, Sklar C. Growth and final height after treatment for childhood Hodgkin disease. J Pediatr Hematol Oncol. 1996;18(3):272-6.
34. Gajjar A, Chintagumpala M, Ashley D, Kellie S, Kun LE, Merchant TE, et al. Risk-adapted craniospinal radiotherapy followed by high-dose chemotherapy and stem-cell rescue in children with newly diagnosed medulloblastoma (St Jude Medulloblastoma-96): long-term results from a prospective, multicentre trial. Lancet Oncol. 2006;7(10):813-20.
35. Ginn KF, Gajjar A. Atypical teratoid rhabdoid tumor: current therapy and future directions. Front Oncol. 2012;2:114.

24

CHAPTER

Radiation Therapy in Gynecologic Cancers

Malolan S Rajagopalan, Sushil Beriwal

INTRODUCTION

Overview

Radiation therapy is an integral component in the management of gynecologic cancers. Using an evidence-based approach, it is estimated that radiation therapy is indicated at least once for 46% of patients with endometrial cancer. It is indicated for 58% of cervical cancer patients, for 34% of those with vulvar cancer, for 100% of those with vaginal cancer, and for 4% of those with ovarian cancer.[1,2]

The past two decades have seen tremendous growth and transformation in the field. The advent and integration of cross-sectional imaging into treatment planning for both external beam radiation therapy (EBRT) and brachytherapy heralds an era of increasingly precise radiation delivery. Intensity-modulated radiation therapy (IMRT) is being increasingly explored and has shown the potential for reduced morbidities while maintaining equivalent tumor control. In this section, we have explored the radiation modalities before delving into their utilization by disease site.

Conformal Radiation Therapy

Conventional EBRT (2DRT) is planned using two-dimensional radiographs. Beams are arranged based on bony anatomy to encompass the presumed areas at risk. While efficient, this technique does not account for variations in soft tissue anatomy and is limited in the ability to protect normal tissue. Conformal radiation therapy refers to the technique of delivering EBRT by achieving a high-dose volume that is shaped to closes match the desired target while minimizing dose to normal tissue. With the development of computed tomography (CT), this has now become possible, and this technique is named three-dimensional conformal radiotherapy (3DCRT).

Three-dimensional conformal radiotherapy is the most widely utilized method of radiation treatment planning and delivery today, and involves a complex process. The first step is the CT simulation in which the patient is positioned in the same fashion as he/she would be for each of the daily treatments. Custom immobilization devices may be utilized and a CT scan is acquired. This creates a virtual image of the patient from which the treatment may be planned. On the planning workstation, other images including magnetic resonance imaging (MRI) and positron emission tomography (PET) and others may co-registered or fused with the planning CT scan. The physician then delineates or contours the tumor and the other regions at risk as well as the normal organs. Each radiation beam is then shaped and multiple beams are cross-fired on the target. 3DCRT continues to be widely implemented in the treatment of gynecologic cancers.

With the availability of greater computing processing power, IMRT is now possible. The process for IMRT is similar to that of 3DCRT, except the optimization process is performed by the computer (inverse planning). The target and normal organs are contoured and the radiation beams are mathematically optimized to create a complex intensity distribution. This technique is able to create highly conformal plans that are able to shape dose to match convex or concave-shaped targets. For gynecologic cancers, this technique affords the ability to dose escalation to the tumor while minimizing dose to normal tissue and thereby decreasing toxicity.

More recent still is the integration of image-guided radiation therapy (IGRT) which refers to the integration of imaging with patient positioning. This ensures that the carefully crafted plans are delivered to the intended target with each fraction.

The advent of advanced and highly conformal techniques does require serious consideration before implementation.

With IMRT, dose gradients are sharp and the potential for marginal and geographic misses of the target does increase. Unlike 3DCRT, which is much more "forgiving" of inaccurate target definition, IMRT is not the same. Additionally, with treatment of pelvic targets, there may be considerable daily variability. For example, variable bladder filling and rectal distension has the potential to move the target several centimeters from the original planning CT (Figs 1A and B). Without proper patient instruction, appropriate margins, and image guidance, the target could be missed entirely. However, when the techniques are performed accurately, there can be a substantial benefit in minimizing toxicity without a decrease in tumor control as has been demonstrated in multiple studies.[3-7]

Brachytherapy

Derived from Greek and referring to therapy delivered from a close distance, brachytherapy is perhaps more integral to the treatment of gynecologic cancers than in any other disease site. Due to the rapid dose fall off as a consequence of the inverse square law, brachytherapy allows for high does to the tumor with sparing of the nearby organs.

Brachytherapy is performed today with an afterloading technique. That is, applicators, needles or catheters are placed first and the radioactive source is later advanced into these devices. Brachytherapy technique may be subdivided based on dose rate. According to the International Commission of Radiation Units (ICRU), low dose rate (LDR) is in the range of 0.4–2 Gy/hr, medium dose rate (MDR) between 2 and 12 Gy/hr and high-dose rate (HDR) is greater than 12 Gy/hr. For LDR therapy, Cesium-137 is most commonly used and for HDR, Iridium-192 is most common.

Low dose rate brachytherapy is typically delivered with one or two insertions over a 2–3 day period. This requires inpatient hospitalization, radiation shielding and radiation precautions for all caretakers and staff. In contrast, HDR brachytherapy is performed in typically 3–5 fractions as an outpatient, with the entire treatment process taking about 2 hours and radiation delivery over just minutes.

In many centers across the world, HDR has supplanted LDR as the treatment of choice. HDR minimizes immobilization times which, in turn, decrease the rates of thromboembolic complications. The use of external applicator fixation devices ensures greater reproducibility. Treatment planning and dosimetry may be better as dose optimization may be achieved through both altering source position but also dwell time. Finally, HDR can be performed as an outpatient procedure, decreasing cost and reducing radiation exposure. Both have been shown to be equally efficacious.[8] However, the delivery of high doses per fraction can increase the risk for late complications. In addition, due to the high doses, meticulous precision is required in applicator placement, planning and delivery as inaccuracies could be potentially devastating.

Pulsed dose rate brachytherapy (PDR) has been explored as a unique technique to harness the advantages afforded by HDR including computer-controlled remote afterloading while mimicking the radiobiology of LDR. With PDR, a pulse delivers about 0.5 Gy over approximately 10 minutes each hour. This technique has been adopted in many centers in Europe and Asia.

Brachytherapy technique for cervical cancer is often performed with a tandem and ovoid or tandem and ring applicator. The tandem is passed through the cervical os into the uterus and the ring or ovoids are placed thereafter.

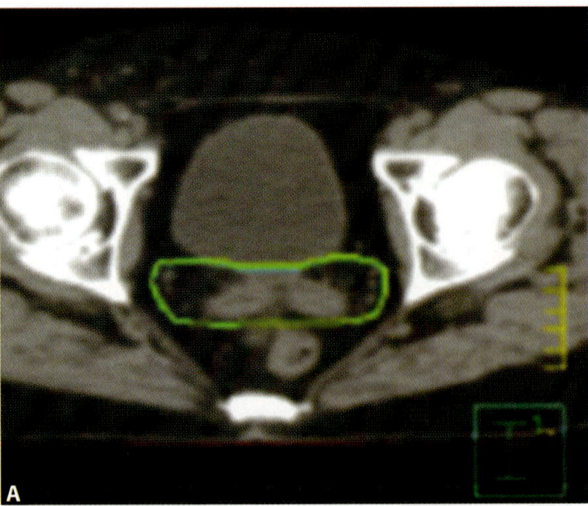

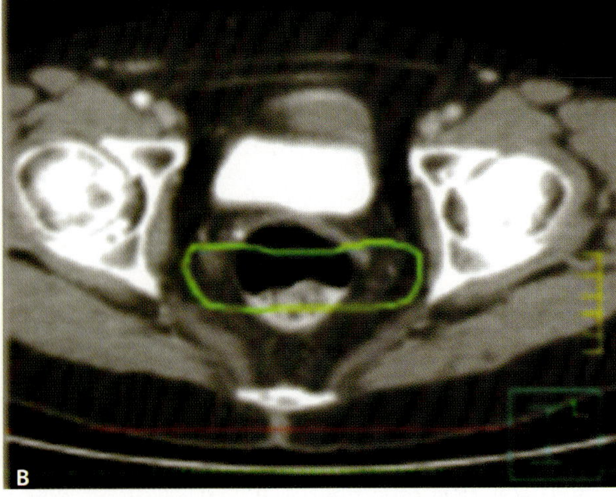

Figs 1A and B Variation of target volume with rectal distension. Panel A demonstrates a CT scan in a patient with an empty rectum. Panel B is a CT scan in the same patient with a distended rectum. Note the degree of motion in the vagina and that with tight margins, the target would be entirely missed due to rectal variation

Following this, either packing or a rectal retractor is required to separate the vagina from the anterior rectal wall. The Manchester System defined Point A, which was intended to correspond to the paracervical triangle, as a point 2 cm superior to the cervical os and 2 cm lateral to the midline. Point B was 5 cm lateral from midline at the same level as Point A. Conventional, two-dimensional planning would involve prescribing the dose to Point A. However, there were a number of limitations with this technique and often led to the underdosing and overdosing based on individual patient anatomy.

The Groupe Européen de Curiethérapie and the European Society for Radiotherapy and Oncology (GEC-ESTRO) have since adopted a 3D image-based treatment planning system.[9] With this approach, an MRI or CT is performed with the applicator in situ and the dose is optimized to a volume and not to a point. MRI is preferred due to superior soft tissue discrimination, and thus more accurate target delineation. With 3D brachytherapy, the volumes include the gross tumor volume (GTV), high-risk clinical target volume (HR-CTV) and intermediate-risk clinical target volume (IR-CTV). In addition, critical organs including the rectum, bladder, sigmoid colon, and small bowel are delineated. Dose is optimized to cover the HR-CTV, which includes the GTV and the entire cervix.

When one utilizes HDR brachytherapy, the HDR dose must be converted to the equivalent dose in 2 Gy fractions (EQD2). That is, the HDR dose cannot be mathematically added to EBRT dose without conversion. A number of resources are available to readily perform this calculation.[10]

Other applicators that are used include the vaginal cylinder, which can be used to treat all or part of the vagina. The tandem and cylinder allows for treatment of the uterus as well as the vagina. Interstitial brachytherapy for gynecologic cancers is achieved by placing needles in the operating room, sometimes with laparoscopic guidance. This may be required if the extent of disease cannot be adequately and safely covered by intracavitary techniques. Many other applicators are available but are beyond the scope of this review. Next we review an evidence-based approach for each disease site.

CERVICAL CANCER

Overview

Cervical cancer is the third most common malignancy in women (following breast and colorectal cancer) and accounts for 530,000 cases annually and 275,000 deaths.[11] Human papilloma virus (HPV) is implicated nearly universally in the development of cervical cancer. In developed countries, there has been a substantial decrease in the incidence and mortality of cervical cancer as a result of screening techniques and, more recently, HPV vaccination. These strategies are not widely adopted in developing countries and, consequently, these countries comprise 85% of new cancers.[11]

The two major histologies of cervical cancer, squamous cell carcinoma and adenocarcinoma, have similar risk factors, which are related to the risk of infection with HPV. Risk factors include early onset of sexual activity, multiple sexual partners, having a high-risk sexual partner, history of sexually transmitted disease and immunosuppression. A weaker association has been suggested with cigarette smoking. The majority of cervical cancers are squamous cell carcinoma, which comprise 70–80% of cases. Adenocarcinoma and adenosquamous comprise 10–20% of cases. Other histologies including neuroendocrine or clear cell carcinoma may occur but are rare.

The staging for cervical cancer is based on the FIGO (International Federation of Gynecology and Obstetrics) system. The staging system is described in Table 1. Of note, due to the prevalence of cervical cancer in developing countries, FIGO has chosen a clinical staging system for this disease. Advanced imaging findings, while influential for therapeutic decisions, are not to change the patient's stage.

Table 1 FIGO staging for cervical cancer

I	Confined to the cervix and uterus
IA	Invasive carcinoma visible by microscopy
IA1	Stromal invasion ≤ 3.0 mm in depth and ≤7.0 mm in horizontal spread
IA2	Stromal invasion > 3.0–5.0 mm in depth and 7.0 mm or less in horizontal spread
IB	Clinically visible lesion, or microscopic lesion >IA2
IB1	Clinically visible lesion, ≤4.0 cm
IB2	Clinically visible lesion, >4.0 cm
II	Invades beyond uterus but not to pelvic wall or lower 1/3 of vagina
IIA	Without parametrial invasion (i.e. involves upper 2/3 of vagina)
IIA1	≤4.0 cm
IIA2	>4.0 cm
IIB	With parametrial invasion
III	Extends to pelvic wall, lower 1/3 of vagina, or causes hydronephrosis
IIIA	Involves lower 1/3 of vagina, no extension to pelvic wall
IIIB	Extends to pelvic wall or causes hydronephrosis or nonfunctioning kidney
IVA	Invades mucosa of bladder or rectum or extends beyond true pelvis
IVB	Distant metastasis

Early Stage

Early stage cervical cancer refers to FIGO stage IA and IB1 disease, based on clinical examination and pathology. For most women with early stage cervical cancer, definitive surgical management is favored over radiation therapy. The surgery of choice usually is radical or modified radical hysterectomy with pelvic lymphadenectomy. A radical hysterectomy includes removal of the uterus, cervix, parametria and upper portion of the vagina.

Surgery has the advantage of preservation of gonadal function and avoidance of early menopause in younger women. Furthermore patients may avoid late toxicities of radiation therapy including shortening and fibrosis of the vagina, bladder and bowel complications and second malignancies. The only study to compare surgery with radiation therapy was performed in Milan in which 343 patients with stage IB–IIA were randomized to radical hysterectomy versus radiation therapy to a median Point A dose of 76 Gy.[12] There was no difference in survival between surgery and radiation at 5 years (87% vs 90%); however, the complication rate (grade 2–3) was higher in the surgical arm (28% vs 12%). This was because of need for postoperative radiation treatment in surgery arm which increased the risk of complications. For patients where pretreatment factors suggest need for postoperative radiation therapy, one should favor treating with definitive radiation therapy to avoid dual modality of treatment and thus decrease the risk of complications. Indications for adjuvant radiation therapy are based on risk factors after pathologic analysis. Intermediate-risk factors (often referred as Sedlis' criteria) were established by the landmark Gynecology Oncology Group (GOG) 92 trial.[13,14] These include lymphovascular space invasion (LVSI), presence of deep stromal invasion and tumor size more than or equal to 4 cm. Women who are found to have two of these criteria are considered to be of intermediate risk and adjuvant therapy in the form of radiation therapy alone is warranted. GOG 92 tested no further therapy versus adjuvant radiation therapy in this cohort of women. Long-term follow-up revealed that adjuvant radiation improved local recurrence (LR) rates (21% vs 14%). Radiation improved the risk of recurrence by 46% (recurrence rate: 31% vs 18%) and demonstrated a trend to improved overall survival, although the study may not have been adequately powered to detect this. Adenocarcinomas were shown to benefit the most from radiation therapy (LR: 44% vs 8%). At this point, the role for adjuvant chemoradiation therapy in patients with intermediate-risk factors has not been clearly established, but it is the subject of ongoing investigation.

Women with cervical cancer treated with radical hysterectomy are considered at high-risk if any of the following criteria (referred to as Peters' criteria) are present: positive surgical margins, positive pelvic lymph node, or parametrial involvement. In these women, the risk of recurrence approaches 40% and adjuvant chemoradiation therapy is indicated. These criteria were established by GOG 109 in which women with these risk factors were randomized after modified radical hysterectomy to radiation therapy alone versus chemoradiation therapy.[15,16] Chemoradiation reduced LR by 50% and distant metastasis by 30%. In the entire cohort, the 4-year overall survival was improved from 71% to 81%. In those with tumors larger than 2 cm and two or more involved lymph nodes, there was absolute survival benefit of about 20%. While GOG 109 used cisplatin and 5-fluorouracil (5-FU) concurrently with radiation, in modern practice, single-agent cisplatin is typically used. The role of additional adjuvant chemotherapy in this subset is part of ongoing randomized study.

Standard techniques for postoperative irradiation include 3D conformal radiation therapy. More contemporary techniques including IMRT have the potential to achieve similar outcomes while improving the toxicity profile. This has been evaluated in phase II trial by the Radiation Therapy Oncology Group (RTOG) 0418 trial. This showed the feasibility and similar disease control rates as conventional treatment techniques with reduction in acute grade 2 bowel toxicity and marrow toxicity. There is ongoing phase III study comparing 3D to IMRT being performed by RTOG to evaluate if there is any difference in morbidity and quality of life.

Locally Advanced Disease

Women with locally advanced cervical cancer (FIGO IB2–IVA) are at a substantially higher risk for recurrence than those with early stage disease. Surgical management may not be appropriate as the tumor may be cut through and the relapse rates are unacceptably high. Chemoradiation is the treatment of choice in these patients and has been established by multiple clinical trials.

The workup in these patients should include lymph node evaluation by PET/CT scans if possible. This will not change staging but will impact radiation fields. If there is urinary tract obstruction, this should be corrected prior to definitive management.

In the 1990s, several clinical trials investigated chemoradiation therapy in locally advanced patients who would be at high-risk for relapse if surgical management were planned.[17] The RTOG 90-01 trial showed a benefit to chemoradiation therapy when compared to radiation alone but a Canadian NCIC trial was negative.[18] A meta-analysis was later performed and showed that chemoradiation was associated with a 12% absolute improvement in survival and 16% absolute improvement in progression-free survival.[19] The National Institutes of Health (NIH) in the United States issued a clinical alert in 1999 indicating that based on these trials, chemoradiation should be implemented as the standard of care in these patients.

Standard chemotherapy in this setting is radiosensitizing cisplatin (40 mg/m^2 weekly). Weekly cisplatin was compared to cisplatin/5-FU in a South Korean trial.[20] This revealed that the single-agent cisplatin was better tolerated and had higher compliance rates while not affecting response and survival rates. Cisplatin has been combined with gemcitabine in a trial from South America as well in an effort to improve efficacy.[21] In this trial, both progression-free survival and overall survival were improved with cisplatin/gemcitabine over cisplatin alone at the cost of increased serious toxicities and hospitalization rates. Furthermore, the role for additional chemotherapy following concurrent chemoradiation has not been well established and is the subject of ongoing clinical trials. At present, the standard remains concurrent single-agent cisplatin with radiation therapy in patients with locally advanced cervical cancer.

The radiation therapy for most women includes two phases of treatment including EBRT and brachytherapy. Brachytherapy is an integral component of care which allows for the safe escalation of dose while shortening the overall treatment time. The time to completion of chemoradiation is particularly important in cervical cancer. For all women undergoing chemoradiation therapy, the treatment should be completed within 8 weeks. Prolongation of treatment is associated with higher rates of pelvic disease progression.

Radiation Technique: EBRT

Classical field borders for pelvic EBRT are: L4/L5 superiorly, below the obturator foramen inferiorly or at least 2–3 cm below vaginal extent of disease, 2 cm lateral to the bony pelvis, 1 cm anterior to the pubic symphysis and posteriorly to cover the sacrum until S2/S3. In our practice, we perform 3D and IMRT-based planning with volumetrically defined targets based on vessel anatomy.

A description of the technique for 3D or IMRT is provided here, and we encourage the reader to refer to the published consensus guidelines and atlases for 3D and IMRT target delineation.[22] CT simulation with full and empty bladder is performed with IV contrast and fleet enema to keep rectum empty. The contours are performed on the full bladder scan with utilization of the empty bladder scan to create an internal target volume (ITV) to account for variation in bladder filling. We instruct patients to present for treatment with a comfortably full bladder.

The CTV1 includes the entire uterus, cervix, parametrium, ovaries and proximal vagina with appropriate ITV margins to account for organ motion based on full bladder and empty bladder scans (Figs 2A to D). If single CT is performed then at least 1 cm of the posterior bladder is included to account for changes in bladder filling. We also delineate 1 cm margin beyond the uterus to account for motion.

The CTV2 (nodal CTV) includes the lymph node stations at risk. For all cervical cancer patients, this volume include the common iliac, internal iliac, external iliac, obturator and presacral (to S2/S3) lymph node groups. When a high pelvic or common iliac lymph node is positive, one should consider including para-aortic station up to the renal vessels as well due to risk of microscopic disease spread. We have published guidelines on contouring the para-aortic region and emphasize that this volume should not be defined by a fixed circumferential margin around the vessels (Figs 3A to C).[23] CTV1 and CTV2 are then summed and adequate planning target volume (PTV) margins are added (typically 0.5–1 cm for CTV2 and 1.0–1.5 cm for CTV1).

The University of California San Diego group assessed interfractional motion in women with cervical cancer by obtaining daily cone beam CT.[24] The researchers contoured the CTV to include the cervix only (without inclusion of the posterior bladder). They found that a PTV margin of 1.5 cm would still fail to encompass the CTV in 32% of fractions but volume of CTV that was missed was small. This provides objective evidence of the large interfraction motion of the cervix and reinforces the importance of adequate margins and image-guided approaches for IMRT therapy of cervical cancer.

In the postoperative setting, this pelvis is treated to 50.4 in 28 fractions. Vaginal cylinder brachytherapy is indicated as a boost in the adjuvant setting if there was a positive vaginal margin. In the definitive setting, the external beam dose to the volume described above is typically 45 Gy and all patients undergo brachytherapy. If nodes are involved then total nodal dose is taken for equivalent dose to approximately to 60 Gy. At our institution, we utilize simultaneous integrated boost to involved lymph nodes with 5–10 mm margin to a dose of 55 Gy in 25 fractions (at 2.2 Gy/fraction) using IMRT. For IMRT planning, critical organs including the small bowel, duodenum, rectum, bladder, femoral heads, bone marrow and kidneys are constrained.

Radiation Technique: Brachytherapy

Brachytherapy is integral to the definitive treatment of cervical cancer. Various schedules for EBRT and brachytherapy are available and utilized. We prefer to interdigitate brachytherapy weekly in the last 1–2 weeks of EBRT depending on tumor size and response to EBRT and continue brachytherapy twice weekly until complete. Regardless of the schedule chosen, it is integral that the treatment package is complete within 8 weeks so that outcomes are not compromised by accelerated repopulation of tumor clonogens.[25]

As described previously, both HDR and LDR techniques are performed. Due to the advantages afforded by HDR, many institutions now prefer this technique. This may be performed using a tandem and ring or tandem and ovoid applicator. Classical dosimetric technique indicates that the dose to Point A should receive a dose an EQD2 of 80–90 Gy.

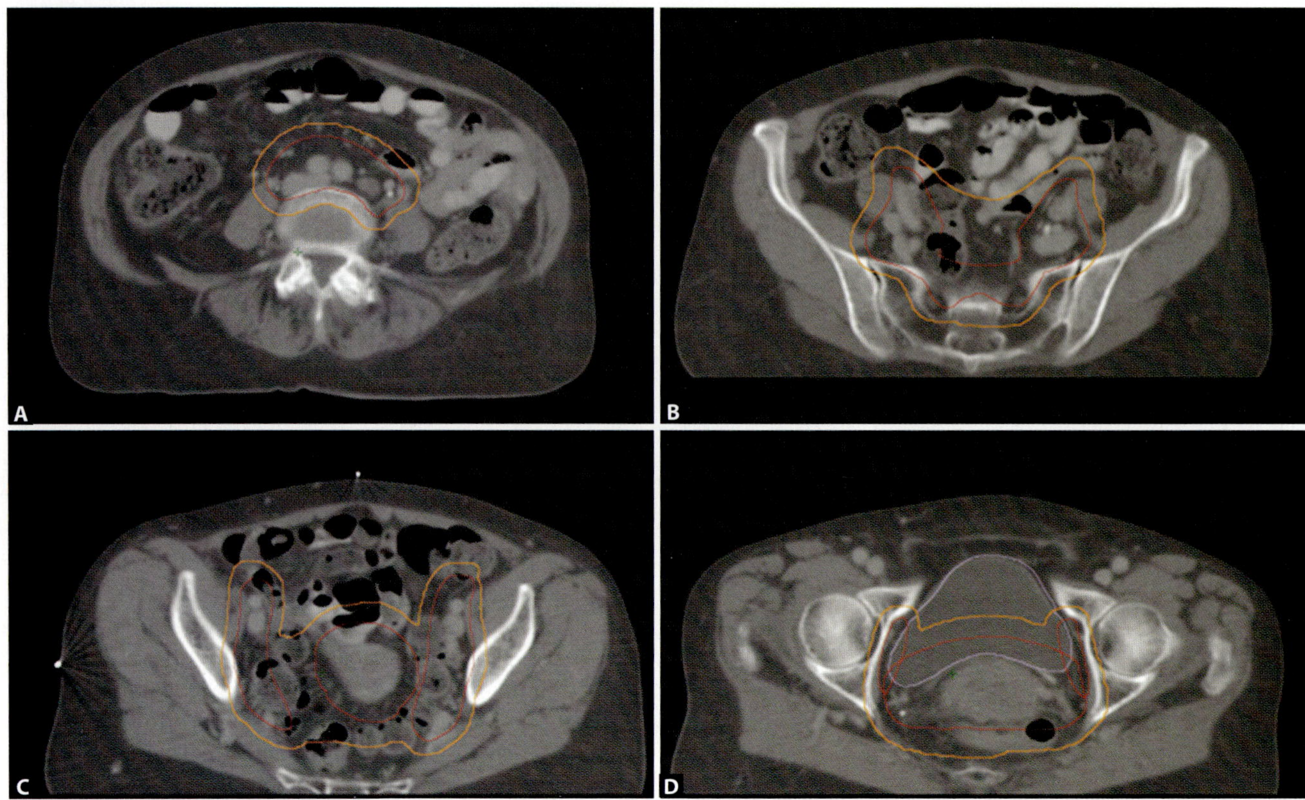

Figs 2A to D Representative contours from a patient with stage IIB cervical cancer. Representative slices from superior to inferior; the red outline is the CTV and the orange outline is the PTV. (A) Panel is obtained from the proximal common iliac chain; (B) Panel shows contouring at the level of the external and internal iliac chain with inclusion of the presacral lymph node region; (C) In the panel, internal and external iliac nodes are included as well as the entire uterus with adequate margins to account for motion; (D) Panel demonstrates the required margins anteriorly to account for variation in bladder filling. The CTV includes the posterior 1 cm of the bladder and the PTV is formed by expanding this by another 1 cm

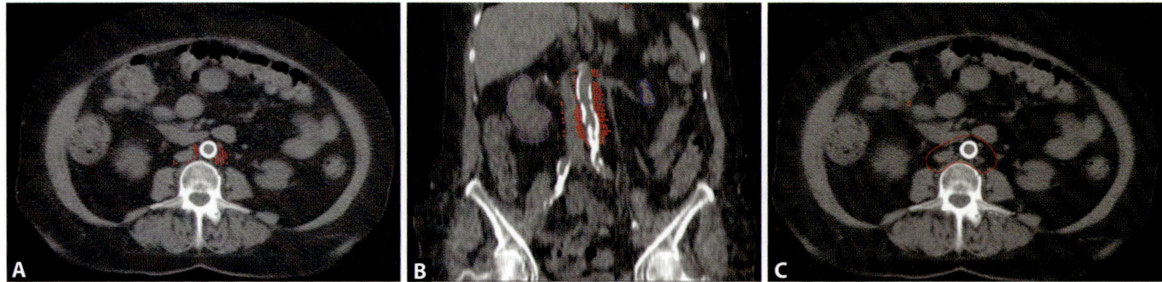

Figs 3A to C Para-aortic lymph node contouring guidelines. The University of Pittsburgh Cancer Institute has published guidelines for contouring the para-aortic lymph node region. (A and B) Panels demonstrate the location of para-aortic lymph nodes in a series of 46 patients on axial and coronal views respectively. Uniform marginal expansion beyond the vessels may inadequately cover the space between the aorta and the psoas muscle where lymph nodes are frequently found; (C) Panel is a representative contouring based on our guidelines. The anatomic boundaries are as follows: laterally, the medial border of left and right iliopsoas muscles; posteriorly, the anterior border of the vertebral body; and anteriorly, and at least 0.75 cm margin in soft tissue around vessels

With image-based brachytherapy, plans are optimized to the HR-CTV which includes the GTV and the entire cervix (Fig. 4). The EQD2 dose to the HR-CTV is in the range of 80–90 Gy depending on response to EBRT. Plans are optimized such that the dose to 90% of the HR-CTV is 100%. Critical organ dosimetry can be carefully monitored and optimized with image-guided techniques. The GEC-ESTRO guidelines are to limit the dose to 2 cm^3 of the rectum, sigmoid colon and bladder to 70–75 Gy, 70–75 Gy and 90 Gy, respectively.[26,27]

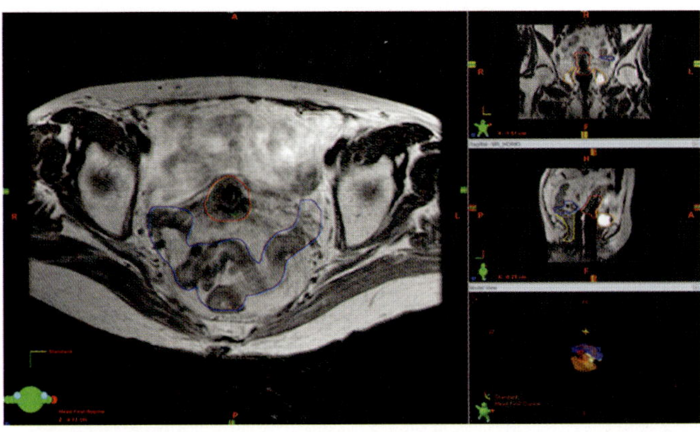

Fig. 4 HDR brachytherapy plan in a patient with cervical cancer. This is a patient with stage IIB cervical cancer who underwent an MRI with ring and tandem applicator in situ to facilitate image-based brachytherapy. The HR-CTV (red), rectum (yellow), sigmoid colon (blue), and bladder (orange) are contoured

Table 2 FIGO staging for endometrial cancer

I	Confined to corpus
IA	Limited to endometrium or invades <½ of myometrium
IB	Invades ≥½ of myometrium
II	Invades stromal tissue of the cervix but does not extend beyond uterus (endocervical glandular involvement only is Stage II)
IIIA	Involves serosa and/or adnexa
IIIB	Vaginal involvement or parametrial involvement
IIIC1	Pelvic lymph node metastasis
IIIC2	Para-aortic lymph node metastasis
IVA	Invades bladder mucosa and/or bowel mucosa
IVB	Distant metastasis (includes inguinal LN, intraperitoneal disease, lung, liver or bone)

Fletcher's conditions of acceptable brachytherapy require (1) adequate geometry and technique to prevent underdosing of the cervix, (2) acceptable dose to the paracervical region and, (3) respect for the tolerances of the critical structures. In some cases, these conditions are unable to be met and interstitial brachytherapy is required. This may occur if the disease is extensive or a narrow vaginal apex precludes optimal intracavitary applicator positioning. HDR interstitial brachytherapy may be delivered by a variety of fractionation schemes. A common fractionation schedule following 45 Gy of EBRT is 5 Gy × 5 fractions delivered twice daily with a 6 hour interfraction interval.

ENDOMETRIAL CANCER

Overview

The worldwide annual incidence of endometrial cancer is about 288,000 with approximately 74,000 deaths.[28] There are two major histologic types. Type I endometrial cancers are of endometrioid histology and are grade 1 or 2. These comprise about 80% of cancers and generally have a more favorable prognosis than the type 2 tumors. The type 2 tumors account for about 15% of cancers and include grade 3 endometrioid tumors as well as non-endometrioid histologies (serous, clear cell, mucinous, squamous, undifferentiated, etc.).

Risk factors for type 1 cancers are related to exogenous or endogenous estrogen exposure. Thus, risk factors include age, obesity, early menarche, late menopause and nulliparity. Unopposed estrogen therapy (without opposing progestin) markedly increases risk of endometrial cancer. Tamoxifen is also known to increase the risk of endometrial cancer in postmenopausal women. Genetic syndromes may predispose certain populations to endometrial cancer. Lynch syndrome or hereditary nonpolyposis colorectal cancer is due to a germline mutation in DNA mismatch repair. Women with this syndrome are at increased risk of endometrial cancer as well as colon and ovarian cancers.

Women often present with abnormal postmenopausal bleeding. Initial workup should include pelvic examination and ultrasonography to assess the endometrial thickness. The diagnosis is confirmed with an outpatient endometrial biopsy if possible. Otherwise a dilation and curettage can be performed for histological diagnosis.

Endometrial cancer is a surgically staged disease. The staging system is detailed in Table 2. The standard staging procedure is a total extrafascial hysterectomy with bilateral salpingo-oophorectomy with pelvic and para-aortic lymph node dissection. Practice patterns do vary regarding the extent and utilization of lymph node dissection. The benefit of lymph node dissection is that it may be potentially therapeutic and accurately directs adjuvant therapy. However, dissection is associated with increased toxicity including lymphedema, symptomatic lymphocysts, deep vein thrombosis and bowel obstruction. The MRC ASTEC trial evaluated this question in 1,400 patients and showed equivalent outcome with or without pelvic lymph node dissection.[29] Thus, controversy does exist regarding its utilization but the standard of care in the United States remains to perform a pelvic and para-aortic lymphadenectomy.

Adjuvant Therapy Overview

Following surgical staging, determination for adjuvant therapy is based upon the risk of relapse. Factors that influence the risk of relapse include depth of invasion into the myometrium, grade, cervical stromal invasion, LVSI, age and nodal status. Other risk factors include lower uterine segment involvement and positive peritoneal cytology (which is no longer included in the staging schema).

Low-risk disease is defined as low-grade (1 or 2) endometrioid cancer with no invasion of the myometrium (a subset of IA). Intermediate-risk disease is classified as cancer that invades the myometrium (stage IA or IB) or demonstrates occult cervical stromal invasion (stage II). This group of patients can be further subdivided into high-intermediate and low-intermediate risk (Table 3). Based on GOG criteria, the adverse factors analyzed include: (1) outer 1/3 myometrial invasion, (2) grade 2 or 3 differentiation and (3) LVSI. Patients of any age with all three risk factors, 50–69 years of age with two risk factors or more than 70 years of age with one risk factor meet GOG criteria for high-intermediate risk.[30] The Post-Operative Radiation Therapy in Endometrial Cancer (PORTEC) group has defined high-intermediate risk as disease which meets 2/3 factors: (1) age more than 60 years, (2) outer half myometrial invasion (stage IB), and (3) grade 3 histology.[31] High-risk patients are those with stage III disease or with adverse histology (serous or clear cell) of any stage.

Low-risk

Women with low-risk disease (low grade and lack of invasion of the myometrium) have an excellent outcome following surgery. Adjuvant therapies in this setting have not been shown to improve outcome. Pelvic radiation therapy is not indicated for these patients. The risk of metastatic disease to the lymph nodes is very low and treatment only increases the morbidity rate. In a recent meta-analysis, pelvic EBRT is associated with worse disease-free survival.[32]

Vaginal brachytherapy enables the local delivery of radiation while sparing surrounding normal tissue. In the low-risk population, there is no statistical benefit to vaginal brachytherapy over observation. In a European study of women with stage IA, grade 1–2 endometrial cancer randomized to surgery followed by observation or vaginal brachytherapy, there were no differences in disease-specific or overall survival. However, there was an increase in genitourinary morbidity (0.6% vs 2.8%).[33] Thus, the recommendations are for observation following definitive surgical management in low-risk disease.

Table 3 GOG and PORTEC criteria for high-intermediate risk endometrial cancer

GOG	*PORTEC*
Risk factors • Outer 1/3 myometrial invasion • Grade 2–3 • Lymphovascular space invasion *Criteria* • Age >70 years with 1 factor • Age 50–69 years with 2 factors • Any age with 3 factors	2 of 3 factors: • Age >60 years • Stage IB • Grade 3

Abbreviations: GOG, Gynecology Oncology Group trial; PORTEC, Post-Operative Radiation Therapy in Endometrial Cancer

Intermediate Risk

Adjuvant treatment options for intermediate-risk endometrial cancer typically involve observation or radiation therapy, depending on the risk factors present. For patients with low-intermediate risk, both observation or adjuvant vaginal brachytherapy are acceptable options. Vaginal brachytherapy carries minimal morbidity and reduces the risk of locoregional recurrence. Observation with salvage therapy for the minority that fails is also reasonable alternative.[34]

For those with high-intermediate risk, adjuvant therapy is indicated. Multiple clinical trials have been conducted in this group of patients. PORTEC 1 randomized patients between observation and adjuvant pelvic radiation.[35] This revealed a decrease in locoregional recurrence at 15 years (16% vs 6%) with no difference in overall survival. Approximately, 75% of recurrences were found in the vaginal vault. This lead to PORTEC 2 which randomized high-intermediate risk patients between pelvic EBRT and vaginal brachytherapy.[31] Of note, patients with IB grade 3 disease were specifically excluded from this trial as they were felt to be at too high of a risk for pelvic failure and were recommended to undergo pelvic EBRT. This trial demonstrated no difference in the two techniques with LR rates at 5 years to be 1.6% and 1.8% for EBRT and brachytherapy, respectively. There was no difference in isolated pelvic recurrence (0.5% vs 1.5%), locoregional relapse (2.1% vs 5.1%) or survival. However, there was substantially less toxicity with brachytherapy and this emerged as the standard of care. The role for chemotherapy to address distant disease in this population is unclear but is the subject on ongoing clinical trials. Table 4 provides guidelines for treatment of stage I endometrial cancer.

High-risk

Data for management of high-risk patients is somewhat limited. For those with stage III disease, chemotherapy is the mainstay of treatment. GOG 122 evaluated whole abdominal radiation versus chemotherapy and found

Table 4 Recommendations for treatment of stage IA and IB endometrial cancer. Risk factors may be determined by GOG or PORTEC criteria for high-intermediate risk as described in Table 3

Stage IA	*Stage IB*
No risk factors G1–2: Observation G3: VCBT or observation	*No risk factors* G1–G2: VCBT G3: EBRT + VCBT
+ Risk factors G1–2: VCBT G3: VCBT or EBRT + VCBT	*+ Risk factors* G1-2: VCBT G3: EBRT + VCBT

Abbreviations: EBRT, external beam radiation therapy; G#, represents grade of disease; VCBT, vaginal cuff brachytherapy

that the chemotherapy arm improved survival.[36] Whole abdomen therapy has since been abandoned. A Japanese and Italian trial has explored adjuvant chemotherapy versus adjuvant pelvic radiation therapy in high-risk patients. Both found no difference in survival between the two arms. Sequential therapy was explored by two trials, the NSGO-9501/EORTC-55991 and MaNGO ILIADE-III.[37] The trials had some differences in inclusion criteria but both randomized high-risk patients to adjuvant radiation therapy or adjuvant chemotherapy and radiation. The pooled results showed improved progression-free survival at 5 years with combined therapy (69% vs 78%) with a trend to improved survival. Our preference is to perform adjuvant sequential chemotherapy and radiation therapy in women with stage III disease. For those with adverse histology, a similar approach with sequential chemotherapy and radiation is utilized, with awareness that there is limited data to support this approach. Phase II data appears to show promising results with a "sandwich" approach with chemotherapy-radiation-chemotherapy for patients with papillary serous carcinoma.[38] There are ongoing randomized studies by GOG and PORTEC to define optimal adjuvant treatment for high-risk endometrial cancer patients including concurrent chemoradiation and the addition of radiation therapy with adjuvant chemotherapy.

Inoperable Endometrial Cancer

Approximately, 3% of patients are medically inoperable due to comorbidities. For these patients, primary radiation therapy is indicated. MRI should be done as part of evaluation. Pelvic radiation followed by brachytherapy is recommended for those with grade 3 disease or large volume of disease by imaging or cervical involvement. For those who appear to have a clinical stage I disease and/or grade 1 or 2 and low volume on MRI imaging, brachytherapy alone is an acceptable approach. We utilize a tandem and cylinder approach or Y applicator brachytherapy with HDR brachytherapy to a dose of 7.5 Gy × 5 fractions for patients treated with brachytherapy alone.[39]

Recurrent Endometrial Cancer

Management of locoregional recurrent endometrial cancer is highly individualized and depends on the extent of recurrence. For those with isolated vaginal recurrence, salvage therapy is fairly effective. Based on the PORTEC trial, the 3-years survival rate for those with isolated vaginal recurrence was 73% and this substantially higher than that following pelvic relapse (8%).[34]

For isolated vaginal relapse in patients who have not had prior radiation therapy, the treatment of choice includes pelvic irradiation and vaginal brachytherapy. Depending on the depth of recurrence, either interstitial or intracavitary brachytherapy may be utilized. In those who have had prior irradiation, the treatment options are limited and re-irradiation may be considered based upon the normal tissue tolerances.

Radiation Technique: EBRT

For postoperative treatment of the whole pelvis for endometrial cancer, both 3DCRT and IMRT techniques may be utilized. Conventional field borders are L5/S1 (superior) to below obturator foramen with inclusion of the upper vagina (inferior). The lateral border is 2 cm lateral to the pelvic brim. Anterior border is the pubic symphysis and the posteriorly to the sacrum until S2/S3.

We define the target volumetrically and utilize IMRT to reduce bowel toxicity (Figs 5A to D). A brief overview is provided, but the reader is encouraged to refer the published consensus guidelines for target delineation.[40] CT simulation with full and empty bladder is performed with intravenous contrast and fleet enema for empty rectum as previously described for cervical cancer. The CTV1 includes the vaginal cuff, paravaginal tissue, proximal half of the vagina. On the full bladder scan, this include 1.0–1.5 cm of the posterior bladder, and the empty bladder scan can be compared to ensure that the target is still included. The CTV2 includes the lymph nodes at risk and includes the low common iliac, internal iliac, external iliac, obturator and presacral (to S2/S3 inferiorly) lymph nodes. For those with positive para-aortic lymph nodes or positive pelvic lymph nodes without para-aortic dissection, we treat an extended field volume with inclusion of the para-aortic lymph nodes; the superior border in this circumstance is the level of the renal vessels. We have published our detailed recommendations for contouring of the para-aortic lymph nodes (Figs 3A to C).[23] Both CTV1 and CTV2 are combined with appropriate margins for PTV and this is taken to a dose of 45–50.4 Gy in 1.8 Gy fractions. This may be followed by vaginal brachytherapy boost to the vaginal cuff especially for high-risk endometrial cancer. For IMRT planning, critical organs including the small bowel, duodenum, rectum, bladder, femoral heads, bone marrow and kidneys are constrained.

Radiation Technique: Brachytherapy

For the adjuvant treatment of the vaginal cuff, we recommend utilization of a vaginal cylinder. The largest diameter cylinder tolerated by the patient is utilized to reduce the vaginal mucosal dose. The target length is proximal 3–4 cm of vagina. Various dose and fractionation schedules are utilized. Our preference is for a dose of 7 Gy × 3 fractions prescribed to a depth of 0.5 cm when vaginal brachytherapy is utilized alone as per the PORTEC2 trial. When utilized as a boost following EBRT, we prescribe 5 Gy × 2 fractions to a depth of 0.5 cm. However, various dose fractionation schemes are acceptable, and we refer the reader to the guidelines

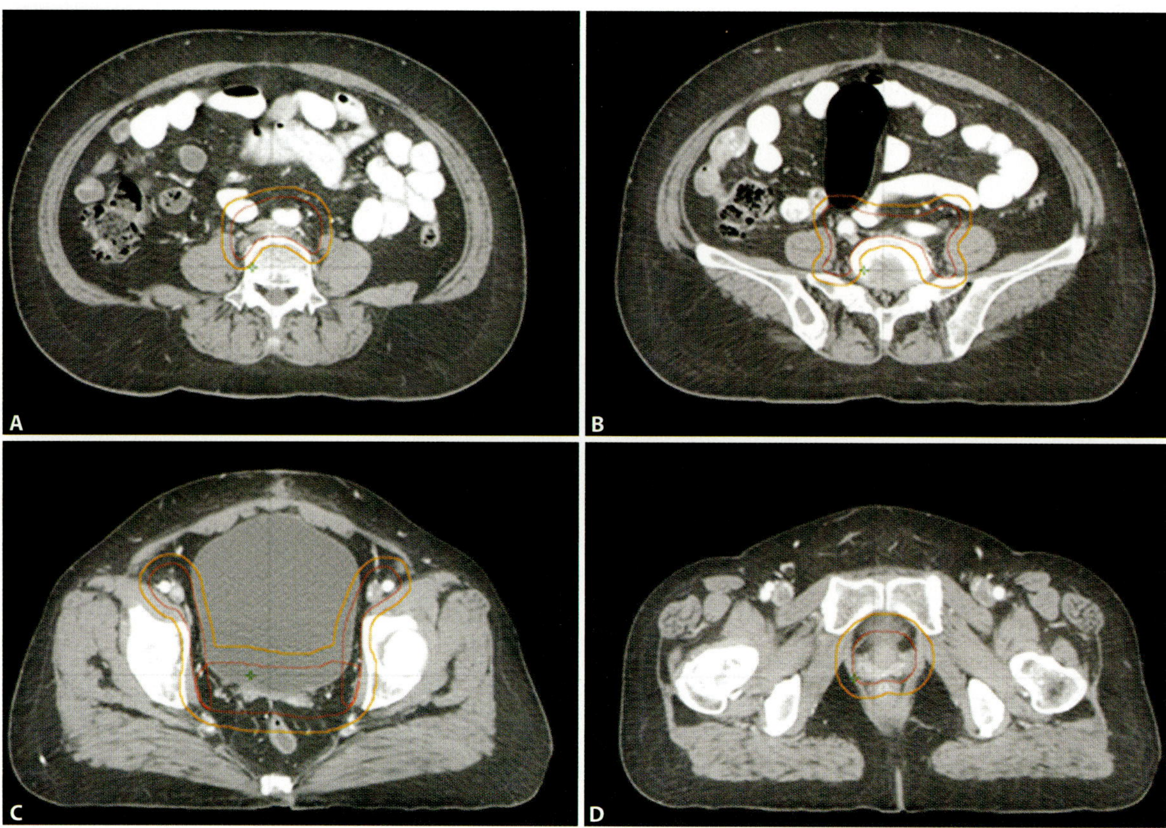

Figs 5A to D Representative contours for the postoperative pelvic radiation treatment from a woman with IB, Grade III endometrial cancer. Panels are representative slices from superior to inferior; the red outline is the CTV and the orange outline is the PTV. (A) Panel is obtained from the proximal common iliac vessels; (B) Panel shows contouring at the level of the common iliac immediately superior to its division into the external and internal iliac chain; (C) In the panel, the internal and external iliac nodes are included as well as the vagina with adequate margins to account for variation in bladder filling; (D) Panel demonstrates the inferior extent of the contouring, including the vagina with adequate margins

published by the American Brachytherapy Society (ABS).[41] We utilized CT-based planning for the first fraction for confirmation of position of applicator up to the apex and permit 3D dosimetry. We have published our experience with this technique and have demonstrated 3D planning enables for lower doses to the bladder and rectum without compromising CTV coverage.[42] For subsequent fractions, we confirm reproduction of positioning by anterior-posterior and lateral x-rays or scout film by the CT scanner and deliver the same plan. Repeat planning does not appear to achieve a significant difference in dosimetry.[43]

VULVAR CANCER

Overview

Vulvar cancer comprises 5% of malignancies of the female genital tract.[44] It is typically a cancer of postmenopausal women with the average age of diagnosis of 65 years. Risk factors include tobacco, prior history of lichen sclerosis, HPV infection and immunodeficiency. HPV is thought to account for about 60% of vulvar cancers and may be contributing to a trend of decreasing average age of diagnosis of vulvar cancer.

The vast majority of vulvar cancers are of squamous cell histology. Melanoma is uncommonly found on the vulva and accounts for the about 5% of primary vulvar cancers. Basal cell carcinomas and sarcoma may also present with a primary vulvar cancer both these are uncommon.

Prior to 1988, vulvar cancer was clinically staged, but it is now a surgically staged disease. The new staging system allows for more accurate lymph node assessment to impact treatment decisions. The staging system is described in Table 5.

Early Stage Disease

For early stage disease (Stage I–II), surgical management is preferred. The surgical management includes modified radical

Table 5 FIGO staging for vulvar cancer

I	Continued to the vulva or perineum
IA	≤2 cm in size and ≤1 mm depth of stromal invasion
IB	>2 cm in size, or any size with >1 mm depth of stromal invasion
II	Extension to adjacent perineal structures (distal 1/3 urethra, distal 1/3 vagina, or anal involvement)
IIIA	1–2 LN mets, each <5 mm 1 LN met, ≥5 mm
IIIB	3 or more LN, each <5 mm 2 or more LN, ≥5 mm
IIIC	LN with extracapsular spread
IVA	Extension to any of the following: proximal 2/3 of urethra, proximal 2/3 of vagina, bladder mucosa, rectal mucosa, or fixed to pelvic bone or fixed or ulcerated LN
IVB	Distant metastasis (includes pelvic LN met)

Abbreviation: LN, lymph node

vulvectomy with an inguinofemoral lymphadenectomy. Recent years have seen changes in surgical paradigm with an increase interest in sentinel lymph node biopsy.

An inguinofemoral lymphadenectomy carries significant morbidity risks including infection, lymphedema, wound healing issues and others. For those with clinically negative groin examination and tumor size 4 cm or less, sentinel lymph node biopsy is considered standard of care is considered. The GROINSS-V trial was an observational study to identify the feasibility of sentinel lymph node biopsy.[45] The study was able to demonstrate feasibility of the technique in a multicenter trial and demonstrated a 2.3% groin failure rate in those with negative sentinel lymph node. In this trial, if the sentinel lymph node was positive, groin dissection was performed. The GROINSS-VII trial is a second observation trial which investigates adjuvant radiation for women with positive sentinel lymph nodes in place of nodal dissection. The final results are still pending; however, interim analysis has revealed that in those with macrometastases, the risk of nodal relapse is high with adjuvant radiation therapy. The protocol has now been amended and patients with macrometastases undergo inguinofemoral nodal dissection with or without adjuvant radiation based on risk factors and final pathology.

The "heaps risk factors" are utilized to assess the need for adjuvant radiation therapy.[46] The most important predictor for recurrence following surgical management is the margin status and those with margins less than 8 mm were found to have a 50% recurrence rate. Other factors include size greater than 4 cm, LVSI and depth greater than 5 mm. Adjuvant radiation to the primary site is indicated when the margins are less than 8 mm or positive or if multiple of the previously listed heaps factors are present.

Indications for adjuvant inguinal and pelvic nodal radiation are based on GOG 37.[47,48] In this trial, women underwent radical vulvectomy and bilateral groin dissection. Those with positive inguinal nodes were randomized to bilateral pelvic lymph node dissection or bilateral inguinal and pelvic radiation. Of those with positive groin nodes, approximately 28% had pelvic lymph node involvement and about 20% had contralateral groin involvement. In the trial, the radiation arm demonstrated superior overall adjuvant radiation therapy was in those with 2 or more involved lymph nodes or one lymph node with extracapsular extension. We also consider nodal positivity in the setting of inadequate dissection (<6 nodes) as another factor for bilateral inguinal and pelvic radiation therapy.

GOG 88 explored the use of bilateral inguinal radiation to replace bilateral inguinal lymph node dissection in those with clinically N0 disease.[49] This trial showed an overall survival benefit to the surgical arm; however, the trial carries a number of flaws. In the surgical arm, up to 20% were found to have positive lymph nodes and underwent adjuvant radiation. Thus, many in this arm underwent multi-modality therapy, biasing the results. Furthermore, the surgical arm included assessment of the pelvic and inguinal lymph nodes while radiation arm had no imaging done to assess inguinal nodes, and some patients may have had involved nodes but were treated for microscopic disease. Finally, the radiation technique was inadequate using low energy electrons with dose prescribed at 3 cm depth and thus under-dosed the region at risk in many patients. In contrast to these results, multiple retrospective series have shown low recurrence rates if adequate radiation techniques are utilized.[50-52]

In the sentinel lymph node era, those with positive micrometastases can complete radiation therapy to the groin. However, based on the early data from GROINS-VII, those with macrometastases by sentinel lymph node biopsy should undergo completion dissection and adjuvant radiation therapy as indicated by pathologic factors. If patient is not suitable for dissection or declines dissection then adjuvant radiation therapy with or without chemotherapy should be delivered to bilateral inguinal and pelvic regions.

Locally Advanced and Unresectable

For those in which a wide local excision is not possible due to the presence of disease in close proximity to critical organs including urethra and anal canal, definitive or preoperative chemoradiation therapy is indicated. Dose escalation and chemotherapy has steadily shown improved response rates and survival. GOG 101 included patients who were unresectable due to either advanced T stage or N stage. Patients were treated with a split course of radiation to a dose of 47.6 Gy with concurrent cisplatin and 5-FU. Among those with unresectable primaries, 48% achieved a complete clinical response (cCR), of which 70% had a complete pathologic response (pCR). Four-year survival was 55%.[53] In the cohort with unresectable nodal disease, 90% were converted to resectable status and the pCR rate for the nodes was about 40%.[54] Beriwal et al. at the University of Pittsburgh Medical Center have published experience utilizing an IMRT technique with a modified GOG 101 protocol and have demonstrated feasibility and excellent outcomes with cCR of 72% and pCR of 64%.[7]

GOG 205 explored dose escalation to 57.6 Gy with concurrent cisplatin and eliminated the treatment break.[55] This demonstrated a 64% cCR rate of which 78% had pCR. The currently ongoing GOG trial explores further dose escalation to 65 Gy, allows for IMRT, and intensifies chemotherapy by combing cisplatin with gemcitabine. The results of this trial are awaited.

Radiation Treatment Planning

Patients undergo CT simulation with contrast. Prior to the study, the vulva, anus, scars and palpable nodes should be wired. The patient is placed in frog-leg position to decrease skin toxicity. We perform CT-based planning and utilize IMRT to decrease toxicity to the skin, femoral heads, bone marrow, bowel, bladder and rectum.

In definitive or preoperative therapy, the primary CTV includes the entire vulva and nodes including bilateral external iliac, internal iliac, obturator and inguinofemoral lymph nodes. If pelvis nodes are involved, the entire common iliac chain should also be included. The pelvic lymph nodes are typically found within 0.7 cm from the blood vessels. The inguinal lymph nodes are contoured as a compartment and may be as far as 2 cm from the vessels (Fig. 6). A recently published guideline is instructive in inguinal

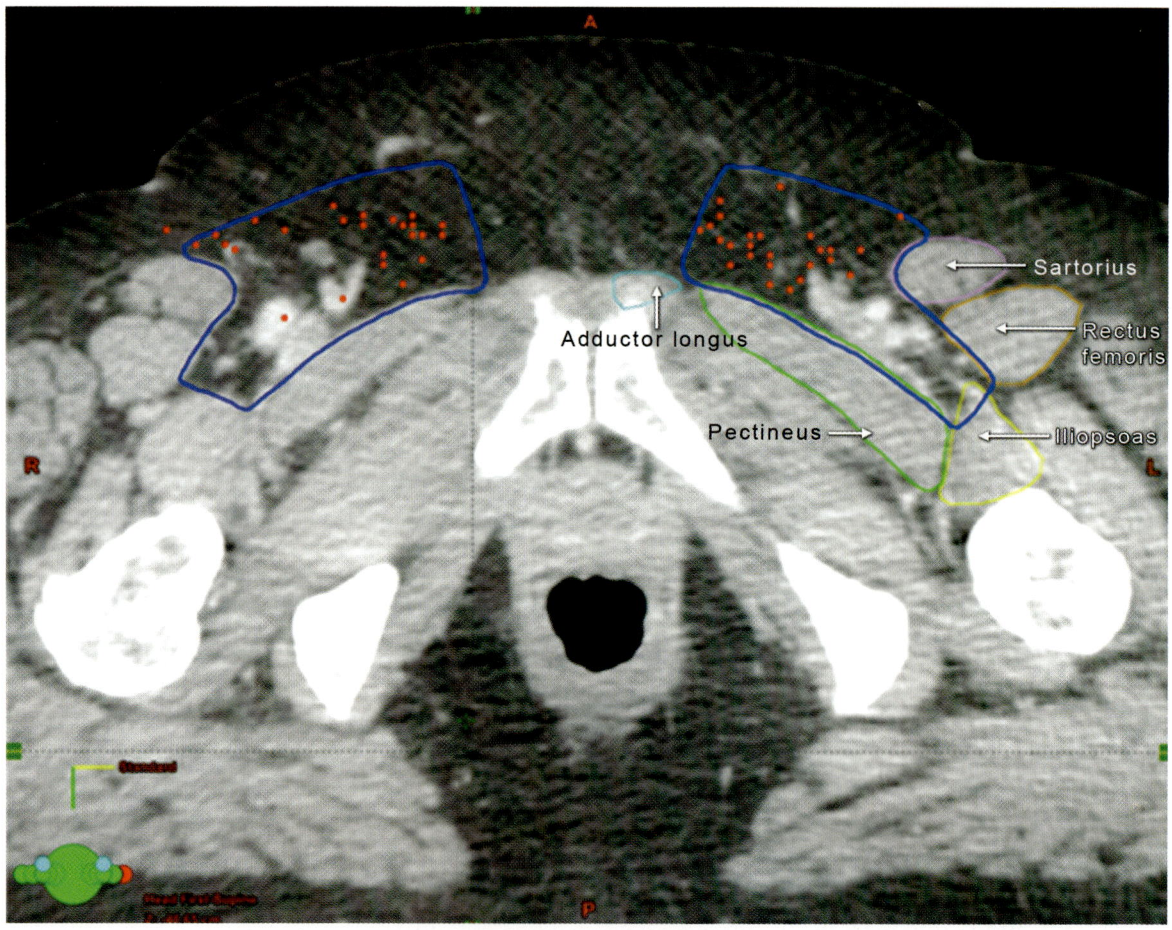

Fig. 6 Inguinal lymph node region contours. The University of Pittsburgh Cancer Institute has published guidelines for contouring the inguinal lymph node region. Inguinal nodes may be found as far as 2 cm from the vessels and the contours must reflect this. The red dots represent the position of inguinal nodes in a series of 22 patients published by the University of Pittsburgh Cancer Institute. Based on our guidelines, the inguinal nodes should be contoured as a compartment, bounded by the adductor longus, pectineus, iliopsoas, rectus femoris and sartorius

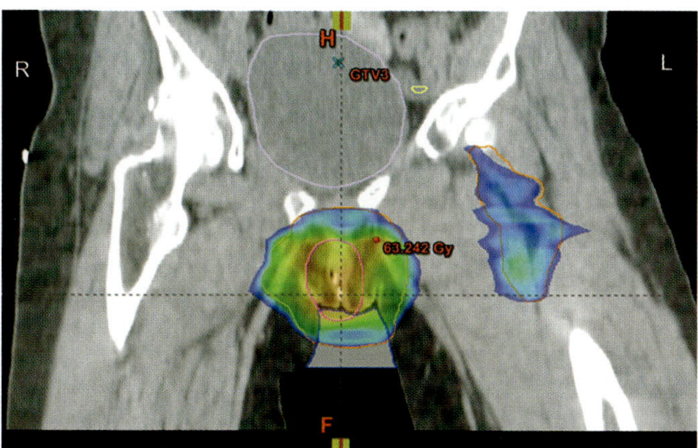

Fig. 7 Bolus for vulvar cancer. A representative coronal slice of a patient with vulvar cancer is shown. The bolus is necessary and must be integrated from the first treatment to ensure adequate dose to the vulva. Also noteworthy is that the CTV (and corresponding dose cloud) are expanded into air. This technique account for the edema that invariably follows once treatment starts

target delineation.[56] A bolus is required to ensure adequate dose to the vulva and should be integrated from the first treatment (Fig. 7). For patients with vaginal involvement, entire vagina should be included in CTV and if disease extends to anal canal then entire anal canal and mesorectum should also be included. For lesions which are posteriorly placed, the perineum should also be included in the primary CTV along with entire vulva.

For preoperative management, concurrent cisplatin and radiation can be performed as per GOG 205. As per this trial, the dose is to 45 Gy to the entire volume described above with a subsequent 12.6 Gy boost to the primary tumor with generous margin for a final dose of 57.6 Gy. Surgery or biopsy of residual disease can be performed in 6–8 weeks. For definitive treatment, dose would be between 60 Gy and 70 Gy based on response and tolerance. For postoperative therapy, the dose is 50.4 Gy with an additional boost, if required, to areas of positive margin or extracapsular extension for the total dose to 55.4–59.4 Gy.

VAGINAL CANCER

Overview

Primary vaginal cancer comprises about 3% of cancers of the female genital tract.[44] The majority of these are squamous cell carcinomas, but other histologies including adenocarcinoma, melanoma, sarcoma and others may also occur. Metastatic cancer to the vagina is more common than primary vaginal cancer and may occur by direct extension or hematogenous or lymphatic spread. The staging system for vaginal cancer is clinical and is described in Table 6.

Table 6 FIGO staging for vaginal cancer

I	Confined to vagina
II	Invades paravaginal tissues but not to pelvic wall
III	Extends to pelvic wall or pelvic or inguinal lymph node metastasis
IVA	Invades mucosa of bladder or rectum or extends beyond the true pelvis
IVB	Distant metastasis

Treatment Overview

Due to the paucity of data, there is variation in the management of vaginal cancer. Treatment is highly individualized based on the size and location of disease and other clinical factors. Early stage disease may be treated with surgery if located in the upper vagina. Otherwise, the management typically includes radiation therapy.

Typically treatment entails EBRT to cover the primary and the regional lymph node groups. This is followed by brachytherapy to achieve a total dose of approximately 70–85 Gy. For those with stage II and greater disease, combined modality therapy with weekly cisplatin, cisplatin/5-FU, or mitomycin C is utilized based on extrapolation from other disease sites including cervical and anal cancer.

Radiation Treatment Planning

External beam radiation therapy fields are designed to cover the primary tumor and draining lymphatics. For most cases, this would include the internal and external iliac lymph nodes and obturator nodes. The inguinal lymph nodes are to be included if the vaginal disease extends into the distal vagina.

Brachytherapy may be delivered using an interstitial or intracavitary technique. Following EBRT, if the disease is nonpalpable or has regressed to less than 5 mm thickness then intracavitary technique could be utilized. Otherwise, interstitial brachytherapy is required to ensure adequate coverage.

There are multiple applicators available for intracavitary brachytherapy. The single-channel vaginal cylinder has traditionally been used. This delivers a uniform dose around the applicator to all four vaginal walls. In recent years, a multi-channel vaginal cylinder has come to market. This enables the dose to be tailored specifically to one of the vaginal walls. This is able to achieve better dosimetry and better spare critical organs. For both techniques, we recommend an image-guided technique and placement of a gold seed marker at the site of disease. Interstitial brachytherapy involves the placement of needles in the vagina to achieve optimal dose distribution. We recommend performing a CT or MRI scan for 3D planning and optimization of the dose distribution thereafter.

REFERENCES

1. Delaney G, Jacob S, Barton M. Estimation of an optimal radiotherapy utilization rate for gynecologic carcinoma: part I—malignancies of the cervix, ovary, vagina and vulva. Cancer. 2004;101:671-81.
2. Delaney G, Jacob S, Barton M. Estimation of an optimal radiotherapy utilization rate for gynecologic carcinoma: part II—carcinoma of the endometrium. Cancer. 2004;101:682-92.
3. Portelance L, Chao KS, Grigsby PW, et al. Intensity-modulated radiation therapy (IMRT) reduces small bowel, rectum, and bladder doses in patients with cervical cancer receiving pelvic and para-aortic irradiation. Int J Radiat Oncol Biol Phys. 2001;51:261-6.
4. Beriwal S, Gan GN, Heron DE, Selvaraj RN, Kim H, Lalonde R, et al. Early clinical outcome with concurrent chemotherapy and extended-field, intensity-modulated radiotherapy for cervical cancer. Int J Radiat Oncol Biol Phys. 2007;68:166-71.
5. Lian J, Mackenzie M, Joseph K, Pervez N, Dundas G, Urtasun R, et al. Assessment of extended-field radiotherapy for stage IIIC endometrial cancer using three-dimensional conformal radiotherapy, intensity-modulated radiotherapy, and helical tomotherapy. Int J Radiat Oncol Biol Phys. 2008;70:935-43.
6. Beriwal S, Jain SK, Heron DE, Kim H, Gerszten K, Edwards RP, et al. Clinical outcome with adjuvant treatment of endometrial carcinoma using intensity-modulated radiation therapy. Gynecol Oncol. 2006;102:195-9.
7. Beriwal S, Coon D, Heron DE, Kelley JL, Edwards RP, Sukumvanich P, et al. Preoperative intensity-modulated radiotherapy and chemotherapy for locally advanced vulvar carcinoma. Gynecol Oncol. 2008;109:291-5.
8. Wang X, Liu R, Ma B, Yang K, Tian J, Jiang L, et al. High dose rate versus low dose rate intracavity brachytherapy for locally advanced uterine cervix cancer. Cochrane Database Syst Rev. 2010:CD007563.
9. Potter R, Haie-Meder C, Van Limbergen E, Barillot I, De Brabandere M, Dimopoulos J, et al. Recommendations from gynaecological (GYN) GEC ESTRO working group (II): concepts and terms in 3D image-based treatment planning in cervix cancer brachytherapy-3D dose volume parameters and aspects of 3D image-based anatomy, radiation physics, radiobiology. Radiother Oncol. 2006;78:67-77.
10. Society AB. HDR Radiobiologic Dose Equivalent Worksheets #1. 2013 [cited 2013 July 4]; Available from http://www.americanbrachytherapy.org/guidelines/ [Accessed April, 2015].
11. International WCRF. Cervical Cancer Rates. 2013 [cited 2013 July 4]; Available from: http://www.wcrf.org/int/cancer_facts-figures/data-specific-cancers/cervical-cancer-statistics.
12. Landoni F, Maneo A, Colombo A, Placa F, Milani R, Perego P, et al. Randomised study of radical surgery versus radiotherapy for stage Ib-IIa cervical cancer. Lancet. 1997;350:535-40.
13. Sedlis A, Bundy BN, Rotman MZ, Lentz SS, Muderspach LI, Zaino RJ. A randomized trial of pelvic radiation therapy versus no further therapy in selected patients with stage IB carcinoma of the cervix after radical hysterectomy and pelvic lymphadenectomy: A Gynecologic Oncology Group Study. Gynecol Oncol. 1999;73:177-83.
14. Rotman M, Sedlis A, Piedmonte MR, Bundy B, Lentz SS, Muderspach LI, et al. A phase III randomized trial of postoperative pelvic irradiation in Stage IB cervical carcinoma with poor prognostic features: follow-up of a gynecologic oncology group study. Int J Radiat Oncol Biol Phys. 2006;65: 169-76.
15. Peters WA, 3rd, Liu PY, Barrett RJ, 2nd, Stock RJ, Monk BJ, Berek JS, et al. Concurrent chemotherapy and pelvic radiation therapy compared with pelvic radiation therapy alone as adjuvant therapy after radical surgery in high-risk early-stage cancer of the cervix. J Clin Oncol. 2000;18:1606-13.
16. Monk BJ, Wang J, Im S, Stock RJ, Peters WA 3rd, Liu PY, et al. Rethinking the use of radiation and chemotherapy after radical hysterectomy: a clinical-pathologic analysis of a Gynecologic Oncology Group/Southwest Oncology Group/Radiation Therapy Oncology Group trial. Gynecol Oncol. 2005;96:721-8.
17. Eifel PJ, Winter K, Morris M, Levenback C, Grigsby PW, Cooper J, et al. Pelvic irradiation with concurrent chemotherapy versus pelvic and para-aortic irradiation for high-risk cervical cancer: an update of radiation therapy oncology group trial (RTOG) 90-01. J Clin Oncol. 2004;22:872-80.
18. Pearcey R, Brundage M, Drouin P, Jeffrey J, Johnston D, Lukka H, et al. Phase III trial comparing radical radiotherapy with and without cisplatin chemotherapy in patients with advanced squamous cell cancer of the cervix. J Clin Oncol. 2002;20: 966-72002E.
19. Green JA, Kirwan JM, Tierney JF, Symonds P, Fresco L, Collingwood M, et al. Survival and recurrence after concomitant chemotherapy and radiotherapy for cancer of the uterine cervix: a systematic review and meta-analysis. Lancet. 2001;358:781-6.
20. Kim YS, Shin SS, Nam JH, Kim YT, Kim YM, Kim JH, et al. Prospective randomized comparison of monthly fluorouracil and cisplatin versus weekly cisplatin concurrent with pelvic radiotherapy and high-dose rate brachytherapy for locally advanced cervical cancer. Gynecol Oncol. 2008;108:195-200.
21. Duenas-Gonzalez A, Zarba JJ, Patel F, Alcedo JC, Beslija S, Casanova L, et al. Phase III, open-label, randomized study comparing concurrent gemcitabine plus cisplatin and radiation followed by adjuvant gemcitabine and cisplatin versus concurrent cisplatin and radiation in patients with stage IIB to IVA carcinoma of the cervix. J Clin Oncol. 2011;29: 1678-85.
22. Lim K, Small W Jr, Portelance L, Creutzberg C, Jürgenliemk-Schulz IM, Mundt A, et al. Consensus guidelines for delineation of clinical target volume for intensity-modulated pelvic radiotherapy for the definitive treatment of cervix cancer. Int J Radiat Oncol Biol Phys. 2011;79:348-55.
23. Kabolizadeh P, Fulay S, Beriwal S. Radiation Therapy Oncology Group Para-aortic Contouring Guidelines for Pancreatic Neoplasm Applicable to Other Malignancies-Assessment of Nodal Distribution in Gynecological Malignancies. Int J Radiat Oncol Biol Phys. 2013;87(1):106-10.
24. Tyagi N, Lewis JH, Yashar CM, Vo D, Jiang SB, Mundt AJ, et al. Daily online cone beam computed tomography to assess interfractional motion in patients with intact cervical cancer. Int J Radiat Oncol Biol Phys. 2011;80:273-80.

25. Perez CA, Grigsby PW, Castro-Vita H, et al. Carcinoma of the uterine cervix. I. Impact of prolongation of overall treatment time and timing of brachytherapy on outcome of radiation therapy. Int J Radiat Oncol Biol Phys. 1995;32:1275-88.
26. Viswanathan AN, Beriwal S, De Los Santos JF, Demanes DJ, Gaffney D, Hansen J, et al. American Brachytherapy Society consensus guidelines for locally advanced carcinoma of the cervix. Part II: high-dose-rate brachytherapy. Brachytherapy. 2012;11:47-52.
27. Dimopoulos JC, Petrow P, Tanderup K, Petric P, Berger D, Kirisits C, et al. Recommendations from Gynaecological (GYN) GEC-ESTRO Working Group (IV): Basic principles and parameters for MR imaging within the frame of image based adaptive cervix cancer brachytherapy. Radiother Oncol. 2012;103:113-22.
28. International WCRF. Endometrial Cancer Rates. 2013 [cited 2013 July 4]; Available from: http://www.wcrf.org/int/cancer-facts-figures/data-specific-cancers/endometrial-cancer-cancer-lining-womb-statistics.
29. Kitchener H, Swart AM, Qian Q, et al. Efficacy of systematic pelvic lymphadenectomy in endometrial cancer (MRC ASTEC trial): a randomised study. Lancet. 2009;373:125-36.
30. Keys HM, Roberts JA, Brunetto VL, Zaino RJ, Spirtos NM, Bloss JD, et al. A phase III trial of surgery with or without adjunctive external pelvic radiation therapy in intermediate risk endometrial adenocarcinoma: a Gynecologic Oncology Group study. Gynecol Oncol. 2004;92:744-51.
31. Nout RA, Smit VT, Putter H, Jürgenliemk-Schulz IM, Jobsen JJ, Lutgens LC, et al. Vaginal brachytherapy versus pelvic external beam radiotherapy for patients with endometrial cancer of high-intermediate risk (PORTEC-2): an open-label, non-inferiority, randomised trial. Lancet. 2010;375:816-23.
32. Johnson N, Cornes P. Survival and recurrent disease after postoperative radiotherapy for early endometrial cancer: systematic review and meta-analysis. BJOG. 2007;114:1313-20.
33. Sorbe B, Nordstrom B, Maenpaa J, Kuhelj J, Kuhelj D, Okkan S, et al. Intravaginal brachytherapy in FIGO stage I low-risk endometrial cancer: a controlled randomized study. Int J Gynecol Cancer. 2009;19:873-8.
34. Creutzberg CL, van Putten WL, Koper PC, Lybeert ML, Jobsen JJ, Wárlám-Rodenhuis CC, et al. Survival after relapse in patients with endometrial cancer: results from a randomized trial. Gynecol Oncol. 2003;89:201-9.
35. Creutzberg CL, van Putten WL, Koper PC, Lybeert ML, Jobsen JJ, Wárlám-Rodenhuis CC, et al. Surgery and postoperative radiotherapy versus surgery alone for patients with stage-1 endometrial carcinoma: multicentre randomised trial. PORTEC Study Group. Post Operative Radiation Therapy in Endometrial Carcinoma. Lancet. 2000;355:1404-11.
36. Randall ME, Filiaci VL, Muss H, Spirtos NM, Mannel RS, Fowler J, et al. Randomized phase III trial of whole-abdominal irradiation versus doxorubicin and cisplatin chemotherapy in advanced endometrial carcinoma: a Gynecologic Oncology Group Study. J Clin Oncol. 2006;24:36-44.
37. Hogberg T, Signorelli M, de Oliveira CF, Fossati R, Lissoni AA, Sorbe B, et al. Sequential adjuvant chemotherapy and radiotherapy in endometrial cancer—results from two randomised studies. Eur J Cancer. 2010;46:2422-31.
38. Einstein MH, Frimer M, Kuo DY, Reimers LL, Mehta K, Mutyala S, et al. Phase II trial of adjuvant pelvic radiation "sandwiched" between combination paclitaxel and carboplatin in women with uterine papillary serous carcinoma. Gynecol Oncol. 2012;124:21-5.
39. Wegner RE, Beriwal S, Heron DE, Richard SD, Kelly JL, Edwards RP, et al. Definitive radiation therapy for endometrial cancer in medically inoperable elderly patients. Brachytherapy. 2010;9:260-5.
40. Small W, Jr., Mell LK, Anderson P, Creutzberg C, De Los Santos J, Gaffney D, et al. Consensus guidelines for delineation of clinical target volume for intensity-modulated pelvic radiotherapy in postoperative treatment of endometrial and cervical cancer. Int J Radiat Oncol Biol Phys. 2008;71:428-34.
41. Small W, Jr., Beriwal S, Demanes DJ, Dusenbery KE, Eifel P, Erickson B, et al. American Brachytherapy Society consensus guidelines for adjuvant vaginal cuff brachytherapy after hysterectomy. Brachytherapy. 2012;11:58-67.
42. Kim H, Houser C, Beriwal S. Is there any advantage to three-dimensional planning for vaginal cuff brachytherapy? Brachytherapy. 2012;11:398-401.
43. Holloway CL, Macklin EA, Cormack RA, et al. Should the organs at risk be contoured in vaginal cuff brachytherapy? Brachytherapy. 2011;10:313-7.
44. Jemal A, Siegel R, Ward E, Hao Y, Xu J, Murray T, et al. Cancer statistics, 2008. CA Cancer J Clin. 2008;58:71-96.
45. Van der Zee AG, Oonk MH, De Hullu JA, Ansink AC, Vergote I, Verheijen RH, et al. Sentinel node dissection is safe in the treatment of early-stage vulvar cancer. J Clin Oncol. 2008;26:884-9.
46. Heaps JM, Fu YS, Montz FJ, et al. Surgical-pathologic variables predictive of local recurrence in squamous cell carcinoma of the vulva. Gynecol Oncol. 1990;38:309-14.
47. Homesley HD, Bundy BN, Sedlis A, Yordan E, Berek JS, Jahshan A, et al. Prognostic factors for groin node metastasis in squamous cell carcinoma of the vulva (a Gynecologic Oncology Group study). Gynecol Oncol. 1993;49:279-83.
48. Kunos C, Simpkins F, Gibbons H, et al. Radiation therapy compared with pelvic node resection for node-positive vulvar cancer: a randomized controlled trial. Obstet Gynecol. 2009;114:537-46.
49. Stehman FB, Bundy BN, Thomas G, Varia M, Okagaki T, Roberts J, et al. Groin dissection versus groin radiation in carcinoma of the vulva: a Gynecologic Oncology Group study. Int J Radiat Oncol Biol Phys. 1992;24:389-96.
50. Manavi M, Berger A, Kucera E, Vavra N, Kucera H. Does T1, N0-1 vulvar cancer treated by vulvectomy but not lymphadenectomy need inguinofemoral radiation? Int J Radiat Oncol Biol Phys. 1997;38:749-53.
51. Petereit DG, Mehta MP, Buchler DA, et al. Inguinofemoral radiation of N0,N1 vulvar cancer may be equivalent to lymphadenectomy if proper radiation technique is used. Int J Radiat Oncol Biol Phys. 1993;27:963-7.
52. Katz A, Eifel PJ, Jhingran A, et al. The role of radiation therapy in preventing regional recurrences of invasive squamous cell carcinoma of the vulva. Int J Radiat Oncol Biol Phys. 2003;57:409-18.

53. Moore DH, Thomas GM, Montana GS, Saxer A, Gallup DG, Olt G. Preoperative chemoradiation for advanced vulvar cancer: a phase II study of the Gynecologic Oncology Group. Int J Radiat Oncol Biol Phys. 1998;42:79-85.
54. Montana GS, Thomas GM, Moore DH, Saxer A, Mangan CE, Lentz SS, et al. Preoperative chemoradiation for carcinoma of the vulva with N2/N3 nodes: a gynecologic oncology group study. Int J Radiat Oncol Biol Phys. 2000;48:1007-13.
55. Moore DH, Ali S, Koh WJ, Michael H, Barnes MN, McCourt CK, et al. A phase II trial of radiation therapy and weekly cisplatin chemotherapy for the treatment of locally-advanced squamous cell carcinoma of the vulva: a gynecologic oncology group study. Gynecol Oncol. 2012;124:529-33.
56. Kim CH, Olson AC, Kim H, et al. Contouring inguinal and femoral nodes; how much margin is needed around the vessels? Practical Radiation Oncology. 2012;2:274-8.

25 CHAPTER

Prostate Cancer

Ajaypal Sandhu, Steve Davis

INTRODUCTION

Prostate cancer is the most common cancer diagnosis in men, by itself accounting for 33% of nonskin cancers in males.[1] Worldwide, there were 899,000 reported cases of prostate cancer in 2008. Over 75% of those cases were reported in developed countries where screening is performed, making the true incidence likely much higher. There is a 25-fold geographic disparity in prostate cancer rates with the highest rates occurring in North America and Northern Europe (104 per 100,000), where screening is common, but also in undeveloped regions of South America and Sub-Saharan Africa. Rates are lowest in South Central Asia (4.1 per 100,000). Despite the high prevalence, mortality from prostate cancer is less common. Worldwide, an estimated 258,000 deaths from prostate cancer occurred in 2008. The variability in mortality rates is not quite as high as in the incidence rates; however, the highest mortality rates are generally in areas with predominantly black populations (18–26 per 100,000 in the Caribbean and Sub-Saharan Africa) and lowest in Asia (2.5 per 100,000).[1]

There are several reasons for the disparity between incidence and mortality. It may be due to widespread use of screening with prostate-specific antigen (PSA), leading to a shift toward earlier diagnosis. This is supported by the fact that the overall incidence of disease has doubled since 1985 without a corresponding increase in mortality. Also important, however, is the natural history of prostate cancer. In the majority of cases, the cancer will grow slowly and stay confined to the prostate gland. Most men with prostate cancer will die with their disease, not of their disease. Despite this, there is a subset of prostate cancer that does behave aggressively and leads to mortality. Identifying cases of the disease that will behave aggressively has proved challenging. An important part of management of care in prostate cancer patients is to understand which patients are at the most risk, who should be treated more or less aggressively, and what treatment choices are best suited to which patients.

DIAGNOSIS AND PROGNOSIS

The most important risk factor for prostate cancer continues to be age, with 68 years being the average age of diagnosis. Age plays an important role in management of disease. In the developed world where screening is practiced, life expectancy has become a determining factor in making a treatment decision. According to several guidelines, including those published by the National Comprehensive Cancer Network (NCCN), patients with a life expectancy of greater than 10 years or 20 years may be managed differently than those with a short life expectancy. Older patients with a life expectancy of less than 10 years are more likely to have their disease managed expectantly. Screening and biopsy of this population is discouraged by many. Despite published guidelines, there is considerable variation in the treatment approach to many cancer patients, and other confounding factors such as medical comorbidities, performance status and bias among physicians regarding outcomes[3,4] all affect decision making. Currently, prognosis and treatment decisions are based on risk stratification using variables such as tumor stage, Gleason score and PSA.

Most prostate cancers are asymptomatic until very advanced stages and screening has been an important aspect of diagnosis and prognosis. The bedrock of screening is the combination of palpation of the prostate through a digital rectal examination (DRE) and a PSA serum test. DRE has been practiced for several decades and continues to factor into staging, but has both relatively low sensitivity and low specificity. With a sensitivity of 70% and a specificity of 50%, only half of those men with abnormal DRE will have cancer on biopsy.[5] Thus, the addition of PSA to screening methodology has been the factor most responsible for our increased sensitivity in detecting prostate cancer much earlier. Exactly who, at what age, and how often to screen populations with PSA testing is a subject of debate, but there is no doubt that higher levels of PSA are an important aspect of risk assessment. Additional refinement of PSA testing such as measurements of percentage of free PSA, PSA velocity, or PSA doubling time are also helpful in identifying patients with high risk disease.

The second major factor that influences risk categorization is the histology of the prostate cancer, universally reported as a Gleason score. Gleason scoring is a method of grading disease based on the architecture of the tumor and the differentiation or likeness to normal glands that the tumor displays. The more regular the architecture and better the differentiation, the lower the number assigned as a Gleason score; a number between 1 and 5. Since a single cancer can display more than one pattern of disease, the two most frequent patterns are identified and added together to give the overall score used in risk assessment; a value between 2 and 10. The third factor that influences risk is the stage of disease, which looks at how far the tumor has spread at the time of diagnosis. Stage takes into account the extent of disease. For example, stage changes if the tumor has spread outside of the prostate capsule, or to the seminal vesicles, it is assigned a higher stage; if the tumor has spread to the draining lymph nodes or distant sites such as bone, the tumor is assigned an even higher stage.[2]

Several authors have taken risk stratification even further to try and calculate individual patient risk. There are well-developed nomograms that help classify different aspects of prostate cancer prognosis. For example, a group of formulas developed by Dr Roach can predict seminal vesicle involvement, extracapsular extension and lymph node spread based on age, PSA and Gleason score (ref?). The Kattan nomograms predict chance of treatment success based on pretreatment factors or biochemical response (ref?). Other factors have also been identified as possible risk factors and include race, geography, family history and dietary fat intake. Because of the multifactorial nature of prostate cancer and the variable natural history of the disease itself, optimum management remains an individual decision.

Finally, since the long-term survival is high in prostate cancer, it has been imperative to develop validated health-related quality of life (HRQOL) measures to optimize the decision-making process.[6] Urinary patterns and continence, sexual function and bowel habits can all be affected by prostate cancer treatments and it is important to weigh the risks of these effects with any decisions that are made. This is particularly true in older patients. Although concerns for toxicity among the older population are legitimate, it is important not to confuse older age with chronic illness and frailty. As life expectancies continue to lengthen, it is important to know that treatment, particularly radiation therapy (RT), is well tolerated by even very elderly patients. Some authors have reported undertreatment among older patients and underutilization of RT.[7] Often, education and methodologies used to acquire health-related information prove the most important factors in assuring patients get the optimal management.

Based on all the above factors, a risk stratification algorithm is recommended for decision making in prostate cancer.

- Low risk (stage T1-2aN0M0, Gleason score 2–6, PSA < 10 ng/mL)
  - Active surveillance (especially for patients > 70 or life expectancy < 10 years)
  - Definitive brachytherapy [either low-dose rate (LDR) seeds or high-dose rate (HDR)]
  - External beam radiation therapy (EBRT) (prostate only)
  - Radical prostatectomy (RP)
- Low-intermediate risk (stage T2b-T2c, Gleason score 7, PSA 10–20 ng/mL, volume of disease < 50% of cores or < 50% any individual core involvement)
  - External beam radiation therapy (prostate and low seminal vesicle)
  - Radical prostatectomy
  - Definitive brachytherapy (only if prostate volume < 50 cc)
- High-intermediate risk (stage T2b-T2c, Gleason score 7, PSA 10–20 ng/mL, volume of disease > 50% of cores or > 50% any individual core involvement, or combination of 2 or 3 of 3 first criteria)
  - External beam radiation therapy (with seminal vesicle coverage)
  - Radical prostatectomy
  - External beam radiation therapy with brachytherapy boost (HDR)
  - Six-months of adverse drug reaction (ADR) (beginning 2 months preradiation therapy) recommended
- High risk (stage T3, Gleason score 8–10, PSA > 20 ng/mL)
  - External beam radiation therapy (with seminal vesicle and consideration of pelvic irradiation)
  - Radical prostatectomy with adjuvant radiation (not favored)
- Clinical and laboratory workup for a freshly diagnosed cancer prostate, follow-up after treatment of prostate cancer.
- All suspected prostate cancer
  - Digital rectal examination
  - Prostate-specific antigen
  - Six-targeted core biopsies of left and right prostate lobes
- If intermediate risk
  - Add bone scan [If risk of nodal disease greater than 10% (usually PSA > 20, T3a or T3b disease)]
  - Add computed tomography (CT) or magnetic resonance imaging (MRI) of abdomen/pelvis
- Follow-up
  - First visit between 2 months and 4 months to assess chronic toxicities

- Then follow-up visits every 6–12 months for 5 years
- Prostate-specific antigen every 6–12 months for 5 years then annually thereafter.

SURVEILLANCE

Under certain circumstances, no treatment may be a reasonable approach to the patient with prostate cancer. Also known as watchful waiting, observation, active surveillance, or deferred treatment, this approach takes into account the indolent natural history of many forms of prostate cancer. Surveillance means active observation utilizing serial DREs and PSA testing. This usually means screening every 6 months for patients with a life expectancy of more than 10 years and every 6–12 months for patients with a life expectancy of less than 10 years. Benefits of this approach include avoiding definitive therapy side effects, preserving quality of life, avoiding treating indolent cancer, and decreased upfront cost. Downsides include possible increased risk of metastases, missed cure opportunities, subsequent therapies becoming more intense, anxiety for the patient and need for frequent examinations and/or biopsy. A large study with long follow-up out of Sweden showed that while the incidence of metastatic disease was similar for patients under surveillance and undergoing surgery for the first 5 years, after 15 years, the incidence of patients followed with active surveillance developing distant disease started to increase.[8] There is an important risk association with higher stage disease (i.e. with extracapsular extension). Large population-based studies have shown longer 5 and 10 year survival rates of treatment groups, whether with surgery or radiation, when compared to observation. These improvements where maintained irrespective of treatment type or age group.[9,10] *Therefore, treatment is usually recommended for most patients with a projected survival of 10 years, and even many patients with higher risk disease who may have older age or other comorbidities.* However, randomized data are lacking comparing different treatment modalities. Nevertheless, there is a generalized approach to consider active surveillance in those patients with low-risk disease and a life expectancy of less than 10 years.

SURGERY

Radical prostatectomy has been the backbone of management for prostate cancer for decades. Large studies have shown that very few patients who undergo RP will die of disease.[11] Surgical techniques have continued to evolve and are improving rapidly. Laparoscopic prostatectomy, and more recently, robotic-assisted prostatectomy have helped reduce complication rates and recovery times. However, even with these newer techniques, there has been recognition that surgery comes with risks and has an HRQOL impact. Given the indolent course in the majority of cases of prostate cancer, the risks of undergoing major surgery may outweigh the benefits for many patients. In fact, a recent widely cited study in the New England Journal of Medicine compared HRQOL data between surgery and RT. In comparison to radiation therapy, patients who undergone surgery had been in good health, had a lower median age, higher education and income. Thus, better overall HRQOL was reported in surgically treated patients. However, their urinary and sexual functions were lower, and there was no difference in outcomes or satisfaction with care when compared to RT.[12] It is unclear why there were these differences in demographics, but it underlines the importance of educating patients about the differences between surgical and radiation techniques in terms of not only effectiveness but also HRQOL impact.

ANDROGEN DEPRIVATION THERAPY

Several large randomized trials have showed the benefit of RT combined with androgen deprivation in high-risk prostate cancer.[13,14] Remaining, however, are questions regarding the best timing and duration of RT with androgen deprivation therapy (ADT). Some studies have suggested a synergistic effect of ADT with RT, which appear to be supported by radiobiologic models of cell kill through increased apoptosis and decreased hypoxia. The reduced volume of the prostate with ADT also can result in a decreased target size with improved dosimetry. Following these studies, ADT usually precedes radiation by several weeks.

The use of androgen deprivation in low-intermediate risk patients is not as clear and there are costs to the use of ADT in combination with RT. The impact on HRQOL can be substantial. Weight gain, night sweats, hot flashes and muscle loss are frequent adverse effects. There are also some studies, though refuted by the recent Radiation Therapy Oncology Group (RTOG) studies, that suggest an increased risk of cardiovascular death in ADT. Although most side effects are reversible, the duration of therapy can mean months or years of these adverse effects.[15,16] D'Amico and colleagues looked at patients with significant comorbidities and showed some detrimental effects of treatment.[17] This is not to suggest that ADT should not be considered standard of care for high and intermediate high-risk patients, but that there are toxicities involved with treatment that have to be balanced with patient goals. Moreover, in the modern era of dose escalation (to be discussed later), the synergistic effects of combined therapy may not be as necessary and current studies are addressing the role of ADT with current, higher doses of radiation.

BRACHYTHERAPY

Prostate brachytherapy has gained popularity due to the need for only a single insertion and the higher biologic doses that can be delivered to the prostate. The procedure is done by inserting dozens of small radioactive seeds, often with iodine-125 or palladium-103, into the prostate using various implantation and mapping schemes. A variable number of seeds are inserted using needles through the perineum which emit radiation for a set period of time, usually a few months. Alternatively, the use of temporary HDR brachytherapy approaches, which include temporary seed placement measured in minutes with iridium-192, have also been reported and appear to show similar efficacy. The rapid falloff of the emitting seeds or HDR source is ideal for sparing surrounding organs at risk like the bladder and rectum. More difficult is sparing the urethra, and in men with a history of urinary retention, side effects can be significant for several months. Indications for *monotherapy are low-risk disease with a small prostate, minimal baseline lower urinary tract symptoms, and for combined EBRT and brachytherapy, intermediate-risk disease with prostate size less than 50 cc.*

Brachytherapy offers several advantages over fractionated external beam radiation. A single seed insertion or a small number of HDR treatments compares favorably to several weeks of external beam irradiation. Compared to surgery, there are potentially fewer complications and recovery times are more rapid (Fig. 1). There is some concern in

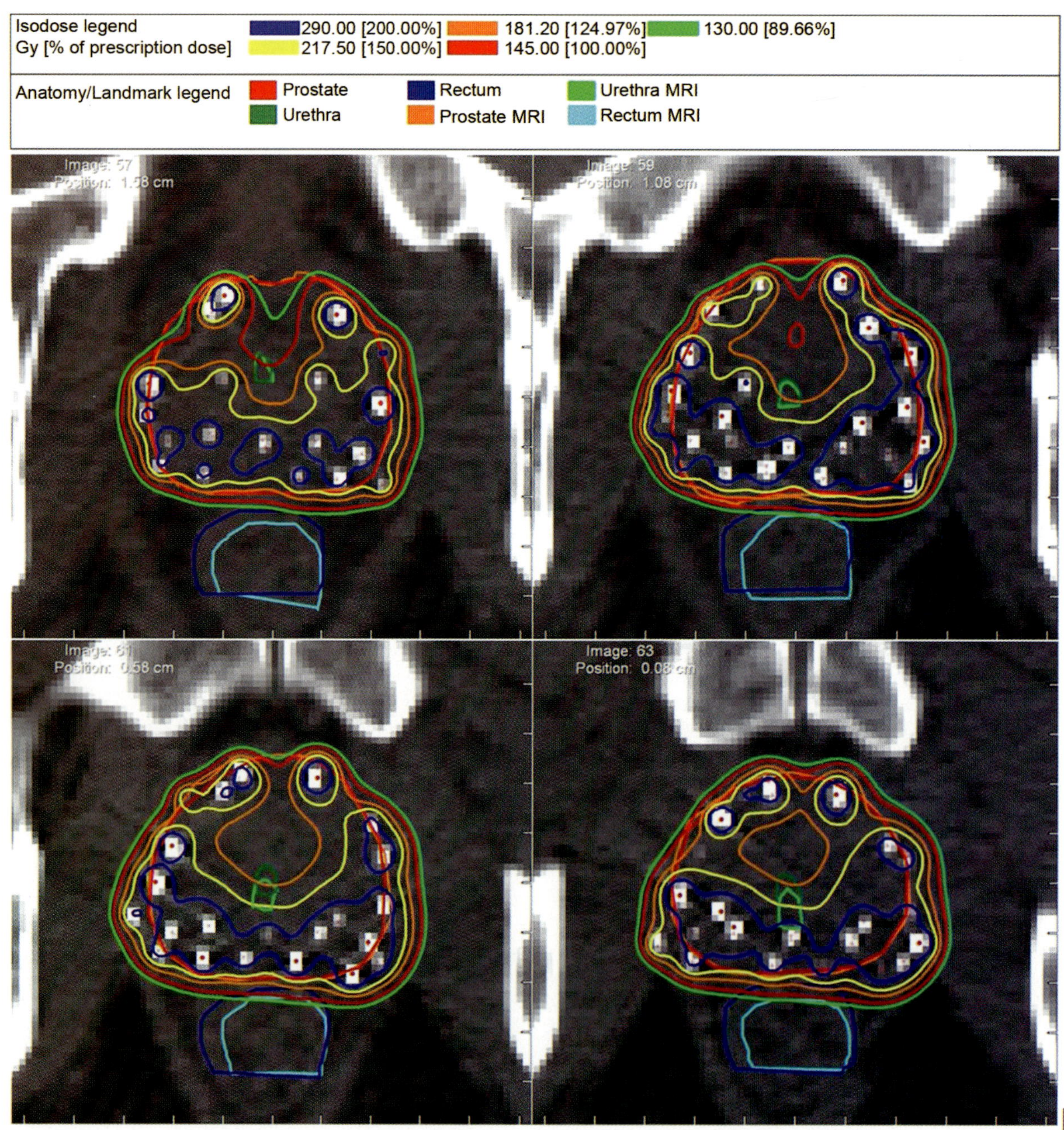

Fig. 1 Seed brachytherapy with isodose distribution—prescription dose 145 Gy

Courtesy: Dr Ajaypal Sandhu, Moores Cancer Center, University of San Diego, USA using brachytherapy in men with significant comorbidities or advanced age. Protracted urinary symptoms and bowel toxicities are potentially increased in elderly men.[18]

Thus, patients should be carefully selected for brachytherapy. It is important to be cautious and identify predictors of higher toxicity before considering brachytherapy as a treatment option. Typically, permanent seed implantation as monotherapy is reserved for lower risk disease.

A dose of 90 Gy (as a combined modality with EBRT) to 140 Gy (as a monotherapy) is prescribed with LDR brachytherapy, and this can achieve cure in greater than 95% of carefully selected cases.

However, inconvenience and trauma resulting from implants should be taken into account as well. Patients with a large prostate or pretreatment urinary symptoms do not form optimal candidates for brachytherapy. Several groups have reported their results with the use of combined EBRT with LDR brachytherapy for patients with intermediate- and high-risk disease and the results are quite good.[19-21] However, the question of when to add external beam to brachytherapy remains a controversy. Even though biochemical control may be similar with different RT approaches, quality of life end points are important to consider in treatment decision making.

DOSE ESCALATION AND INTENSITY-MODULATED RADIATION THERAPY

One of the most important advancements in the treatment of prostate cancer over the last two decades has been the introduction of intensity-modulated radiation therapy (IMRT). With the advancement in computer processing power and optimization software, IMRT is able to use reverse planning to create highly conformal radiation therapy. The use of multileaf collimator (MLC) that creates highly customizable fields, coupled with this software optimization, is the heart of IMRT. By allowing more conformal radiation in three dimensions, the surrounding organs at risk are further spared[22] (Fig. 2). There have now been several dosimetric and clinical reports of decreased toxicity in prostate patients using IMRT in both the definitive and adjuvant/salvage setting.[23-25]

Given these lower toxicity profiles, IMRT has rapidly been adopted as the gold standard in EBRT.

The other benefit of more conformal therapy is the ability to safely deliver higher overall doses of radiation. Where for several years doses of less than 70 Gy were utilized, there are now several published trials that have showed that higher doses (> 70 Gy) delivered with more fractions, so-called dose escalation, are not only safe, but more effective with higher rates of local control and lower biochemical failure.[26-29]

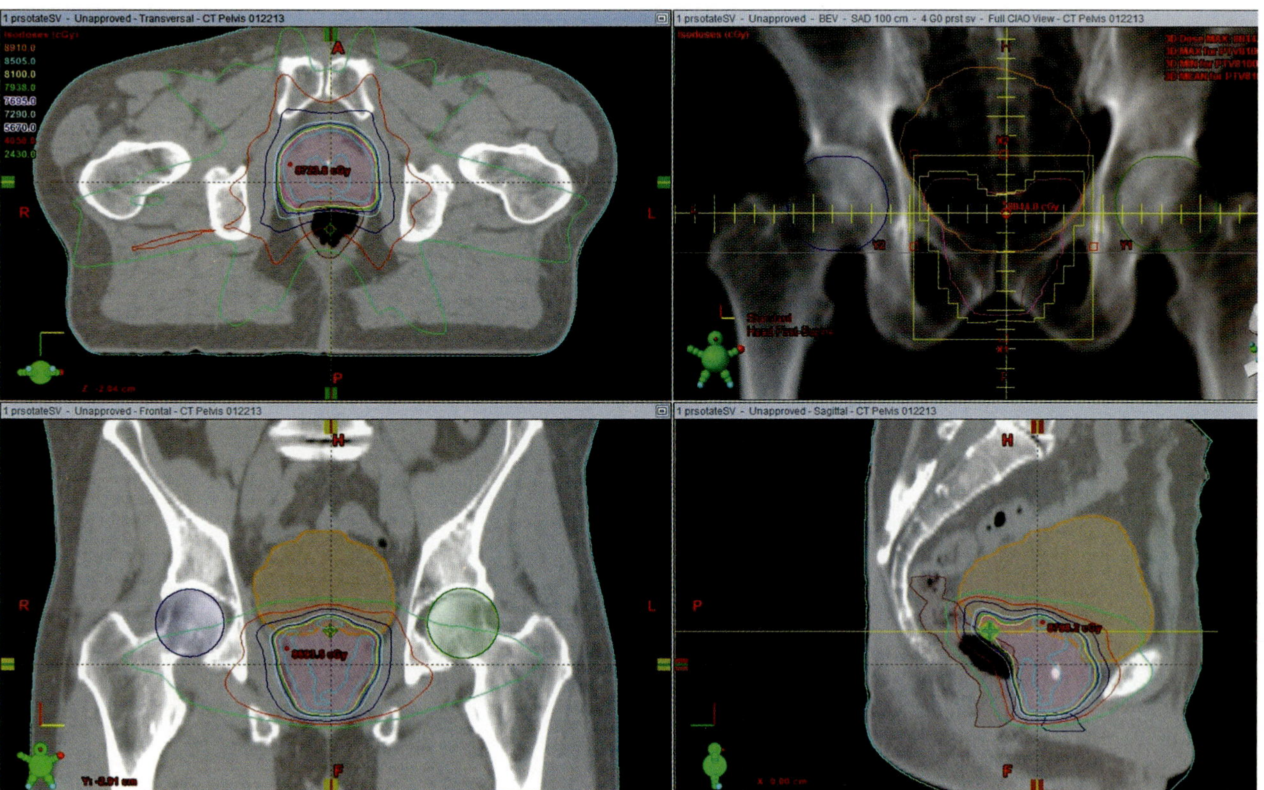

Fig. 2 Intensity-modulated radiation therapy (IMRT) dose distribution

Courtesy: Dr. Ajaypal Sandhu, Moores Cancer Center, University of San Diego, USA

One study from MD Anderson looked at 301 patients with stage I–III disease. They were randomized to receive either 70 Gy or 78 Gy. At 10 years, they found that freedom from biochemical failure increased to 78% from 59% in the 78 Gy group. The results were most notable for patients who presented with a PSA greater than 10 (78% vs 39%) although the benefit applied to all risk groups.[30] One large study by Zelefsky and coworkers reported the results of dose escalation to 81 Gy in 561 prostate cancer patients using IMRT. At 7 years, they showed an actuarial risk of grade 2 or higher toxicity of only 1.6%. Moreover, failure rates were extremely low and the treatment was well tolerated even in elderly patients.[31] The group at the Memorial Sloan Kettering Cancer Center, New York, did a retrospective review of 478 men treated between 1997 and 2004 to a dose of 86.4 Gy with IMRT. They found a 99% freedom from biochemical failure at 5 years for low-risk prostate cancer, and for all patients, the risk of grade 3 toxicity was only 0.6%.[32]

IMAGE-GUIDED RADIATION THERAPY

Another breakthrough in the delivery of RT in the treatment of prostate cancer is image-guided radiation therapy (IGRT). IGRT uses advances in image technology to directly visualize the target at the time of treatment to improve patient set-up, eliminate errors of positioning, and even potentially adapting target fields to changes in the size and shape of the prostate or pelvic nodal volumes. In-room techniques are various and have used ultrasound localization, two-dimensional (2D) imaging, the placement of radiopaque fiducial markers before treatment, or real-time three-dimensional (3D) imaging using cone-beam computed tomography (CBCT).[33,34] Several studies have shown the movement of the prostate with variable filling of the bladder and rectum, and it is an ideal organ to track daily to assure consistent localization. IGRT fills this need and not only assures that the target is not undertreated, but assures that the surrounding organs at risk are not overtreated.

At our institution, we routinely use IGRT in prostate cancer patients undergoing IMRT, both in patients undergoing definitive therapy and those undergoing postprostatectomy RT. We looked at 100 consecutively treated patients with T1c-T4 disease between 2005 and 2008. We found no grade 3 or higher toxicity, and only 16% and 2% of genitourinary (GU) and gastrointestinal (GI) late grade 2 toxicity, respectively.[35] For men with intact prostate, three to five radiopaque markers are placed for kilovoltage X-ray localization on a daily basis (Fig. 3). However, increasingly we are decreasing the logistical complications of fiducial placement and using in-room CBCT for daily prostate localization. Treatment fields are adjusted daily to conform to changes in rectal and bladder filling. For patients treated adjuvantly or in the salvage setting, surgical clips can be used to accurately track the target volume. The other benefit of IGRT is that tighter planning target volume (PTV) can be utilized. Several studies have now emerged that validate lower toxicity and excellent control using IGRT.[36,37] Also emerging are the uses of transponders that are implanted like fiducials, but allow for not only interfraction movement,

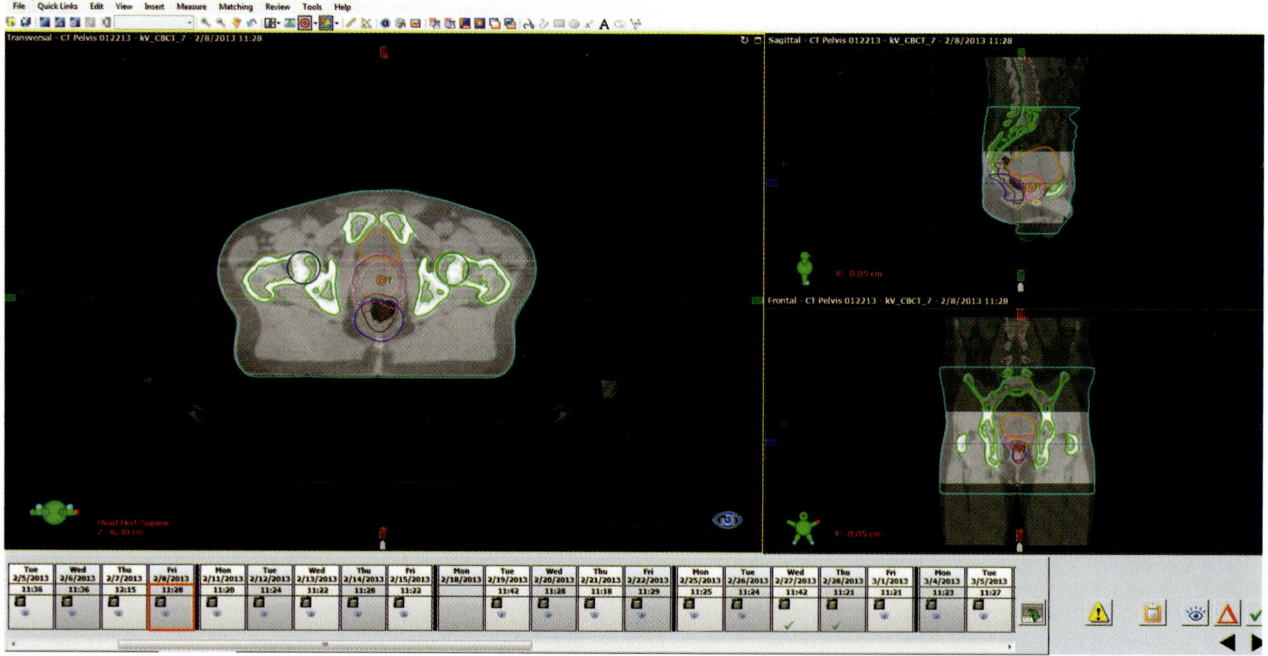

Fig. 3 Kilovoltage CT image guidance [image-guided radiation therapy (IGRT)]
Courtesy: Dr. Ajaypal Sandhu, Moores Cancer Center, University of San Diego, USA

but intrafraction monitoring of prostate movement during the respiratory cycle using gating techniques.[38] In all cases, IGRT methods are improving the conformality and efficacy of EBRT.

HYPOFRACTIONATION AND STEREOTACTIC BODY RADIATION THERAPY

Technologic advancements such as IMRT and IGRT have led some investigators to explore the delivery of higher than conventional doses per fraction in prostate cancer patient, an approach known generally as hypofractionation. A specific technique of hypofractionation, known as stereotactic body radiation therapy (SBRT), is also under investigation. Although hypofractionated treatments are now routinely done without stereotaxis, the name has come to represent large doses delivered in a small number of fractions. This approach is especially appealing in elderly patients, where social support and transportation may be lacking to provide the 9 weeks of treatment required for dose-escalated IMRT. Overall treatment can be reduced by several weeks[39] and delivered in as few as 5–7 days in the case of SBRT.[40]

Although hypofractionation reduces the clinic visits for the patient, the compelling reason supporting the use of hypofractionation is radiobiological.[41] It has been postulated that schedules with fewer and larger fractions of RT should improve the therapeutic ratio in patients with prostate cancer. The concern, however, is that high doses per fraction may also significantly increase late toxicity. Most trials to date have reported safety of these schedules with at least equal efficacy.[42] There are several randomized clinical trials that are ongoing to evaluate this approach. One trial from Fox Chase Cancer Center is looking at 2.7 Gy per fraction versus conventional 2.0 Gy per fraction thereby reducing the treatment time to 5.2 weeks. Another from the United Kingdom, Medical Research Council (MRC) trial, is looking at 2,100 patients randomized to 57 Gy in 3 Gy fractions, 60 Gy in 3 Gy fractions or 74 Gy in 2 Gy fractions. Preliminary data from both these trials shows no difference in toxicities between the arms.[43,44] For the time being, however, hypofractionated RT still should be considered experimental until mature results of ongoing randomized trials become available.

PROTON THERAPY

Treatment of the prostate has also been at the forefront in the emergence of proton beam RT. The physical characteristics of protons make them an ideal modality to treat prostate cancer. The low entry and exit doses of protons with the ability to control the depth of high-dose areas (called the "Bragg peak") reduce the collateral radiation exposure to surrounding normal tissues. Protons have similar biological properties as photons, and therefore, have similar impact on tumor kill. However, they offer a sharper peripheral penumbra and no exit dose that have the potential to further spare surrounding organs at risk. Dosimetric studies have shown both good target homogeneity, a potential weakness of protons, and excellent sparing of surrounding organs, even when compared to IMRT.[45] More recently, proton delivery methods have advanced that allow dose painting techniques that combine the best features of both proton therapy and IMRT, so-called intensity-modulated proton therapy (IMPT) (Fig. 4).[46]

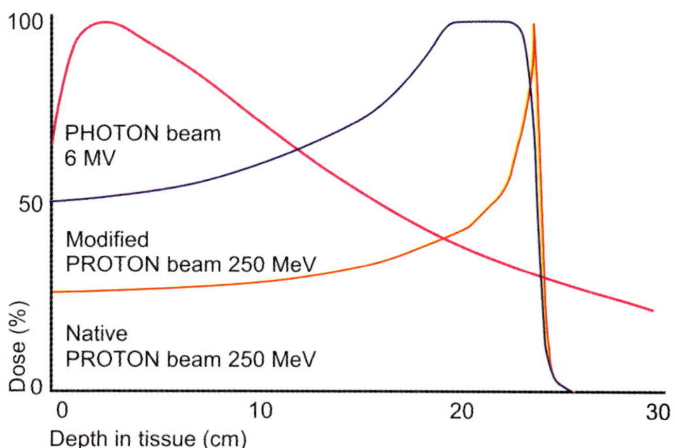

Fig. 4 Bragg peak effect with protons versus photon attenuation curve

Source: Wikipedia. (2014). Bragg Peak. [online] Available from http://upload.wikimedia.org/wikipedia/commons/1/12/BraggPeak.png [Accessed on May, 2015].

The idea of using proton beams for cancer therapy is not new and has been used at Massachusetts General Hospital, United States, since the 1970s. These early treatments involved the use of a fixed beam with very limited treatment fields. Regardless, Massachusetts General Hospital and investigators at Loma Linda University, California, have reported long-term results that have shown the safety and efficacy of proton beam therapy. For example, Loma Linda University reported grade 3 or higher toxicity of less than 1%.[47] The Proton Radiation Oncology Group (PROG) reported a prospective phase III multi-institutional study of combined photon and proton therapy using a proton boost technique. They showed low morbidity and low rates of biochemical failure.[48] Like in photons, studies of dose escalation of up to 82 Gy have also been shown to be safe.[49] The potential low toxicity profile of protons is seen as especially important in prostate cancer therapy where quality of life measures (HRQOL) are an important aspect of determining the best treatment course. Despite these studies and the theoretic benefits, recent population-based studies have not shown protons to be clearly superior to conventional photons in terms of disease control or toxicity. This may be due to the large improvements over the last decade in photon therapy using IMRT and IGRT as discussed above. In addition, a substantial downside of proton therapy is the cost and capital expenditures required to perform the treatment. There are still relatively few proton centers, and most are concentrated within the United States. The expense to build this type of facility maybe becoming prohibitive, especially in today's cost-sensitive medical care climate.

POSTPROSTATECTOMY RADIATION THERAPY

For many patients who choose to undergo RP for treatment of their prostate cancer, RT after surgery may still be advised. Careful attention to pathologic features and adverse factors on evaluation of the removed prostate is needed to assess risk of recurrence. From several studies, certain risk factors for local recurrence have been identified. These include extracapsular extension, involvement of the seminal vesicles, and positive margins of the surgically resected specimen.[50-52] The Southwest Oncology Group (SWOG) 8794 study confirmed that patterns of failure after prostatectomy are local which further supports that idea of RT for improved local control. Importantly, the timing of postprostatectomy treatment is important, as delaying therapy until biochemical failure has been shown to be less effective and may result in a higher risk of distant metastases.[53] Fortunately, the toxicity of adjuvant RT is low, and its efficacy should be further improved using novel RT approaches as discussed above such as IMRT and IGRT.[54]

In other situations, risk factors that lead to an immediate need for adjuvant radiation are not present, and patients present for radiation only after biochemical failure, a situation known as salvage radiotherapy. Stephenson and colleagues looked at over 1,500 patients treated with radiation after biochemical failure post-RP. They saw an overall 6-year freedom from progression after radiation of 45%. They showed that factors that were associated with post-RT progression were a pre-RT PSA greater than 2.0, a Gleason score of 8–10, negative surgical margins or a PSA doubling time less than 10 months. They also noted that early salvage was better than late salvage.[55] Trock and associates analyzed the use of hormonal therapy with salvage RT. They retrospectively compared 160 patients treated with RT alone versus 78 patients treated with RT and hormonal therapy versus 39 patients that were observed. They saw no benefit to adding hormonal therapy but a threefold reduction in prostate cancer-specific mortality when compared to the observation group.[56]

PALLIATIVE RADIATION

Despite all of advances in the treatment of prostate cancer, advanced disease persists and management of the symptoms of advanced disease, to include local pelvic pain, hematuria, lower urinary obstructive symptoms and pain from metastatic lesions continue to be an important area where RT can play a role. Palliative RT is effective in controlling local pelvic symptoms such as hematuria, pain and obstruction. Hindson et al. evaluated the role of pelvic treatment in metastatic disease and found that in 35 hormonally refractive prostate cancer patients, treated with a median dose of 60 Gy in 20 fractions, complete and partial responses in 8.6% and 51.4% were achieved.[57]

For osseous metastases in prostate cancer, pain can be debilitating. Palliative RT has been shown to be very effective in controlling the pain causes by osseous metastases. Treatment regimens range from as short as 8 Gy in a single fraction to 30 Gy over the course of 2 weeks.[58] Another approach involves the injection of radiopharmaceuticals including strontium-89 and samarium-153.[59,60]

SUMMARY AND CONCLUSION

Prostate cancer continues to be a major cause of disease, especially among older men. While active surveillance, surgery, brachytherapy and EBRT are viable treatment options, physician and patient education is vital to assure that proper treatment decisions are made. Modern techniques, including dose-escalated IMRT, IGRT and proton therapy, are making it possible to deliver better therapy with less side effects. These technologies provide new opportunities to limit the dose to normal tissues, thereby decreasing the treatment-related toxicity as well as shorter treatment durations improving HRQOL as well as treatment efficacy.

REFERENCES

1. Globocan 2008 Cancer fact sheet. International Agency for Research on Cancer (IARC), Section of Cancer Information, 2010. 150 Cours Albert Thomas, 69372 Lyon CEDEX 08, France.
2. American Joint Committee on Cancer. Prostate cancer. In: Greene FL, Page DL, Fleming ID (Eds). AJCC Cancer Staging Manual, 6th edition. New York: Springer-Verlag; 2003. pp. 309-16.
3. Extermann M. Measurement and impact of comorbidity in older cancer patients. Crit Rev Oncol Hematol. 2000;35(3):181-200.
4. Sandhu A, Mundt AJ. Radiation therapy for older cancer patients. Aging Health. 2(6):919-30.
5. Catalona WJ. Prostate Cancer. Orlando, FL: Grune & Stratton; 1984.
6. Dandapani SV, Sanda MG. Measuring health-related quality of life consequences from primary treatment for early-stage prostate cancer. Semin Radiat Oncol. 2008;18(1):67-72.
7. Vulto AJ, Lemmens VE, Louwman MW, Janssen-Heijnen ML, Poortmans PH, Lybeert ML, et al. The influence of age and comorbidity on receiving radiotherapy as part of primary treatment for cancer in South Netherlands, 1995 to 2002. Cancer. 2006;106(12):2734-42.
8. Johansson JE, Andrén O, Andersson SO, Dickman PW, Holmberg L, Magnuson A, et al. Natural history of early, localized prostate cancer. JAMA. 2004;291(22):2713-9.

9. Barry MJ. Words of wisdom: re: survival associated with treatment vs observation of localized prostate cancer in elderly men. Wong Y, Mitra N, Hudes G, et al. JAMA 2006;296:2683-93. Eur Urol. 2007;51(6):1751.
10. Tward JD, Lee CM, Pappas LM, Szabo A, Gaffney DK, Shrieve DC. Survival of men with clinically localized prostate cancer treated with prostatectomy, brachytherapy, or no definitive treatment: impact of age at diagnosis. Cancer. 2006;107(10):2392-400.
11. Stephenson AJ, Kattan MW, Eastham JA, Bianco FJ Jr, Yossepowitch O, Vickers AJ, et al. Prostate cancer-specific mortality after radical prostatectomy for patients treated in the prostate-specific antigen era. J Clin Oncol. 2009;27(26):4300-5.
12. Sanda MG, Dunn RL, Michalski J, Sandler HM, Northouse L, Hembroff L, et al. Quality of life and satisfaction with outcome among prostate-cancer survivors. N Engl J Med. 2008;358(12):1250-61.
13. Bolla M, Collette L, Blank L, Warde P, Dubois JB, Mirimanoff RO, et al. Long-term results with immediate androgen suppression and external irradiation in patients with locally advanced prostate cancer (an EORTC study): a phase III randomised trial. Lancet. 2002;360(9327):103-6.
14. Pilepich MV, Winter K, John MJ, Mesic JB, Sause W, Rubin P, et al. Phase III radiation therapy oncology group (RTOG) trial 86-10 of androgen deprivation adjuvant to definitive radiotherapy in locally advanced carcinoma of the prostate. Int J Radiat Oncol Biol Phys. 2001;50(5):1243-52.
15. Valicenti RK, Winter K, Cox JD, Sandler HM, Bosch W, Vijayakumar S, et al. RTOG 94-06: is the addition of neoadjuvant hormonal therapy to dose-escalated 3D conformal radiation therapy for prostate cancer associated with treatment toxicity? Int J Radiat Oncol Biol Phys. 2003;57(3):614-20.
16. Efstathiou J, Bae K, Shipley W, et al. Goserelin not related to increased risk for CV death (Abstract 11). Proceedings of the 2008 Genitourinary Cancers Symposium; San Francisco, CA, 2008.
17. D'Amico A, Chen M, Renshaw A, et al. Comorbidities affect benefit of combined radiation, androgen suppression (Abstract 13). Proceeding of the 2008 Genitourinary Cancers Symposium; San Francisco, CA, 2008.
18. Chen AB, D'Amico AV, Neville BA, et al. Patient and treatment factors associated with complications after prostate brachytherapy. J Clin Oncol. 2006;24(33):5298-304.
19. Critz FA, Levinson K. 10-year disease-free survival rates after simultaneous irradiation for prostate cancer with a focus on calculation methodology. J Urol. 2004;172(6 Pt 1):2232-8.
20. Bittner N, Merrick GS, Galbreath RW, Butler WM, Wallner KE, Allen ZA, et al. Primary causes of death after permanent prostate brachytherapy. Int J Radiat Oncol Biol Phys. 2008;72(2):433-40.
21. Burri RJ, Ho AY, Forsythe K, Cesaretti JA, Stone NN, Stock RG. Young men have equivalent biochemical outcomes compared with older men after treatment with brachytherapy for prostate cancer. Int J Radiat Oncol Biol Phys. 2010;77(5):1315-21.
22. Xing L, Wu Q, Yang Y, et al. Physics of IMRT. In: Mundt AJ, Roeske JC, (Eds). Intensity Modulated Radiation Therapy: A Clinical Perspective. Hamilton, Ontario: BC Decker, 2005. pp. 20-52.
23. De Meerleer G, Vakaet L, Meersschout S, Villeirs G, Verbaeys A, Oosterlinck W, et al. Intensity-modulated radiotherapy as primary treatment for prostate cancer: acute toxicity in 144 patients. Int J Radiat Oncol Biol Phys. 2004;60(3):777-87.
24. Zelefsky MJ, Fuks Z, Happersett L, Lee HJ, Ling CC, Burman CM, et al. Clinical experience with intensity modulated radiation therapy (IMRT) in prostate cancer. Radiother Oncol. 2000;55(3):241-9.
25. Teh BS, Mai WY, Augspurger ME, Uhl BM, McGary J, Dong L, et al. Intensity modulated radiation therapy (IMRT) following prostatectomy: more favorable acute genitourinary toxicity profile compared to primary IMRT for prostate cancer. Int J Radiat Oncol Biol Phys. 2001;49(2):465-72.
26. Dearnaley DP, Sydes MR, Graham JD, Aird EG, Bottomley D, Cowan RA, et al. Escalated-dose versus standard-dose conformal radiotherapy in prostate cancer: first results from the MRC RT01 randomized controlled trial. Lancet Oncol. 2007;8(6):475-87.
27. Peeters ST, Heemsbergen WD, Koper PC, van Putten WL, Slot A, Dielwart MF, et al. Dose-response in radiotherapy for localized prostate cancer: results of the Dutch multicenter randomized phase III trial comparing 68 Gy of radiotherapy with 78 Gy. J Clin Oncol. 2006;24(13):1990-6.
28. Pollack A, Zagars GK, Smith LG, Lee JJ, von Eschenbach AC, Antolak JA, et al. Preliminary results of a randomized radiotherapy dose-escalation study comparing 70 Gy with 78 Gy for prostate cancer. J Clin Oncol. 2000;18(23):3904-11.
29. Zietman AL, DeSilvio ML, Slater JD, Rossi CJ Jr, Miller DW, Adams JA, et al. Comparison of conventional-dose vs high-dose conformal radiation therapy in clinically localized adenocarcinoma of the prostate: a randomized controlled trial. JAMA. 2005;294(10):1233-9.
30. Pollack A, Zagars GK, Starkschall G, Antolak JA, Lee JJ, Huang E, et al. Prostate cancer radiation dose response: results of the M. D. Anderson phase III randomized trial. Int J Radiat Oncol Biol Phys. 2002;53(5):1097-105.
31. Zelefsky MJ, Chan H, Hunt M, Yamada Y, Shippy AM, Amols H. Long-term outcome of high dose intensity modulated radiation therapy for patients with clinically localized prostate cancer. J Urol. 2006;176(4 Pt 1):1415-9.
32. Cahlon O, Zelefsky MJ, Shippy A, Chan H, Fuks Z, Yamada Y, et al. Ultra-high dose (86.4 Gy) IMRT for localized prostate cancer: toxicity and biochemical outcomes. Int J Radiat Oncol Biol Phys. 2008;71(2):330-7.
33. Song WY, Schaly B, Bauman G, et al. Evaluation of image-guided radiation therapy (IGRT) technologies and their impact on the outcomes of hypofractionated prostate cancer treatments: a radiobiological analysis. Int J Radiat Oncol Biol Phys. 2006;64(1):289-300.
34. Smitsmans MH, de Bois J, Sonke JJ, Betgen A, Zijp LJ, Jaffray DA, et al. Automatic prostate localization on cone-beam CT scans for high precision image-guided radiotherapy. Int J Radiat Oncol Biol Phys. 2005;63(4):975-84.
35. Nath SK, Sandhu AP, Rose BS, Simpson DR, Nobiensky PD, Wang JZ, et al. Toxicity analysis of postoperative image-guided intensity-modulated radiotherapy for prostate cancer. Int J Radiat Oncol Biol Phys. 2010;78(2):435-41.

36. Jani AB, Gratzle J, Muresan E, et al. Analysis of acute toxicity with the use of transabdominal ultrasonography for prostate positioning during intensity-modulated radiotherapy. Urology. 2005;65(3):504-8.
37. Nichol A, Chung P, Lockwood G, Rosewall T, Divanbiegi L, Sweet J, et al. A phase II study of localized prostate cancer treated to 75.6 Gy with 3D conformal radiotherapy. Radiother Oncol. 2005;76(1):11-7.
38. Kupelian P, Willoughby T, Mahadevan A, Djemil T, Weinstein G, Jani S, et al. Multi-institutional clinical experience with the Calypso system in localization and continuous, real-time monitoring of the prostate gland during external radiotherapy. Int J Radiat Oncol Biol Phys. 2007;67(4):1088-98.
39. Kupelian PA, Willoughby TR, Reddy CA, et al. Hypofractionated intensity-modulated radiotherapy (70 Gy at 2.5 Gy per fraction) for localized prostate cancer: Cleveland Clinic experience. Int J Radiat Oncol Biol Phys. 2007;68(5):1424-30.
40. Pawlicki T, Cotrutz C, King C. Prostate cancer therapy with stereotactic body radiation therapy. Front Radiat Ther Oncol. 2007;40:395-406.
41. Fowler JF, Ritter MA, Chappell RJ, et al. What hypofractionated protocols should be tested for prostate cancer? Int J Radiat Oncol Biol Phys. 2003;56(4):1093-104.
42. Miles EF, Lee WR. Hypofractionation for prostate cancer: a critical review. Semin Radiat Oncol. 2008;18(1):41-7.
43. Pollack A, Hanlon AL, Horwitz EM, Feigenberg SJ, Konski AA, Movsas B, et al. Dosimetry and preliminary acute toxicity in the first 100 men treated for prostate cancer on a randomized hypofractionation dose escalation trial. Int J Radiat Oncol Biol Phys. 2006;64(2):518-26.
44. Intensity-Modulated Radiation Therapy in Treating Patients with Localized Prostate Cancer. Clinical Trials.gov Identifier: NCT00392535.
45. Vargas C, Fryer A, Mahajan C, Indelicato D, Horne D, Chellini A, et al. Dose-volume comparison of proton therapy and intensity-modulated radiotherapy for prostate cancer. Int J Radiat Oncol Biol Phys. 2008;70(3):744-51.
46. Trofimov A, Nguyen PL, Coen JJ, Doppke KP, Schneider RJ, Adams JA, et al. Radiotherapy treatment of early stage prostate cancer with IMRT and protons: a treatment planning comparison. Int J Radiat Oncol Biol Phys. 2007;69(2):444-53.
47. Slater JD, Rossi CJ Jr, Yonemoto LT, Bush DA, Jabola BR, Levy RP, et al. Proton therapy for prostate cancer: the initial Loma Linda University experience. Int J Radiat Oncol Biol Phys. 2004;59(2):348-52.
48. Zietman AL, Bae K, Slater JD, Shipley WU, Efstathiou JA, Coen JJ, et al. Randomized trial comparing conventional-dose with high-dose conformal radiation therapy in early-stage adenocarcinoma of the prostate: long-term results from Proton Radiation Oncology Group/American College of Radiology 95-09. J Clin Oncol. 2010;28(7):1106-11.
49. Rossi CJ. Conformal proton beam radiation therapy for prostate cancer: concepts and clinical results. Commun Oncol. 2007;4:235-40.
50. Thompson IM Jr, Tangen CM, Paradelo J, Lucia MS, Miller G, Troyer D, et al. Adjuvant radiotherapy for pathologically advanced prostate cancer: a randomized clinical trial. JAMA. 2006;296(19):2329-35.
51. Bolla M, van Poppel H, Collette L, van Cangh P, Vekemans K, Da Pozzo L, et al. Postoperative radiotherapy after radical prostatectomy: a randomized controlled trial (EORTC trial 22911). Lancet. 2005;366(9485):572-8.
52. Wiegel T, Bottke D, Willich N, et al. Phase III results of adjuvant radiotherapy (RT) vs, wait and see (WS) in patients with pT3 prostate cancer following radical prostatectomy (RP) J Clin Oncol. 2005;23:381.
53. Swanson GP, Hussey MA, Tangen CM, Chin J, Messing E, Canby-Hagino E, et al. Predominant treatment failure in postprostatectomy patients is local: analysis of patterns of treatment failure in SWOG 8794. J Clin Oncol. 2007;25(16):2225-9.
54. Sandhu A, Sethi R, Rice R, Wang JZ, Marcus L, Salem C, et al. Prostate bed localization with image-guided approach using on-board imaging: reporting acute toxicity and implications for radiation therapy planning following prostatectomy. Radiother Oncol. 2008;88(1):20-5.
55. Stephenson AJ, Scardino PT, Kattan MW, Pisansky TM, Slawin KM, Klein EA, et al. Predicting the outcome of salvage radiation therapy for recurrent prostate cancer after radical prostatectomy. J Clin Oncol. 2007;25(15):2035-41.
56. Trock BJ, Han M, Freedland SJ, Humphreys EB, DeWeese TL, Partin AW, et al. Prostate cancer-specific survival following salvage radiotherapy vs observation in men with biochemical recurrence after radical prostatectomy. JAMA. 2008;299(23):2760-9.
57. Hindson B, Turner S, Do V. Palliative radiation therapy for localized prostate symptoms in hormone refractory prostate cancer. Australas Radiol. 2007;51(6):584-8.
58. Steenland E, Leer JW, van Houwelingen H, Post WJ, van den Hout WB, Kievit J, et al. The effect of a single fraction compared to multiple fractions on painful bone metastases: a global analysis of the Dutch Bone Metastases Study. Radiother Oncol. 1999;52(2):101-9.
59. Quilty PM, Kirk D, Bolger JJ, Dearnaley DP, Lewington VJ, Mason MD, et al. A comparison of the palliative effects of strontium-89 and external beam radiotherapy in metastatic prostate cancer. Radiother Oncol. 1994;31(1):33-40.
60. Resche I, Chatal JF, Pecking A, Ell P, Duchesne G, Rubens R, et al. A dose-controlled study of 153Sm-ethylenediaminetetramethylenephosphonate (EDTMP) in the treatment of patients with painful bone metastases. Eur J Cancer. 1997;33(10):1583-91.

26

CHAPTER

Castration-resistant Prostate Cancer

Sandeep Batra, Vikash Kumar, Tejinder Kataria

INTRODUCTION

Androgen deprivation therapy is the first-line treatment of all newly diagnosed metastatic prostate cancer despite response rates as high as 80–90%, nearly all men eventually develop disease progressed while still on androgen deprivation.[1] Various different terms have been used to describe prostate cancers that relapse after initial hormonal ablation therapy, including hormone-refractory prostate cancer (HRPC), androgen-independent cancers, and hormone-independent cancers.[2] It is important to differentiate castration-resistant prostate cancer (CRPC) from true HRPC. Although CRPC responds to secondary hormonal manipulations, true HRPC resists all hormonal measures. The key defining factors of CRPC are:

- Castrate serum levels of testosterone (< 50 ng/dL)
- Three consecutive rises of prostate-specific antigen (PSA), 1 week apart, resulting in two 50% increases over the nadir
- Antiandrogen withdrawal for at least 4 weeks for flutamide and for at least 6 weeks for bicalutamide
- Prostate-specific antigen progression despite consecutive hormonal manipulations and progression or appearance of two or more lesions on bone scan or soft tissue lesions using Response Evaluation Criteria in Solid Tumors and with nodes greater than 2 cm in diameter.[3]

RATIONALE AND MOLECULAR PATHWAYS

Androgen-based pathways continue to have a clinically significant role in the progression of CRPC. In addition to the androgen production by the adrenal gland and testes, several of the enzymes involved in the synthesis of testosterone and dihydrotestosterone including cytochrome P450 17-alpha-hydroxysteroid dehydrogenase (CYP17) are highly expressed in tumor tissue.[4] This understanding has led to the development of drugs that act by inhibition of the enzymes responsible for androgen production as well as agents that inhibit the androgen receptor.

Second-line Hormonal Therapy

Androgen Synthesis Inhibitors

Ketoconazole (an antifungal drug) is a potent inhibitor of the side chain cleavage enzyme, which plays a critical role in adrenal steroidogenesis.

Abiraterone was developed through screening chemical derivatives of a parent structure of pregnenolone and in preclinical studies this is ten times more potent than ketoconazole. The structural changes in abiraterone account potent and irreversible inhibition of CYP17.[5]

Patients treated with either of these agents are at risk for adrenal insufficiency and require steroid replacement therapy.

Androgen Receptor Antagonists

Progression of CRPC in some patients may not be effectively treated by a focus safely on ligand-directed therapy. Some metastatic and primary prostate tumors retain activation of the androgen receptor in processes that are entirely independent of the androgen ligand. Amplification of the androgen receptor gene,[6] increased androgen receptor sensitivity is the proposed mechanisms and may coexist.[7] Enzalutamide, a small molecule antagonist of the androgen receptor, has important clinical activity and a role in the management of CRPC.

Immumotherapy for CRPC

Prostate acid phosphatase (PAP), prostate-specific membrane antigen (PSMA) and PSA are the tumor-associated antigens expressed by prostate cancer cells that can serve as targets for immunotherapy. Decreased immunogenicity of surface antigens by defective presentation of antigen to effector cells has been attributed to poor in vivo immune response to prostate cancer. Autologous dendritic cells can be used to deliver prostate cancer antigens for effective in vivo immune response.

Chemotherapy for CRPC

Prior to the development of the taxanes, chemotherapy was considered relatively ineffective in men with CRPC. Taxane-based regimens have been associated with higher rates of objective tumor regression, biochemical response and longer overall survival (OS).

Abiraterone

- An orally administered small molecule, irreversibly inhibits CYP17A1 enzymes 17-alpha-hydroxylase and C17, 20-lyase and blocks the synthesis of androgen in testes, tumor cells and adrenal glands.
- Delays disease progression and improves survival in CRPC patients. Efficacy proven both in chemotherapy naive and docetaxel-exposed patients.
- In a randomized phase III trial, the progression-free survival (PFS) and OS were significantly increased with abiraterone plus prednisolone compared with placebo plus prednisolone (16.5 vs 8.3 months and 35.3 vs 30.1 months) in chemotherapy naive patients.[8,9]
- Radiological PFS, PSA response rate and OS were statistically significantly improved (5.6 vs 3.6 months, 29.5 vs 5.5 months and 15.8 vs 11.2 months) in patients who had been previously treated with docetaxel.[10,11]

Enzalutamide: Androgen Receptor Antagonist

- Inhibits nuclear translocation of androgen receptor thus inhibiting association of androgen receptor with DNA.
- Overall survival significantly increased with enzalutamide (18.4 vs 13.6 months) compared with placebo in phase III AFFIRM trial.[12]
- Well-tolerated drug with consistent benefits across all subgroups.
- Additional clinical studies are underway to determine the efficacy of second-line hormonal therapies sequential or in combination.

Sipuleucel-T

- Autologous dendritic cell therapeutic vaccine
- Enhances immune T-cell response to PAP
- Prepared from peripheral blood mononuclear cells obtained by leukapheresis[13]
- Significant OS benefits (25.8 vs 21.7 months) were seen in phase III IMPACT trial[14]
- It is an option for men with CRPC having asymptomatic or minimally symptomatic disease.

Docetaxel

- Overall survival benefit (19.2 vs 16.3 months) with docetaxel plus prednisolone versus mitoxantrone plus prednisolone TAX 327 trial.[15]
- Higher PSA response rate (45 vs 32%).
- Three-weekly and 2-weekly schedules well tolerated with comparable results.
- Weekly docetaxel as good as 3-weekly mitoxantrone.
- No upper limit of number of cycles of docetaxel may be continued until disease progression or intolerance.
- Three-weekly docetaxel plus daily prednisolone (5 mg twice a day) is the standard of care for men with CRPC.

Cabazitaxel

- Semisynthetic taxane.
- Only indicated for use in combination with prednisolone for patients with previously treated and progressed on docetaxel.
- Overall survival benefit (15.1 vs 12.7 months) and PFS benefit (2.8 vs 1.4 months) as established by TROPIC trial.[16]
- Significantly more toxic than mitoxantrone.

Other chemotherapy drugs having activity in CRPC are mitoxantrone, estramustine, paclitaxel. Limited actively has also been seen with fluorouracil, gemcitabine, cyclophosphamide, platinum analogs, etc.

CONCLUSION

Castration-resistant prostate cancer (CRPC) is a heterogeneous disease and patient subgroups exist that are benefitted with either of any hormonal, immunological or cytotoxic therapies. Indentifying right drug for right patient should hopefully improve the chances of treatment response and survival.

REFERENCES

1. Goodin S, Rao KV, DiPaola RS. State-of-the-art treatment of metastatic hormone-refractory prostate cancer. Oncologist. 2002;7(4):360-70.
2. Scher HI, Halabi S, Tannock I, Morris M, Sternberg CN, Carducci MA, et al. Design and end points of clinical trials for patients with progressive prostate cancer and castrate levels of testosterone: recommendations of the Prostate Cancer Clinical Trials Working Group. J Clin Oncol. 2008;26(7):1148-59.
3. Mottet N, Bellmunt J, Bolla M, Joniau S, Mason M, Matveev V, et al. EAU guidelines on prostate cancer. Part II: Treatment of

advanced, relapsing, and castration-resistant prostate cancer. Eur Urol. 2011;59(4):572-83.

4. Barrie SE, Potter GA, Goddard PM, Haynes BP, Dowsett M, Jarman M. Pharmacology of novel steroidal inhibitors of cytochrome P450(17) alpha (17 alpha-hydroxylase/C17-20 lyase). J Steroid Biochem Mol Biol. 1994;50(5-6):267-73.
5. Potter GA, Barrie SE, Jarman M, Rowlands MG. Novel steroidal inhibitors of human cytochrome P45017 alpha (17 alpha-hydroxylase-C17,20-lyase): potential agents for the treatment of prostatic cancer. J Med Chem. 1995;38(13):2463-71.
6. Visakorpi T, Hyytinen E, Koivisto P, Tanner M, Keinänen R, Palmberg C, et al. In vivo amplification of the androgen receptor gene and progression of human prostate cancer. Nat Genet. 1995;9(4):401-6.
7. Gregory CW, Johnson RT Jr, Mohler JL, French FS, Wilson EM. Androgen receptor stabilization in recurrent prostate cancer is associated with hypersensitivity to low androgen. Cancer Res. 2001;61(7):2892-8.
8. Ryan CJ, Smith MR, de Bono JS, Molina A, Logothetis CJ, de Souza P, et al. Abiraterone in metastatic prostate cancer without previous chemotherapy. N Engl J Med. 2013;368(2):138-48.
9. Dana E. Rathkopf, Matthew R. Smith, Johann S. de Bono, Christopher J. Logothetis. Neal D Shore et al. Updated Interim Efficacy Analysis and Long-term Safety of Abiraterone Acetate in Metastatic Castration-resistant Prostate Cancer Patients without Prior Chemotherapy (COU-AA-302). European Urology. 2014;(66): 815–25.
10. de Bono JS, Logothetis CJ, Molina A, Fizazi K, North S, Chu L, et al. Abiraterone and increased survival in metastatic prostate cancer. N Engl J Med. 2011;364(21):1995-2005.
11. Fizazi K, Scher HI, Molina A, Logothetis CJ, Chi KN, Jones RJ, et al. Abiraterone acetate for treatment of metastatic castration-resistant prostate cancer: final overall survival analysis of the COU-AA-301 randomised, double-blind, placebo-controlled phase 3 study. Lancet Oncol. 2012;13(10):983-92.
12. Scher HI, Fizazi K, Saad F, Taplin ME, Sternberg CN, Miller K, et al. Increased survival with enzalutamide in prostate cancer after chemotherapy. N Engl J Med. 2012;367(13):1187-97.
13. Small EJ, Schellhammer PF, Higano CS, Redfern CH, Nemunaitis JJ, Valone FH, et al. Placebo-controlled phase III trial of immunologic therapy with sipuleucel-T (APC8015) in patients with metastatic, asymptomatic hormone refractory prostate cancer. J Clin Oncol. 2006;24(19):3089-94.
14. Kontoff PW, Hegano CS, Shore ND, Berger ER, Small EJ, Penson DF, et al. Sipuleucel-T, immunotherapy for castration-resistant prostate cancer. N Engl J Med. 2010:363(5):411-22.
15. Tannock IF, de Wit R, Berry WR, Horti J, Pluzanska A, Chi KN, et al. Docetaxel plus prednisone or mitoxantrone plus prednisone for advanced prostate cancer. N Engl J Med. 2004;351(15):1502-12.
16. de Bone JS, Oudart S, Ozguroglu M, Hansen S, Machiels JP, Kocak I, et al. Prednisone plus cabazitaxel or mitoxantrone for metastatic castration-resistant prostate cancer progressing after docetaxel treatment: a randomised open-label trial. Lancet. 2010;376(9747):1147-54.

27

CHAPTER

Ocular Malignancies: An Overview

Trinanjan Basu, Tejinder Kataria

INTRODUCTION

The delicate balance between cure of disease and preservation of ocular functions makes intraocular and orbital tumors an important entity among radiation oncologist. Most of them around 75% are choroidal or uveal melanomas and then comes orbital lymphomas. Retinoblastoma being predominately pediatric age group tumor accounts for 20% of cases.[1,2]

Radiation therapy either as external beam or brachytherapy is an effective modality while treating various subsites of ocular structures. Radiotherapy either as primary or as adjuvant resulted in satisfactory outcome over the years. Parallel to the same fear of injuries to various ocular structures has also been a concern especially among ophthalmologists.[3,4] Modern radiotherapy techniques as in other sites of body have led to new paradigm of management.[5,6]

Here, we will briefly address various application of radiotherapy in treating ocular malignancies.

ANATOMY

The human eye can broadly be divided into ocular adnexa and eyeball (Fig. 1). The ocular adnexa consists of the eyelids, cilia, lacrimal glands, lacrimal drainage apparatus, and conjunctiva. The eyeball or globe on the other hand has three layers. The outer coat consists of the clear cornea on the front and the sclera occupying the posterior aspect. The middle coat uvea is formed by the choroid, ciliary body, and iris, all of which contain a high concentration of melanocytes as well as vessels. The innermost sensory layer is called retina which extends from the ora serrata anteriorly to the optic nerve posteriorly.[7,8]

The lens is suspended from the ciliary body and is located posterior to the iris. The orbit is composed of seven bones: frontal, maxilla, lacrimal, palatine, ethmoid, sphenoid and zygomatic and it encloses the ocular globe, vessels, nerves, orbital fat, lacrimal gland, and ocular muscles: four recti and two oblique muscles.

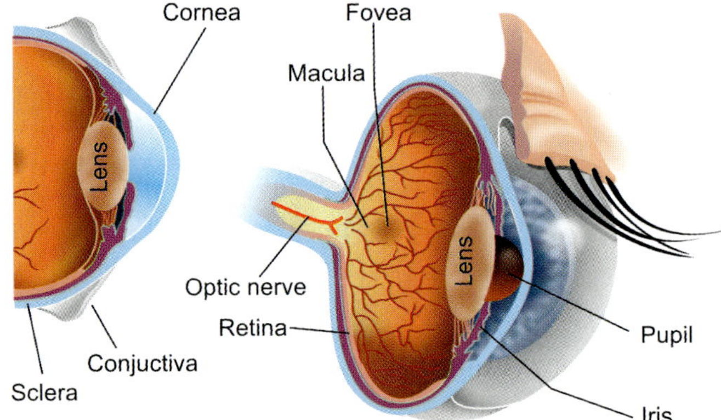

Fig. 1 Anatomy of human eye

(Downloaded from http://www.webmd.com/eye-health/picture-of-the-eyes)

CLASSIFICATION

The main types of ocular malignant tumors are given in Table 1.[9]

METASTATIC CARCINOMA TO THE POSTERIOR UVEA

Tumor metastases to the uvea once considered rare, is now probably the most common malignant disease involving the eye. Uveal metastases most commonly originate from primary breast and lung cancers in women, and lung and gastrointestinal tract cancers in men.[10-12] In an autopsy series of patients with breast cancer, a third of the cases included

Table 1 Ocular malignant diseases as per site of origin

Ocular structure of origin	*Types*
A. Eyelids and lacrimal drainage systems	1. Basal cell carcinoma 2. Squamous cell carcinoma 3. Sebaceous carcinoma of eyelid glands, sweat glands and hair follicles 4. Malignant melanoma
B. Conjunctiva	1. Invasive squamous cell carcinoma 2. Malignant melanoma 3. Ocular syndromes: a. Tuberous sclerosis b. Retinocerebellar capillary hemangiomatosis (von Hippel-Lindau syndrome) c. Encephalofacial cavernous hemangiomatosis (Sturge-Weber syndrome) d. Racemose hemangiomatosis (Wyburn-Mason syndrome)
C. Intraocular tumors	1. Malignant melanoma of iris and choroid 2. Metastatic carcinoma of the choroid 3. Retinal adenocarcinoma 4. Retinoblastoma 5. Glial tumor of the retina 6. Astrocytoma of the optic nerve 7. Histiocytic lymphoma/ reticulum cell sarcoma
D. Orbital tumors	1. Juvenile pilocytic astrocytoma 2. Orbital meningioma 3. Orbital rhabdomyosarcoma (RMS) 4. Leukemia 5. Lymphoma (NHL) 6. Lacrimal gland tumors 7. Metastatic orbital tumors

uveal metastases.[12] Uveal metastases are mostly unifocal but may also be multifocal and bilateral. In an analysis by Shields et al.[12] of 520 eyes containing 950 uveal metastatic tumors, found 88% in the posterior uvea, 9% in the iris, and 2% in the ciliary body.

The aim of therapy is to restore normal vision as far as possible because overall survival may be limited to months. Observation for small lesions can be carried out if patient is already on systemic chemotherapy. If the patient has visual symptoms, treatment should be immediate.

If there are no evidence of systemic metastatic disease or if the uveal metastasis does not respond to systemic therapy, external beam or brachytherapy to the eye is often performed. For patients with uveal metastases and active systemic disease, palliative response is achieved by delivering a 30–40 Gy over 3–4 weeks to the entire ocular structure. Brachytherapy with ^{125}I plaque and a prescribed dose of 40 Gy to the tumor apex is recommended for oligometastatic diseases from breast or colon malignancies where longer survival has been documented.[13-15]

Currently, hypofractionated radiotherapy with CyberKnife (Accuray, Sunnyvale, CA) is being explored for the treatment of uveal metastasis.[16]

MALIGNANT MELANOMA OF THE POSTERIOR UVEA

Uveal melanoma is the most common primary intraocular tumor in adults. The disease is found in all ages and mean age at diagnosis is in the mid-50s.[17,18]

Diagnostic procedures include indirect ophthalmoscopy, fundus photography, autofluorescence photography, fluorescein and indocyanine angiography, ultrasound (both A and B modes), optical coherence tomography (OCT), magnetic resonance imaging (MRI), and CT scan.

By far the most important means of diagnosis is the detection of the ophthalmoscopic examination findings. The classical finding of orange pigment on the surface of the tumor along with a history of a nevus that showed signs of growth over time is characteristic.[18]

In 1942 Callender et al. proposed histopathological classification of malignant uveal melanomas and was subsequently modified by McLean in 1983 that correlated between cell type and mortality.[19,20]

Callender's Classification of Uveal Melanoma

- Spindle A cell (the most benign, < 5% 5-year mortality rate)
- Spindle B cell (mortality rate 40% in 5-year)
- Pure epithelioid cell (most aggressive, mortality rate 69% in 5 years)
- Mixed cell (mortality rate 51% in 5 years)

TNM Classification of Uveal Melanoma (International Union Against Cancer UICC)[21]

T1 < 10 mm greatest dimension, < 3 mm thickness
T1 A < 8 mm greatest dimension, < 2 mm thickness
T1 B > 8–10 mm greatest dimension, > 2 cm and < 3 mm thickness
T2 > 10–15 mm greatest dimension, 3–5 mm thickness
T3 > 15 mm greatest dimension, > 5 mm thickness
T4 Extraocular extension
N1 All sites, regional
M Metastasis

Management of uveal melanoma continues to be controversial with several approaches including periodic observation, laser photocoagulation, thermotherapy, plaque brachytherapy, charged particle radiotherapy, local resection, and enucleation.[17,18] In those cases where there is hope for useful vision, every attempt should be made with an organ-conserving procedure. Tumor size and stage are the major determining factors for deciding the treatment modalities.
Plaque brachytherapy can be administered for medium-size uveal melanomas (3–8 mm in thickness and 10–15 mm in diameter). Large tumors (> 8 mm in thickness and > 15 mm in base) are managed with local resection or plaque brachytherapy. Enucleation is preferred due to ocular intolerance to conservative methods.[22]

Uveal melanoma with involvement of the iris, ciliary body, or the posterior choroid and are managed accordingly. Tumors that are diffuse, display a relatively fast growth pattern, and have extrascleral extension are amenable to be treated with enucleation.[23]

In the United States and Canada, the melanoma treatment controversy has led to the development of the Collaborative Ocular Melanoma Study (COMS).[24-26] COMS is a prospective randomized study that, among other aims, was designed to compare survival in patients treated with either brachytherapy or enucleation.

As per COMS report 28, published in December 2006 which analyzed 1,317 patients with choroidal melanoma between 1987 and 1998 and had randomly assigned treatment like enucleation or to ^{125}I plaque brachytherapy. The conclusion of this study showed that mortality rates following ^{125}I brachytherapy did not differ from those following enucleation through 12 years of follow-up. At present, ^{125}I is predominantly used in the United States, Canada, and the United Kingdom,[27] whereas ^{106}Ru is quite popular in Germany.[28]

The current relative indications for treating a posterior uveal melanoma with plaque radiation therapy are generally as follows: (a) selected small melanomas that are documented to be growing or that show clear-cut signs of activity on the first visit, (b) most medium-sized and some large choroidal and ciliary body melanomas in an eye with potential salvageable vision, or (c) almost all actively growing melanomas that occur in the patient's only useful eye.

If a melanoma exceeds 15 mm in diameter and 10 mm in thickness, one should anticipate visual morbidity from radiation therapy, and enucleation should be strongly advised.[29]

A retrospective analysis of ocular melanoma patients treated with ^{125}I plaque brachytherapy was performed by Jensen et al.[30] at the Mayo Clinic. In that study, 156 patients were treated with episcleral plaques in concordance with COMS design. Excellent tumor control was observed with 5-year overall survival of 83% and 5-year disease-specific survival of 91%. They observed that dose rates more than 90–100 cGy/hour were associated with increased systemic control but worse radiation toxicity.

RETINOBLASTOMA

Retinoblastoma is the most common intraocular malignancy of childhood with approximately 4% of pediatric population affected by the same.[31] The disease is bilateral in 20–30% of patients.[32] Of newly diagnosed children, 10% have a family history of retinoblastoma. The remaining 90% are sporadic. Retinoblastoma can arise in hereditary, nonhereditary, and chromosome-deletion forms, the latter occurring on the long arm of chromosome 13 (13q).[32,33] In general, the hereditary form is diagnosed earlier than the nonhereditary form of the disease. The nonhereditary form is unilateral and it is not associated with an increased risk of other malignancies.[32,33]

As per molecular genetic studies 13q14 mutation which is a tumor suppressor gene termed the RB gene encodes a protein the inhibitory function of which is thought to be on cell growth. When the function is lost, there is increased cellular growth unopposed by any inhibitory signal.[34]

> Although the disease may be present at birth, most children with retinoblastoma are diagnosed around the age 3 or 4 years.[33] The most common presenting signs and symptoms are leukocoria, strabismus, or a mass in the fundus noticed during ocular examination.[31]

Evaluation with an accurate history evaluating prenatal and prematurity, oxygen therapy, history of leukocoria at birth, family habit of pets and family history of retinoblastoma all are important.

It is frequent for the family members to notice a whitish pupillary reflex at a certain angle and light intensity or to observe a white eye instead of red eye.

Slit-lamp biomicroscopy with dilated pupils reveal congenital cataract or a retrolental membrane, suggesting diagnoses other than retinoblastoma. Binocular indirect ophthalmoscopy seeking characteristic ophthalmic features of retinoblastoma or spontaneously regressed retinoblastoma remains the most important diagnostic tool.[35] Retinoblastoma on A-mode ultrasonography shows very intense reflections from calcium deposits. B-mode ultrasonography shows a heterogeneous acoustic solidity with highly reflective intrinsic echoes within the tumor and attenuation of orbital pattern.[36] On CT scan, it usually appears as a dense heterogeneous lesion with hyperdense foci corresponding to calcification. CT is valuable for assessing extraocular extension and invasion of the optic nerve.[36] MRI appears to be most helpful in differentiating retinoblastoma from simulating lesions such as Coats disease, retinal detachment, retinopathy of prematurity, and persistent hyperplastic primary vitreous (PHPV). Involvement of the optic nerve, extraocular extension, and intracranial midline neoplasm in trilateral retinoblastoma are best detected by contrast-enhanced MRI studies.[36]

The final ophthalmologic procedure is accurate mapping and sizing of tumor deposits in both eyes, which is best accomplished by indirect bilateral ophthalmoscopy with the child under general anesthesia. Mapping and sizing permit visual prognostic classification using the system of Reese and Ellsworth.[37] In 2003, International Classification of Retinoblastoma was developed and more recently the American Joint Committee on Cancer (AJCC) and the St. Jude's System have been developed to include extraocular extension and metastasis, which determine survival after treatment (Tables 2 to 4).

Enucleation of the involved globe has been the traditional method of treatment for unilateral disease and early enucleation is the main reason for the marked improvement

Table 2 International classification system for retinoblastoma

	Description	*Specific features*
A	Small tumor	Retinoblastoma < 3 mm[a]
B	Larger tumor	Retinoblastoma > 3 mm[a] or
	Macula	Macular retinoblastoma location (< 3 mm to foveola)
	Juxtapupillary	Juxtapupillary retinoblastoma location (< 1.5 mm to disc)
	Subretinal fluid	Additional subretinal fluid (< 3 mm from margin)
C	Focal seeds	Retinoblastoma with: Subretinal seeds < 3 mm from retinoblastoma Vitreous seeds < 3 mm from retinoblastoma Both subretinal and vitreous seeds < 3 mm from retinoblastoma
D	Diffuse seeds	Retinoblastoma with: Subretinal seeds > 3 mm from retinoblastoma Vitreous seeds > 3 mm from retinoblastoma Both subretinal and vitreous seeds 3 mm from retinoblastoma
E	Extensive retinoblastoma	Extensive retinoblastoma occupying > 50% globe or Neovascular glaucoma Opaque media from hemorrhage in anterior chamber, vitreous, or subretinal space Invasion of postlaminar optic nerve, choroid (> 2 mm), sclera, orbit, anterior chamber

a: 3 mm in basal dimension or thickness.

Table 3 AJCC staging for retinoblastoma

T1/p1	< 25% of retina
T2/pT2	> 25 and < 50% of retina
T3/Pt3	> 50% of retina and/or intraocular beyond retina
T3a/pT3a	> 50% of retina and/or cells in vitreous
T3B	Optic disc
pT3b	Optic nerve up to lamina cribrosa
T3c	Anterior chamber and/or uvea
pT3c	Anterior chamber and/or uvea and/ or intrascleral
T4/pT4	Extraocular
T4a	Optic nerve
pT4a	Beyond lamina cribrosa, not at resection line
T4b	Other extraocular
pT4b	Other extraocular and/or at resection line.
N1/pN1	Regional nodal metastasis
MI	Distant metastases

Table 4 St. Jude staging system for retinoblastoma

Stage I: Tumor (unifocal or multifocal) confined to retina
a. Occupying one quadrant or less
b. Occupying two quadrants or less
c. Occupying more than 50% of retinal surface
Stage II: Tumor (unifocal or multifocal) confined to globe
a. With vitreous seeding
b. Extending to optic nerve head
c. Extending to choroid
d. Extending to choroid and optic nerve head
e. Extending to emissaries
Stage III: Extraocular extension of tumor
a. Extending beyond cut end of optic nerve (including subarachnoid extension)
b. Extending through sclera into orbital contents
c. Extending to choroid and beyond cut end of optic nerve (including subarachnoid extension)
d. Extending through sclera into orbital contents and beyond cut end of optic nerve (including subarachnoid extension)
Stage IV: Distant metastases
a. Extending through optic nerve to brain
b. Blood-borne metastases to soft tissue(s) and bone(s)
c. Bone marrow metastases

in survival during the past half century.[38] The fellow eye, although apparently normal at diagnosis, remains at risk and must be examined at frequent intervals until the child is at least of school age. The therapy of bilateral disease is more complex and traditionally has consisted of enucleation of the eye with more advanced disease and radiation therapy for the less involved eye. Tragically, in some cases, both eyes contain advanced tumors, and there is no hope of retaining useful vision. In such cases, bilateral enucleation has been traditionally recommended.

External Beam Techniques for Retinoblastoma

Retinoblastoma was first successfully treated by X-rays in 1903 as reported by Hilgartner et al.[39] Armstrong and Weiss et al.[40,41] described various techniques including the classic single temporal portal and modifications allowing retinal irradiation while shielding of the lens and anterior chamber. This technique results in underdosing the anterior and posterior chamber and future risk of recurrences.

The modified technique used a lateral portal with the anterior beam edge at the equator of the globe and an anterior portal containing a 7-mm diameter central divergent block hung in a pendulum fashion along the central axis of the beam to protect the lens.[41] Donaldson and Egbert[33] recommended the use of the Comberg contact lens with the field edge at the ora serrata. McCormick et al.[42] compared a lens-sparing technique with a modified lateral technique designed to reduce the lens dose to 50% of the volume dose to the globe. The lens-sparing technique was associated with relapse in about two thirds of the treated eyes compared with 17% with the modified lateral technique.

3D Conformal Radiotherapy Technique

Treatment of unilateral retinoblastoma with four noncoplanar fields like anterior oblique: superior, inferior, medial, and lateral is dependent upon the stage and anatomy.

Caution must be taken to minimize the dose to critical structures such as fellow eye, chiasm, pituitary gland, brainstem, posterior-most upper teeth, and upper cervical spine. The entire retina should be treated, including 5–8 mm of proximal optic nerve. Literature recommended dosage being 42–44 Gy in daily fractions of 1.8 or 2.0 Gy over a period of 4.5–5 weeks.

Since 70–80% of patients are 3 years or younger, conscious sedation is required.

Brachytherapy for Retinoblastoma

Plaque radiation therapy can be used as primary or secondary treatment. Amendola et al.[43] reported their experience with 20 patients treated with brachytherapy as a boost after external beam therapy for very large or locally recurring tumors. 16 of 20 patients (80%) had tumor control; the remaining four patients (20%) required enucleation for failure. Shields et al.[44] reported solitary plaque radiation therapy in 91 cases of recurrent or residual retinoblastoma in which the only other option was enucleation. Tumor control and globe salvage were achieved in 89% of cases with plaque irradiation mean dose to tumor apex of 41 Gy at median follow-up of 52 months.

The conclusion with role of radiotherapy in advanced retinoblastoma being achievement of excellent long-term local control and survival with low rates of treatment-related toxicity and secondary malignancy even after 11 years follow-up.[45]

Second Malignancies in Retinoblastoma

Trilateral retinoblastoma includes the association of bilateral and/or familial retinoblastoma and neuroblastic tumors in the pineal gland or other midline structures. DePotter et al.[46] reported the incidence of trilateral retinoblastoma around 5–8%. The tumor usually occurs in children around 23 months and is highly fatal despite aggressive treatment with chemotherapy, radiation therapy, Gamma Knife therapy, and others.

RADIATION TOXICITIES TO EYE

Traditional radiotherapy has always been feared because of acute and late sequelae to the ocular structures. For dry eye to develop, incidence of injury increases from 0% with doses of 30 Gy to 100% after doses more than or equal to 57 Gy with conventionally fractionated external beam radiotherapy (EBRT). The eyelid also develops transient erythema at doses of 30 Gy, with telangiectasia and loss of eyelashes beginning to occur at 40 Gy. Late squeal like ectropion and entropion are noted if EBRT doses exceed 50 Gy. Chances of corneal perforation increase when the cornea receives EBRT dose in excess of 60 Gy. Cataract is a well-known radiation complication presenting as posterior subcapsular opacification. In general, latency and frequency of cataract is a function of radiation dose and conventionally fractionated EBRT dosage exceeding 12 Gy is held responsible. The complications in inner eye structures like retina and optic nerve is primarily determined by the total radiation dose. None of the patients receiving a dose of less than 50 Gy developed optic neuropathy or chiasm injury. In contrast, the 10-year actuarial incidence of optic nerve-chiasm injury was approximately 5% for patients receiving 50–60 Gy.[5,47]

In the Table 5, these acute and late effects of radiotherapy to ocular structures are being elaborated.[48]

Table 5 Early and late effects of radiotherapy upon ocular structures

Structure	*Early effects*	*Late sequelae*
Eyelid	Erythema, telangiectasia, loss of eyelashes	Trichiasis, ectropion, entropion
Lacrimal system	Dry eye, burning sensation in eyes	Atrophy, stenosis of NLD
Conjunctiva	Conjunctivitis	Conjunctival scarring
Cornea	Keratitis, corneal ulcer	Corneal perforation
Lens		Cataract
Retina and optic nerve	Macular edema, transient visual loss	Optic neuropathy

Abbreviation: NLD: naso-lacrimal duct

REFERENCES

1. Available from http://www.eyecancer.com last accessed on 07.01.2015.
2. Available from http://www.cancerresearchuk.org last accessed on 07.01.2015.
3. Macfaul PA, Bedford MA. Ocular complications after therapeutic irradiation. Br J Ophthalmol. 1970;54(4):237-47.
4. Nakissa N, Rubin P, Strohl R, Keys H. Ocular and orbital complications following radiation therapy of paranasal sinus malignancies and review of literature. Cancer. 1983;51(6):980-6.
5. Jeganathan VS, Wirth A, MacManus MP. Ocular risks from orbital and periorbital radiation therapy: a critical review. Int J Radiat Oncol Biol Phys. 2011;79(3):650-9.
6. Marchand V, Dendale R. Normal tissue tolerance to external beam radiation therapy: eye structures. Cancer Radiother. 2010;14(4-5):277-83.
7. Available from http://www.webmd.com/eye-health/picture-of-the-eyes.
8. Available from http://www.allaboutvision.com/resources/anatomy.htm.
9. Jerry A Shields, and Carol L Shields. Review of Ophthalmic Tumors. Oncology Service, Wills Eye institute, Philadelphia. February 2013.
10. Brady LW, Shields JA, Augsburger JJ, Day JL. Malignant intraocular tumors. Cancer. 1982;49(3):578-85.
11. Ferry AP, Font RL. Carcinoma metastatic to the eye and orbit. I. A clinicopathologic study of 227 cases. Arch Ophthalmol. 1974;92(4):276-86.
12. Shields CL, Shields JA, Gross NE, Schwartz GP, Lally SE. Survey of 520 eyes with uveal metastases. Ophthalmology. 1997;104(8):1265-76.
13. Seregard S, Pelayes DE, Singh AD. Radiation therapy: uveal tumors. Dev Ophthalmol. 2013;52:36-57.
14. Shields CL. Plaque radiotherapy for the management of uveal metastasis. Curr Opin Ophthalmol. 1998;9(3):31-7.
15. Cohen VM. Ocular metastases. Eye (Lond). 2013;27(2):137-41.
16. Vlachostergios PJ, Voutsadakis IA, Papandreou CN. Orbital metastasis of breast carcinoma. Breast Cancer (Auckl). 2009;3:91-7.
17. Margo CE. The Collaborative Ocular Melanoma study: an overview. Cancer Control. 2004;11(5):304-9.
18. Shields JA, Shields CL. Management of posterior uveal melanoma: past, present, and future: the 2014 Charles L. Schepens Lecture. Ophthalmology. 2015:122(2):414-28.
19. Coleman K, Baak JP, van Diest PJ, Mullaney J. Prognostic value of morphometric features and the callender classification in uveal melanomas. Ophthalmology. 1996;103(10):1634-41.
20. McLean IW, Foster WD, Zimmerman LE, Gamel JW. Modifications of Callender's classification of uveal melanoma at the Armed Forces Institute of Pathology. Am J Ophthalmol. 1983;96(4):502-9.
21. Edge SB, Byrd DR, Compton CC, et al. Malignant melanoma of the uvea. AJCC Cancer Staging Manual. 7th edition. New York, NY: Springer; 2010, pp 547-59.
22. Finger PT, Zhou D, Kalach N, Semenova E, Choi W. ^{103}Pd versus ^{125}I ophthalmic plaque brachytherapy: preoperative comparative radiation dosimetry for 319 uveal melanomas. J Radiat Oncol. 2014;3(4):409-16.
23. Liu YC, Tsai CC, Lee FL, Lee SM, Kao SC. Mortality from uveal melanoma treated by enucleation --a 16-year survey in Taiwan. Acta Ophthalmol. 2013;91(7):e583-4.
24. Collaborative Ocular Melanoma Study Group. The COMS randomized trial of iodine 125 brachytherapy for choroidal melanoma: V. Twelve-year mortality rates and prognostic factors: COMS report No. 28. Arch Ophthalmol. 2006;124(12):1684-93.
25. Straatsma BR, Fine SL, Earle JD, Hawkins BS, Diener-West M, McLaughlin JA. Enucleation versus plaque irradiation for choroidal melanoma. Ophthalmology. 1988;95(7):1000-4.
26. Damato B. Progress in the management of patients with uveal melanoma. The 2012 Ashton Lecture. Eye (Lond). 2012;26(9):1157-72.
27. Bell DJ, Wilson MW. Choroidal melanoma: natural history and management options. Cancer Control. 2004;11(5):296-303.
28. Takiar V, Gombos DS, Mourtada F, Rechner LA, Lawyer AA, Morrison WH, et al. Disease control and toxicity outcomes using ruthenium eye plaque brachytherapy in the treatment of uveal melanoma. Pract Radiat Oncol. 2014;4(4):e189-94.
29. Shields JA, Shields CL. Atlas of intraocular tumors. Philadelphia: Lippincott Williams & Wilkins, 1999.
30. Jensen AW, Peterson IA, Kline RW, Stafford SL, Schomberg PJ, Robertson DM. Radiation complications and tumor control after ^{125}I plaque brachytherapy for ocular melanoma. Int J Radiation Oncol Biol Phys. 2005;63(1):101-8.
31. Shields CL, Shields JA. Diagnosis and management of retinoblastoma. Cancer Control. 2004;11(5):317-27.
32. Donaldson SS, Smith LA. Retinoblastoma: biology, presentation and current management. Oncology. 1989;3(4):45-51.
33. Donaldson SS, Egbert PR. Retinoblastoma. In: Pizzo P, Poplack D (Eds). Principles and Practice of Pediatric Oncology. Philadelphia: JB Lippincott; 1989.
34. Weinberg RA. Integration of molecular genetics into cancer management. Keynote presentation at National Conference on

Integration of Molecular Genetics into Cancer Management. Miami, FL; April 10-12, 1991.

35. Shields JA, Stephens RA, Augsburger JJ. Metastatic tumor to the uveal tract. In: Lommatzsch PK, Blodi FC (Eds). Intraocular Tumors. Berlin: Akademie-Verlag; 1983. pp.433-44.
36. DePotter P, Gonzalez CF, Flanders AE, et al. Imaging studies of intraocular tumors. In: Alberti WE, Sagerman RH (Eds). Medical Radiology: Radiotherapy of Intraocular and Orbital Tumors. Berlin: Springer-Verlag; 1993. pp. 295-309.
37. Reese AB, Ellsworth RM. The evaluation and current concept of retinoblastoma therapy. Trans Am Acad Ophthalmol Otolaryngol 1963;67:164-72.
38. Shields JA. Modern techniques in the management of retinoblastoma. Trans Pacific Coast Otolaryngol Ophthalmol Soc. 1979;60:235.
39. Hilgartner HL. Report of a case of double glioma treated with X-ray. 1903. Tex Med. 2005;101(7):10.
40. Armstrong DI. The use of 4-6 MeV electrons for the conservative treatment of retinoblastoma. Br J Radiol. 1974;47(558):326-31.
41. Weiss DR, Cassady JR, Petersen R. Retinoblastoma: a modification in radiation therapy technique. Radiology. 1975;114(3):705-8.
42. McCormick B, Ellsworth R, Abramson D, Haik B, Tome M, Grabowski E, et al. Radiation therapy for retinoblastoma: comparison of results with lens-sparing versus lateral beam techniques. Int J Radiat Oncol Biol Phys. 1988;15(3):567-74.
43. Amendola BE, Markoe AM, Augsburger JJ, Karlsson UL, Giblin M, Shields JA, et al. Analysis of treatment results in 36 children with retinoblastoma treated by scleral plaque irradiation. Int J Radiat Oncol Biol Phys. 1989;17(1):63-70.
44. Shields JA, Shields CL, DePotter P, Hernandez JC, Brady LW. Plaque radiotherapy for residual or recurrent retinoblastoma in 91 cases. J Pediatr Ophthamol Strabismus. 1994;31(4):242-5.
45. Orman A, Koru-Sengul T, Miao F, Markoe A, Panoff JE. The modern role of radiation therapy in treating advanced-stage retinoblastoma: long-term outcomes and racial differences. Int J Radiat Oncol Biol Phys. 2014;90(5):1037-43.
46. DePotter P, Shields CL, Shields JA. Clinical variation of trilateral retinoblastoma: a report of 13 cases. J Pediatr Ophthalmol Strab. 1994;31:26-31.
47. Parsons JT, Bova FJ, Fitzgerald CR, Mendenhall WM, Million RR. Severe dry-eye syndrome following external beam irradiation. Int J Radiat Oncol Biol Phys. 1994;30(4):775-80.
48. Laskar SG, Basu T, Chaudhary S, Chaukar D, Nadkarni M, Gn M. Postoperative interstitial brachytherapy in eyelid cancer: long term results and assessment of Cosmesis After Interstitial Brachytherapy scale. J Contemp Brachytherapy. 2015; 6(4):350-5.

28

CHAPTER

Soft Tissue Sarcoma

Shyam Singh Bisht, Tejinder Kataria, Rahul Patil

INTRODUCTION

Soft tissue sarcomas (STS) are derived from mesenchymal tissue and are a relatively uncommon group of malignancies accounting for approximately 1% of all adult cancers. Median onset of STS is generally from age of 50 years to 55 years. More than 50% of these tumors originate in the limbs (extremities), whereas approximately 40% arise in the retroperitoneum or visceral tissues and trunk and 10% in head and neck. Major prognostic factors are tumor size, pathologic grade, and depth of involvement of the tumor. Lymph node involvement is an adverse characteristic in STS but is rarely encountered except in certain histologic subtypes. The predominant pattern of relapse is to the lungs for most STS, but intra-abdominal lesions will generally relapse within the abdomen, including the liver. Gastrointestinal stromal tumors (GIST) are rare STS that predominantly arise in the stomach or small intestine has favorable response to molecular targeted therapy (imatinib). Clinical examination to evaluate lesion size and mobility and the relationship to the investing fascia deep to the subcutaneous fat (i.e., superficial versus deep) and adjacent neurovascular structures or bone. All soft tissue masses deep to the investing fascia should be considered sarcoma until proven otherwise. Histologic confirmation is necessary. Cross-sectional imaging with computed tomography (CT) or magnetic resonance imaging (MRI) is essential. If the underlying diagnosis is rhabdomyosarcoma, a bone marrow biopsy is necessary as well as cerebrospinal fluid analysis in parameningeal lesions. CT of the retroperitoneum may also be valuable for evaluation of extremity myxoid liposarcoma (MLS). In general, the approach is surgery with or without local radiation therapy (RT). Chemotherapy remains controversial and is generally restricted to established chemoresponsive lesions and high-risk cases. A complete and durable response to systemic chemotherapy is uncommon and generally seen only in histologic subtypes such as liposarcoma and synovial sarcoma. The 5-year survival overall is approximately 60%, but this depends on the site of the primary tumor and other prognostic factors.

ETIOLOGY AND EPIDEMIOLOGY

Environmental Etiologic Factors

Most cases have no clearly defined etiologic factors. Several factors have been identified that either predispose or are associated with the development of STS such as herbicide exposure and constitutional and hormonal factors during childhood, puberty, and adulthood, radiation exposure (accidental, therapeutic, or diagnostic exposure).

Radiation-associated STS have demonstrated inferior survival compared with sporadic STS. One hypothesis is that incomplete damage in normal tissues results in mutagenic responses and disorganized reparative proliferation that can eventually trigger tumor induction. This may provide a basis for the observation that RT-induced sarcomas commonly originate on the perimeter of the previous RT target volume and not necessarily in the high-dose region. Certain conditions in themselves are associated with intrinsic host predisposition to radiation-induced neoplasia, most notably retinoblastoma.

Desmoid tumors are commonly seen in the anterior abdominal wall after pregnancy, although the biologic and traumatic basis for this is unclear. Several chemical carcinogens, including thorotrast, vinyl chloride, and arsenic, are established in the causation of hepatic angiosarcomas. Workers exposed to phenoxy herbicides, chlorophenols, and dioxins had higher mortality rates from cancer compared with controls, and the increase was highest for STS. There have been conflicting reports about occupational exposure to phenoxyacetic acids detectable in chlorophenols (frequent in wood preservatives) and certain herbicides.

Molecular Pathogenetic Mechanisms

Contemporary appreciation of the molecular pathogenesis and behavior of STS suggests that these lesions are divisible into two major genetic groups: (1) those possessing specific genetic alterations and usually simple karyotypes, such as reciprocal chromosomal translocations (e.g., SS18-SSX1 or SS18-SSX2 in synovial sarcoma); and (2) sarcomas with nonspecific genetic alterations and complex unbalanced karyotypes.[1]

PATHOLOGY

Classic Pathology Classification

The most common pathologic classification scheme for STS is based on histogenesis, as described by the World Health Organization (WHO) in which tumors are named according to the normal tissues that they most resemble (Box 1).

However, as the degree of histologic differentiation becomes less apparent, the determination of a putative cellular origin becomes increasingly difficult numerous subtypes are recognized, the most common being the liposarcoma and malignant fibrous histiocytoma or undifferentiated pleomorphic sarcoma subtypes. Although some benign lesions (especially lipomas) may resemble mature differentiated normal tissue, many STS arise in tissues that do not typically possess the putative normal tissues mentioned. For example, synovial sarcomas are only rarely found in synovial tissues. With advances in molecular characterization of STS, and the emerging dissatisfaction with traditional methods of classification, it is not unexpected that recent proposals have explored gene expression profiling for these tumors to attempt to identify a genome-based classification scheme.

Grade

It provides a means to identify cases at greatest risk for distant metastasis when combined with other factors. Several grading schemes have been proposed and validated. The three-tier system proposed by the French Federation of Cancer Centres is precisely defined, easy to use and widely employed. The French system relies on a relatively balanced evaluation of parameters (differentiation score, mitoses, necrosis), but its greatest limitation lies in the assignment of a differentiation score. Roughly defined as the extent to which a lesion resembles normal tissue, differentiation score has little applicability for tumors that ostensibly have no normal tissue counterpart. Some STS do not lend themselves well to grading. These include: (1) those in which grade provides no additional information (e.g., well-differentiated liposarcoma or atypical lipomatous neoplasm, Ewing's sarcoma); (2) "ungradable" histologic subtypes (e.g., epithelioid sarcoma, clear cell sarcoma, angiosarcoma); and (3) sarcomas that have traditionally been graded but where this characteristic does not appear to differentiate these lesions prognostically (e.g., malignant peripheral nerve sheath tumor). The TNM stage classification of the American Joint Committee on Cancer (AJCC) now employs a three-tiered grading system based largely on the wish to incorporate the French system.[2]

Box 1 Histologic classification of soft tissue sarcoma[3]

Fibrous Tumors
- Fibromatoses
- Superficial fibromatoses
- Palmar and plantar (Dupuytren's contracture fibromatoses)
- Penile (Peyronie's fibromatosis)
- Knuckle pads
- Deep fibromatoses
- Abdominal fibromatosis (abdominal desmoid)
- Extra-abdominal fibromatosis (extra-abdominal desmoid)
- Intra-abdominal fibromatosis (intra-abdominal desmoid)
- Mesenteric fibromatosis (including Gardner's syndrome)
- Infantile (desmoid-type) fibromatosis
- Fibrosarcoma
- Adult fibrosarcoma
- Inflammatory fibrosarcoma

Fibrohistiocytic Tumors
- Dermatofibrosarcoma protuberans (including pigmented form, Bednar tumor)
- Heterogeneous tumors without specific differentiation (formerly malignant fibrous histiocytoma)
- Undifferentiated pleomorphic sarcoma
- Myxofibrosarcoma
- Undifferentiated pleomorphic sarcoma with giant cells
- With inflammation
- Angiomatoid "malignant fibrous histiocytoma"

Lipomatous Tumors
- Atypical lipoma
- Liposarcoma
- Well-differentiated liposarcoma
- Lipoma-like liposarcoma
- Sclerosing liposarcoma
- Inflammatory liposarcoma
- Dedifferentiated liposarcoma
- Myxoid/round cell liposarcoma
- Pleomorphic liposarcoma

Smooth Muscle Sarcomas
- Leiomyosarcoma
- Epithelioid leiomyosarcoma

Skeletal Muscle Sarcomas
- Rhabdomyosarcoma
- Embryonal rhabdomyosarcoma
- Botryoid rhabdomyosarcoma
- Spindle cell rhabdomyosarcoma
- Alveolar rhabdomyosarcoma
- Pleomorphic rhabdomyosarcoma
- Rhabdomyosarcoma with ganglionic differentiation (ectomesenchymoma)

Contd...

Contd...

Malignant Tumors of Blood and Lymph Vessels
• Epithelioid hemangioendothelioma
• Angiosarcoma and lymphangiosarcoma
• Kaposi's sarcoma
• Malignant Perivascular Tumors
• Malignant glomus (glomangiosarcoma) tumor
• Malignant hemangiopericytoma
Malignant Synovial Tumors
• Malignant giant cell tumor of tendon sheath
Malignant Neural Tumors
• Malignant peripheral nerve sheath tumor (MPNST) (neurofibrosarcoma)
• Malignant triton tumor (MPNST with rhabdomyosarcoma)
• Glandular MPNST
• Epithelioid MPNST
• Malignant granular cell tumor
• Primitive neuroectodermal tumor
• Neuroblastoma
• Ganglioneuroblastoma
• Neuroepithelioma (peripheral neuroectodermal tumor)
Paraganglionic Tumors
• Malignant paraganglioma
Extraskeletal Cartilaginous and Osseous Tumors
• Extraskeletal chondrosarcoma
• Myxoid chondrosarcoma
• Mesenchymal chondrosarcoma
• Extraskeletal osteosarcoma
Pluripotential Malignant Mesenchymal Tumors
• Malignant mesenchymoma
• Alveolar soft part sarcoma
• Epithelioid sarcoma
• Malignant extrarenal rhabdoid tumor
• Desmoplastic small cell tumor
• Ewing's sarcoma—extraskeletal
• Clear cell sarcoma (melanoma of soft parts)
• Gastrointestinal stromal tumors
• Synovial sarcoma
• Biphasic synovial sarcoma
• Monophasic synovial sarcoma

PATHOLOGIC FEATURES AND NATURAL HISTORY

Malignant Fibrous Histiocytoma

It is the most common STS of middle and late adulthood and is originally described in 1960s, the term was used to describe a group of sarcomas deemed to be derived from a mixed histiocytic and fibroblastic lineage. The existence of "malignant fibrous histiocytoma" as a distinct entity is now considered controversial and at best is regarded as a heterogeneous group of tumors without a specific known line of differentiation. Reclassification of many tumors in this group has afforded better prognostication, and the old term "malignant fibrous histiocytoma" now is generally considered obsolete.[4] Current nomenclature recognizes the entities of undifferentiated high-grade pleomorphic sarcoma (previously storiform-pleomorphic "malignant fibrous histiocytoma") and myxofibrosarcoma (formerly myxoid "malignant fibrous histiocytoma"), which is now the most common sarcoma of older adults, peaking in incidence in the seventh and eighth decades and presenting most frequently in the lower extremity.[5] Most of these tumors are deep seated, developing in fascia and skeletal muscle, and have a high potential for local recurrence. Low-grade myxofibrosarcoma is known to have a particularly infiltrative growth pattern, and imaging evaluation with particular attention to tail-like extensions should be considered for management. The natural history is extraordinarily variable, reflecting the heterogeneity of these lesions. The most common site for metastases from pleomorphic sarcomas is the lung (90%), bone (8%), and liver (1%), with rare regional lymph node metastases.[4]

Angiosarcoma

The majority of angiosarcomas are considered to originate from the endothelium of the blood vasculature. They are typically composed of an accumulation of an irregular or sinusoidal pattern of vessel with vascular spaces lined by a single row of atypical endothelium that may be several layers thick. Particularly unique is the propensity of superficial angiosarcoma to occur in the dermal tissues of the head and neck manifesting typically on the scalp (about 50%) or facial skin.[6] These neoplasms commonly present as purple, bruise-like lesions. The macules usually become nodular, may coalesce, and may ulcerate. Frank bleeding is an ongoing and major problem and often results in chronic oozing through dressings.

The clinical examination must be meticulous because it is the only real means of identifying the deceptive areas of multifocal involvement that may exist. Metastasis is common if patients survive sufficiently long and occur most typically in regional lymph nodes and the lung. On immunohistochemistry, these tumors are usually positive for factor VIII-related antigen, vimentin, CD34, and CD31. It is suggested that angiogenesis and vascular permeability play a central role in the development of angiosarcomas. This is likely influenced by vascular endothelial growth factor A (VEGF-A), which plays a significant role in angiogenesis and vascular permeability. Bevacizumab, a humanized monoclonal antibody to VEGF, is an attractive agent to consider in angiosarcoma, given its ability to inhibit tumor growth. Another rare variant is one complicating the treatment of breast carcinoma, with superficial angiosarcoma appearing extensively within the confines of the previously irradiated volume and a tendency to develop disease in the opposite breast. A further interesting redisposition in angiosarcoma is its tendency to arise in cardiac tissues, where it represents one of the most common pathologic subtypes of a rare presentation of STS.

Rhabdomyosarcoma

Rhabdomyosarcoma is fifth most common cancer in childhood, but it also occurs in the adult, where the outcome is significantly less favorable. The rhabdomyosarcoma classification recognizes embryonal, botryoid, alveolar, and pleomorphic subtypes for both childhood and adult cases. 70% of rhabdomyosarcomas can be classified as embryonal and 20% alveolar, and the remainder are variants, including the uncommon pleomorphic subtype. Embryonal rhabdomyosarcoma has variable amounts of primitive spindle or round cells in a myxoid background.

The botryoid rhabdomyosarcoma is thought to be a variant of the embryonal type and only accounts for 5% of cases. Botryoid tumors have a particularly favorable prognosis. A diagnosis of alveolar rhabdomyosarcoma is made if the tumor has alveolar-like spaces that are filled with round malignant, eosinophilic cells. Presence of any amount of alveolar morphology in the lesion qualifies it to be alveolar rhabdomyosarcoma, and alveolar morphology has been identified as a poor prognosticator.

Today the diagnosis of the less favorable alveolar subtype is generally based on the identification of the characteristic chromosomal translocations t(2;13)(q35;q14) and t(1;13)(p36,q14) and their fusion products.[1] Rhabdomyosarcoma is also one of the sarcomas associated with a risk of lymph node metastasis. Irrespective of age, the alveolar and embryonal subtypes manifest high rates of response to chemotherapy and RT. The initial evaluation of rhabdomyosarcoma includes bone marrow examination. Sampling of cerebrospinal fluid should be considered in patients with parameningeal lesions.

Liposarcoma

Liposarcoma is the second most commonly encountered subtype of STS, and MLS is the most common variant. It also has an unusual pattern of recurrence that includes a predilection for soft tissue metastases. Apparent multifocal presentation or recurrence at two or more anatomically separate soft tissue sites (with predilection for the retroperitoneum and mediastinum) and bone metastases are a striking yet unpredictable feature of MLS and contrasts to other STS.[7] More favorable survival in a large cohort of liposarcoma patients compared with other histologic subtypes has been reported in a series exceeding 1,000 cases. MLS also appears to manifest an unusually sensitive response to RT.[8] This radiosensitivity may explain the propensity for unexpectedly favorable local control (> 95%) after adjuvant RT.[9,10]

Dermatofibrosarcoma Protuberans

Dermatofibrosarcoma protuberans is a superficial tumor that often manifests as deceptive dermal, raised, purple or red lesion(s) in the lower neck, upper chest, and shoulder girdle regions, although any site may be involved. This tumor arises from the dermis and exhibits a characteristic slow but persistent growth over many years. Infiltration can take place along connective tissue septa, between adnexae and interdigitating with lobules of subcutaneous fat. Dermatofibrosarcoma protuberans is composed of densely packed spindle cells arranged in a storiform or cartwheel pattern. CD34 staining is extensively positive in nearly all cases. 10–15% of all dermatofibrosarcoma protuberans lesions contain areas of fibrosarcoma, and such cases tend to exhibit more aggressive behavior. More than 90% of these tumors are characterized by the t(17;22)(q22;q13) reciprocal chromosomal translocation that is now becoming the hallmark feature of the diagnosis.

The recent observations of response to imatinib in dermatofibrosarcoma protuberans predicted by the presence of the t(17;22) translocation provides possibilities for molecular target therapies in the future. Excellent control rates seen with surgery alone or combined with RT; and these targeted approaches are generally applicable to situations in which surgery and RT are not feasible approaches. For inoperable cases, imatinib has demonstrated antitumor effects in advanced disease harboring t(17;22) and is also active in fibrosarcomatous disease.

Synovial Sarcoma

Synovial sarcomas are tumors of pluripotential mesenchymal cells and composed of two morphologically distinct types of cells that form a characteristic biphasic pattern. *The biphasic synovial sarcoma* includes epithelial cells with a surrounding spindle or fibrous component. The spindle cells stain positive for keratin and epithelial membrane antigen. Vimentin is demonstrable in spindle cells but absent in epithelial cell S-100 staining may give positive results. *Monophasic synovial* sarcomas of both fibrous and epithelial types are recognized. Synovial sarcomas contain a characteristic chromosomal translocation that is the gold standard in establishing the diagnosis, with the observation that 100% of biphasic and 96% of monophasic synovial sarcomas possess the specific t(X;18)(p11;q11) translocation. Typically occurring in the para-articular areas of the tendon sheaths and joints of young adults, at least 50% of synovial sarcomas are in the lower limbs (especially the knee), and most of the remainder originate in the upper limbs. There is little resemblance between synovial membranes and synovial sarcoma, and because the tumor rarely arises from synovial tissue it has been suggested that the name of this subtype should be modified. Management includes conservation surgery and RT.[11] The disease also has a reputation for higher risk of lymph node metastasis (< 2–14%), although elective nodal management is not indicated. An increased potential for distant metastases has been observed with larger tumors (> 5 cm), local relapse, and age older than 20 years.

Pathways of Spread

Local Disease

Most STS tend to spread in a longitudinal direction within the muscle groups where they originate, typically an extremity. As they extend, lesions invade muscle and contiguous structures and may envelop major neurovascular structures. The extending border comprises an outer perimeter of edematous tissue intermixed with a reactive zone of neovascularity with interspersed tumor satellites and pseudopodia. This surrounding area is generally termed the pseudocapsule and may encourage erroneous interpretation of anatomic disease containment and encourage enucleation. Such operations, frequently called "shell outs," almost invariably mean that residual disease remains. STS generally respect barriers to tumor spread in the axial plane of the extremity such as bone, interosseous membrane, and major fascial planes, and this feature should be exploited in planning tissue-preserving approaches to management. Thus, the margins of RT should be wide in the cephalocaudal direction but in the cross-section there may be much greater security in defining nontarget structures. Extremity lesions arising in extracompartmental spaces such as the axilla, femoral triangle, sartorial canal, and popliteal space have the ability to extend proximally and distally at considerable distances with less anatomic restraint and early involvement of the neurovascular bundle. The RT margins should reflect this and include undisturbed tissue planes and barriers to tumor incursion. For nonextremity lesions, the direction of sarcoma growth is also along the involved musculature but care must be taken to ensure that the fascial planes are appropriately recognized and encompassed in surgical or RT target volumes.

Regional Lymph Node Involvement

In STS, there is generally no need for any specific regional lymph node treatment. Important exceptions to this generalization include epithelioid sarcoma, synovial sarcoma, clear cell sarcoma, angiosarcoma, and rhabdomyosarcoma.[20] Lymph node involvement has been associated with an adverse prognosis.[13] However, data suggest that isolated lymph node metastasis may not be as deleterious a factor. This is reflected in the most recent version of the TNM staging system.

Distant Metastasis

Most sarcomas present with localized disease, and overt metastasis is present in only 10% of cases at diagnosis. The predominant risk is to the lungs. Spread to bone may be seen after lung metastases but is seen with the greatest regularity in MLS, where it may be the first site of relapse. MLS also has the unusual characteristic of developing isolated soft tissue metastases. In patients with retroperitoneal sarcoma and intra-abdominal visceral sarcomas, the liver is a more common site of first metastasis.

Clinical Manifestations

The presenting feature of extremity and superficial torso STS is most often with a painless mass. If pain or other symptoms are evident, it usually indicates origin from or invasion of neurovascular structures. Larger tumors may ulcerate the skin or invade adjacent compartments and bone, leading to fracture. In general, superficial (or subcutaneous) lesions are smaller than those deep to fascia or in the retroperitoneum.
Growth rate appears to be an important determinant of the clinical course. Low-grade sarcoma (especially low-grade liposarcoma) may grow at an imperceptible rate without symptoms, and the lesion may be enormous at presentation. This is especially the case for massive low-grade liposarcomas of the retroperitoneum. Head and neck sarcomas may originate within the upper aerodigestive tract and present as symptoms of nasal obstruction, cranial nerve dysfunction, proptosis, and associated features of mass effect.

MANAGEMENT

Multidisciplinary teams consisting of surgeons, radiation oncologists, medical oncologists, pathologists, radiologists ideally would see the patient and participate in formulating a treatment plan before implementation of any component of therapy.

Another practical but important factor is that the radiation oncologist should ideally be aware of and preferably have an opportunity to see the patient before any surgery being performed. Otherwise, imaging and pathology details may be lacking or inadequate and precisely appreciating the original tumor characteristic for accurate postoperative adjuvant treatment may not be possible. The consequence of a fragmented RT service with significantly compromised outcome was evident in a study that addressed an extremity subsite of STS in one center where the local failure was 28% compared with that in two other centers (local failure 5–10%) where treatment and consultation were restricted to sarcoma specialist radiation oncologists working in the same multidisciplinary setting as the surgeons.

Initial Assessment

All soft tissue masses deep to the investing fascia should be considered to be sarcoma until proven otherwise. The type of biopsy, or a prior inappropriate excision, may jeopardize the form and outcome of local treatment by contaminating tissues that were uninvolved initially.[14] Prebiopsy cross-sectional imaging is necessary to avoid compromising the planning of management. During examination particular attention to the relationship to the investing fascia deep to the subcutaneous fat (i.e., whether superficial versus deep) and adjacent neurovascular structures or bone and lesion size and mobility.

Imaging

Accurate, highly sophisticated imaging to delineate tumor extent for diagnostic, surgical, and RT planning is essential to the management of sarcoma. CT scan accurately delineates bony anatomy surrounding the tumor. The multiplanar imaging and soft tissue detail rendered by MRI makes this modality ideal for staging and treatment planning of STS, but it continues to be nonspecific. Most STS will appear as low signal intensity on T1-weighted images and high signal intensity on T2-weighted images. These features are nonspecific and require a biopsy for diagnosis. MRI is also essential to evaluate peritumoral edema that is not as apparent with CT. The contribution of PET to routine management is currently uncertain. The most common metastatic spread pattern of sarcoma is to the lungs. Consequently, imaging of the chest is necessary, CT of the chest is always necessary for high-grade tumors.

Biopsy

The biopsy should be carefully designed to facilitate subsequent surgical removal and adjuvant therapy. The biopsy track should be excised afterward or alternatively may be included in the RT target volume of preoperative treatment. Alternatives to open biopsy include fine-needle aspiration biopsy (FNAB) or core needle biopsy. FNAB can be useful, but these tumors are rare, complex, and difficult to diagnose even in experienced hands and FNAB only should be used when a cytopathologist with extensive experience in sarcoma is available. Core needle biopsy under local anesthesia provides a more consistent tissue specimen and cell preparation compared with FNAB. In the event that an open biopsy is required, an incisional biopsy of deep tumors is preferred over excisional biopsy to minimize the difficulty of the "unplanned" excision. This unplanned approach may increase the rate of local recurrence in sarcomas of the extremities.[14]

PRIMARY THERAPY

The 5-year survival of patients with STS overall is approximately 60%. The local control in extremity sarcomas is 90%. An overall approach to the local management of nonmetastatic extremity, head and neck, and superficial trunk (including body wall) STS is confined to surgery with or without RT and chemotherapy is recommended in selected cases, including chemoresponsive lesions and in some high-risk cases.

Local Management

Surgery is the mainstay of the management of STS and was formerly used alone, albeit often in the form of an amputation. The policy in STS surgery is of attempting to achieve negative surgical margins. Better understanding of the fascial containment and routes of spread, as well as advancements in surgical techniques such as microvascular free-flap reconstruction, have led to tissue preservation in most patients. If the deep compartment is involved or has been contaminated, reexcision, RT, or frequently both may be required. In the absence of bone invasion, the periosteum is an adequate surgical margin for STS treated with wide excision and RT. For most superficial STS (the "a" subcategory in the TNM) the clinician's preoccupation should be with margins of resection above the fascia. Having positive margins nearly doubles the risk of local recurrence and increases the risk of distant recurrence and disease-related death.[15]

Two categories of positive surgical margins are associated with a higher risk of local recurrence despite the use of adjuvant RT: (1) patients who present after prereferral unplanned excision and who have a positive margin on subsequent re-excision (local recurrence rate: 31.6%) and (2) those with unanticipated positive margins occurring during primary sarcoma resection (local recurrence rate: 37.5%).[15] Small, isolated positive resection margin, planned with the intention of sparing a critical anatomic structure (e.g., at a major nerve, vessel, or bone), has a favorable outcome, provided adjuvant RT is appropriately applied, compared with the more extensive margin-positive situations noted earlier in which significant local contamination may be present.

Rationale for Adjuvant Radiation Therapy

Adjuvant RT is generally used to permit more conservative tissue resections and therefore less-extensive operations than would have ordinarily been the case. External beam photons delivered preoperatively or postoperatively or by brachytherapy are the usual modes of administration. Strander et al., in a systematic overview involving 4,579 patients, employed data from 5 randomized trials, 6 prospective studies, 25 retrospective studies, and 3 additional articles.[16] Adjuvant RT improved the local control rate in combination with conservative surgery in the treatment of STS of the extremities and trunk in patients with negative, marginal, or minimal microscopic positive surgical margins. A local control rate of 90% is expected. More recently, Kim et al. reported no significant difference between patients who received RT with R0 margins compared with those treated with close or positive margins combined with RT in terms of local failure free and OS and concluded that margin status did not predict for local failure when adjuvant RT is used. For STS in other anatomic sites, such as retroperitoneum, head and neck, breast, and uterus, the benefit in local control with adjuvant RT is less compelling. In the situation in which positive margins remain after surgery, postoperative RT doses greater than 64 Gy, superficial tumor location, and extremity site have been associated with improved local control.[17]

Randomized Trials of Adjuvant Radiation Therapy

Adjuvant RT with conservative surgical resection has been evaluated in two randomized clinical trials.[18,19] Yang et al[19] the NCI randomized high grade extremity lesions after limb-sparing surgery to receive adjuvant RT or no further treatment after the surgery. Concurrent chemotherapy was also used depending on grade. The local control for those receiving RT was 99% compared with 70% in the control group ($p = 0.0001$). The results were similar for high- and low-grade tumors. Adjuvant RT, using brachytherapy, was also evaluated in a randomized trial at Memorial Sloan Kettering Cancer Center with a similar effect in high-grade lesions.[18]

Scheduling: Preoperative versus Postoperative Radiation Therapy

A Canadian randomized trial compared preoperative and postoperative RT in extremity STS. Wound complications were twice as common with preoperative RT as with postoperative RT (35% versus 17%), although the increased risk was almost entirely confined to patients with sarcomas of the lower extremity. RT toxicity rates in the Canadian trial after 2 years differed between the two arms of the study with a tendency to manifest greater fibrosis in the postoperative arm of the study. This analysis suggested strongly that larger treatment volumes were predictive of greater joint stiffness and fibrosis and may also contribute to limb edema. Patients with late treatment responses such as fibrosis, joint stiffness, or limb edema had significantly lower limb function scores at later time points. The 5-year results for preoperative versus postoperative RT, respectively, were as follows: local control, 93% versus 92%; metastatic relapse free, 67% versus 69%; recurrence-free survival, 58% versus 59%; OS, 73% versus 67% ($p = 0.48$); and cause-specific survival, 78% versus 73% ($p = 0.64$).[20] Only resection margins were significant for local control. Tumor size and grade were the only significant factors for metastatic relapse, OS, and cause-specific survival. Grade was the only consistent predictor of recurrence-free survival. Recently, a literature-based meta-analysis of oncologic outcomes of preoperative versus postoperative RT in localized resectable STS analyzed five eligible studies that included a total of 1,098 patients. This analysis suggested that the risk of local recurrence may be lower after preoperative RT and that the risk of metastatic spread is not increased with the delay in surgical resection necessary to complete preoperative RT. A retrospective analysis was conducted using the National Oncology Database and found 1,087 patients who received RT with surgery. OS was significantly improved with preoperative RT versus postoperative RT, with a median survival of 124 months and 90 months, respectively ($p = .02$). Cause-specific survival was also significantly higher with preoperative RT.

Radiation Therapy Alone

Although every effort should be made to attempt resection, there remain patients in whom definitive RT may be considered owing to a combination of unresectability and/or medical comorbidity or to achieve palliation when surgery is not considered appropriate.[21] Tepper et al. treated 51 patients with definitive photon beam irradiation to a total dose of 64–66 Gy. The 5-year local control and survival rates were 33% and 25%, respectively. Local control was better for tumors less than 5 cm (87.5%) than in tumors 5–10 cm (53%) or greater than 10 cm (30%). These researchers also noted a rise in complications at doses of 68 Gy or more, which appears to provide a therapeutic window. Potentially, higher doses of RT with concurrent dose intensified chemotherapy regimens, possibly delivered with conformal RT volumes to further protect normal tissues, provide an opportunity to enhance local control in this setting. Rhomberg et al. prospectively evaluated the radiation sensitizer razoxane in a randomized controlled trial. Among 82 patients with gross disease, RT combined with razoxane demonstrated an increased response rate compared with photon irradiation alone (74% versus 49%) with improved local control (64% versus 30%, $p < 0.05$). Acute skin reactions were enhanced in the "sensitizer" arm, but late toxicity was not increased.

Radiation Therapy Dose

External Beam Dose Fractionation for Resectable Disease

Postoperative radiotherapy is considered to be the standard approach for nearly all intermediate or high-grade STS. This allows preservation of function with similar local control rates and survival to radical resection (i.e., compartmental excision or amputation).[22] The majority of patients with low-grade tumors will not require radiotherapy, however, it should be considered for those with large, deep tumors that are incompletely resected, especially if adjacent to vital structures that could limit further surgery in the future. External beam radiation therapy (EBRT) prescriptions for postoperative RT depend on the tumor grade and involvement of the surgical margin but typically employ 60 and 66 Gy for low- and high-grade tumors, respectively, with a "shrinking field" technique after 50 Gy at 1.8–2.0 Gy per fraction.[23] Not infrequently, doses may need to be limited to 45–50 Gy in certain anatomic areas containing critical structures (e.g., head and neck, intra-abdominal sites) to minimize morbidity. In these situations the preoperative approach probably has an advantage. For preoperative RT, encompass gross tumor, including peritumoral edema where possible, to a dose of 50 Gy in 25 fractions over 5 weeks to be followed by surgery 4–6 weeks later.

External Beam Dose Fractionation for Unresectable Disease

Unresected disease treated with the goal of long-term control should receive at least 70 Gy in 35 fractions or equivalent when this is anatomically feasible, bearing in mind adjacent normal tissues that may demand dose modification.

Brachytherapy Dose

The optimal adjuvant doses for postoperative brachytherapy remain undefined. Doses will vary depending on the dose rate and whether it is being used as a sole modality or in conjunction with EBRT. The prescription point for the implant may also vary but is generally recommended at an isodose line 5–10 mm from the plane of the implant. There is general agreement about the dose for low-dose rate (LDR) monotherapy and doses of 45–50 Gy at about 0.45 Gy/hour seem acceptable with the skin dose not exceeding 20–25 Gy when large areas of skin are treated. When LDR brachytherapy is used with EBRT (typically 45–50 Gy) doses of 15–25 Gy are generally administered over 2–3 days. Fractionated high-dose rate (HDR) brachytherapy is more problematic.[24] In general, doses of approximately 36 Gy in 10 fractions using a 6-hour interfraction interval have been suggested, although some authors have used higher doses.

Radiation Target Volume

The existence of a zone of uncertain size and location that may contain subclinical disease "risk zone" depends on a number of factors. They include the amount of disturbance of tissue planes and barriers to tumor incursion that may already have taken place, including scars and drain sites. Such areas will need to be included with an appropriate margin. In the preoperative setting the gross tumor volume (GTV) is typically represented by the radiologically defined tumor but the acceptable volume margin remains problematic, depending on the nature of the prior biopsy, the anatomic containment of the lesion, and the imaging characteristics of the lesion. The local growth characteristics of STS have suggested that tumor cells may be located in the surrounding soft tissues at some distance from the main tumor mass. In a study, sarcoma cells were identified histologically in the tissues beyond the tumor in 10 of 15 patients who had not received previous RT. In six cases, tumor cells were located within 1 cm of the tumor margin, and in four cases malignant cells were found at a distance greater than 1 cm and up to a maximum of 4 cm. The location of tumor cells beyond the margin did not correlate with tumor size, nor did it correlate with the location or extent of peritumoral changes.[25]

External Beam Volumes

Within the framework of uncertainty 4-cm CTV margin [approximating a 5-cm field margin after the planning target volume (PTV) and penumbra are considered] beyond any imaging abnormalities, including "peritumoral edema," or areas of surgical disruption irrespective of grade or size of the tumor may be appropriate. Above is based on randomized trial that provided very acceptable 5-year local control rates.[26] Other work in this area includes the description by Kim and colleagues 212 of a preoperative three-dimensional RT volume for extremity STS. The CTV included the T1-weighted post-gadolinium-defined GTV with 1.0–1.5 cm radial and 3.5 cm longitudinal margins. The PTV expansion was 5–7 mm where 95% of the prescribed dose was delivered with acceptable local control, disease-free survival (DFS), and overall survival (OS). In addition, the recently completed RTOG-0630 trial defined the preoperative RT volume with slightly smaller margins. For intermediate- to high-grade tumors greater than or equal to 8 cm, the CTV included the gross tumor and clinical microscopic margins with suspicious edema as defined by MRI T2-weighted imaging, plus 3 cm margins in the longitudinal dimension. The volume could be shortened to include the end of a compartment. The radial margin was defined as 1.5 cm, including any portion of the tumor not confined by an intact barrier to spread. For lower-grade tumors, the CTV still included the GTV and suspicious edema, plus 2 cm margins in the longitudinal directions. The radial margin from the lesion was 1 cm, including any portion of the tumor not confined by an intact barrier to tumor spread. A randomized phase III trial of volume of postoperative RT given to adult patients with extremity STS is underway by the United Kingdom National Cancer Research Network (NCRN) that is comparing a 5 cm longitudinal margin from GTV or 1 cm from the surgical scar, whichever is longer in the craniocaudal direction, and a 2 cm axial margin (standard arm) versus a 2-cm longitudinal margin to GTV and a 2 cm axial margin (experimental arm) to assess if a reduced volume of postoperative RT will increase limb function without compromising local control. Patients in both arms of the study will receive 66 Gy over 6.5 weeks with a volume reduction after 25 fractions (50 Gy) in the standard arm to the same volume as used from the outset in the experimental arm. Limb function is to be assessed using the Toronto Extremity Salvage Score (TESS).

Combined Preoperative Chemotherapy and Radiation Therapy

Enhancing the local effect of RT with concurrent chemotherapy while also promptly addressing the distant metastasis risk before the surgery is an attractive concept. Strategies include the use of perfusion techniques as well as a sequential intravenous chemotherapy and RT strategy in patients with localized, high-grade, large (> 8 cm) extremity STS. The protocol involved three courses of doxorubicin (adriamycin), ifosfamide, mesna, and dacarbazine (MAID) interdigitated with two 22-Gy courses of RT (11 fractions each) for a total preoperative radiation dose of 44 Gy. This was followed by surgical resection. An additional 16 Gy (8 fractions) boost dose was delivered if the surgical margins were microscopically positive. The outcomes of 48 patients treated with this regimen appeared superior to those of a matched cohort of historical controls. The 5-year OS were 87% versus 58% (p = .0003) for the MAID versus control patients cohorts with the difference linked to an improvement in the distant metastases rate (5-year freedom from distant metastasis rate of 75% versus 44% (p = .0016), and the local control was similar in both groups. Because of the promising results seen in this single institution pilot study, the RTOG initiated a phase II trial to evaluate this neoadjuvant regimen in a multi-institutional intergroup setting. Kraybill and colleagues reported the short-term results of this phase II study in the management of high-risk, high-grade STS of the extremities and body wall. Patients received neoadjuvant modified MAID, interdigitated preoperative RT (44 Gy administered in split courses), and three cycles of postoperative modified MAID. Estimated 3-year rates for DFS, distant DFS, and OS were 56.6%, 64.5%, and 75.1%, respectively. There were three deaths associated with this protocol (5%). Two were secondary to acute myelogenous leukemia, and the third patient died secondary to leukopenic sepsis and respiratory failure. Grade IV toxicity was experienced by 84% of patients. Five patients required amputations, two of which were related to treatment toxicity. The authors noted the substantial toxicity of this trial, precluding its unmodified use outside of a clinical trial setting. Additional protocols have been developed with adjuvant and neoadjuvant chemotherapy because of the biology of STS and poor outcome. However, concern remains regarding efficacy and toxicity issues concerning these protocols.

REFERENCES

1. Antonescu CR: The role of genetic testing in soft tissue sarcoma. Histopathology. 2006;48(1):13-21.
2. The American Joint Committee on Cancer: the 7th edition of the AJCC cancer staging manual.
3. Fletcher CDM, Unni K, Mertens K (Eds). World Health Organization Classification of Tumours: Pathology and Genetics of Tumours of Soft Tissue and Bone. Lyon, France, IARC Press (International Agency for Research on Cancer); 2002.
4. Nascimento AF, Raut CP. Diagnosis and management of pleomorphic sarcomas (so-called "MFH") in adults. J Surg Oncol. 2008;97(4):330-9.
5. Nakayama R, Nemoto T, Takahashi H, Ohta T, Kawai A, Seki K, et al. Gene expression analysis of soft tissue sarcomas: characterization and reclassification of malignant fibrous histiocytoma. Mod Pathol. 2007;20(7):749-59.
6. Sturgis EM, Potter BO: Sarcomas of the head and neck region. Curr Opin Oncol. 2003;15(3):239-52.
7. Antonescu CR, Elahi A, Healey JH, Brennan MF, Lui MY, Lewis J, et al. Monoclonality of multifocal myxoid liposarcoma: confirmation by analysis of TLS-CHOP or EWS-CHOP rearrangements. Clin Cancer Res. 2000;6(7):2788-93.
8. Pitson G, Robinson P, Wilke D, Kandel RA, White L, Griffin AM, et al. Radiation response: an additional unique signature of myxoid liposarcoma. Int J Radiat Oncol Biol Phys. 2004;60(2):522-6.
9. Guadagnolo BA, Zagars GK, Ballo MT, Patel SR, Lewis VO, Benjamin RS, et al. Excellent local control rates and distinctive patterns of failure in myxoid liposarcoma treated with conservation surgery and radiotherapy. Int J Radiat Oncol Biol Phys. 2008;70(3):760-5.
10. Chung PW, Deheshi BM, Ferguson PC, Wunder JS, Griffin AM, Catton CN, et al. Radiosensitivity translates into excellent local control in extremity myxoid liposarcoma: a comparison with other soft tissue sarcomas. Cancer. 2009;115(14):3254-61.
11. Italiano A, Penel N, Robin YM, Bui B, Le Cesne A, Piperno-Neumann S, et al. Neo/adjuvant chemotherapy does not improve outcome in resected primary synovial sarcoma: a study of the French Sarcoma Group. Ann Oncol. 2009;20(3):425-30.
12. Riad S, Griffin AM, Liberman B, Blackstein ME, Catton CN, Kandel RA, et al. Lymph node metastasis in soft tissue sarcoma in an extremity. Clin Orthop Relat Res. 2004;(426):129-34.
13. Behranwala KA, A'Hern R, Omar AM, Thomas JM. Prognosis of lymph node metastasis in soft tissue sarcoma. Ann Surg Oncol. 2004;11(7):714-9.
14. Mankin HJ, Mankin CJ, Simon MA. The hazards of the biopsy, revisited. Members of the Musculoskeletal Tumor Society. J Bone Joint Surg Am. 1996;78(5):656-63.
15. Gerrand CH, Wunder JS, Kandel RA, O'Sullivan B, Catton CN, Bell RS, et al. Classification of positive margins after resection of soft-tissue sarcoma of the limb predicts the risk of local recurrence. J Bone Joint Surg Br. 2001;83(8):1149-55..
16. Strander H, Turesson I, Cavallin-Ståhl E. A systematic overview of radiation therapy effects in soft tissue sarcomas. Acta Oncol. 2003;42(5-6):516-31.
17. Delaney TF, Kepka L, Goldberg SI, Hornicek FJ, Gebhardt MC, Yoon SS, et al. Radiation therapy for control of soft-tissue sarcomas resected with positive margins. Int J Radiat Oncol Biol Phys. 2007;67(5):1460-9.
18. Pisters PW, Harrison LB, Leung DH, Woodruff JM, Casper ES, Brennan MF, et al. Long-term results of a prospective randomized trial of adjuvant brachytherapy in soft tissue sarcoma. J Clin Oncol. 1996;14(3):859-68.
19. Yang JC, Chang AE, Baker AR, Sindelar WF, Danforth DN, Topalian SL, et al. Randomized prospective study of the benefit of adjuvant radiation therapy in the treatment of soft tissue sarcomas of the extremity. J Clin Oncol. 1998;16(1):197-203.

20. Davis AM, O'Sullivan B, Turcotte R, Bell R, Catton C, Chabot P, et al. Late radiation morbidity following randomization to preoperative versus postoperative radiotherapy in extremity soft tissue sarcoma. Radiother Oncol. 2005;75(1):48-53..
21. Kepka L, Delaney TF, Suit HD, Goldberg SI. Results of radiation therapy for unresected soft-tissue sarcomas. Int J Radiat Oncol Biol Phys. 2005;63(3):852-9.
22. Yang JC, Chang AE, Baker AR, Sindelar WF, Danforth DN, Topalian SL, et al. Randomized prospective study of the benefit of adjuvant radiation therapy in the treatment of soft tissue sarcomas of the extremity. J Clin Oncol. 1998;16(1):197-203.
23. University of Birmingham. (2015). VORTEX Trial. [online] Available from http://www.vortex.bham.ac.uk/VORTEX Protocol version 5.1 18.05.2009.pdf. [Accessed April 2015].
24. Nag S1, Shasha D, Janjan N, Petersen I, Zaider M; American Brachytherapy Society. The American Brachytherapy Society recommendations for brachytherapy of soft tissue sarcomas. Int J Radiat Oncol Biol Phys. 2001;49(4):1033-43.
25. White LM, Wunder JS, Bell RS, O'Sullivan B, Catton C, Ferguson P, et al. Histologic assessment of peritumoral edema in soft tissue sarcoma. Int J Radiat Oncol Biol Phys. 2005;61(5):1439-45.
26. O'Sullivan B, Davis AM, Turcotte R, Bell R, Catton C, Chabot P, et al. Preoperative versus postoperative radiotherapy in soft-tissue sarcoma of the limbs: a randomised trial. Lancet. 2002;359(9325):2235-41.

29

CHAPTER

Drug Discovery and Clinical Trial Process

Dinesh Chand Doval, Sanjay Gupta

INTRODUCTION

Diseases are the major cause of death, disability and sufferings worldwide. Emergence of new diseases without effective prevention or control as well as growing ineffectiveness of available medicines pose a serious threat to mankind and may potentially be the end of road for modern medical treatments. According to World Health Organization (WHO) 2004, global burden of disease report the leading global risk for the mortality are high blood pressure (13% death globally), tobacco use (9% death globally), high blood glucose (6% death globally), physical inactivity (6% death globally), overweight and obesity (5% death globally). It is predicted that for low-income countries, noncommunicable diseases (NCDs) will contribute half of the total disease burden in 2030 making human immunodeficiency virus (HIV)/acquired immunodeficiency syndrome (AIDS) a major cause of death (12%) followed by prenatal disease (6%), depression (4%) and ischemic heart disease (4%). It is also predicted that lung, stomach and liver cancer will appear as a leading causes of death in 2020. Almost 79% of all death caused by NCD occurs in low-income countries. Hence, there is a need to provide newer, safer and effective medicines to almost 5.6 billion people of the world in a single segment of NCD. Apart from this, emerging new infectious disease such as severe acute respiratory syndrome, Ebola, avian flu, swine flu as well as antibiotic-resistant strains of already known bacteria and various other diseases require the availability of newer and effective medicines on an urgent basis.

WHY DO WE NEED CLINICAL TRIALS?

Clinical trials are the mainstay for bringing out newer, better and safe medicines to serve the mankind. It is the most expensive and time-consuming component of the drug discovery process and constitute approximately 70% of the total time and money spent in the overall development process. Typically it takes approximately 12 years and US$ 900 million to bring one new drug from conception to market out of which 6–7 years are spent in various phases of clinical trials. The first documented evidence of clinical trial dates back to 1747 when James Lind discovered citrus fruit as a cure for scurvy. In the modern world, clinical trials are conducted in four different phases (I, II, III, and IV), where each phase is aimed at addressing a scientific question. While the initial safety of a new drug is established in phase-I of clinical trial, the later phases establishes the efficacy of the drug along with the safety. As clinical trials moves in a phase-wise manner, the next phase is initiated only if the drug passes the earlier phase.

DRUG DISCOVERY PROCESS—A LONG JOURNEY

The drug discovery process begins with the generation of a new idea that is targeted towards chemically modifying a disease process via a drug. The idea is usually generated from a comprehensive understanding of a disease process and a continuing involvement with research in specific therapeutic area of interest. The first step is selection and validation of a "target" which is followed by selection of "drug" that has the ability to interact with the target (Flow chart 1).

- *Target selection* involves choosing a disease to treat and then developing a model for that disease. Thus, researcher first select or discover a biological target such as a particular enzyme, receptor or ion channel that the scientific team believes may be linked to a pathologic process. It is estimated that up to 10 genes contribute to multifactorial diseases. These disease genes are further linked to another five to ten gene products in physiological and pathophysiological pathways leading to an availability of approximately 10,000 potential drug targets.

Flow chart 1 Drug discovery process

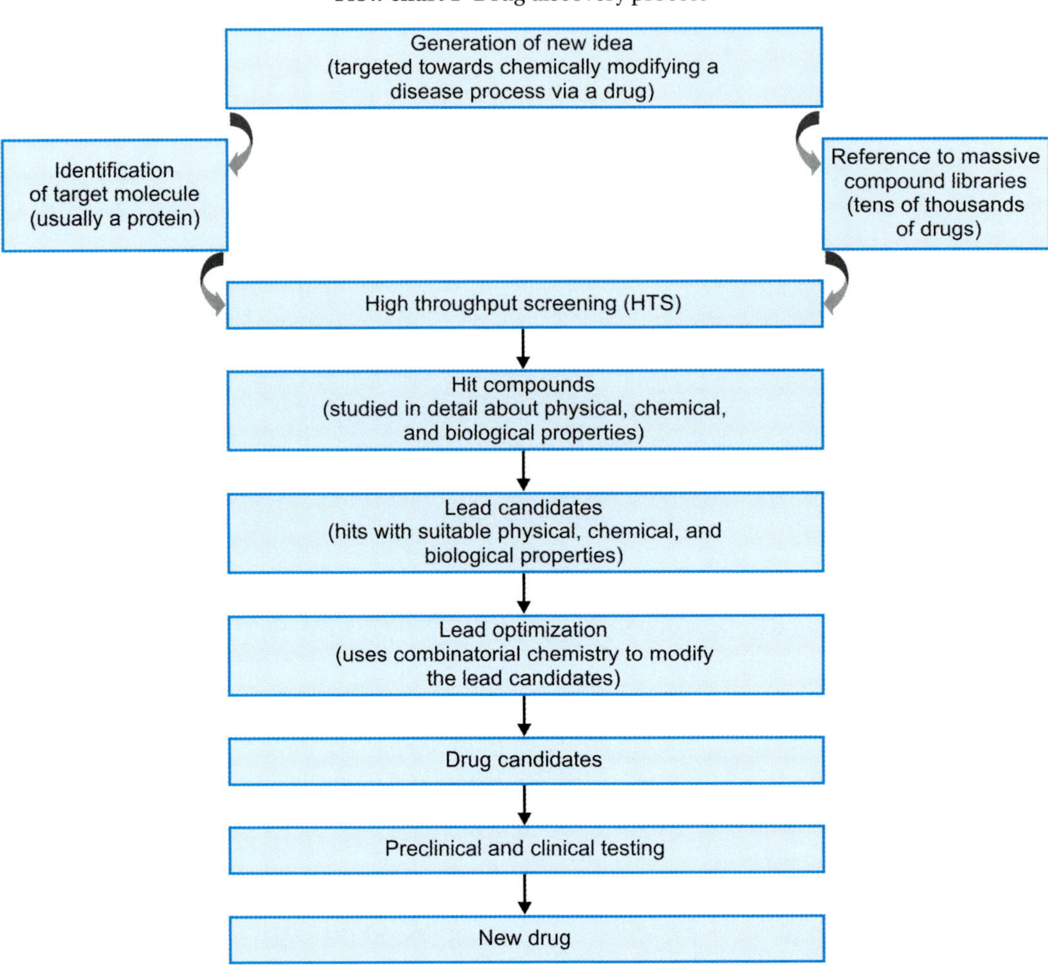

- *Target validation* involves demonstration of relevance of the target protein in a disease process.
- *Drug selection or lead selection* is a process that involves finding a drug or group of drugs which has the ability to interact with target protein and modulate its activity. Tens of thousands of potential drug substances (obtained from massive compound libraries) are tested against the target proteins in a robotic process called high throughput screening (HTS).
- High throughput screening yields hit compounds that are further studied in detail for their physical, chemical and biological properties. Hit compounds with suitable physical, chemical and biological properties are called *lead candidates.*
- Lead candidates are then chemically modified and pharmacologically characterized to obtain compounds with suitable pharmacodynamic and pharmacokinetic properties to become a drug in a process called *lead optimization.*

The compound with best profile is then chosen for further investigation in the form of *preclinical* and *clinical* testing.

PRECLINICAL TESTING

Preclinical tests are performed in the laboratory, using a wide array of chemical and biochemical assays, cell-culture models and animal models. The pharmacological activity of every new compound is carefully analyzed. As the experience with the compound increases, experimental steps and methods can be modified. Preclinical testing involves:

- Pharmacological testing
- Toxicology testing (acute, subacute, chronic, reproductive and mutagenic)
- Animal pharmacokinetic testing.

CLINICAL TESTING

Clinical testing of a drug is done in four phases (I, II, III and IV) of clinical trials. The knowledge gained from one phase is assessed before progressing to the next phase. However, research in a particular phase may continue after the drug has progressed to further stages of development (Table 1).

Table 1 Four phases of clinical trials for clinical testing of a drug

Phase-I	To establish initial safety and maximum tolerance, pharmacokinetics, etc. in 20–80 healthy human volunteers. Also called as "first in man".
Phase-II	Universally accepted as a standard requirement for the evaluation of efficacy and safety of the drug. Careful observations are made to determine the dose and adverse reactions in 100–200 patients with the relevant indication, e.g. randomized, placebo-control, blinded, etc.
Phase-III	Final premarketing phase; multicentric, several patients; safety and efficacy data to establish a drug's risk-benefit relationship; the basis of regulatory submissions.
Phase-IV	Additional safety data; tests the approved drug for additional conditions; expand to much larger patient population.

1. *Phase-I:* Clinical trials are conducted to establish initial safety, maximum tolerance and pharmacokinetics of a new drug in 20–80 healthy human volunteers (with the exception of cancer drugs where phase-I trials are done on cancer patients). These are also called as "first in man" and acts as a basis of validating the findings from preclinical testing into human beings. Usually phase-I trials are initiated with a very low dose (1/10th of the optimal animal dose) which is gradually increased to determine the maximum tolerated dose. During phase-I trials, sufficient information about the drug's pharmacokinetics and pharmacological effects is obtained to plan a well-controlled, phase-II trial. An investigational new drug (IND) application is filed to regulatory authorities for seeking the permission to initiate phase-I clinical trials.
2. *Phase-II:* Clinical trials are universally accepted as a standard requirement for the evaluation of efficacy and safety of a new drug. Careful observations are made to determine the dose and adverse reactions in 100–200 patients with the relevant indication. If a new drug is found to be effective and safe in phase-II trials, it is moved to next phase of development. In case of lack of efficacy the development of drug is stopped at this phase itself.
3. *Phase-III:* Clinical trials are the final premarketing phase of clinical trials. These are large, multicentric trials to establish the safety and efficacy of a new drug vis-à-vis existing standard of care/placebo to form the basis for regulatory submission. If a new drug is found to be safe and effective in phase-III trials, a new drug application (NDA) is filed to regulatory authorities for seeking marketing permission.
4. *Phase-IV:* Clinical trials are postmarketing studies that are conducted for generating additional safety data on a drug once it is marketed. Regulatory authorities can withdraw the marketing authorization of a drug anytime if there are safety concerns on its usage.

It is estimated that for every 10,000–30,000 drug molecules screened, only 250–300 enters the preclinical testing, 5 enters the clinical testing and 1 reaches to the market.

CLINICAL TRIAL ENDPOINT/OUTCOME

A clinical trial endpoint/outcome is a measure of the clinical benefit to the participants. It could be either clinical or surrogate endpoint. While efficacy, safety and quality of life (QoL) are widely accepted clinical endpoints, a laboratory measurement or physical sign could constitute a surrogate endpoint.

Efficacy: It is a measure of the effectiveness of the investigational product in eliminating or reducing the symptoms of the medical condition under study.

Safety: It is an estimate of the adverse reaction or events associated with the use of an investigational product.

Quality of life: The issue of QoL is very important for the management of chronic diseases like cancer especially when the patients present with advanced diseases requiring aggressive treatment that leaves them functionally disabled. Therefore, it has become an important determinant of demand for care, compliance with treatment regimen and overall treatment satisfaction. Generally, QoL measures physical, mental and social well-being in addition to the absence of disease or illness. A number of instruments have been created and adopted for assessing the QoL in different patient populations. Although there is no consensus as yet, the European Organisation for Research and Treatment of Cancer (EORTC) questionnaires have been widely implemented and utilized in international clinical trials.

Surrogate endpoint: A surrogate endpoint is a laboratory measurement or physical sign used as a substitute for a clinically meaningful endpoint that measures directly how a participant feels, functions or survives. Surrogate endpoints are used because they can be measured earlier, are convenient or less invasive, can be measured more frequently and may reduce the sample size as well as the duration of clinical trials.

GENERAL ENDPOINT CONSIDERATIONS IN ONCOLOGY CLINICAL TRIALS

In oncology clinical trials, following endpoints are generally considered while designing the clinical study:

- Overall survival (OS)
- Endpoints based on tumor assessments
  - Disease-free survival (DFS)
  - Objective response rate
  - Time to progression (TTP)

  - Progression-free survival (PFS)
  - Time-to-treatment failure
- Endpoints involving symptom assessment
  - Specific symptom endpoints
  - Quality of life
- Biomarkers.

MOLECULAR BIOLOGY AND GENETICS IN ONCOLOGY

Advances in molecular technology have resulted in the discovery of biomarkers relevant to various cancers that can play an important role in the assessment of risk in addition to screening, surveillance, prognosis and monitoring of the disease. Over the years, several groups have attempted to establish the molecular classification of various cancers. The modern technology such as next generation sequencers (NGS) is paving the way for the advancement in the field of cancer genomics. It is estimated that a detailed study of more than 25,000 cancer genomes is required at the levels of genomic, epigenomic and transcriptomic in order to make an outline of a reliable atlas or map of oncogenic mutations and to uncover the mutagenic influences on most relevant human cancers and their subtypes. Cancer genomics is a subset of personalized medicine that involves application of patient-specific profiles containing genomic, clinical and environmental factors to assess individual risks for the prevention as well as for the personalized disease management strategies. Gene expression profiles (GEPs) is currently being used in a variety of cancers. Some of the notable example includes:

- *Breast cancer*:
  - BRCA1 and BRCA2 in hereditary breast and ovarian cancer syndromes
  - 21 Gene Recurrence Score (Oncotype Dx)
  - Amsterdam 70 gene profile (Mammaprint) in hormone receptor negative and HER-2 positive early stage breast cancer
  - Predictor Analysis of Microarray 50 (PAM50)
- *Colorectal cancer*:
  - Screening: MicroSatellie Instability Testing (MSI)
  - KRAS mutations
- *Nonsmall cell lung cancer*: Epidermal growth factor receptor (EGFR) mutations, ALK translocations, activating KRAS mutations, ROS1 translocation, HER-2 mutation
- *Malignant melanoma*: BRAF mutation, MAPK pathway (MEK inhibitors) P13K/AKT pathway inhibitors
- *Gastrointestinal stroma tumors (GIST)*: Activating mutations in KIT or the platelet derived growth factor receptor alpha (PDGFRA).

The discovery of various genes has triggered the development of a novel approach for the management of various cancers in the form of targeted therapies. Targeted therapy refers to a medication or drug that targets a specific pathway in the growth and development of a tumor thereby providing a biological solution to the problem. The various targeted approaches for the management of cancer that are currently being explored include monoclonal antibodies, EGFR inhibitors, antiangiogenesis, proteasome inhibitors, tyrosine kinase inhibitors, farnesyl transferase inhibitors, gene therapy, immunotherapy, etc.

CLINICAL RESEARCH MARKET (SIZE AND TRENDS)

Site ClinicalTrials.gov (a registry and results database of publicly and privately supported clinical studies of human participants conducted around the world) enlists a total of 144,308 clinical trials across 182 countries by the end of April 2013. Of the 144,308 studies the open and closed studies constitutes 31.5% and 68.5%, respectively. In terms of number of clinical trials, United States tops the list with 47% of all clinical studies followed by Canada and Germany with 7% each and France and United Kingdom with 6% and 5% studies, respectively. India is ranked at 23rd position both under "All Studies" as well as "Open Studies" category.

India has a listing of 2,212 clinical trials of which 548 studies are currently in the enrolment phase. Of the 2,212 studies, 45% are phase-III, 21% are phase-II and 12% are phase-I clinical trials (Fig. 1). Oncology tops the therapeutic area list with 24% share followed by infectious diseases (17%), cardiovascular disease (CVD) (12%), diabetes (10%), central nervous system (CNS) diseases (8%), and others (28%), respectively (Fig. 2).

India clearly provide strategic advantage due to the availability of large patient populations, highly educated manpower, a wide spectrum of disease, lower operational costs, English-speaking population and a favorable economic and intellectual property environment.

CLINICAL TRIALS—DR DC DOVAL'S EXPERIENCE

Between April 1997 and June 2013, the author had personally conducted a total of 93 studies in the capacity of principal

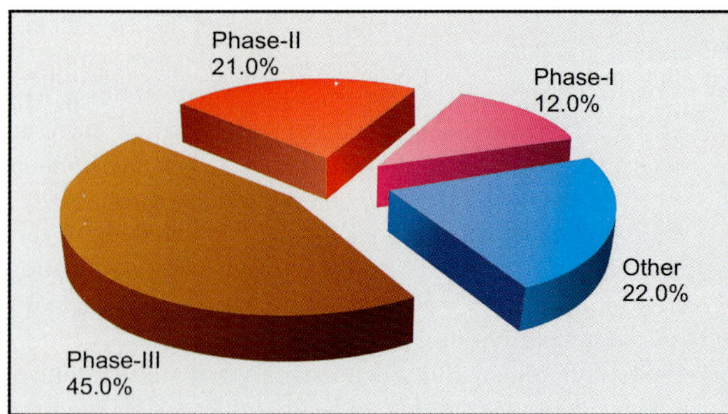

Fig. 1 Phase-wise distribution of clinical trials outsourced to India

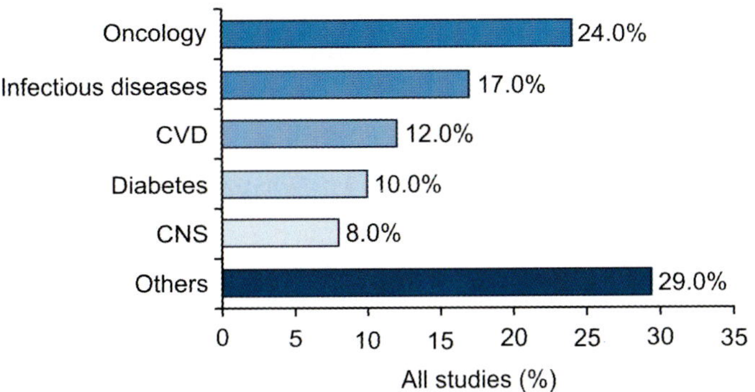

Fig. 2 Therapeutic area-wise distribution of clinical trials outsourced to India

Table 2 Distribution of 93 studies based on type of study and phase

Type of study/phase	*Number of studies*
I	5
II	21
III	37
IV	7
Basic research	4
Others	19

investigator. The distribution of these studies based on type of study and phase is depicted in Table 2.

The distribution of 93 studies based on tumor type is depicted in Table 3.

Table 3 Distribution of 93 studies based on tumor type

Tumor type	*Number of studies*
Breast cancer	32
Lung cancer	
• NSCLC	15
• SCLC	1
• Bronchioloalveolar carcinoma	1
Pancreatic cancer	5
Renal cell carcinoma (RCC)	4
Gall bladder cancer	4
Colorectal cancer	4
Gastric cancer	3
Hepatocellular cancer (HCC)	2
Head and neck cancer	2
Multiple myeloma	2
Prostate cancer	1
Biliary tract cancer	1
Ovarian cancer	1
Non-Hodgkin lymphoma (NHL)	1
CLL	1
Bladder cancer	1
Other	12

Abbreviations: NSCLC, nonsmall cell lung cancer; SCLC, small cell lung cancer; CLL, chronic lymphocytic leukemia

Emergence of new diseases as well as growing resistance to the available medicine poses a serious threat to the mankind that needs to be addressed on a priority basis. Since clinical trial is the only way to make newer treatment options available to the mankind, no one can imagine a world without it unless we feel that available treatment options are adequate and we no longer need any new medicine or therapy for the current or future generations. Imagine a world when a person will survive a complex surgical procedure but will die of postsurgical infections caused by the microorganism that are resistant to the available antibiotics. Hence, there is an unmet medical need to develop newer drugs or therapies. Like other developing countries, some key barriers exists in India that includes limited technical know-how on drug discovery, poor compliance to the regulatory framework, patient's rights and safety, lack of training at the level of various stakeholders, infrastructural challenges, etc. and needs to be addressed in a similar fashion.

Ethical companies set globally consistent standards and conduct trials only in the countries where good clinical practice (GCP) compliance is assured and where they can market the product on a later date. Indian investigators and clinical research professionals have already demonstrated their medical and scientific competence by participating in several global registration trials as well as by publishing their research work in peer-reviewed scientific medical journals of repute. Over the years, thousands of patients in India have benefited by participating in clinical trials and there is no reason why we should not make newer treatment options available to them through participation in clinical trials especially for diseases like cancer.

BIBLIOGRAPHY

1. ClinicalTrials.gov. Homepage. [online] Available from www.clinicaltrials.gov/. [Accessed April, 2015].
2. Julka PK. Clinical trials in India-Dilemmas for Developing Countries. The Monitor. 2007;21(2):69-71.
3. World Health Organization. The Global Burden of Disease. 2004 Update. [online] Available from www.who.int/healthinfo/global_burden_disease/GBD_report_2004update_full.pdf. [Accessed April, 2015].
4. World Health Organization. The World Medicines Situation Report. [online] Available from www.who.int/medicines/areas/policy/world_medicines_situation/en/. [Accessed April, 2015].

30 CHAPTER

Quality Assurance of High Dose Rate: Brachytherapy (Remote Afterloading Unit)

Karrthick KP, Ramu Mahendran, Samba Siva Selli R, Senni Andaver

INTRODUCTION

The term quality assurance (QA) is "all those planned and systematic actions necessary to provide adequate confidence that a product or a service will satisfy given requirements for quality".[1]

For radiation oncology, a QA program is essentially a set of policies and procedures to maintain the quality of patient care. The general criteria or standards of quality are usually set collectively by the professional experts. It is expected that a QA program designed specifically for an institution will meet those standards.

The goal of a QA program for linear accelerators (Linac) is to ensure that the machine characteristics do not deviate significantly from their baseline values acquired at the time of acceptance and commissioning.

Many of these baseline values are entered into the treatment planning systems (TPS) to characterize and/or model treatment machine, and therefore can directly affect treatment plans calculated for every patient treated on that machine. Deviation from the baseline values could thus results in suboptimal treatment of patients.

Machine parameters can deviate from their baseline values as a result of many reasons. There can be unexpected changes in machine performance due to machine malfunction, mechanical breakdown.

Physical accidents or component failure—major component replacements like the waveguide, bending magnet, etc. may also alter machine performance from its original parameters. In addition there can be gradual changes as a result of aging of the machine components. These patterns of failure must be considered when establishing a periodic QA program.

NEED FOR QUALITY ASSURANCE IN RADIOTHERAPY

An assessment of clinical requirements in radiotherapy shows that a high degree of accuracy is necessary to produce the desired result of tumor control rates that are as high as possible, along with acceptable complication rates. QA procedures in radiotherapy can be characterized as follows:

- Quality assurance reduces the uncertainties and errors in dosimetry, treatment planning, equipment performance and treatment delivery, thereby improving dosimetric accuracy, geometric accuracy and the precision of dose delivery. This improves radiotherapy results (treatment outcomes), raising tumor control rates as well as reducing complication and recurrence rates.
- Quality assurance not only reduces the likelihood of accidents and errors, it also increases the probability that they will be recognized and rectified sooner if they do occur, thereby reducing their consequences for patient treatment. This is the case not only for larger incidents but also for the higher probability minor incidents.
- Quality assurance allows a reliable intercomparison of results among different radiotherapy centers, ensuring a more uniform and accurate dosimetry and treatment delivery. This is necessary for clinical trials and also for sharing clinical radiotherapy experience and transferring it between centers.

QUALITYASSURANCEFORLINEARACCELERATORS

TEST FREQUENCIES

Depend on vulnerability of QA parameters:

- Daily
- Weekly

- Monthly
- Yearly
- On major repair and servicing.

The recommended QA tests for Linac are summarized in the following tables as per the AAPM Task Group 142 report: Quality assurance of medical accelerators (2009),[1] Table 1 (daily), Table 2 (monthly), Table 3 (annual).

The daily (or in some cases weekly) *tests* include parameters that can affect dose to the patient by dosimetric (output constancy) or geometric (lasers, optical distance indicator, field size) means.

- The daily safety tests include audiovisual monitoring of the patient and testing of the door interlock. With respect to electronic portal imaging devices (EPID) and kV imaging, the operation and functionality are tested daily as well as collision interlocks.
- The daily tests are typically performed by the morning warm-up therapist, who should be trained by a qualified medical physicist with a well-defined policy and procedure to follow, if any of the tests are found to be out of tolerance.
- *Monthly tests* include those that have a lower likelihood of changing over a month (e.g. tray position or profile consistency, which also serves as an energy check for photons). These tests are typically more detailed and are performed by the medical physicist.
- *The annual tests* are a subset of the tests performed during acceptance testing and commissioning procedures. During the annual review of dosimetry systems, constancy factors are established, reconfirmed, or updated.

Table 1 Daily quality assurance in Linac (Infinity/Synergy-S)

Sl. no.	*General checks*	*Action level*
1	TV viewing system	Functional
2	Audiovisual monitor	Functional
3	Door light radiation indicator	Functional
4	Door interlock	Functional
5	Field light	Functional
6	Hand pendants	Functional
7	Machine interlock	Functional
Sl. no.	*Mechanical checks*	*Action level (mm)*
1	Optical distance indicator verification	<2
2	Laser alignment	<2
3	Field size matching (10 × 10 cm)	<2
Sl. no.	*Radiation checks*	*Action level (%)*
1	X-ray output constancy	<3
2	Electron output constancy	<3
3	Photon beam energy check (TPR 20/10)	<3
4	Electron beam energy check (R 50)	<3
Sl. no.	*Imaging test (cone-beam CT)*	*Action level*
1	Isocenter check	<2 mm
2	Image quality	Satisfactory

Table 2 Monthly quality assurance in Linac (Infinity/Synergy-S)

Sl. no.	*Mechanical checks*	*Action level*
1	Safety interlocks	Functional
2	Emergency OFF switch	Functional
3	Applicator position	Functional
4	Latching of cones to collimator	Functional
5	Gantry angle indicator	±0.5°
6	Couch isocenter	1 mm radius
7	Treatment couch position indicator	<1 mm
8	Coincidence of couch, collimator and gantry isocenter	1 mm radius
9	Jaw position indicators	<2 mm
10	Optical distance indicator	1 mm
11	Cross hair centering	1 m
Sl. no.	*Radiation checks*	*Action level*
1	Backup monitor unit check	Satisfactory
2	Optical and radiation field congruence	±1 mm each side
3	Photon output constancy	2%
4	Electron output constancy	2%
5	Photon beam profile constancy	1%
6	Electron beam profile constancy	1%
7	Photon beam energy constancy	1%
8	Electron beam energy constancy	1%
Sl. no.	*Multileaf collimator tests*	*Action level*
1	Setting versus radiation field	2 mm
2	Backup diaphragm settings	2 mm
3	Travel speed	>0.5 cm/s
4	Leaf speed stability	1 mm
Sl. no.	*Imaging test*	*Action level*
1	Uniformity and noise	<1.5%
2	Geometric distortion	<2 mm
3	Spatial resolution	10 line pairs
4	Contrast	1.50%
5	Scaling	<2 mm
6	HU constancy	<1%

Table 3 Annual quality assurance for Linac (Infinity/Synergy-S)

Sl. no.	*Mechanical checks*	*Action level*
1	Collimator rotation isocenter	±1 mm from baseline
2	Gantry rotation isocenter	±1 mm from baseline
3	Couch rotation isocenter	±1 mm from baseline
4	Electron applicator interlocks	Functional
5	Coincidence of radiation and mechanical isocenter	±2 mm from baseline
6	Table top sag	2 mm from baseline
7	Table angle	1°
8	Table travel maximum range movement in all directions	±2 mm
Sl. no.	*Radiation checks*	*Action level*
1	Backup monitor unit check	Satisfactory
2	Optical and radiation field congruence	±1 mm each side
3	Photon output constancy	2%
4	Electron output constancy	2%
5	Photon beam profile constancy	1%
6	Electron beam profile constancy	1%
7	Photon beam energy constancy	1%
8	Electron beam energy constancy	1%
9	X-ray beam quality (PDD or TPR 20/10)	±1%
10	Electron beam quality (R 50)	±2%
11	X-ray monitor unit linearity	±2% >5 MU
12	Electron monitor unit linearity	±2% >5 MU
13	Output factors for electron applicators	±2% from baseline
14	Electron/X-ray off-axis factor	±1% from baseline
15	TBI/TSET output calibration	2% from baseline
16	TBI/TSET accessories	2% from baseline
17	TBI/TSET mode	Functional
Sl. no.	*Multileaf collimator tests*	*Action level*
1	Setting versus radiation field	2 mm
2	Backup diaphragm settings	2 mm
3	Travel speed	>0.5 cm/s
4	Leaf speed stability	1 mm
5	Leaf position repeatability	±1 mm
6	Leaf position accuracy	±1 mm
7	MLC transmission	±1%
8	Qualitative test (picket fence)	Visual inspection

Contd...

Contd...

Sl. no.	*Imaging test (CBCT kV and planar MV)*	*Action level*
1	Uniformity and noise	<1.5%
2	Geometric distortion	<2 mm
3	Spatial resolution	10 line pairs
4	Contrast	1.50%
5	Scaling	<2 mm
6	HU constancy	<1%
7	Imaging dose	baseline
8	Beam quality/energy	baseline

Daily Quality Assurance

Quality Assurance Beam Checker Plus

Daily output checks and verification of output constancy, beam energy, flatness and symmetry can be done by Beam Checker Plus (Fig. 1).

Features:

- It automatically determines which energy was delivered (photons and/or electrons).
- Verifying that the beam energy, flatness, symmetry, output constancy and other parameters of the beam are not changing over time.
- It has an inherent buildup—for photons = 3.5 cm, and for electrons = 1.5 cm.
- It has an onboard sensor—for temperature and pressure corrections.

Setup and measurement:

- Place the Beam Checker on treatment couch and set field size = 20 × 20 cm^2.
- Set source-surface distance (SSD) = 100 cm for infinity, SSD = 125 cm for Synergy-S, to get field size of 20 × 20 cm^2.
- Make alignment using cross hairs and room lasers.
- Power ON the Beam Checker, and select the machine (Infinity/Synergy-S).
- Delivered monitor units (MU) = 100, dose rate = 400–600 MU/min.
- Expose it to the beam with any baseline energy, and the front panel display will identify the energy, give a pass/fail indication based on preconfigured action levels.
- Save this measurement to internal memory, and automatically reset for the next exposure.
- At a later time, all measurement data can be transferred to the PC for analysis and trending.

Isocenter Align Device

It is a useful device to check whether the room lasers are properly aligned or not (Fig. 2).

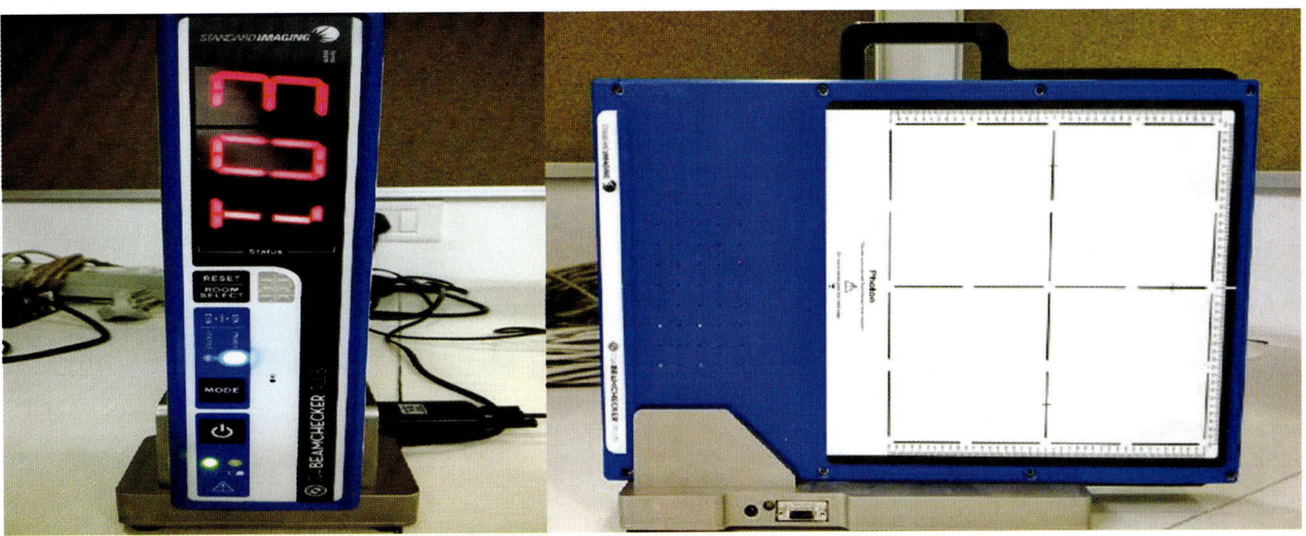

Fig. 1 Quality assurance Beam Checker Plus—standard imaging

Source: Division of Radiation Oncology, Medanta—The Medicity, Haryana, India

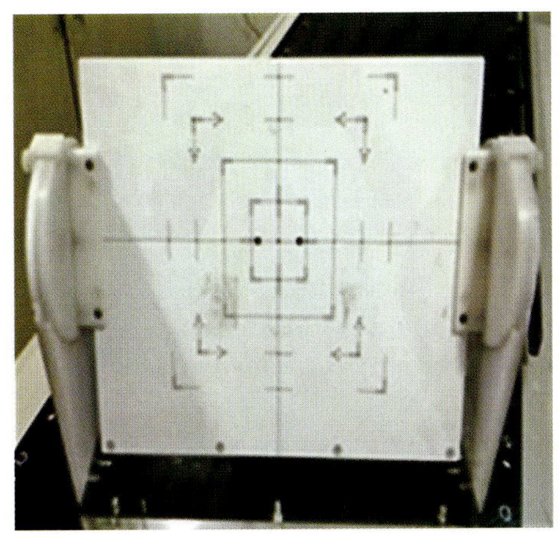

Fig. 2 Isocenter align device—standard imaging

Source: Division of Radiation Oncology, Medanta—The Medicity, Haryana, India

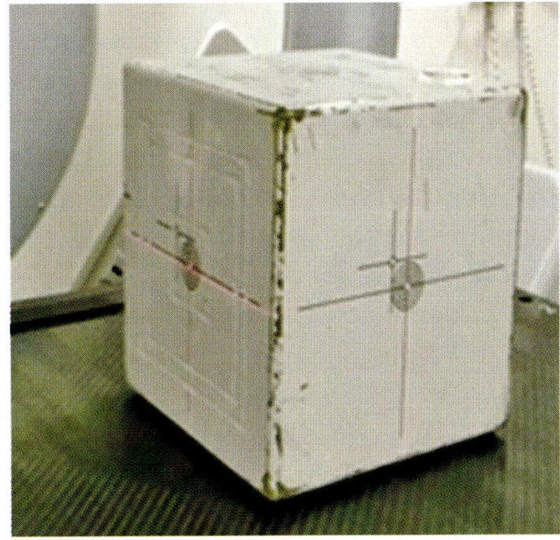

Fig. 3 QUASAR penta-guide phantom

Source: Division of Radiation Oncology, Medanta—The Medicity, Haryana, India

- A precision alignment device for routine quality control of lasers, Linac and simulators.
- Place the tool on the Linac couch and use the laser alignment marks with the room lasers to align the device at the isocenter.
- Check the laser alignment marks to ensure that the room lasers are properly aligned or not.
- The positions between two laser points (horizontal and vertical) correspond to ±1 mm.

The QUASAR Penta-guide Phantom

The penta-guide phantom is designed for daily QA of Linac-based cone-beam computed tomography (CBCT) imaging systems. Tests include the registration alignment of crossed kV and MV imaging systems and isocenter alignment of CBCT (Fig. 3).

Tests are related to:

- System safety,
- Geometric accuracy, that is agreement of the CBCT imaging isocenter with the isocenter of the MV treatment beam,
- Registration and correction accuracy, that is how accurately can the system position a patient,
- Image quality and
- X-ray tube and generator performance (dose to the patient).

Setup and measurement:

- The QUASAR penta-guide phantom ensures the accuracy of Linac-mounted image-guidance systems, including

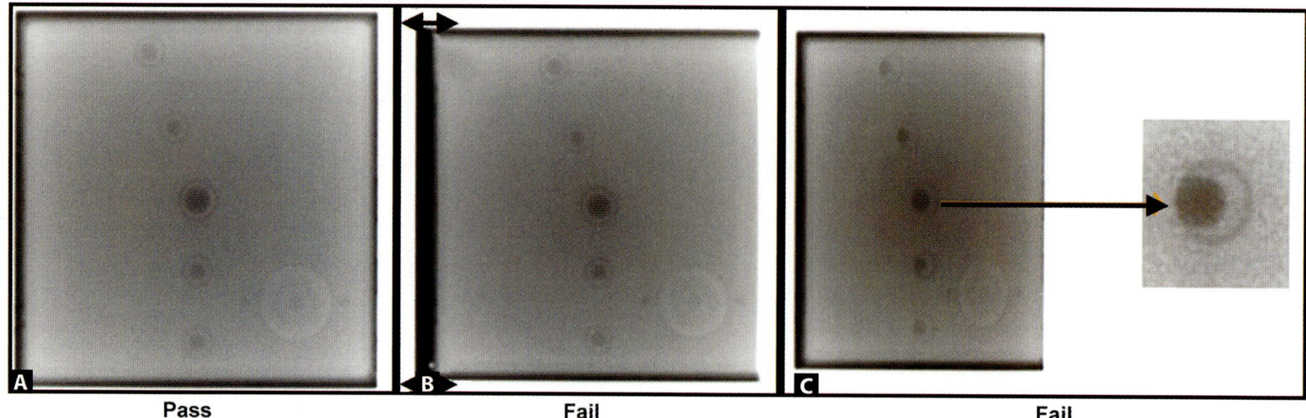

Figs 4A to C Examples for pass/fail criteria. (A) Phantom centered in field of view, spheres centered in rings; (B) Example for translation misalignment; (C) Example for rotational misalignment

Source: Division of Radiation Oncology, Medanta—The Medicity, Haryana, India

CBCT and X-ray volume imaging (XVI) by enabling daily tests.

- Tests include the registration and alignment of crossed kV and MV imaging systems and isocenter alignment of CBCT.
- Within the phantom there are five air-filled spheres (Figs 4A to C) and five low-density rings are placed.
- The use of air-filled spheres ensures sufficient image contrast without high-density streak artifacts. The spheres and rings are designed to appear on kV and MV projection images of the phantom.
- The CBCT tests make use of a CT image of the phantom and these reference images are the standard against which the daily anteroposterior (AP), right lateral and CBCT images are compared.
- Place the phantom at the isocenter of the CT scanner and acquire a CT scan of the phantom.
- Export the CT scan images to the TPS. Within the TPS place the isocenter at the center of the phantom (center of the central sphere).
- Export the plan to mosaiq and CT image to the CBCT imaging system and save it for daily QA.
- Place the phantom on the Linac couch and use the laser alignment marks within the room lasers to align the phantom with the isocenter.
- Acquire AP and right lateral kV projection images of the phantom.
- Use automatic 2D image matching tool for registration of the CBCT image with the reference CT scan of the phantom.
- The registration tool will determine the x, y, z discrepancy between the CBCT and TPS isocenter.
- Record these values, typically this offset should be *less than 2 mm* in each direction.

Monthly Quality Assurance in Linac (Infinity/Synergy-S)

Mechanical Isocenter

Mechanical isocenter is the intersection of axis of rotation of collimator, gantry and couch.

Purpose: To check the coincidence of collimator, gantry and couch rotation axis with isocenter.

Procedure:
Collimator rotation: Fix a graph paper on the couch such that the front pointer should match at a point on the graph. Then mark the front pointer tip at a regular interval of collimator rotation. This procedure can be done with the help of cross wire and the tolerance of alignment is *2 mm diameter circle.*

Gantry rotation: A horizontal rod with pointer is fixed on the couch such that the front pointer tip is as close as possible with horizontal rod tip. The gantry is rotated 360° and the displacement between the two tips is visually noted and measured.

The tolerance of displacement of the isocenter is ±*1 mm (2 mm diameter circle).*

Couch rotation: The procedure is similar to that of collimator rotation check. The intersection points are marked for different couch angles at fixed collimator position. The tolerance is 2 mm diameter circle.

Radiation Isocenter Check (Spoke Test)

Purpose: To check the uncertainty produced in the position of central axis of radiation beam and also with respect to mechanical isocenter.

Procedure:
Collimator rotation: With the gantry in the vertical position, place a film on the table top at isocenter (SSD = 100 cm). Place a buildup (1.5 cm for 6 MV) on the film. Open the upper jaws (X-axis) of the collimator wide open and close the lower jaws (Y-axis) to obtain a narrow slit of about 2–3 mm at isocenter. Expose the film at regular intervals of collimator rotation (at least 6–7 exposures). The process is repeated with upper jaw closed and lower jaw open in another film.

Gantry rotation: The film is placed perpendicular to the table top and is exposed at different gantry angles. The gantry is rotated around the film with jaws slit perpendicular to the film edge.

Couch rotation: The setup is similar as in collimator rotation check. The collimator and gantry will be fixed at 0° and the couch is rotated with different jaws slits to expose the films.

The processed film will show star pattern (spokes) with a dark (star) central region. The intersection points of the dark lines are marked and they should fall inside a *2 mm diameter circle*. The cross hairs are marked on the film using pinprick method. The distance between the dark line center and cross hair center should be within *2 mm*.

Light/Radiation Field Coincidence (Congruence Test)

Purpose: To check that the field light is coincident with the radiation field.

Procedure: Film is fixed on the table top at the isocenter (SSD = 100 cm). The edges of the field light and cross hairs are marked using pinprick method. Place a buildup (1.5 cm for 6 MV) on the top of the film and expose it. The procedure is repeated for different field sizes of 5 × 5 cm, 10 × 10 cm and 30 × 30 cm, and this test should be performed at four gantry angles (0°, 90°, 180°, 270°), to check the jaw sag due to gravity.

The coincidence of the field light and radiation beam is visually analyzed in the processed film. The field size and penumbra of the radiation field are measured using scanner and analyzing software or densitometer. The separation between optical field edge and 50% isodose line shall not exceed *2 mm*.

Photon Beam Quality Index

Purpose: To check the photon beam energy is stable (Fig. 5).

Procedure: The ratio of the ionization (J20/J10) measured at 20 cm and 10 cm depths, respectively, for field size of 10 × 10 cm at the detector level and with a constant source-to-detector distance (SDD) (100 cm) is called quality index. It is also termed as tissue phantom ratio (TPR).
The quality index (QI) is defined as:

QI = J20/J10

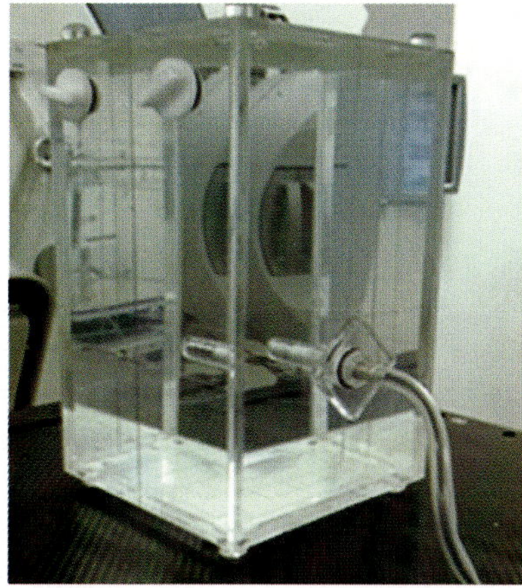

Fig. 5 TPR 20/10 phantom—standard imaging

Source: Division of Radiation Oncology, Medanta—The Medicity, Haryana, India.

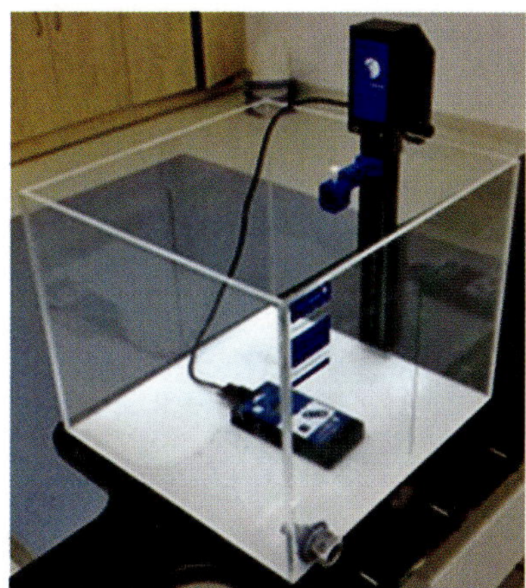

Fig. 6 1D Water Phantom—Sun Nuclear

Source: Division of Radiation Oncology, Medanta—The Medicity, Haryana, India.

Where,
J20 = Absorbed dose at 20 cm depth,
J10 = Absorbed dose at 10 cm depth.

Output Calibration for Photons and Electrons

Purpose: To check the consistency of photon and electron beam output periodically.

Procedure: Following the standard dosimetry formalism, IAEA Technical Reports Series (TRS) No. 398,[2] the output calibration of the Linac for all available beam energies and field sizes in photon and electron beams are checked periodically with the help of *1D Water Phantom* and *FC65-G Farmer Type Chamber* for photon output measurement and NACP parallel plate ionization chamber for electron output measurement (Fig. 6).

The tolerance of output variation should be within ±2%.

Radiation Field Analyzer Blue Phantom 2

Purpose: Percentage depth dose (PDD) and beam profile measurement help for characterizing the photon and electron beam energy and also for treatment time calculation (Fig. 7).

Procedure:

- Percentage depth dose and beam profile measurements are done with the help of radiation field analyzer (RFA).
- The PDD and profiles at different depths (D_{max}, 5 cm and 10 cm) are measured for a reference field size ($10 \times 10\ cm^2$).
- Percentage depth dose normalizes dose at depth with respect to D_{max} and determines how much dose can be delivered at depth relative to the D_{max}.
- The acceptance criteria are the variance for a 10 × 10 cm field size, 100 cm SSD at 10 cm depth. Acceptable difference is ±2%.

Beam profile:

Flatness: The flatness of profile is calculated using the guidelines set in AAPM TG 45.[3] Obtain maximum (V_{max}) and minimum (V_{min}) values of dose in the central 80% region of the respective beam profiles, and calculate the field flatness parameter V using the following equation:

$$V = (V_{max} - V_{min}/V_{max} + V_{min}) \times 100$$

The values should be within ±3%.

Symmetry: The profile plot may be folded imaginarily at the field center and the two halves of the profiles are compared within the central 80% flattened beam area. The tolerance value is *2%*.

The flatness and symmetry of profiles at different gantry angles can be measured using the exposed films.

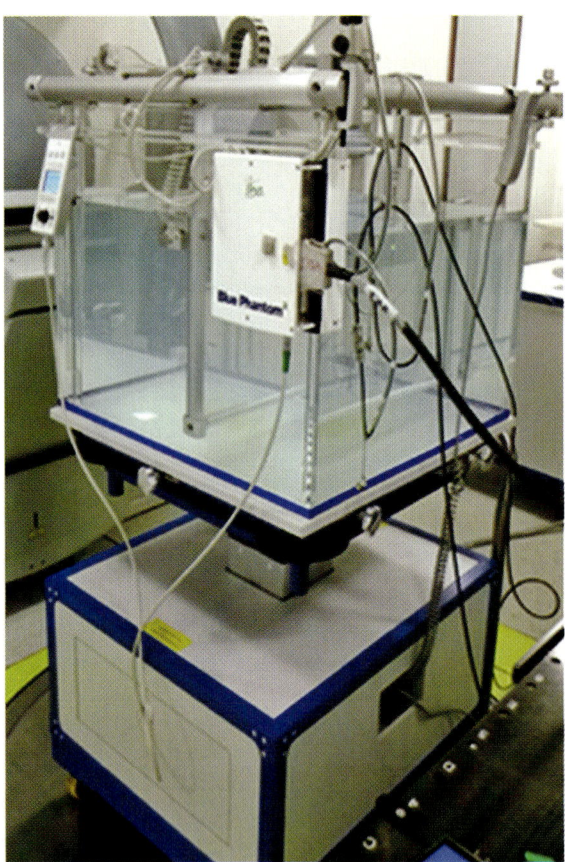

Fig. 7 Radiation field analyzer Blue Phantom 2—IBA

Source: Division of Radiation Oncology, Medanta—The Medicity, Haryana, India.

Quality Assurance of Multileaf Collimator

Purpose: To assure the delivery of treatment beams using multileaf collimator (MLC) is accurate.

Procedure: Quality assurance procedure will vary depending upon the intensity-modulated radiation therapy (IMRT) system like step and shoot, sliding window or dynamic mode.

Hence, it is essential to check that the speed, acceleration and position of leaves are controlled and accurate as per the plan by the TPS.

Static multileaf collimator: A standard shape like rectangular or diamond is created using MLC in shaped software or in TPS. This shape is transferred to the treatment unit and a film at isocenter is exposed for analysis.

Dynamic multileaf collimator: In the shaped software, 2 mm gap slits are created between the opposing leaves. Keeping all the leaves in fixed steps (2 cm) and creating the gaps at the stop positions will give rise to a pattern of straight dark lines on the irradiated films. This pattern is termed as *"garden fence"*. Any variation or width of the dark lines would indicate positional error of a leaf. This test should be performed at four gantry angles (0°, 90°, 180°, 270°), to check the MLC sag due to gravity.

Multileaf collimator carriage (bank): The accuracy of the carriage movement and MLC leaf positioning in producing the subfields is determined by the reproducibility in positioning. "*Picket fence*" film is irradiated by multiple strip exposures by consecutive leaf movements of a 5 cm wide rectangular field spaced at 5 cm intervals.

The processed films were analyzed using software to check the positional error within ±*1 mm*.

Quality Assurance of Imaging (XVI System)

Purpose: Imaging QA test to verify that the XVI system is within the given specification.

The following imaging tests are done with the help of *Catphan (CTP 600) Phantom* as per the AAPM Task Group142 report: Quality assurance of medical accelerators (2009) (Fig. 8).[1]

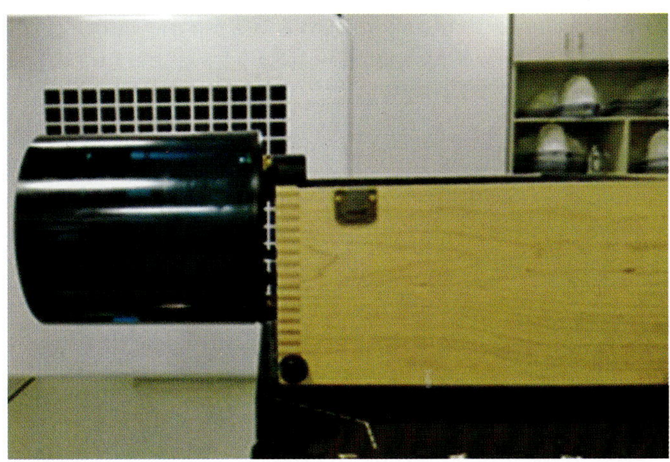

Fig. 8 Catphan (CTP 600) Phantom-Elekta, Phantom Laboratory

Source: Division of Radiation Oncology, Medanta—The Medicity, Haryana, India

- Three-dimensional image quality,
- Transverse uniformity,
- Low-contrast visibility,
- Spatial resolution,
- Transverse vertical scale,
- Transverse horizontal scale, and
- Sagittal geometric.

Patient Specific Quality Assurance (IMRT/VMAT)

Purpose: Patient specific QA is a method used to ensure that the correct amount of radiation is being delivered to the correct location. The accuracy of any treatment plan [IMRT/volumetric modulated arc therapy (VMAT)] can only be guaranteed through patient specific QA and this QA program encompasses machine-related parameters such as beam flatness and energy stability, MLC accuracy and accurate modeling of the TPS.

Patient specific quality assurance has several purposes:

- Ensures that the TPS has accurately calculated the dose for the planned treatment.
- Patient specific QA verifies that the large amount of treatment data involved has been faithfully transferred from the TPS to the record and verification system.
- Patient specific QA ensures that the delivery system is capable of delivering the fields as planned.
- IMatriXX Evolution and combination of IMatriXX and multicube phantom (Fig. 9).

IMatriXX Evolution:

- The dosimetric device is an ionization chamber array consisting of 1,020 single air-vented plane-parallel cylindrical ionization chambers. Arranged in a 32 × 32 matrix.
- A maximum field of view of 24 × 24 cm^2 can be achieved. The 2D array detectors (IMatriXX Evolution) are capable of providing real-time measurement and it can be easily connected to a PC with a standard ethernet cable. The dose can be measured directly, after calibration of 2D array.

Procedure:

- The treatment plans are typically copied onto a phantom geometry in which dosimetric measurements can be taken.
- The treatment is delivered to the phantom and measured doses are compared to calculated doses from the TPS.

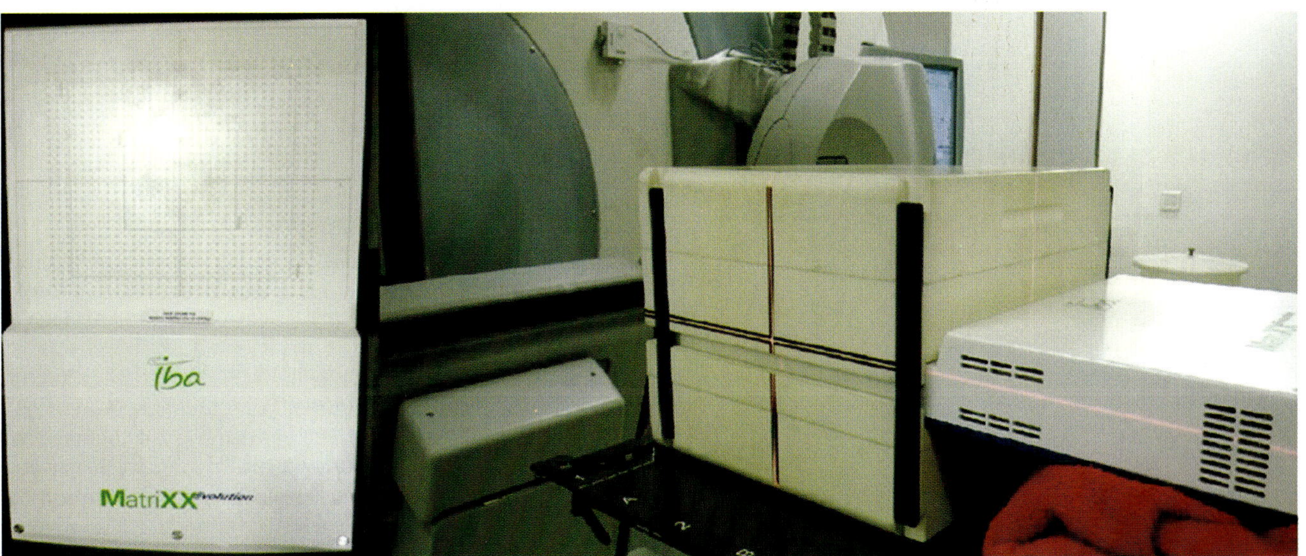

Fig. 9 IMatriXX Evolution—standard imaging

Source: Division of Radiation Oncology, Medanta—The Medicity, Haryana, India

- A common approach is to export the energy fluence or the dose in a specific plane from the TPS for single field or multiple field arrangements and compare this to the measured data.
- For planar (beam-by-beam) verification, measurement is performed using a zero gantry angle.

Point dose analysis:
The percentage difference between calculated and measured dose is determined, and the QA passes if the difference is within some predetermined threshold (3 mm and 3%).

Delta dose: 3%,
Delta distance: 3 mm,
Gamma: Less than one.

Gamma analysis:

- To overcome the potential problems with the binary test, a numerical method called gamma analysis is used like a binary pass/fail method.
- The gamma method uses a set of criteria for testing (3% difference and 3 mm distance).
- A point is said to pass the gamma test if the gamma value at the point is less than one.
- Gamma analysis is a suitable quantitative method of determining the level of agreement between two dose distributions.

COMPASS 3D dosimetry:

- COMPASS is a continuous patient safety monitoring system. It is used for QA and plan verification in IMRT and VAMT.
- It computes dose three-dimensionally in a geometrical representation of a patient or a phantom.
- Quality assurance system consists of COMPASS software which can be used for pure dose calculation or together with a 2D array detector (IMatriXX with the gantry angle sensor) for a measurement-based dose reconstruction, this is called indirectly measured dose.

QUALITY ASSURANCE OF HIGH DOSE RATE: REMOTE AFTERLOADING UNIT[3]

DAILY QUALITY ASSURANCE

- Door interlocks
- Lights and alarms
- Console functions
- Switches
- Batteries
- Printer
- Visual inspections of indicators on the control console
- Treatment units and entrance to the treatment room
- Source guide and
- Source positioning accuracy check using source position check roller.

Monthly Quality Assurance (At the Time of Source Replacement or Source Calibration)

Autoradiograph

Purpose: To verify the positioning accuracy and uniformity of source as planned.

Procedure:

- In an X-Omat film with graph sheet two parallel lines are drawn at 10 cm distance and a horizontal line is drawn bisecting these two parallel lines at one end.
- A flexible catheter with X-ray marker is placed on one-line in such a way that the first marker is in coincidence with the reference line.
- Another catheter is placed on the other line in such a way that the tip of the catheter is 5 mm above the reference line.
- Standard dwell positions of source are configured with equal intervals (one source at each centimeter) and dwell time (0.3 seconds for 10 Ci).
- The treatment is executed and a radiograph of the film is taken. In the developed film, the dummies and the exposed source of the film are taken and the coincidence of dummy and source position is verified.

Calibration of Source (Ir-192)

Purpose: To find the strength of high dose rate (HDR) Ir-192 source and compare it with the specified value.

Procedure:

- Source dosimetry system employs a well-type ionization chamber (HDR 1000 Plus Well Chamber), especially designed for the calibration of HDR Ir-192 (Fig. 10).
- The source is driven into the polymethylmethacrylate (PMMA) tube insert adapter to a reference position (maximum current reading).
- The radiation of the source ionizes the air in the chamber. This results in a small current. The amount of current is related to the activity of the source.

The source strength is calculated from the measurement readings with the following formula:

$$Si = M \times Ni \times K_{TP}$$

Where,

Si = Source strength of the Ir-192 source depending on Ni, the output Si is available in Air Kerma Strength in $cGym^2/h$ or Ci.

M = Measurement reading in nA.

Ni = Calibration factor for Air Kerma Strength or Ci.

K_{TP} = Environmental factor, the chamber is vented to the atmosphere, the currents are normalized to 20° and 1,013 mbar.

$$K_{TP} = [(273.15 + T)/293.15] \times (1{,}013/P)$$

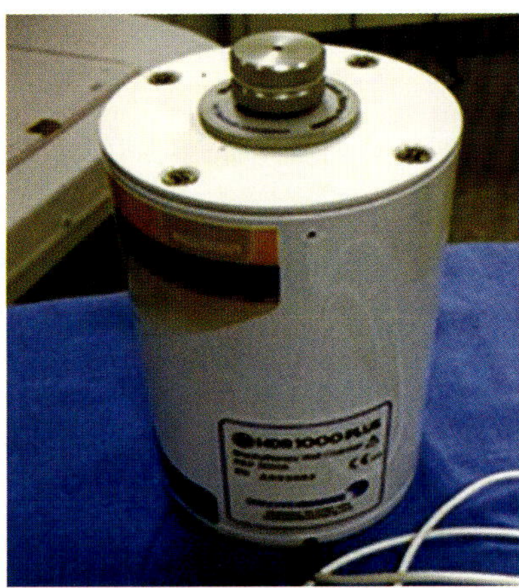

Fig. 10 HDR 1000 Plus Well Chamber—standard imaging

Source: Division of Radiation Oncology, Medanta—The Medicity, Haryana, India

Deviation between Specified and Measured Source Strength = (Measured Activity - Quoted Activity) × 100/ Quoted Activity

Timer Linearity, End Error and Timer Error

Timer error

Purpose: To determine the timer error occurring during transit of source.

Procedure: A treatment with reference distance for 60 seconds (t) at maximum dwell position is programmed and executed. The charge accumulated in the dosimeter (R1) is noted.

Again, the same treatment is executed with interruptions in midway (30 seconds) during the treatment. The charge accumulated from the dosimeter (R2) is noted.

Timer error = (R2 - R1)t/(2R1 - R2) seconds

%Timer error = (Timer error in seconds × 100)/60%.

Timer linearity and end error

Purpose: To check that the timer is linear and to determine the end error in the linearity.

Procedure: A treatment with reference distance for 320 seconds at maximum dwell position is programmed and executed. The charge accumulated in the dosimeter is noted for 300 seconds.

Swipe test

Purpose: To check if the catheter is contaminated by radioactive material.

Procedure: A flexible catheter is connected with the treatment unit and a treatment with multiple source dwell positions is executed. Then the catheter is tested for contamination using a contamination monitor.

QUALITY ASSURANCE IN CYBERKNIFE[4-6]

DAILY QUALITY ASSURANCE

- System status check
- Safety interlocks check
- Laser alignment check
- Treatment manipulator perch position laser check
- Linac output constancy check using FC65-G Farmer chamber
- Robot positioning accuracy using automated quality assurance (AQA) phantom
- Beam data measurements such as beam flatness, symmetry, beam center, penumbra width, field size, laser and light field coincidence—using SRS Profiler and
- Dose rate check (MU/min).

MONTHLY QUALITY ASSURANCE

- Beam parameters check
- Dose delivery verification check
- Linac laser and radiation coincidence check
- Robot targeting accuracy [end-to-end test (E2E)].
- Robot positioning accuracy
- Imaging system alignment check
- Treatment couch positioning check and
- Quality assurance of the Irish collimator.

System Status Checks

Perform a daily status check to ensure that the Cyberknife system is within specifications and monitor any drift in operating parameters.

Prestart-up checks during system off condition:

- Check that all emergency stop positions (E-stop) are in pulled out position
- Check that the treatment manipulator teach pendant is in the proper mode
- Check the pressure at 30 ± 2 Psi and 2.1 kg/cm of SF_6 gas and recharge if needed
- Verify that the key (ESCC) is not turned to service mode
- Now ready to power on the Cyberknife system.

Poststart-up checks during system on condition:

- Check the SF_6 gas pressure range: it should be 28–32 Psi
- Check the Linac gun heater voltage: it should be 5.2 ± 0.5 V
- Check the Linac magnetic heater voltage: it should be 9.3 ± 0.5 V
- Check the chiller water temperature range: it should be 19 ± 1°C
- Check that all mechanical interlocks are active
- Verify that the treatment manipulator is positioned in its perch position

- Verify that the door interlocks and E-stops are enabled and
- Check water flow rate is more than 3 liter/min.

Safety Interlocks Checks

Purpose: Check the treatment door interlock and the operator control panel E-stop button daily.

Procedure

- In physics mode, deliver 400 MU.
- While the beam is ON, open the treatment room door.
- The radiation should terminate and a red E-stop message should be displayed on the treatment delivery computer describing the error.
- Close the treatment room door, recover from the error, and continue to deliver the radiation.

Linac Output Constancy Checks

Purpose: The daily output constancy check confirms that the dosimetry electronics and all additional factors that have the potential to influence dose output accuracy are evaluated.

Procedure

- Place the Farmer chamber (FC65-G) with 1 cm (6 MV) buildup cap in Birdcage Connect.
- The chamber is connected with superMAXX electrometer.
- Make sure that the Linac has fixed collimator (60 mm).
- Measure atmospheric temperature and pressure (K_{TP}).
- Set bias voltage (±300 V) and readout in continuous mode.
- Deliver MU = 100.
- Measure the meter readings and correct with temperature and pressure.
- Finally compare with baseline readings and the difference should be equal to or less than 2%.

Beam Parameters Check

Check the beam characteristics such as field symmetry, field flatness, field size, beam center, penumbra width and light-radiation coincidence with the help of Sun Nuclear SRS Profiler (Figs 11A and B).

SRS Profiler

- Quality assurance tool for stereotactic radiosurgery fields measuring multiple beam parameters such as beam flatness, symmetry, field size, beam center, penumbra width and light-radiation coincidence in a single exposure.
- It has 125 Sun point diode detectors (0.000019 cm^3) and 4 mm detector spacing with 2 mm radial spacing.

Setup and measurement

- The SRS Profiler is fitted in the Cyberknife "birdcage" and is firmly positioned at 80 cm SSD.
- The SRS Profiler has field marks for 10, 20, 40, 60, 80, 100 and 120 mm circular fields.
- A computer with software is required to communicate with the SRS Profiler and displays the data.
- The cable connects the SRS Profiler to the power data interface (PDI + 18 V DC).
- Software automatically detects the attached device and configures the appropriate display.

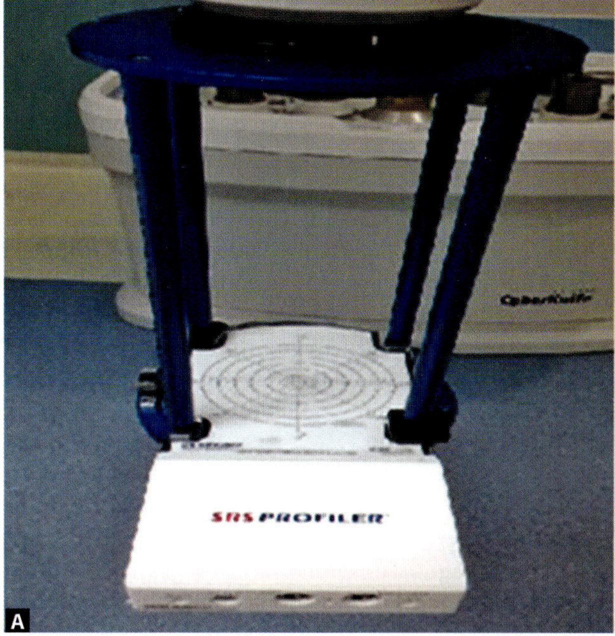

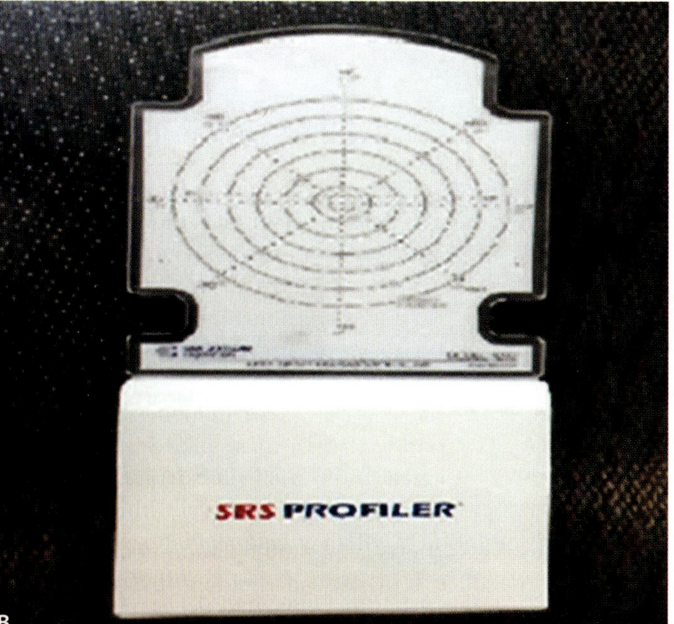

Figs 11A and B (A) SRS profiler placed at birdcage; (B) Sun nuclear SRS profiler

Source: Division of Radiation Oncology, Medanta—The Medicity, Haryana, India

- The SRS Profiler is exposed to radiation; the software instantly displays the acquired dose on the monitor; frame capture (up to 20 frames/s) is done and played back.
- It measures the beam measurements such as central axis dose (CAD), flatness, symmetry, beam center, field size, light and radiation coincidence, penumbra width, etc.
- The penumbra width is calculated and displayed in the analysis panel in the penumbra region (i.e. 20–80% intensity).

Photon Beam Calibration

Purpose: Checks the beam characteristics such as beam quality, energy stability, symmetry, flatness and penumbra with the help of RFA and stereotactic diode detectors (SFD/RFD).

Procedure

- Place the RFA at proper location.
- Using the teach pendant, position the Linac so the radiation beam central axis (CAX) is perpendicular to the floor.
- Ensure the water phantom is level.
- Fill the tank to the height necessary to obtain reading at a depth of 300 mm.
- Mount the stereotactic diode detector in the water phantom.
- Setup the measurement for 800 mm source-axis distance (SAD) and 50 mm depth.
- Insert a 40 mm fixed collimator.
- Measure the beam profile along two orthogonal directions.
- Analyze beam parameters such as flatness (<3%), symmetry (<2%) and penumbra (<4.5 mm).

Imaging System Alignment Check

Purpose: Check the mechanical alignment of the imaging system to document that it is performing according to specification.

Procedure:

- Attach the isopost to the camera stand.
- Use treatment mode to acquire an image of the isopost.
- Acquire an image and verify that the crystal is at less than one pixel from the baseline where it was last calibrated.
- Record results.

Automated Quality Assurance Test

Purpose:

- Automated quality assurance test should be performed daily to check robot mastering of the treatment manipulator and alignment of the imaging system.
- It is a targeting reproducibility test performed using the AQA phantom, a small plastic phantom that contains Fiducial (Fig. 12A and B).
- The AQA test checks the reproducibility of targeting two beams (vertical and horizontal).
- The AQA phantom is made of acrylic (1.18 g/cm^3) with tungsten ball (3.5 cm diameter) under the cube for attenuation [eccentricity (e) of the beam and shadow].
- It works under the principle of eccentricity. "Eccentricity is a number that describes the degree of roundness of the ellipse".

Performing the automated quality assurance test

- Place two orthogonal film (Gafchromic EBT3) (AS and LS) in phantom. Label two pieces of unexposed EBT3 film and load them into the AQA phantom.

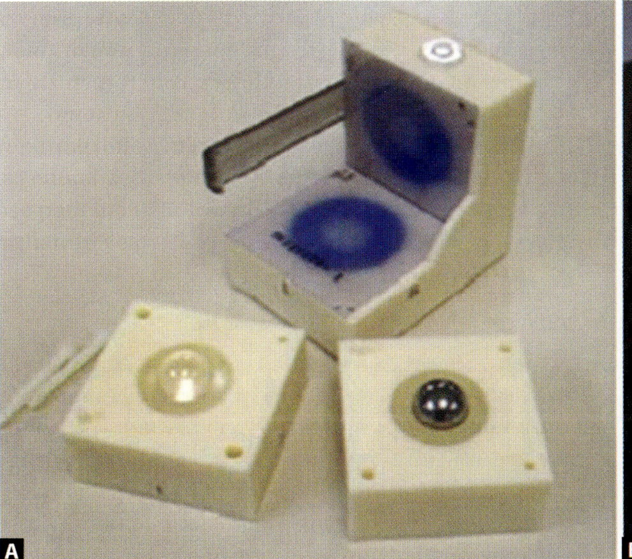

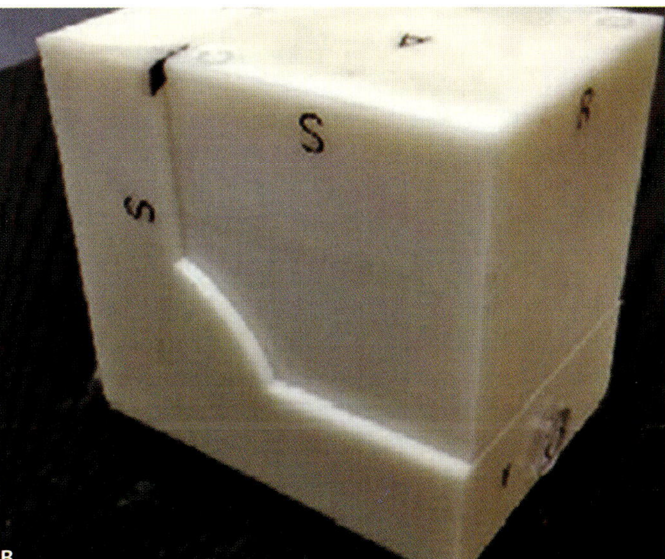

Figs 12A and B AQA Phantom—Accuray

Source: Division of Radiation Oncology, Medanta—The Medicity, Haryana, India

- Orient the AQA phantom on the treatment couch and coarsely align the AQA phantom using room lasers.
- Acquire X-ray image and use the treatment couch to align the AQA phantom. Ensure the phantom aligned to within 0.5 mm and 0.5°.
- Deliver the AQA test plan.
- Remove the AQA phantom from the treatment couch and unload the exposed films.
- Scan the film and import into the AQA software.
- The radial error should not exceed 1 mm.
- Print and save the analysis results for documentation.

End-to-end Test

Purpose

- End-to-end test is a targeting test designed to demonstrate the geometric targeting accuracy of the Cyberknife system throughout all phases of treatment planning and treatment delivery.
- The E2E test is used to determine the total positional error for each stationary tracking mode and motion tracking mode installed on a Cyberknife system.
- Stationary tracking modes include the 6D skull tracking system, the Fiducial tracking system, Xsight spine tracking system, Xsight lung tracking system and synchrony respiratory tracking system.
- Targeting accuracy is quantified based on radiation delivered to a ball cube phantom.
- End-to-end test is a targeting test designed to demonstrate the geometric targeting accuracy of the Cyberknife system throughout all phases of treatment planning and treatment delivery.
- Dose distributions are recorded on films inserted into the ball cube and analyzed.
- The total error should be below 0.9 mm for skull tracking and Xsight spine tracking.
- The total error should be less than 1.5 mm for tracking using synchrony.

Phantoms used in End-to-end Tests

The phantoms used in end-to-end tests are shown in Table 4.

Head and Neck Phantom

- The head and neck phantom is used in E2E tests for 6D skull tracking system, Fiducial tracking system and Xsight spine tracking system.
- The phantom has skull and spine features that are suitable for accurate tracking.
- A ball cube containing film is inserted into a cavity in the phantom.
- There are two cavities, one for ball cube, and one for the mini ball cube.

Table 4 Phantoms used in end-to-end tests

Mode	*Phantom*
6D skull tracking	Cyberknife head and neck phantom with ball cube
Fiducial tracking system	Cyberknife head and neck phantom with ball cube
Xsight spine tracking system	Cyberknife head and neck phantom with mini ball cube
Fiducial tracking with synchrony system	Ball cube with synchrony QA tool
Xsight lung tracking system	Motion phantom with thorax body and low density lung tumor film insert

Procedure:

- The head phantom is imaged using CT.
- A treatment plan is developed with the goal of conforming the 70% isodose line to the target ball.
- After the delivery, the orthogonal films are scanned and analyzed using software for accuracy that determines the shift between the centroid of the 70% isodose curve and the center of the film.
- Test is repeated for each tracking technique: skull tracking, Fiducial tracking, spine tracking, and synchrony-based tracking (Figs 13A to C).

Synchrony Quality Assurance Tool for Motion Tracking

- The synchrony QA tool for motion tracking is used in E2E tests for the synchrony system.
- The ball cube containing film is inserted inside the dome of the synchrony QA tool (Figs 14A and B).

Motion Phantom (Xsight Lung Tracking System)

- The motion phantom includes thorax phantoms and moving rods for testing the Xsight lung tracking system.
- The motion phantom does not use a ball cube-film cast, instead, it uses low, medium and high-density inserts containing film (Figs 15A and B).

Patient Specific Quality Assurance in Cyberknife

Purpose:

- Ensures that the TPS has accurately calculated the dose for the planned treatment.
- Verifies that the large amount of treatment data involved has been faithfully transferred from the TPS to the record and verification system.
- Ensures that the delivery system is capable of delivering the fields as planned (Figs 16A and B).

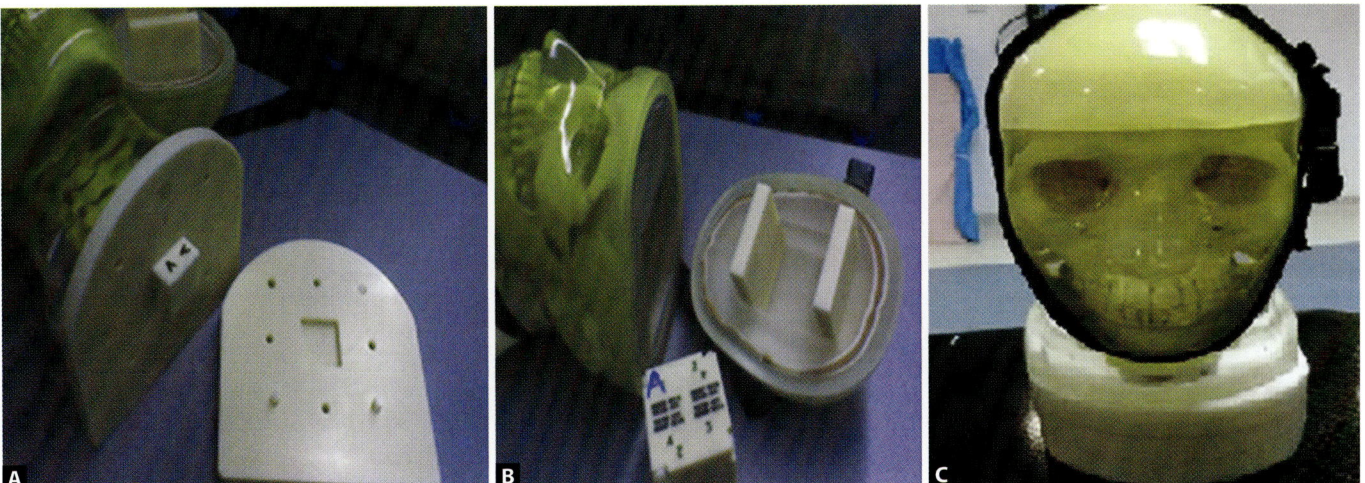

Figs 13A to C (A) A 3.12-cm ball cube in neck for Xsight spine QA; (B) A 6.25-cm ball cube in cranium for fiducial and skull tracking QA; (C) Anthropomorphic head and neck phantom—Accuray

Source: Division of Radiation Oncology, Medanta—The Medicity, Haryana, India

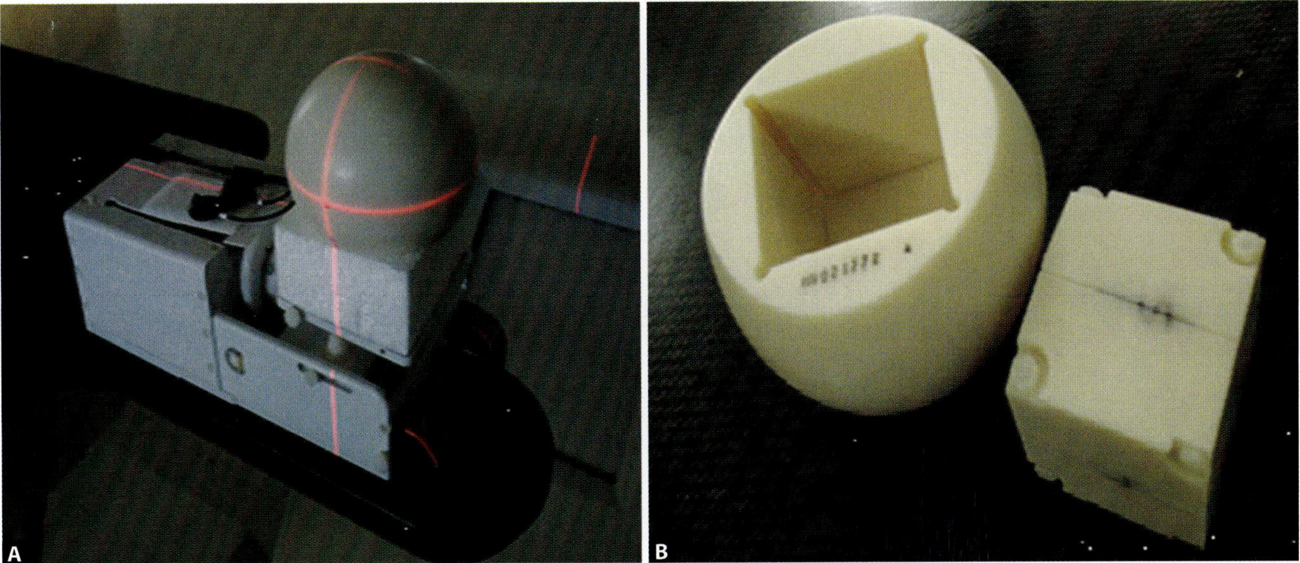

Figs 14A and B (A) Synchrony respiratory tracking system QA; (B) Ball phantom and ball cube, Accuray

Source: Division of Radiation Oncology, Medanta—The Medicity, Haryana, India

Procedure:

- Quality assurance plan is generated using the baby blue phantom studysets, once the treatment plan is authorized in multiplan system.
- The tracking modality is changed to Fiducial as default for phantom. The target volume is merged with the ionization chamber volume.
- Dose calculation is done with high resolution ray tracing algorithm.
- Mean dose in the chamber volume of interest (VOI) is taken as the reference TPS calculated dose, since the volume of the chamber is 0.007 cm^3.
- The total MU is rescaled to 0.5 to reduce the delivery time.
- Quality assurance plan is saved as a deliverable plan and a fractionation is added in plan administration module.
- In Cyberknife machine, QA plan is measured with the baby blue phantom.
- For measurement, A16 Exradin chamber and superMAXX electrometer are used.
- Room temperature and pressure are noted. Warm-up to the chamber is given in physics mode. Two thousand monitor units are given as warm-up.
- In plan QA mode, the selected patient plan is loaded.
- Fiducial tracking is used for the accurate positioning of phantom.

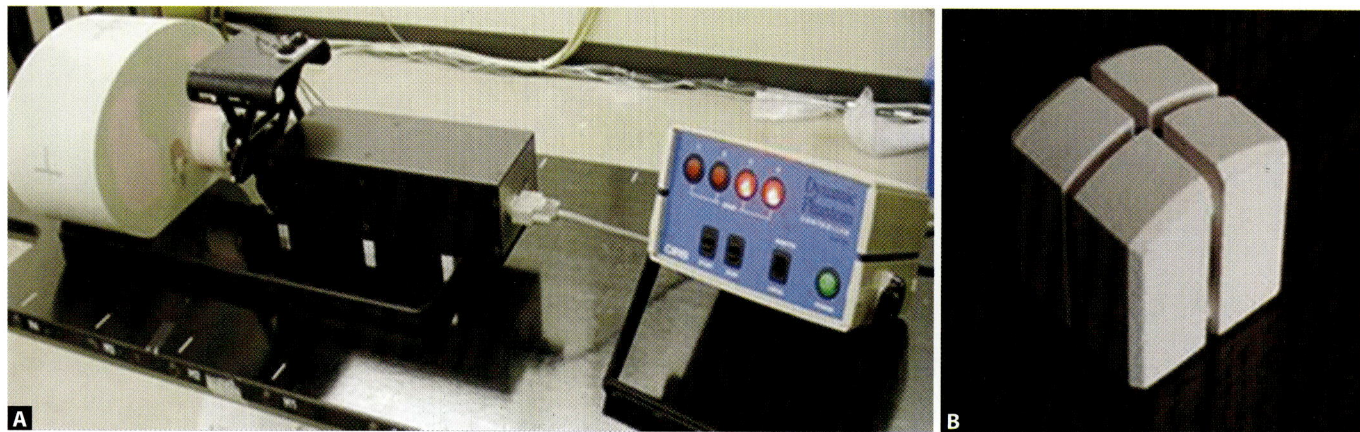

Figs 15A and B (A) Xsight lung tracking system QA; (B) Invisible lung density moving ball cube, accuray

Source: Division of Radiation Oncology, Medanta—The Medicity, Haryana, India

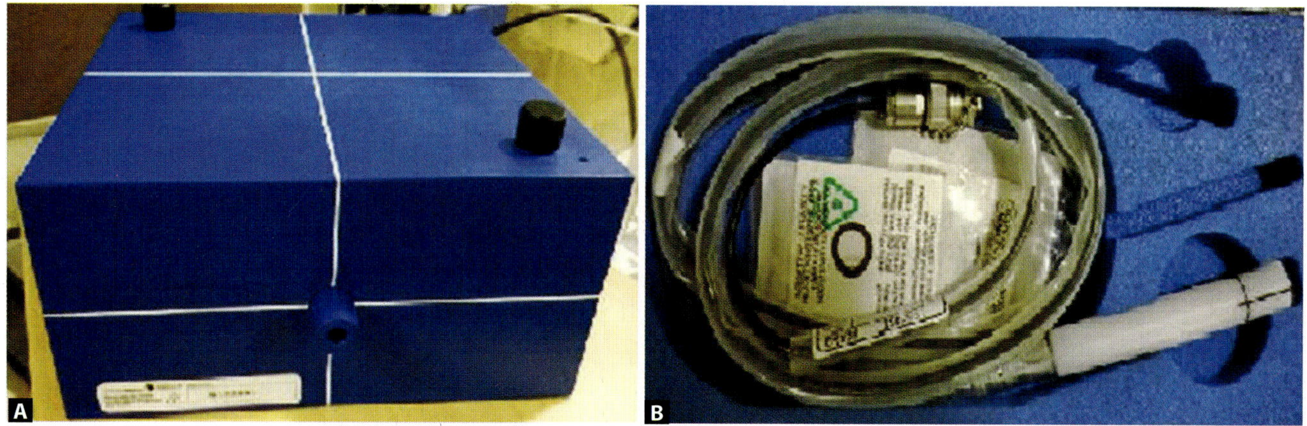

Figs 16A and B (A) Baby blue phantom (Accuray); (B) FC65-G ion chamber (standard imaging)

Source: Division of Radiation Oncology, Medanta—The Medicity, Haryana, India

- QA plan is delivered in the phantom. Meter reading is taken and correction factors are applied. Measured dose is determined from the corrected meter reading.
- The percentage deviation of TPS calculated dose and measured dose is determined.

REFERENCES

1. Klein EE, Hanley J, Bayouth J, Yin FF, Simon W, Dresser S, et al. Task Group 142 report: quality assurance of medical Accelerators. Med Phys. 2009;36(9):4197-212.
2. IAEA. Absorbed dose determination in external beam radiotherapy: an International code of practice for dosimetry based on standards of absorbed dose to water, Technical Reports Series No. 398. Vienna: IAEA; 2000.
3. Rivard et al. Update of AAPM Task Group No. 43 Report: A Revised AAPM protocol for Brachytherapy dose calculation. Med. phy: 2005;31(3).
4. Accuray Inc. Physicsessential guide. VolP/N023699A-ENG. Sunnyvale, CA: Accuray, Inc; 2006.
5. Dieterich et al. Report of AAPM TG 135: Quality Assurance for Robotic radiosurgery. Medical physics. 2011
6. Dieterich, Pawlicki et al. Cyberknife Image-guided delivery and Quality Assurance. Int J Radiation Oncology Biol Phys 2008;71(1).

31

CHAPTER

Pain Management in Cancer Patients

Kuldeep Sharma, Tejinder Kataria

INTRODUCTION

The International Association for the Study of Pain (IASP) defines pain as "an unpleasant sensory and emotional experience associated with actual or potential tissue damage, or described in terms of such damage".[1]

At least two-thirds of cancer patients experience pain at some time during the course of their illness, and most need opioid analgesics.[2] For many patients, physical pain is the only symptom of cancer. Pain involves physical, mental and spiritual aspects, all of which need to be addressed.

Dame Cicely Saunders' concept of "total pain" was first described in the 1960s.[3] This concept is now understood in terms of the sophisticated interaction of physical and emotional aspects, which make up the subjective feeling of pain.

Our understanding of the basic mechanisms of pain has improved considerably over the past few years. We now know that physical injury, pain pathways, and our emotional processing of this information are interlinked in the nervous system. Anxiety, fear and sleeplessness modify the perception of pain.

COMMON TERMINOLOGIES AND CONCEPTS IN PAIN

Pain can be nociceptive or neuropathic. Nociceptive pain is caused by stimulation of peripheral nerve fibers that respond only to stimuli approaching or exceeding harmful intensity.

Nociceptive pain is further classified into "visceral", "deep somatic" and "superficial somatic" pain. Visceral structures are very sensitive to stimulus like stretch, ischemia and inflammation, while it is relatively insensitive to stimuli like burning and cutting which otherwise evokes pain. *Visceral pain* is poorly locatable, diffuse, and often referred to superficial structure located away from the actual point of origin of pain. It may be accompanied by processes like nausea and vomiting and usually described as sickening, deep, squeezing and dull.[4] *Deep somatic pain* is initiated by stimulation of nociceptors located in muscles, ligaments, tendons, bones, blood vessels, fasciae, etc., and is described as dull, aching and poorly localized. *Superficial pain* is initiated by activation of nociceptors lying superficially in skin and surrounding tissues, and is sharp, well-defined and clearly located. Examples of injuries evoking superficial somatic pain include superficial wounds and first-degree burns.[5]

Neuropathic pain is caused by actual or potential damage to the peripheral or central nervous system. It is often reported as burning, shooting, or stabbing pain and is occasionally associated with abnormal sensations like perception of normal touch as pain (allodynia). It may be caused by tumor invasion, compression, surgery, radiotherapy and chemotherapy. In many instances, neuropathic pain does not respond to opioids, and in such situation patients may require additional measures.

The term *episodic pain* is used to describe an acute pain that is transient, severe and has intensity that is above baseline. Episodic pain thus encompasses breakthrough pain and incidental pain. *Breakthrough pain* includes pain returning before the next dose of opioid or an acute exacerbation of pain occurring on the background of pain which is otherwise controlled by an opioid regimen. Incidental pain is usually defined as that occurring due to a defined and voluntary action like body movement or passing urine or stool.

MANAGEMENT OF PAIN

With proper assessment and a systematic approach using the World Health Organization (WHO) three-step analgesic ladder, about 80% of cancer patients can be treated for their pain using inexpensive drugs.[6] About 10% patients will require more complex, sometimes invasive, treatment to control their pain, and in another 10% patients with cancer pain, the pain may not be treated fully.[7] Such pain is often termed as "difficult pain".

Assessment of Pain

Assessment of pain is the first and foremost step in pain management but this step is often overlooked. In general, the health care system does a poor job in assessing pain. In literature recording of pain symptoms by physicians and nurses in medical records has been observed to be poor.[8] There are various reasons behind this.

Observation, studies have documented that many patients do not report pain unless specifically asked.[9] Patients may under-report pain for various known reasons[10] (Table 1).

Failure to assess pain is another major cause of untreated pain. In a study involving physicians caring for cancer patients, 76% participants reported failure to conduct routine pain assessment as the single most important reason for inadequate pain management.[11] It has been found in studies that when pain assessment is based on a caregiver's estimation, there is a poor correlation between actual pain and perceived pain. Such discrepancy between physician's perception and patients' report of pain intensity has been shown to be responsible for inadequate pain management.[12] In general, oncologists and other physicians are often under-trained in using standardized, patient-reported pain measures in their clinical practice.[13]

The National Comprehensive Cancer Network (NCCN) practice guidelines for cancer pain base all therapeutic recommendations on a quantitative pain assessment.[14] The Joint Commission on Accreditation of Healthcare Organizations (JCAHO) announced all outpatient clinics to "recognize the right of patients to appropriate assessment and management of pain; assess the existence and intensity of pain in all patients; and record the results of the assessment in a way that facilitates regular reassessment and follow-up".[15] The JCAHO mandate that "pain is considered the 'fifth' vital sign," and that "pain intensity ratings are recorded along with temperature, pulse, respiration and blood pressure".[16] Despite these directives, little is known about the frequency or method of pain assessment in outpatient oncology practice.

Pain management has been shown to improve when routine pain assessment is based on a quantitative pain rating scale.[12] Various types of pain assessment scales are available for clinical use (Table 2).

Different institutions prefer a different scale as per the patient profile, availability of time and other resources and the level of information intended in the department. Some of these scales are very comprehensive, require more time to complete and hence become impractical in busy oncology units. Numerical rating scale (NRS) (0–10, 11-point scale) provides a reliable and valid measure of pain intensity and is very quick to administer and easy to use.[17]

The assessment of pain in children poses a specific challenge to the oncologists as there is no ideal method to assess pain in them and there is ambiguity regarding the choice of tool for pain assessment. A study demonstrated excellent correlations between scores based on numeric rating scale, visual analog scale and pictorial faces pain scale, supporting the validity for using numeric rating scale in children above 7 years of age.[18] They also observed that children reported an increased frequency of scores near the lower anchor (i.e. toward "no pain") while using visual analog scale but not with the NRS, suggesting a tendency for children to shift scores when only end-point descriptors are available. These data suggest a potential advantage for using the numeric rating scale, which offers more meaningful and salient numerical points along the scale.[18] Recent studies

Table 1 Reasons for under-reporting of pain

• Perception that pain is a natural part of having advanced cancer
• Fear that reporting pain will draw the doctor's attention away from the primary disease
• Belief that increasing pain means progressive cancer and patient wants to remain in "denial"
• Fear of potential side effects of analgesics
• Fear of being perceived as a constant "complainer"
• Fear of "using up" opioids too early in the course of illness, leaving no means for relief in future
• Concern about the additional cost of pain management
• Wish to avoid disturbing family members

Table 2 Types of scales commonly used to assess cancer pain

Unidimensional pain scales
• Visual analog scale (VAS)
• Numerical rating scale (NRS)
Ancillary unidimensional pain scales
• Pain relief scale
• Patient satisfaction scale
• Pain management index
Multidimensional pain scales
• McGill pain questionnaire
• Memorial pain assessment card
• Wisconsin brief pain questionnaire
Quality-of-life based scales
• Functional living index-cancer
• Spitzer uniscale
• Rotterdam symptom checklist
• European QLQ-C30
• Functional assessment of cancer therapy
• Edmonton symptom assessment system

have thus impress upon a need for further study of this tool in children in future.[18,19]

Medical Management of Pain

A combined approach including pharmacological and non-pharmacological measures can lead to optimum analgesia with minimum side effects in most patients. Data suggest that most cancer pain can be controlled well with oral analgesics and along with supplemental therapeutic modalities; approximately, 95% of patients can be free of significant pain.[17] However, despite the publication and widespread distribution of guidelines for pain management over last three decades, many cancer patients still receive inadequate analgesia.[20]

Pharmacological Management of Pain: WHO Analgesic Ladder

The WHO analgesic ladder, which has been extensively validated, is a framework of principles for pain management which allows flexibility in the choice of analgesics.[2,21] Since its inception in 1986, analgesic ladder remains the mainstay of approach to analgesia WHO (Fig. 1).

Twycross and Wilcock stated that for effective pain control, analgesics should be given "by the mouth, by the clock, by the ladder".[22] The same principle applies when WHO analgesic ladder is adopted.

For mild pain, nonsteroidal anti-inflammatory drugs are the agents of choice. The choice of a particular drug depends on the patient's profile, the properties and side effects associated with the drug, cost and preference of the

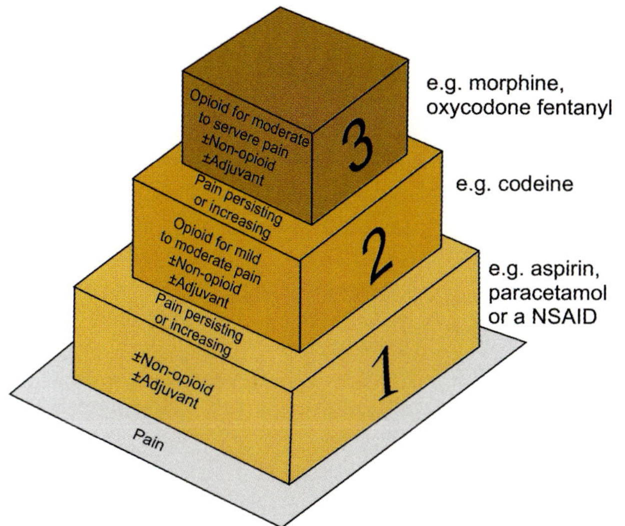

Fig. 1 WHO analgesic ladder

prescribing physicians. For managing moderate to severe pain, weak and strong opioids hold the key. There is no strong evidence in literature to support the superiority of one opioid over another. However, the clinical profile regarding benefits and side effects varies significantly among opioids because of variable factors like pharmacokinetics, routes of administration and genetic variability.

Morphine is the most commonly used opioid for severe pain. The systemic bioavailability of oral morphine lies between 15% and 60%. This explains the wide variation in effective analgesic dose of morphine between patients.[23] The rectal bioavailability of morphine is similar to its oral bioavailability and the same dose at same frequency as that taken orally should be given rectally if indicated by this route. The oral dose of morphine should be halved to get the equianalgesic dose by subcutaneous route and is divided by two or three, depending on the clinical situation when given as parenteral diamorphine. Patients rarely require intravenous administration of morphine except for those with an indwelling central line, particularly children. Intramuscular opioid injections are not recommended in patients receiving palliative care. Transdermal fentanyl may be prescribed as an alternative to oral morphine for patients who require stable opioid doses. Patients with deranged renal functions require special attention as any opioid can accumulate in patients with renal dysfunction. Opioids like fentanyl, alfentanil, hydromorphone, or buprenorphine are usually safer to use in patients with compromised renal function but still warrants careful monitoring.[23]

Dose titration: While starting pain management with morphine, normal release formulation with a rapid onset and short duration of action, is preferred for dose titration. Whenever possible, it should be given by mouth, with the prescribed dose repeated at regular intervals such that the pain does not return. The commonly recommended and simplest method is to prescribe a 4-hourly dose with an extra dose of same strength for "breakthrough pain" as often as necessary. After 24 or 48 hours, the daily requirements can be reassessed and the regular dose can be titrated accordingly. This process is continued until pain relief is stabilized. The regular 4-hourly dose ranges from 5 mg to 250 mg. Most patients require less than 200 mg a day but there is no arbitrary upper limit for morphine dosage.

Maintenance dose: Once the pain is controlled and dose is established, maintenance should be with a controlled release preparation. Controlled release morphine is available as a once daily or twice daily preparation, lasting 24 or 12 hours. The 12-hourly dose is calculated by summing the daily 4-hourly dose and dividing it by 2.

Common adverse effects of opioids (Table 3)

Sedation: Mild to moderate sedation is one of the most common side effects at the start of treatment, but in most cases, it resolves within a few days. Ability to drive does not seem to be significantly impaired in alert patients receiving a stable opioid dose but patients should be cautioned regarding such activities.[24]

Nausea and vomiting: Nausea is more common than vomiting in patients taking oral morphine. This side effect also resolves over a few days of treatment, and can easily be controlled with metoclopramide (10 mg 8 hourly) or haloperidol (1.5 mg at night or twice daily) in majority of patients.

Constipation: It develops in almost all patients and should be treated prophylactically with laxatives. Opioid related constipation persists even when all other side effects are settled.

Dry mouth: It is sometimes the most troublesome adverse effect of morphine. Patients should be advised simple measures like plenty of fluids to combat this. Other measures like frequent sips of iced drinks, saliva replacements, or saliva stimulants may also help.

Respiratory depression: It is uncommon unless doses much higher than prescribed have been given.

Opioid toxicity induced agitation and confusion may be misinterpreted as uncontrolled pain and further opioids are sometimes given. A vicious cycle follows, in which patient is given sedation and may become dehydrated, resulting in the accumulation of opioid metabolites resulting in further toxicity. Before the more sophisticated use of opioids, toxicity was often mislabeled as terminal agitation (Table 3).

If toxicity occurs, opioid analgesia needs to be withheld. The patient may need to miss one or several 4-hourly doses, and then it can be started at a reduced dose or converted to an alternative opioid at a lower dose. Treatment of agitation should be with haloperidol 1.5–3 mg orally or subcutaneously, repeated hourly as needed. Consider using the opioid antagonist naloxone, if life-threatening respiratory depression occurs. It should be used with care, however, as it may increase the patient's pain.

If the pain is not controlled with a dose of morphine which causes intolerable side effects, the possible measures include exploring unreported psychosocial issues, treating the side effects, changing the dose and/or route of opioid, or changing to an alternative opioid. The use of drugs called adjuvants or co-analgesics may be appropriate in such situation.[25]

Table 3 Opioid toxicity

Reasons for opioid toxicity
• Rapid dose escalation • Pre-existing renal impairment • Opioid resistant pain • Use after therapeutic pain relieving intervention, for example, chemotherapy, radiotherapy, or nerve block.
Common warning signs
• Pinpoint pupils • Hallucinations • Vomiting • Drowsiness • Confusion • Myoclonic jerks • Microsleeps

Adjuvant Analgesics

An adjuvant analgesic is a drug whose primary indication is not pain but that has an analgesic effect in some painful conditions when used with other analgesics. Examples include antidepressants, steroids, antiepileptics, etc. (Table 4).

Tricyclic antidepressants are recommended in relieving neuropathic pain. Strong evidence for use of selective serotonin reuptake inhibitors (SSRIs) in neuropathic pain is lacking. However, anticonvulsants like carbamazepine, phenytoin,

Table 4 Adjuvant analgesics and their use

Common adjuvant analgesics for cancer pain	*Dose*	*Drugs indications*
Nonsteroidal anti-inflammatory drugs (NSAIDs), e.g. diclofenac	50 mg oral 8-hourly (SR 75 mg 12-hourly)	Bone pain Soft tissue infiltration Inflammatory pain
Corticosteroids	8–16 mg per day; morning use; titrate down to lowest effective dose	Raised intracranial pressure Soft tissue infiltration Nerve compression Hepatomegaly
Gabapentin	100–300 mg at bedtime (starting dose) (titrate to 600 mg 8-hourly; may need higher dose)	Nerve compression or infiltration Paraneoplastic neuropathies
Antidepressants, e.g. amitriptyline	12.5– 25 mg nocte (starting dose) 10 mg nocte (elderly)	Nerve pain of any etiology
Anticonvulsants, e.g. carbamazepine	100–200 mg nocte (starting dose)	Nerve pain of any etiology
Bisphosphonates	Various regimens (commonly 4 mg IV infusion 4 weekly)	Bone pain

sodium valproate, clonazepam, gabapentin, or pregabalin are partially effective in managing neuropathic pain.[6] There is no specific measurable difference in the analgesic potential of tricyclic antidepressants and anticonvulsants in neuropathic pain but gabapentin potentially causes lesser adverse effects. Gabapentin and pregabalin are now routinely prescribed for neuropathic pain. While, *pregabalin* has a similar pharmacological profile to gabapentin, it seems more potent than later. Studies have shown better efficacy of pregabalin against neuropathic pain and an improved sleep pattern. Moreover, the titration of dose is easier than with gabapentin. At present, there is no evidence for combining two or more adjuvants. If titration has reached a limit and pain has partially responded, a second adjuvant may be added by replacing the first one or reducing its dose.

Non-pharmacological Management

There are several non-pharmacological techniques for management of pain. Non-pharmacological treatments, along with interventions such as surgery, radiotherapy, bisphosphonates, chemotherapy and other tumoricidal treatments, should be integrated with analgesic approach, whenever appropriate.[26]

Psychological techniques: Psychological techniques, such as cognitive behavioral therapies, include simple relaxation exercises, hypnosis and biofeedback. These methods modify the overt behavior and underlying cognitions and train the patient in coping strategies and behavioral techniques.

Acupuncture: This is an old technique used and described extensively in eastern medicine for centuries. Its application is believed to act by releasing endogenous analgesics within the spinal cord. Acupuncture is particularly useful for myofascial pain, which is a common phenomenon in many cancer pain syndromes.

Transcutaneous electrical nerve stimulation (TENS): It may have a similar mechanism of action to acupuncture. There is evidence to support its use in both acute and chronic pain situations.

Herbal medicine and homeopathy: These are widely used for pain, but often with little evidence for efficacy. Regulations on safety for these treatments are limited compared with those for conventional drugs, and doctors should be careful about unrecognized side effects.

Invasive analgesic techniques: Invasive techniques are often recommended for "difficult pain" in clinical practice (Table 5) but before considering them, it is important to exclude untreated causes like depression, general anxiety and distress (though untreated pain may also lead to any or all of these). A basic guideline is to use the technique with the least likelihood of severe side effects. In general, neurodestructive techniques should be reserved for situations when other measures have failed or when life span is obviously limited.

Table 5 Invasive techniques for analgesia

Peripheral techniques
• Peripheral nerve blocks - Intercostal block - Femoral block - Sciatic block • Major nerve block - Brachial plexus block - Psoas/paravertebral sensory nerve root ablation - Celiac plexus block
Central techniques
• Nondestructive - Epidural - Intrathecal • Neurosurgical/destructive - Rhizotomy - Cordotomy - Intrathecal phenol

Spinal routes of drug delivery: With improvements in catheter and pump technology, use of spinal route is becoming commoner in pain management. There is a concern for safety in routine practice; however, it has been seen that if trained staff carries out the technique, complication rates are low. These techniques allow flexible, long-term analgesia that can be used in an outpatient setting. Catheters can be inserted either into the epidural space or into the subarachnoid (intrathecal) space, as per the clinical situation. The line may be tunneled subcutaneously to reduce risks of infection and movement of the catheter. The choice of technique depends on several factors, which need to be reviewed before considering the patients for these novel procedures.

Some Practical Key Points for Managing Cancer Pain

- Pain assessment needs to be conducted initially at baseline and repeated to gauge response at regular intervals or whenever new therapy is initiated.
- If pain is not controlled, increase the dose in the range of 30–50%.
- A baseline recording of pain intensity in excess of 30 mm on a visual analog scale (or > 3 on 0–10 scale) is usually equivalent to moderate pain on a categorical scale.[27] A consistent 13 mm change in pain severity on a 100 mm visual analog scale is clinically significant.[28]
- The choice of drug should be based on the intensity or severity of the pain rather than the disease stage.
- Likewise, the decision to use an opioid for severe pain should be based on severity of pain and not on prognosis.
- When a non-opioid drug is used with an opioid for moderate pain, often combination formulations are

preferred by patients for increased convenience. Care must be taken with the dose of each component in the formulation as some combinations contain subtherapeutic doses of the opioid.[6]

- Increase the rescue dose at the same time and to the same level in line with the regular 4-hourly dose. Rescue treatment can be repeated hourly if necessary.[17]
- Give a rescue dose before any procedure or movement which is likely to exacerbate pain.
- Antidepressants and anticonvulsants may occasionally be prescribed simultaneously, although it is recommended to use one drug at a time in view of their overlapping side effects.
- Development of tolerance to opioids is rare in cancer patients. Requirements for increasing dose of morphine can usually be explained by progressive disease rather than tolerance.
- Psychological dependence or addiction for opioids is not an actual problem in oncology practice, except in some cases with pre-existing addiction.
- Physical dependence can occur, and this physiological response can manifest itself as a flu-like illness in some patients if an opioid is discontinued suddenly.
- "No news is good news" does not apply in pain management practice as many patients do not want to "bother" the physician by reporting pain.

REFERENCES

1. Bonica JJ. The need of a taxonomy. Pain. 1979;6(3):247-8.
2. World Health Organization. Cancer Pain Relief with a Guide to Opioid Availability, 2nd edition. Geneva: WHO; 1998.
3. Saunders C. A personal therapeutic journey. BMJ. 1996; 313(7072):1599-601.
4. Urch CE, Suzuki R. Pathophysiology of somatic, visceral, and neuropathic cancer pain. In: Sykes N, Bennett MI, Yuan CS. Clinical Pain Management: Cancer Pain, 2nd edition. London: Hodder Arnold; 2008. pp. 3-12.
5. Spanswick CC, Main CJ. Pain management: an Interdisciplinary Approach. Edinburgh: Churchill Livingstone; 2000. p. 93.
6. Fallon M, Hanks G, Cherny N. Principles of control of cancer pain. BMJ. 2006;332(7548):1022-4.
7. Fallon M, McConnell S. The principles of cancer pain management. Clin Med. 2006;6(2):136-9.
8. Strömgren AS, Groenvold M, Pedersen L, Olsen AK, Spile M, Sjøgren P. Does the medical record cover the symptoms experienced by cancer patients receiving palliative care? A comparison of the record and patient self-rating. J Pain Symptom Manage. 2001;21(3):189-96.
9. Cleeland CS. The impact of pain on the patient with cancer. Cancer. 1984;54(11 Suppl):2635-41.
10. Davis MP, Walsh D. Cancer pain: how to measure the fifth vital sign. Cleve Clin J Med. 2004;71(8):625-32.
11. Van Roenn JH, Cleeland CS, Gonin R, et al. Physician attitudes and practice in cancer pain management. A survey from the Eastern Cooperative Oncology Group. Ann Intern Med. 1993;119(2):121-6.
12. Au E, Loprinzi CL, Dhodapkar M, Nelson T, Novotny P, Hammack J, et al. Regular use of a verbal pain scale improves the understanding of oncology inpatient pain intensity. J Clin Oncol. 1994;12(12):2751-5.
13. Wu AW, Cagney KA, St John PD. Health status assessment. Completing the clinical database. J Gen Intern Med. 1997; 12(4):254-5.
14. Grossman SA, Benedetti C, Payne R, et al. NCCN practice guidelines for cancer pain. Oncology. 1999;13:33-44.
15. Joint Commission focuses on pain management. Oakbrook Terrace, IL: Joint Commission on Accreditation of Healthcare Organizations; 1999.
16. Joint Commission on Accreditation of Healthcare Organizations: 1999-2000 Comprehensive Accreditation Manual for Ambulatory Care (CAMAC): Patient Rights and Organization Ethics. 1999.
17. Levy MH. Pharmacologic treatment of cancer pain. N Engl J Med. 1996;335(15):1124-32.
18. von Baeyer CL, Spagrud LJ, McCormick JC, Choo E, Neville K, Connelly MA. Three new datasets supporting use of the numerical rating scale (NRS-11) for children's self-reports of pain intensity. Pain. 2009;143(3):223-7.
19. von Baeyer CL. Children's self-report of pain intensity: what we know, where we are headed. Pain Res Manag. 2009;14(1):39-45.
20. Cleeland CS, Gonin R, Hatfield AK, Edmonson JH, Blum RH, Stewart JA, et al. Pain and its treatment in outpatients with metastatic cancer. N Engl J Med. 1994;330(9):592-6.
21. Zech DF, Grond S, Lynch J, et al. Validation of World Health Organization guidelines for cancer pain relief: a 10-year prospective study. Pain. 1995;63(1):65-76.
22. Twycross R, Wilcock A. Symptom Management in Advanced Cancer, 3rd edition. Oxford: Radcliffe Medical Press; 2001.
23. Twycross R, Wilcock A, Charlesworth S, et al. Palliative Care Formulary, 2nd edition. Oxford: Radcliffe Medical Press; 2002.
24. Vainio A, Ollila J, Matikainen E, et al. Driving ability in cancer patients receiving long-term morphine analgesia. Lancet. 1995;346(8976):667-70.
25. Colvin L, Forbes K, Fallon M. Difficult pain. BMJ. 2006; 332(7549):1081-3.
26. World Health Organisation. Cancer Pain Relief and Palliative Care, 2nd edition. Geneva: WHO; 1996.
27. Collins SL, Moore RA, McQuay HJ. The visual analogue pain intensity scale: what is moderate pain in millimetres? Pain. 1997;72(1-2):95-7.
28. Todd KH, Funk KG, Funk JP, et al. Clinical significance of reported changes in pain severity. Ann Emerg Med. 1996; 27(4):485-9.

Index

Page numbers followed by *f* refer to figure, and *t* refer to table

S

T

U

V

W

X

Y